Clinical Advances in Ophthalmology

Clinical Advances in Ophthalmology

Editor: Anastasia Maddox

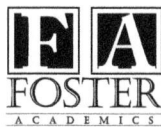

FA FOSTER
ACADEMICS

www.fosteracademics.com

www.fosteracademics.com

FA FOSTER
A C A D E M I C S

Cataloging-in-Publication Data

Clinical advances in ophthalmology / edited by Anastasia Maddox.
    p. cm.
Includes bibliographical references and index.
ISBN 978-1-63242-944-5
1. Ophthalmology. 2. Eye--Diseases. 3. Eye--Diseases--Treatment. I. Maddox, Anastasia.
RE46 .C55 2020
617.7--dc23

Foster Academics,
118-35 Queens Blvd., Suite 400,
Forest Hills, NY 11375, USA

ISBN 978-1-63242-944-5 (Hardback)

Contents

Preface

A branch of surgery and medicine that involves the diagnosis and treatment of eye disorders and diseases is known as ophthalmology. There are many changes in the eye and its surrounding areas due to various disorders and diseases, and aging. It branches into various sub-specialties like ocular oncology, ophthalmic pathology, pediatric ophthalmology, etc. These specialties are classified according to the disease or diseases of certain parts of the eye. Some of the common eye diseases are cataract, diabetic retinopathy, macular degeneration and glaucoma, among others. Optical coherence tomography, ultrasonography and fluorescein angiography are some of the tests used for diagnosing eye diseases. This book contains some path-breaking studies in the field of ophthalmology. It includes some of the vital pieces of work being conducted across the world, on various topics related to this field of study. This book is meant for students who are looking for an elaborate reference text on ophthalmology.

Various studies have approached the subject by analyzing it with a single perspective, but the present book provides diverse methodologies and techniques to address this field. This book contains theories and applications needed for understanding the subject from different perspectives. The aim is to keep the readers informed about the progresses in the field; therefore, the contributions were carefully examined to compile novel researches by specialists from across the globe.

Indeed, the job of the editor is the most crucial and challenging in compiling all chapters into a single book. In the end, I would extend my sincere thanks to the chapter authors for their profound work. I am also thankful for the support provided by my family and colleagues during the compilation of this book.

Editor

Tear Ferning Test and Pathological Effects on Ocular Surface before and after Topical Cyclosporine in Vernal Keratoconjunctivitis Patients

Marcella Nebbioso ⓘ,[1] Marta Sacchetti ⓘ,[1] Guia Bianchi,[1] Anna Maria Zicari ⓘ,[2] Marzia Duse,[2] Paola Del Regno,[1] and Alessandro Lambiase ⓘ[1]

[1]Department of Sense Organs, Sapienza University of Rome, p. le A. Moro 5, 00185 Rome, Italy
[2]Department of Pediatrics, Faculty of Medicine and Odontology, Sapienza University of Rome, p. le A. Moro 5, 00185 Rome, Italy

Correspondence should be addressed to Marcella Nebbioso; marcella.nebbioso@uniroma1.it

Academic Editor: Gonzalo Carracedo

Background. Vernal keratoconjunctivitis (VKC) is a rare ocular surface inflammatory disease that affects mainly boys in the first decade of life. Clinical observations show that it generally regresses spontaneously with the onset of puberty, but therapeutic measures must be taken before then to control the course of the disease. *Purpose.* To evaluate the role of the lacrimal mucous component in VKC patients and compare tear ferning test (TFT) modifications, MUC5AC levels in tears, and density of conjunctival goblet cells to clinical characteristics before and after treatment with cyclosporine A (CY) in eye drops. *Methods.* Forty-seven patients affected by VKC and 30 healthy subjects aged between 3 and 16 years of life were enrolled. All individuals were submitted to complete eye examination and skin prick test (SPT) for the most common allergens. Then, they were subjected to collection of the tears and to impression cytology to evaluate TFT, MUC5AC levels, and conjunctival goblet cell density, before and after treatment with CY in eye drops. *Results.* Comparing the VKC group vs. the control group at baseline, a significant alteration in the degree of the ferns was found, indicating a pathological condition of the lacrimal mucous layer. In addition, an increased number of goblet cells were observed in the patients. The concentration of lacrimal secretory mucins (MUC5AC) did not show significant differences between the 2 groups. Patients treated with CY have reported improvements of some signs and symptoms of disease activity, including TFT, and a tendency of conjunctival goblet cell density to normalise. *Conclusions.* The results obtained demonstrated for the first time a significant alteration of the lacrimal mucin component evaluated in the VKC group, and an improvement of the latter after CY therapy.

1. Introduction

Vernal keratoconjunctivitis (VKC) is an ocular chronic inflammation that mainly affects children (males/females = 3/1) in the first decade of life and tends to regress generally in puberty [1, 2]. This form is relatively rare and is more frequent in warm, dry, and windy climates, such as the Mediterranean, Central Africa, India, and South America. Type I hypersensitivity linked to immunoglobulin E (IgE) and mediated Th2 lymphocytes appears to be, in fact, only one of the cofactors of the disease in which environmental, hormonal, hereditary, and immune-allergological factors interact; so, the etiopathogenesis of this disease is multifactorial [2, 3]. The typical ocular symptoms are conjunctival hyperemia, itching, tearing, photophobia, and foreign body sensation. The recent literature distinguishes this disease into 4 types [3–5]:

(1) Tarsal form: small, medium, and/or giant papillae on the tarsal conjunctiva are visible with the eversion of the upper eyelid

(2) Limbal form: nodules or Horner–Trantas dots are present on the corneal limbus

(3) Corneal form: alterations of the corneal stroma and nerves are associated with intense hypersensitivity and photophobia

(4) Mixed form which has intermediate characteristics of the 3 types

Though called "vernal", VKC often has a chronic course throughout the year with seasonal outbreaks, in spring and summer, characterised by a worsening of symptoms, and frequent corneal involvement, ranging from superficial punctate keratitis with corneal ulcers that compromise visual function [3–5]. Diagnosis is based on clinical features, age, familiarity, disease progression, and the presence of typical clinical signs and symptoms. Allergic mediators such as histamine, leukotrienes, and prostaglandins directly stimulate secretory activity of conjunctival goblet cells, while inflammatory cytokines may regulate the secretion, proliferation, and apoptosis of the many cells involved. In fact, alterations in the expression of mucins on the ocular surface are associated with numerous pathologies, and it has been observed that a reduction or a dysfunction of the conjunctival caliciform cells results in instability of the tear film [6, 7].

In particular, several transmembrane mucins (MUC1, MUC4, and MUC16), and secretion mucins have been identified (MUC2 and MUC5AC) on the ocular surface [6–8]. MUC5AC is the major secretory mucin of the tear film, and its concentration in human tears ranges from 1 to more than 200 ng/mL. Moreover, the production of MUC5AC by the goblet cells is a target of regulation for allergic and inflammatory mediators produced by innate and adaptive immunity cells. Secretory mucous membranes remove allergens and pathogens from the ocular surface and play an important lubricating activity in epithelial cells. In fact, in patients with VKC, there is an increase in the number of conjunctival goblet cells; following the use of antihistamines and anti-inflammatory topical drugs with VKC, there is a reduction in the number of conjunctival caliciform cells to normal values [9–11]. Moreover, the expression of MUC5AC mRNA derived from goblet cells is reduced in eyes with corneal shield ulcers. At the same time, MUC1, MUC2, and MUC4 expression increases as a possible defense mechanism to compensate for the reduced protective effect of MUC5AC [8–10].

Cyclosporine A (CY) is a neutral, hydrophobic, cyclic polypeptide calcineurin inhibitor which was first purified in 1979 from cultures of the fungus *Tolypocladium inflatum* gams and from other imperfect fungi. Topical CY does not penetrate ocular tissues due to its poor water solubility and acts on conjunctiva as an immunomodulator, causing a reduction of inflammatory cells, particularly T cells, HLA-DR+ cells, and plasma cells [5–7, 12].

The purpose of this study was to evaluate the role of the lacrimal mucous component in VKC patients. In particular, the mucous component of the tear film was evaluated by tear ferning test (TFT), dosing of MUC5AC levels, and density of conjunctival goblet cells. In addition, modifications of TFT, MUC5AC levels in tears and conjunctival goblet cell density were compared to clinical features and evaluated prior and after treatment with topical CY.

2. Materials and Methods

We enrolled 47 children (38 males and 9 females) between 3 and 16 years of age with clinical diagnosis of VKC. They were submitted to ophthalmology clinic study by the Department of Allergology and Pediatric Immunology of the "Sapienza University of Rome". Also, we enrolled 30 healthy controls (20 males and 10 females) aged 5–16 years. Inclusion criteria for the children in the study were as follows:

(i) Diagnosis of VKC based on the child's history and the presence of some signs and symptoms, including itching, photophobia, and tearing in the spring/summer

(ii) Age between 3 and 16 years

(iii) Symptoms associated with the presence of tarsal conjunctival papillae and/or limbal nodules, and mucous secretion

(iv) Persistent or recurrent symptoms of VKC with little or no response to common pharmacological products for allergies

(v) No use of contact lenses

Exclusion criteria were as follows:

(i) Diagnosis of ocular pathologies such as glaucoma, blepharitis, ocular infections, cheratoconus, iritis, cataract, and other corneal or conjunctivitis pathologies

(ii) Diagnosis of systemic pathologies such as cancer, arteriosa hypertension, diabetes, cardiophathies, etc.

(iii) Ocular surgery in the six months prior to inclusion in the study

(iv) Systemic or local therapy for other pathologies

In accordance with the Helsinki Declaration, all parents were informed about the use of their data, and informed consent was obtained. The study also fully complied with the Good Clinical Practice guidelines and was approved by the Ethics Committee of our Hospital, Sapienza University of Rome (Authorization Rif. CE: 2336/26.01.2012-23/11/2015).

For each patient, the following anamnestic data were collected: age, sex, family history of atopy, and autoimmune diseases, presence of associated atopic conditions, age of VKC onset, perennial or seasonal course, and prior topical therapy. All patients underwent a skin prick test (SPT) for the most common inhaled and food allergens: dog and cat epithelium, parietary, grass and olive pollen, dust mites, pine, birch, plane and cypress, cow's milk proteins, eggs, fish, wheat, and soy. Patients were also subjected to a complete eye examination with visual acuity measurement, front and back biomicroscopy, indirect ophthalmoscopy, and a clinical technique to evaluate the ocular tear film by the Schirmer I test, break-time test (BUT), fluorescein test, etc. Some clinical signs and symptoms of pathological activity to baseline were evaluated with a score from 0 to 3. The total score of the signs (TSS) was calculated as the sum of the score of conjunctival hyperemia and chemosis, conjunctival serous and mucosal secretion, large and small tarsal papillae, limbal dots or nodules, and superficial wound corneal epithelium or corneal ulceration, obtaining a TSS from 0 to 18. The total score of the symptoms (TSyS) was calculated as the sum of the score of itching, photophobia, tearing, and foreign body sensation obtaining a TSyS from 0 to 12. The tears and conjunctival cells of the patients were collected to perform: TFT, impression cytology, and MUC5AC levels. All investigations were carried out by the same physician. In the past, 33 patients (70.21%) had previously been treated with antiallergic and/or anti-inflammatory topical therapy, but without symptom control except for short periods. All patients were prescribed a multidose bottle of galenic preparation containing 1% CY in 15 mL of 0.1% sodium hyaluronate to be applied 3 times/day (Vismed Light®, Medivis Srl Catania, Italy, and 1% CY). Patients were re-evaluated 3 months after the start of topical therapy.

2.1. Procedure

2.1.1. Tear Ferning Test (TFT). All patients and controls were subjected to TFT. The technique was performed by drawing tears from the lower marginal lacrimal meniscus with a glass microcapillary tube. The collection of the material was performed at the beginning of the ophthalmic examination to avoid any contamination or dilution by topical anesthetics or colorants such as fluorescein. The sample thus obtained was placed on an optical microscopy slide and left to dry by evaporation at room temperature; slides were then evaluated at the optical microscope to classify the response to the sifting test [13–15]. Thus, qualitative TFT was used for assessment of protein denaturation according to some authors [13–15] (Figure 1).

> *Type I,* continuous. Large, uniform, and thickly branched ferns without the presence of free spaces between the ferns for the right amount of protein.
>
> *Type II,* discontinuous. Abundant felcization but with empty spaces between branches; decreased film stability.
>
> *Type III,* reduced. Sparse ferns with empty spaces and mucin accumulations.
>
> *Type IV,* no ferns, presence of clusters of degenerate substances. Typical signs of dry eye. Tear film altered by stability, pH, firmness, and osmolarity.

Type I was considered normal to indicate good mucous efficiency and hence indirectly good tear film. Types II and III were considered as a transition form to indicate a state of difficulty in the mucus to maintain its integrity and functions. In types II and III, it is possible to find needle-like ferns instead of arboriforms due to the presence of an abundant protein mat rich in sugars and salts which alters the fern structure. Precipitated glycoproteins are antibodies such as IgM, IgG, and IgE, and in allergic subjects, IgE takes on the appearance of a small cross. Type IV was indicated as corresponding to a profound mucosal alteration. Qualitative TFT was evaluated with a score of 1 to 4 and calculated as type I to IV in both patients and controls, before and after topical therapy.

2.1.2. Conjunctival Impression Cytology. The patients were also subjected to conjunctival impression cytology, taking four samples per patient, two specimens per eye, at the level of the nasal and temporal conjunctiva. Impression cytology was obtained after the administration of topical anaesthesia with 2 drops of 4% ossibuprocain. The filters used for the collection were special nitrocellulose filters (Millicell-®CM Culture Plate Insert, 0.4 μm, Ø 12 mm, PICM 012 50, Millipore). The operator kept the membrane on the conjunctiva for 5 seconds using the plastic support.

The preparations were then fixed with the Bio-Fix cytological fixator (Kaltek s.r.l.), placed in its original container and numbered for subject, eye, area, and date of exam. The samples were stored in a freezer at −80°C, pending semi-Schiff (PAS) staining.

PAS colouration was performed by applying the following procedure to all cytology samples:

(i) periodic acid at 0.5% for 2 min; washing in distilled water

(ii) Schiff reagent for 10 min; washing in running water trays for 5 minutes

(iii) Pure haematoxylin for 2 min; washing in running water trays for 5 minutes

The samples were then observed under NIKON Eclipse E600 optical microscope to perform caliciform-forming cell counts. The density of the goblet cells was defined as the average of the cells per field in 3 different random fields.

2.1.3. Dosing of MUC5AC Levels. The tears of the patients were collected by inserting Microsponges (Alcon Laboratory, Fort Worth, Texas) into the inferior tarsal conjunctiva of both eyes for 60 seconds. The sponges were removed and put in a 1.5-mL Eppendorf vial containing the subject's identification number, the eye examined, and the date of withdrawal. So prepared, the sample was centrifuged, 12000 revolutions per minute (rpm) for 5 minutes, and stored in a freezer at −80°C. The immunoenzymatic test (ELISA) was performed on the samples collected to search for MUC5AC (Abbexa). The exam was a direct Sandwich test. The tear sample diluted at 30 : 1 was added to prefilled wells with the anti-MUC5AC antibody and left to incubate. A second antibody conjugated to an enzyme such as peroxidase was used to observe the positivity of the reaction. After washing to remove excess substances, the chromogenic substrate, tetramethylbenzidine, was added. Then, a colourimetric reaction was developed to allow quantification of the reagent indirectly bound to the enzyme by means of a suitable spectrophotometer.

2.2. Statistical Analysis. Qualitative variables were summarised by percentages and counts. The differences between groups were evaluated by Fisher's test or chi-square test. Quantitative variables were summarised by mean and standard deviation (SD). The differences between the groups were evaluated by nonparametric test by Mann–Whitney. TFT scores, the number of conjunctival goblet cells, and

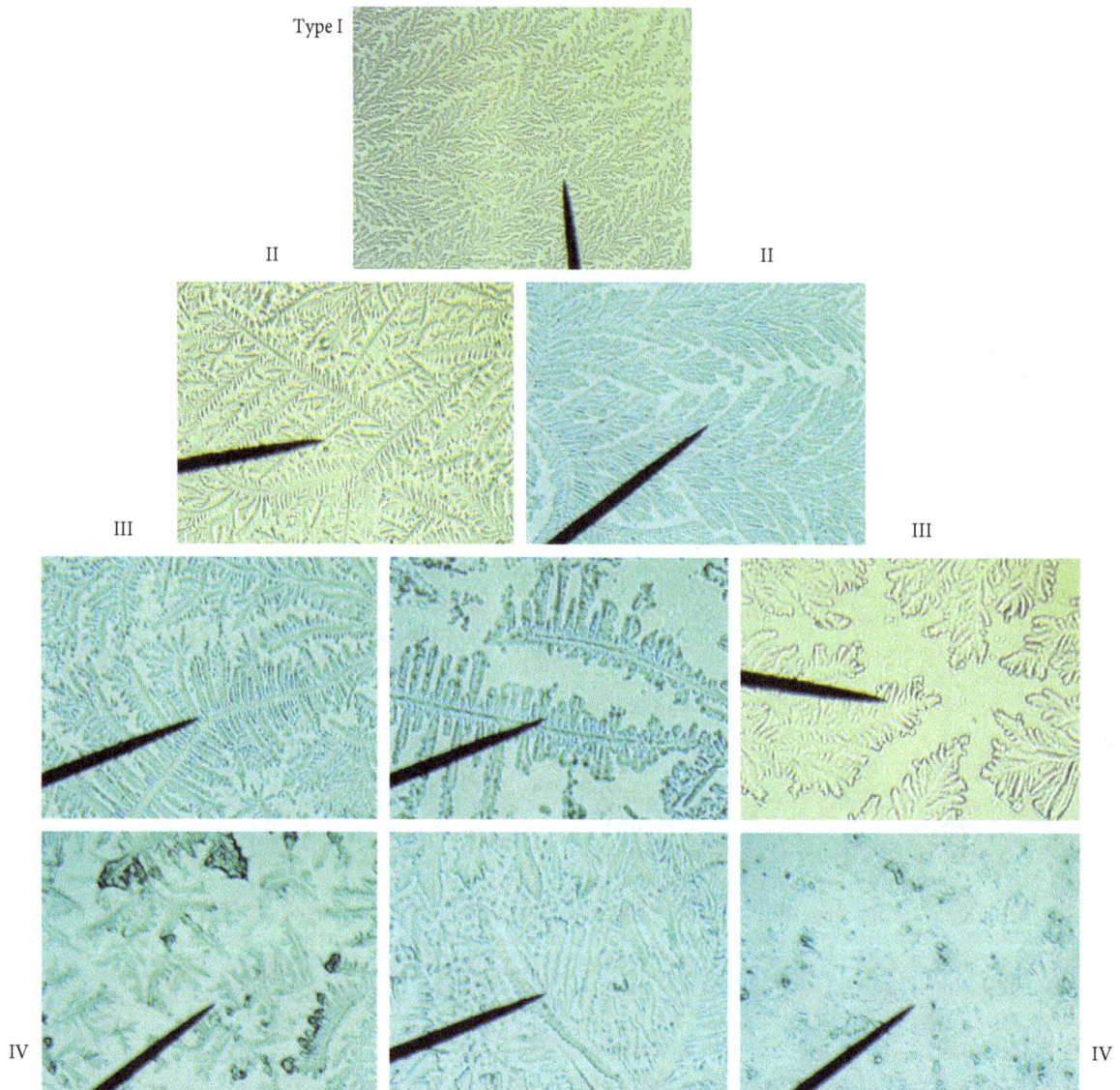

FIGURE 1: Tear ferns (100×magnification). Type I (control): uniform and compact branched fern. Type II: the number of branches decreased, while the interval increased. Type III: the number of branches decreased significantly, and the interval space increased significantly. Type IV: the number of ferns is low, and the pattern is indefinite.

lacrimal MUC5AC levels were compared at baseline and after therapy in the different groups by the t-test for independent samples and the Wilcoxon test for paired samples. The correlations between clinical, demographic, and biological parameters were performed by Spearman rho. Values of $p < 0.05$ were considered statistically significant. Statistical analysis was conducted with the SPSS 18.0 software (Statistical Package of Social Sciences, Chicago, IL, USA).

3. Results

The study included 47 patients (38 males, 9 females) aged 3 to 16 (mean age 8.8 ± 4.7 SD years) with VKC, and 30 healthy, nonallergic controls (20 males, 10 females), aged 5 to 16 (mean age 11.3 ± 4.2 SD years). According to the literature, VKC prevalence was higher in males than in females (79.85% vs 20.15%) in the population we studied.

Fifty-seven percent of patients had a family history of allergic diseases, and 12% had a parent with autoimmune disease. Two patients had VKC in the family (cousin/father). Forty-six percent of the patients were positive for the allergen SPT. Thirty percent of the sample tested had a positive allergic history (25% rhinitis; 5% atopic dermatitis). The average onset of VKC was 2.7 ± 1.3 SD years before. Thirty patients (63.83%) were affected by tarsal form, 12 (25.53%) by limbal form, 3 (6.38%) by mixed form, and 2 (4.26%) by corneal form. The VKC patients instilled 1% CY in 0.1% sodium hyaluronate 3 times at day. Then, they were re-evaluated 3 months after the start of topical therapy. The clinical and demographic characteristics of the sample being studied are summarised in Table 1.

The mean ages between the different groups were not statistically significant. The test results were found to be normal in the control group and abnormal in the VKC group.

Comparing the VKC group vs. healthy controls at baseline, we found a significant increase in the degree of the TFT that was 2.43 ± 0.80 SD in VKC subjects and 1.17 ± 0.40 SD in healthy subjects ($p < 0.001$) (Figure 2(a)). This indicated a pathological alteration of the lacrimal mucous layer. In addition, VKC patients had an increased number of goblet cells, 30 ± 20 SD cells/field, compared to healthy controls, 25 ± 11 SD cells/field, although this was not statistically significant (Figure 2(b)). The concentration of MUC5AC did not show significant differences between patients with VKC and healthy controls: VKC: 4,103.33 ± 286.35 SD pg/mL vs. healthy: 3,795.40 ± 837.44 SD pg/mL (Figure 2(c)).

Probably, this indicates a pathological alteration of the lacrimal mucous layer related to the production of fibroblastic material. An irritation of the goblet cells without statistically significant variation of their number and of the concentration of MUC5AC is present.

By correlating the clinical and biological parameters, the TFT score showed a direct correlation with mucous secretion severity ($p = 0.004$, $R = 0.373$) and conjunctival chemosis ($p = 0.031$, $R = 0.278$), indicating that in patients with secretion and severe chemosis, TFT also demonstrates poor quality of the lacrimal mucous component (Figures 3(a) and 3(b)).

The greatest number of conjunctival goblet cells correlated significantly with the greater severity of the tarsal papillae ($p = 0.005$, $R = 0.499$) and limbal nodules ($p = 0.047$, $R = 0.328$). In addition, a statistically significant inverse correlation between the number of goblet cells and the duration of the chronic disease was demonstrated ($p = 0.048$, $R = -0.465$) for probable chronic damage to the conjunctival tissue (Figures 4(a)–4(c)).

The lacrimal MUC5AC levels correlated inversely with TSS ($p = 0.042$, $R = -0.356$) (Figure 5(a)) and with TFT score ($p = 0.047$, $R = -0.427$) (Figure 5(b)) of VKC patients. These data indicated that a higher concentration of MUC5AC correlated with a less severe VKC and with a better quality of the tear mucous component.

Patients were re-evaluated 3 months after the start of 1% CY topical therapy, and no side effect attributable to the use of topical drug was found (Figures 6(a)–6(c) and 7(a)–7(c)) Some signs and symptoms of pathological activity improved after CY if compared to baseline, such as the following:

(1) Conjunctival hyperemia/chemosis, baseline 2.5 (±0.5 SD) score, and posttherapy 0.40 (±0.49 SD) score ($p = 0.001$)

(2) Tarsal papillae, baseline 2.3 (±0.5 SD) score, and posttherapy 1.61(±0.2 SD) score ($p = 0.016$)

(3) Lacrimation, baseline 2.3 (±0.7 SD) score, and posttherapy 0.65 (±0.06 SD) score ($p = 0.045$)

(4) TFT, baseline 2.43 (±0.80 SD) score, and posttherapy 1.93 (±0.67) score ($p = 0.044$)

(5) Improved density of conjunctival goblet cells, baseline 30 (±20 SD) cells/field, and posttherapy 23 (±8 SD) cells/field ($p = 0.044$)

TABLE 1: Clinical and demographic characteristics of 47 VKC patients.

Age range	3–16 years
Age (average ± SD)	8.8 ± 4.7 years
VKC onset (average ± SD)	2.7 ± 1.3 years
Sex: male and female	38 (79.85%) 9 (20.15%)
Forms of VKC	Tarsal: 30 (63.83%)
	Limbal: 12 (25.53%)
	Mixed: 3 (6.38%)
	Corneal: 2 (4.26%)
Total score of signs	12.5 ± 2.0 SD
Total score of symptoms	8.1 ± 2.1 SD
TFT score (average ± SD)	2.43 ± 0.80
Lacrimal MUC5AC (pg/ml)	4,103.33 ± 286.35 SD
Density goblet (cells/field)	30.0 ± 20.0 SD
Score of signs (TSS)	*Average ± SD*
Hyperemia/chemosis conjunctival	2.5 ± 0.5
Mucous and serious secretions	2.3 ± 0.7
Tarsal papillae < 3 mm	2.3 ± 0.5
Tarsal papillae > 3 mm	2.2 ± 0.4
Horner–Trantas nodules	2.5 ± 0.2
Epithelial keratitis	0.5 ± 0.02
Score of symptoms (TSyS)	*Average ± SD*
Itching and photophobia	4.0 ± 0.7
Tearing	2.1 ± 0.8
Foreign body sensation	2.0 ± 0.6

VKC: vernal keratoconjunctivitis; SD: standard deviation; TFT: tear ferning test.

There were no changes in lacrimal MUC5AC levels, baseline 4,103.33 (±286.35 SD) pg/mL, and posttherapy 3,909.18 (±606.01 SD) pg/mL.

4. Discussion

In our study, we evaluated the clinical and structural modifications of the lacrimal mucinic component in patients affected by VKC. In particular, the results obtained demonstrated for the first time that there was a significant alteration of the lacrimal mucus in subjects with VKC compared to controls, and moreover, the degree of alteration of the lacrimal mucin component correlated significantly with the severity of the pathology. In addition, the parameters of the disease showed a significant improvement after immunomodulatory therapy with topical CY.

Tabbara and Okumoto were the first to report the use of ferning as a qualitative test for ocular tear discomfort in 91% of patients with several forms of conjunctivitis [16]. Beside, Norn (1994) believes, after having examined for various ocular disorders 225 subjects, that the ferning method has a sensitivity and a specificity of the same order as the commonly used tests for qualitative and quantitative lacrimal film (Schirmer I, BUT, rose bengale, lactoferrin) [15]. Other authors suggest that TFT could be used as a simple, inexpensive, and low-invasive test to clinically evaluate the tear film [13]. Both the BUT and TFT tests reflect the dysfunction of tear mucin indirectly [17]. Our research shows that TFT could be useful in the objective evaluation of tear film and also be a marker of

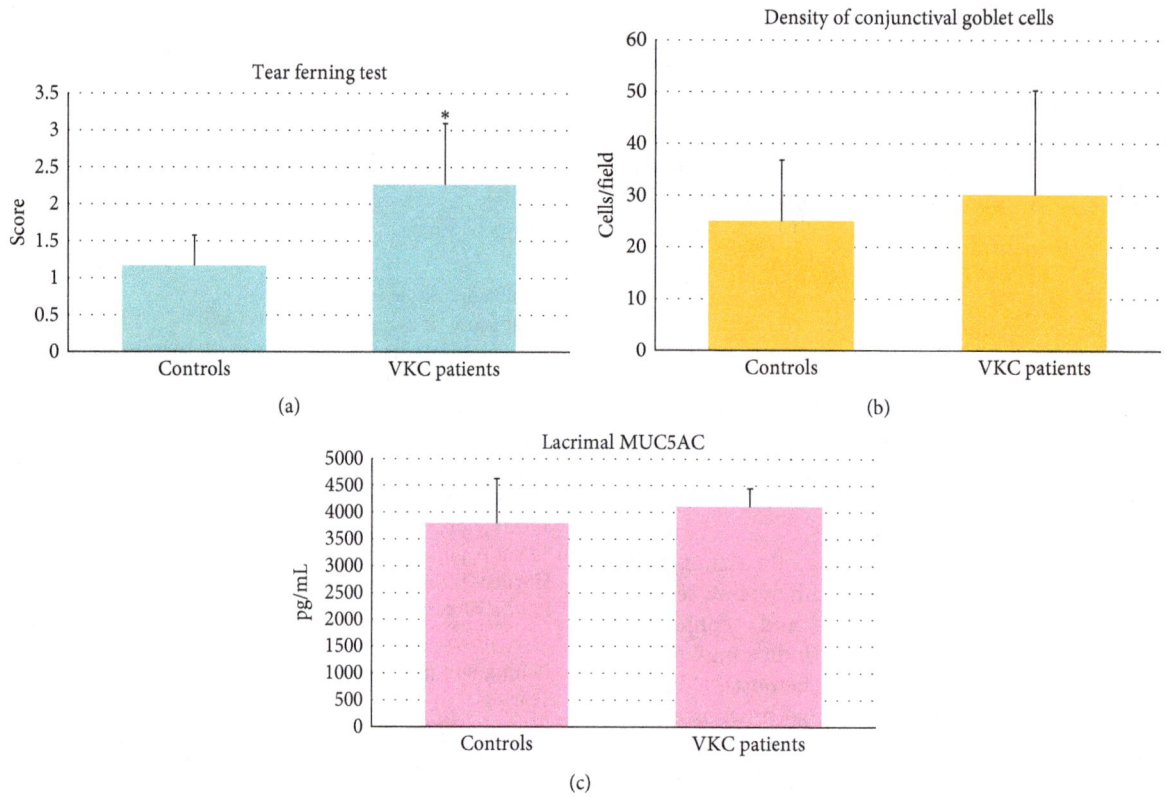

Figure 2: Significant increase of the TFT (tear ferning test) score in VKC (vernal keratoconjunctivitis) patients, 2.43 ± 0.80 SD, vs. controls, 1.17 ± 0.40 SD ($p < 0.001$) (a). Increase in the goblet cells density, though not statistically significant, 30 ± 20 SD cells/field in VKC patients, vs. controls, 25 ± 11 SD cells/field (b). The concentration of MUC5AC does not show significant differences between VKC patients, 4,103.33 ± 286.35 SD pg/mL, and controls, 3,795.40 ± 837.44 SD pg/mL (c).

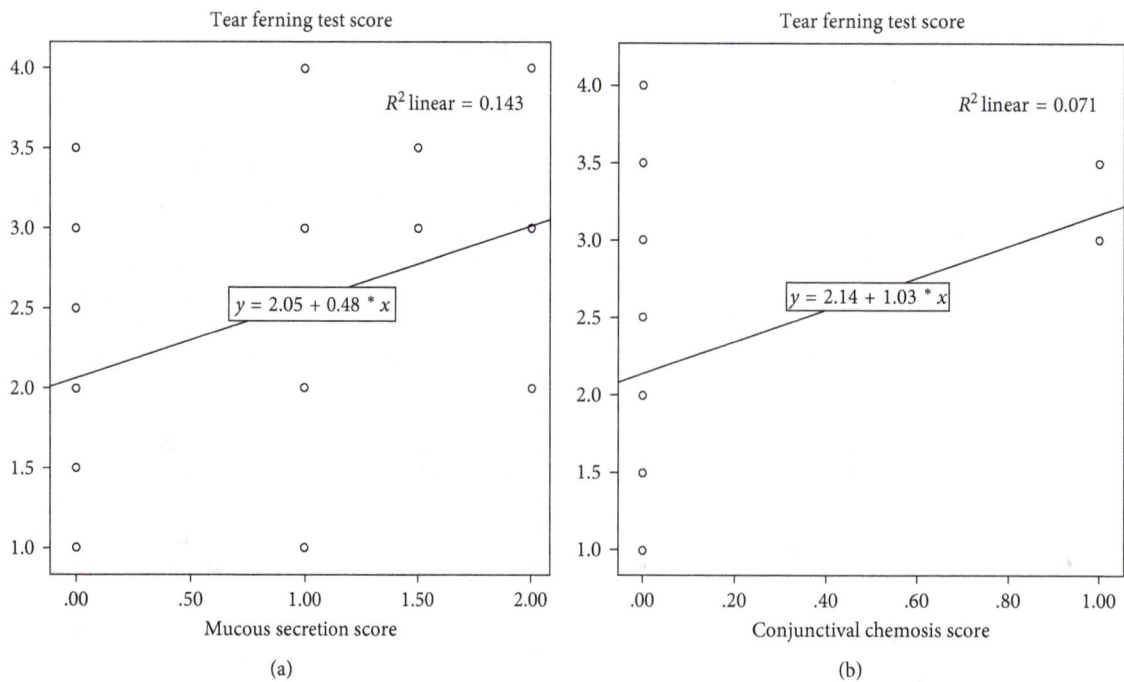

Figure 3: The tear ferning test (TFT) score shows direct correlation with mucous secretion severity ($p = 0.004$, $R = 0.373$) (a) and conjunctival chemosis ($p = 0.031$, $R = 0.278$) (b), indicating altered quality of the lacrimal mucous component.

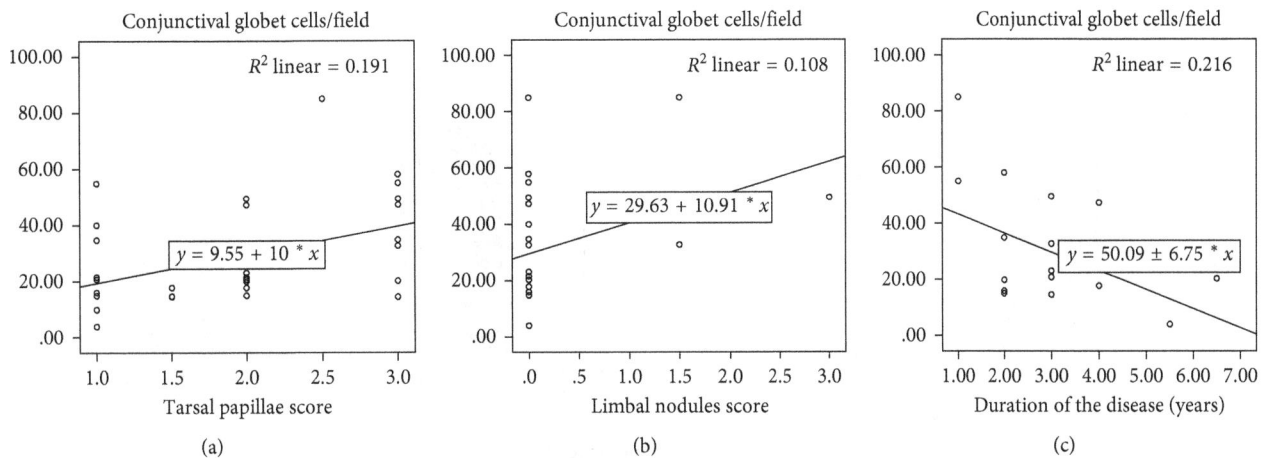

FIGURE 4: The greatest number of conjunctival goblet cells correlates significantly with the greater severity of the tarsal papillae ($p = 0.005$, $R = 0.499$) (a), and limbal nodules ($p = 0.047$, $R = 0.328$) (b). In addition, inverse correlation between the number of goblet cells and the duration of the chronic disease was demonstrated ($p = 0.048$, $R = -0.465$) for probable chronic damage to the conjunctival tissue (c).

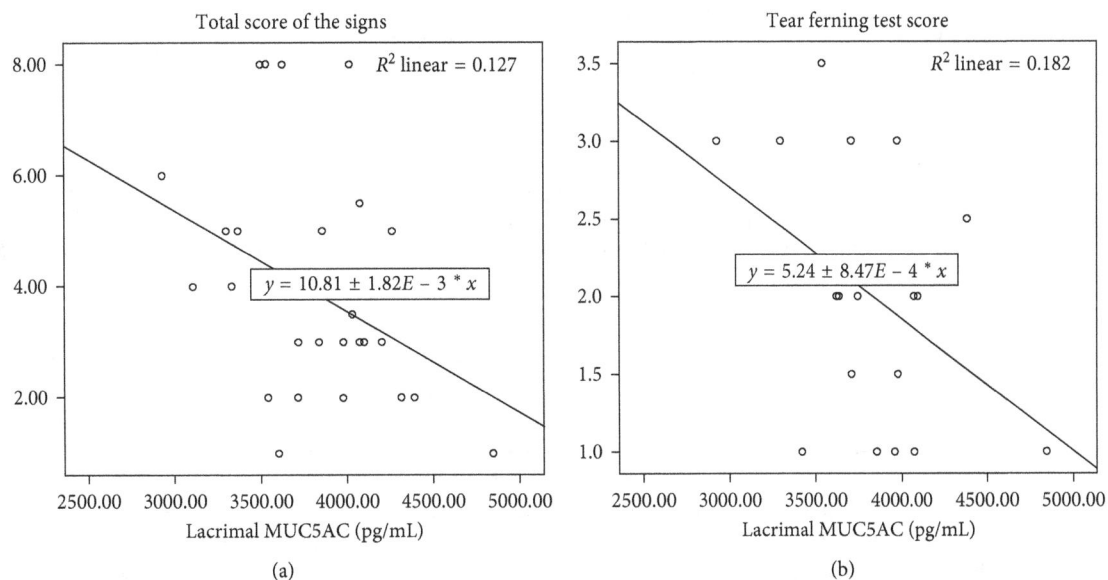

FIGURE 5: Lacrimal MUC5AC levels correlates inversely with TSS (total score of the signs) ($p = 0.042$, $R = -0.356$) (a) and with TFT (tear ferning test) score ($p = 0.047$, $R = -0.427$) (b) of VKC (vernal keratoconjunctivitis) patients for less severe VKC and better quality of the tear mucous component.

therapeutic efficacy in patients with VKC. Indeed, there are some factors that may change TFT, and the exact nature of what determines the pattern is still not fully understood [13]. In fact, rapid crystallisation of the tears, evaporation, temperature, humidity, impurities, role of electrolytes, spatial location of organic molecules, etc. play a role in the formation of the ferns under the microscope [13]. Precisely for these reasons, according to other authors, it could be more useful to use other tests like counting the number of goblet cells, or rose bengal 1% stain, or lissamine green 2% stain score [18, 19]. For now, the recent literature (Zeev, 2014) asserts that the numerous diagnostic tests used are not yet widely accepted and are often not reproducible [20].

Data of our research were accompanied by the demonstration of an increased density of goblet cells in the conjunctival epithelium of VKC patients with a more severe score of tarsal and limbal papillae, both of which are indexes of disease severity [21]. Aragona et al. demonstrated that, in the conjunctival epithelium of VKC patients, there were alterations in calcium density, intercellular junctions, the amount of nuclear chromatin, and the degree of cellular keratinization with a higher number of goblet cells, but smaller in shape than in healthy controls [22]. In addition, we observed under optical microscope that the goblet cells appeared to be clustered and sometimes clotted in mucine clusters associated with the presence of metaplasic cellular specimens with some pyknotic nuclei [22] (Figure 8).

(a)

(b)

(c)

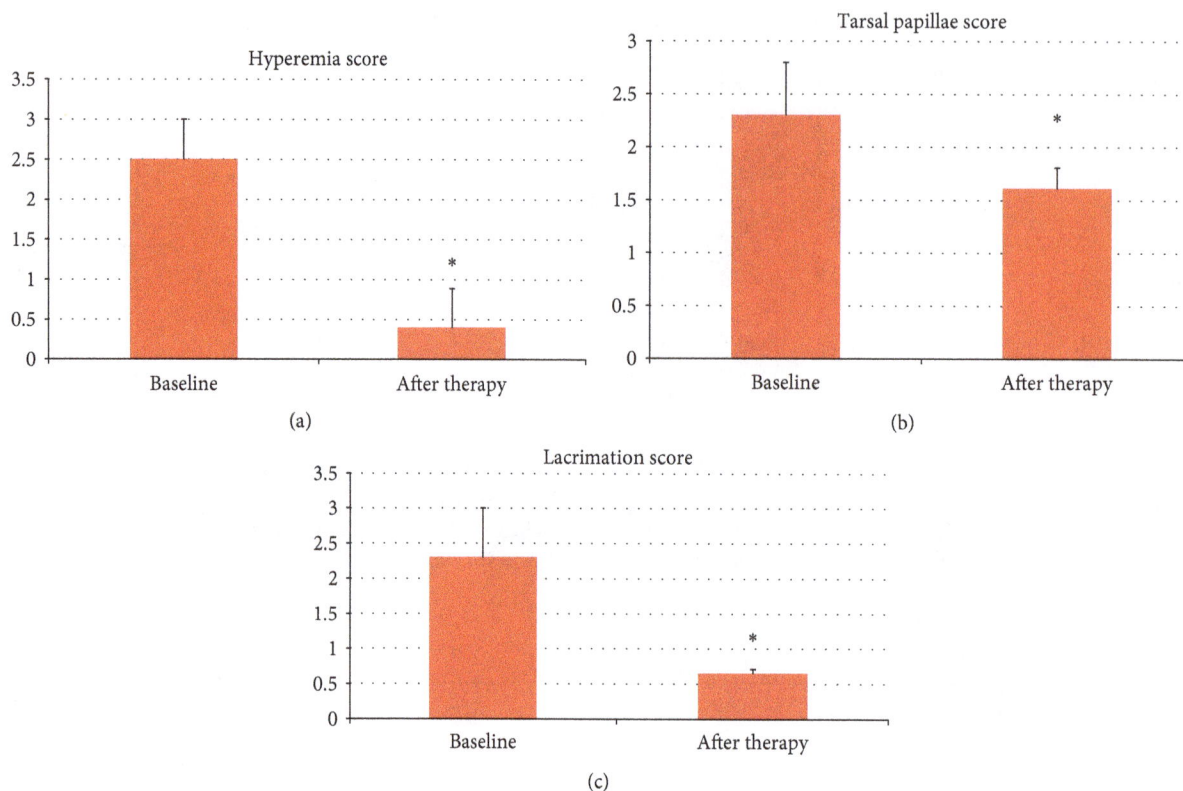

FIGURE 6: Some signs of pathology improvement 3 months after the start of CY (cyclosporine) therapy, such as: conjunctival hyperemia/chemosis, baseline 2.5 (± 0.5 SD) score, and posttherapy 0.40 (± 0.49 SD) score ($p = 0.001$) (a); tarsal papillae, baseline 2.3 (± 0.5 SD) score, and posttherapy 1.61 (± 0.2) score ($p = 0.016$) (b); and lacrimation, baseline 2.3 (± 0.7 SD) score, and posttherapy 0.65 (± 0.06 SD) score ($p = 0.045$) (c).

Conjunctival epithelium, therefore, reacts to the inflammatory stimulus with structural changes that can be considered partly as defense mechanisms and partly as degenerative signs. On the contrary, in both type-1, IgE-mediated, and type-4 hypersensitivity reactions, T-lymphocytes play a role in the development of VKC disease. Subsequently, the increase in mucus secretion could also play an important role in the pathogenesis of the disease by providing a network on which allergens may bind, stressing inflammatory stimulation. This could indicate a pathological alteration of the lacrimal mucous layer related to infiltration of conjunctival, limbal, and corneal inflammatory cells with production of fibroblastic material. In fact, the conjunctiva is characterised by an infiltration of inflammatory cells, especially eosinophils, mast cells, and T-lymphocytes [3, 21–23]. Patients with VKC have been shown to have increased levels of activated CD4+, Th2-lymphocites, and of inflammatory cytokines IL-3, IL-4, IL-5, and IL-6, indicating that there is a hypersensitivity reaction to an unknown pathogen [3, 21–23]. Inflammatory cytokines may regulate the secretion, proliferation, and apoptosis of goblet cells [24–26], while allergic mediators such as histamine, leukotrienes, and prostaglandins directly stimulate the secretory activity of these cells [24–27].

Our patients showed only an irritation of the goblet cells without a statistically significant variation of their number and of MUC5AC concentration. This aspect would represent the first phase of conjunctival inflammatory response. With the persistence of the inflammatory stimulus, the degenerative cell phenomena would manifest themselves as the sign of persistent damage to the ocular surface [22].

Moreover, we showed that, in patients with long-term disease, the density of conjuntival goblet cells is lower (Figure 4(c)), indicating a progressive squamous metaplasia of the conjunctiva associated with the duration of chronic inflammation. This could be due to the fact that inflammatory mediators initially stimulate a hyperplasia of conjunctival goblet cells while the persistence of the inflammation could cause a reduction in the density of goblet cells [21–23]. In our study, we also evaluated the tendency of the number of conjunctival goblet cells to normalise in patients with VKC after topical CY therapy. Although these data do not reach statistical significance, they stimulate a reflection on the immunoregulatory properties of drug treatment. Therapeutic activity could be useful to stimulate the still viable cells that in just 3 months of topical therapy have recovered their functionality [28, 29].

As is well known, CY is an immunomodulator that reduces the proliferation of CD4+ lymphocytes through interleukin-2 (IL-2) transcription blockade; it reduces conjunctival fibroblasts and IL-1 production [2, 30, 31]. CY also has an inhibitory effect on the activation of eosinophils, basophils, and mast cells and on the release of histamine, and inflammation mediators [30, 32]. We noticed a significant

(a)

(b)

(c)

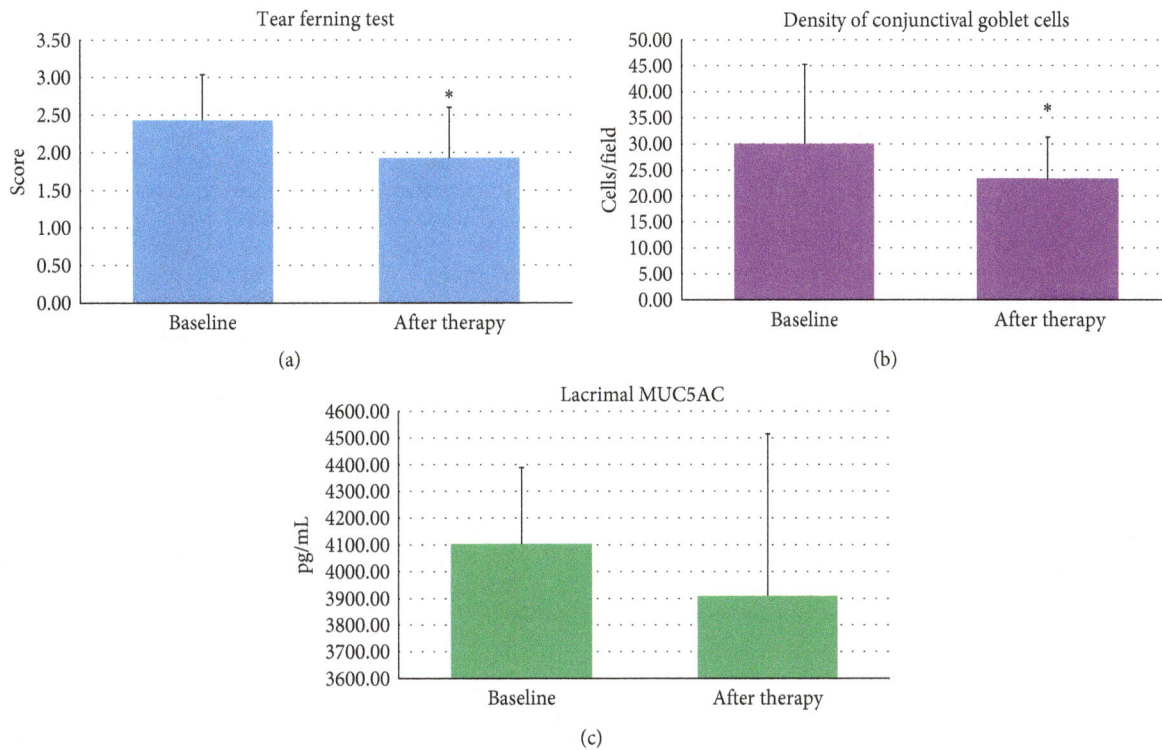

FIGURE 7: Some signs of pathology improvement 3 months after the start of CY (cyclosporine) therapy, such as TFT (tear ferning test), baseline 2.43 ($\pm$0.80 SD) score, and posttherapy 1.93 ($\pm$0.67) score ($p = 0.044$) (a); density of conjunctival goblet cells, baseline 30 ($\pm$20 SD) cells/field, and posttherapy 23 ($\pm$8 SD) cells/field ($p = 0.044$) (b). There are no changes in the MUC5AC levels before (4,103.33 $\pm$ 286.35 SD pg/ml) and after therapy (3,909.18 $\pm$ 606.01 SD pg/ml) (c), even because a 3-month treatment period is too short to evaluate the possible functional improvement of the conjunctiva in patients with chronic VKC (vernal keratoconjunctivitis).

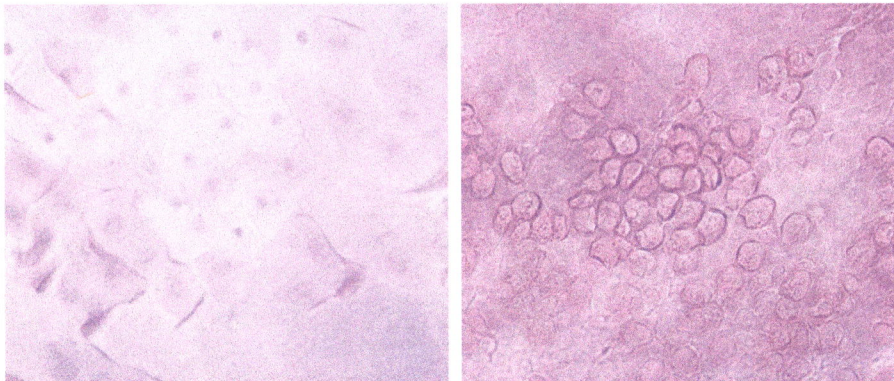

FIGURE 8: Observation of conjunctival cytogenes by an optical microscope. The goblet cells appear to be clustered and clotted in mucine clusters associated with the presence of metaplasic cellular specimens with some pyknotic nuclei.

improvement in the signs and symptoms of patients with VKC after 3 months of 1% CY topical therapy [32, 33]. Our data did not reveal differences in the concentration of lacrimal MUC5AC between patients with VKC and healthy controls, but correlations with clinical data showed a greater concentration of MUC5AC in the tears of less severe patients and with a better quality of mucus (Figures 5(a) and 5(b)). Such evidence suggests a protective role of MUC5AC, where a higher concentration of lacrimal MUC5AC is associated with better quality of the tear mucus component. In fact, we know that MUC5AC contributes to making the tear film

a non-Newtonian viscoelastic structure, capable of modifying its viscosity depending on the size of the applied force, thereby reducing the friction between the eye and eyelid [24, 27].

5. Conclusions

This research confirmed the data of the literature on efficacy of topical CY therapy in patients with VKC, demonstrating a statistically significant improvement in clinical and structural ocular inflammation. The results also showed, for the first time, a significant alteration of the lacrimal mucinic component evaluated by TFT in subjects with VKC compared with healthy controls, before and after CY topical therapy. These observations encourage to consider a possible use of TFT in daily clinical practice, and the density of conjunctival goblet cells in VKC patients could be a marker of duration of the disease.

A larger study population and an increase in observation time by at least 12 months after therapy will be necessary to better understand the role of mucins in maintaining the integrity of the mucus barrier and of the ocular surface. All this, in order to lead to a therapeutic strategy to reduce the signs and symptoms, avoid conjunctival fibrosis, and allow, when possible, healing from the disease.

Conflicts of Interest

The authors have no conflicts of interest and have no proprietary interest in any materials or methods described within this article.

Authors' Contributions

M. Nebbioso and A. Lambiase participated in the study design. M. Sacchetti performed the literature search. M. Duse and A.M. Zicari helped in data interpretation. G. Bianchi and M. Nebbioso wrote the paper. P. Del Regno contributed equally to this study.

References

[1] L. Bielory, "Allergic and immunologic disorders of the eye. Part II: ocular allergy," *Journal of Allergy and Clinical Immunology*, vol. 106, no. 6, pp. 1019–1032, 2000.

[2] S. Bonini, M. Coassin, S. Aronni, and A. Lambiase, "Vernal keratoconjunctivitis," *Eye*, vol. 18, no. 4, pp. 345–351, 2004.

[3] P. C. Donshik, W. H. Ehlers, and M. Ballow, "Giant papillary conjunctivitis," *Immunology and Allergy Clinics of North America*, vol. 28, no. 1, pp. 83–103, 2008.

[4] M. Nebbioso, A. M. Zicari, V. Lollobrigida, M. Marenco, and M. Duse, "Assessment of corneal alterations by confocal microscopy in vernal keratoconjunctivitis," *Seminars in Ophthalmology*, vol. 30, no. 1, pp. 40–43, 2015.

[5] M. Nebbioso, A. M. Zicari, C. Celani, V. Lollobrigida, R. Grenga, and M. Duse, "Pathogenesis of vernal keratoconjunctivitis and associated factors," *Seminars in Ophthalmology*, vol. 30, no. 5-6, pp. 340–344, 2015.

[6] F. Mantelli and P. Argüeso, "Functions of ocular surface mucins in health and disease," *Current Opinion in Allergy and Clinical Immunology*, vol. 2008, no. 8, pp. 477–483, 2008.

[7] R. McKenzie, J. Jumblatt, and M. Jumblatt, "Quantification of MUC2 and MUC5AC transcripts in human conjunctiva," *Investigative Ophthalmology and Visual Science*, vol. 41, no. 3, pp. 703–708, 2000.

[8] M. Jumblatt, R. McKenzie, and J. Jumblatt, "MUC5AC mucin is a component of the human precorneal tear film,"

[9] M. Dogru, N. Okada, N. Asano-Kato et al., "Atopic ocular surface disease: implications on tear function and ocular surface mucins," *Cornea*, vol. 24, no. 1, pp. S18–S23, 2005.

[10] M. Dogru, N. Okada, N. Asano-Kato et al., "Alterations of the ocular surface epithelial mucins 1, 2, 4 and the tear functions in patients with atopic keratoconjunctivitis," *Clinical and Experimental Allergy*, vol. 36, no. 12, pp. 1556–1565, 2006.

[11] I. Corum, B. Yeniad, L. K. Bilgin, and R. Ilhan, "Efficiency of Olopatadine hydrochloride 0.1% in the treatment of vernal keratoconjunctivitis and goblet cell density," *Journal of Ocular Pharmacology and Therapeutics*, vol. 21, no. 5, pp. 400–405, 2005.

[12] M. Nebbioso, V. Fameli, M. Gharbiya, M. Sacchetti, A. M. Zicari, and A. Lambiase, "Investigational drugs in dry eye disease," *Expert Opinion on Investigational Drugs*, vol. 25, no. 12, pp. 1437–1446, 2016.

[13] A. M. Masmali, C. Purslow, and P. J. Murphy, "The tear ferning test: a simple clinical technique to evaluate the ocular tear film," *Clinical and Experimental Optometry*, vol. 97, no. 5, pp. 399–406, 2014.

[14] M. Rolando, F. Baldi, and G. Calabria, "Tear mucus crystallinzation in children with cystic fibrosis," *Ophthalmologica*, vol. 197, no. 4, pp. 202–206, 1988.

[15] M. Norn, "Quantitative tear ferning. Clinical investigations," *Acta Ophthalmologica*, vol. 72, no. 3, pp. 369–372, 2009.

[16] K. F. Tabbara and M. Okumoto, "Ocular ferning test. A qualitative test for mucus deficiency," *Ophthalmology*, vol. 89, no. 6, pp. 712–714, 1982.

[17] X.R. Zhang, Q.S. Li, M.H. Xiang, R.X. Cai, and Z. Yu, "Analysis of tear mucin and goblet cells in patients with conjunctivochalasis," *Spektrum der Augenheilkunde*, vol. 24, no. 4, pp. 206–213, 2010.

[18] M. J. Doughty, "Goblet cells of the normal human bulbar conjunctiva and their assessment by impression cytology sampling," *Ocular Surface*, vol. 10, no. 3, pp. 149–169, 2012.

[19] V. Valim, V. F. Trevisani, J. M. de Sousa, V. S. Vilela, and R. Belfort Jr, "Current approach to dry eye disease," *Clinical Reviews in Allergy and Immunology*, vol. 49, no. 3, pp. 288–297, 2015.

[20] M. S. Zeev, D. D. Miller, and R. Latkany, "Diagnosis of dry eye disease and emerging technologies," *Clinical Ophthalmology*, vol. 20, no. 8, pp. 581–590, 2014.

[21] S. Bonini, S. Bonini, A. Lambiase et al., "Vernal keratoconjunctivitis: a model of 5q cytokine gene cluster disease," *International Archives of Allergy and Immunology*, vol. 107, no. 1-3, pp. 95–98, 1995.

[22] P. Aragona, G. F. Romeo, D. Puzzolo, A. Micali, and G. Ferreri, "Impression cytology of the conjunctival epithelium in patients with vernal conjunctivitis," *Eye*, vol. 10, no. 1, pp. 82–85, 1996.

[23] D. A. Dartt and S. Masli, "Conjunctival epithelial and goblet cell function in chronic inflammation and ocular allergic inflammation," *Current Opinion in Allergy and Clinical Immunology*, vol. 14, no. 5, pp. 464–470, 2014.

[24] P. R. Burgel, S. C. Lazarus, D. C. Tam et al., "Human eosinophils induce mucin production in airway epithelial cells via epidermal growth factor receptor activation," *Journal of Immunology*, vol. 167, no. 10, pp. 5948–5954, 2001.

[25] A. M. Zicari, M. Nebbioso, A. Zicari et al., "Serum levels of IL-17 in patients with vernal keratoconjunctivitis," *European Review for Medical and Pharmacological Sciences*, vol. 17, no. 9, pp. 1242–1244, 2013.

Investigative Ophthalmology and Visual Science, vol. 40, no. 1, pp. 43–49, 1999.

[26] A. M. Zicari, B. Mora, V. Lollobrigida et al., "Immunogenetic investigation in vernal keratoconjunctivitis," *Pediatric Allergic and Immunology*, vol. 25, no. 5, pp. 508–510, 2014.

[27] M. Korsgren, J. S. Erjefalt, O. Korsgren, F. Sundler, and C. G. Persson, "Allergic eosinophil-rich inflammation develops in lungs and airways of B cell-deficient mice," *Journal of Experimental Medicine*, vol. 185, no. 5, pp. 885–892, 1997.

[28] U. Keklikci, S. I. Soker, Y. B. Sakalar, K. Unlu, S. Ozekinci, and S. Tunik, "Efficacy of topical cyclosporin A 0.05% in conjunctival impression cytology specimens and clinical findings of severe vernal keratoconjunctivitis in children," *Japanese Journal of Ophthalmology*, vol. 52, no. 5, pp. 357–362, 2008.

[29] K. S. Kunert, A. S. Tisdale, and I. K. Gipson, "Goblet cell numbers and epithelial proliferation in the conjunctiva of patients with dry eye syndrome treated with cyclosporine," *Archives of Ophthalmology*, vol. 120, no. 3, pp. 330–337, 2002.

[30] D. Faulds, K. L. Goa, and P. Benfield, "Cyclosporin. A review of its pharmacodynamic and pharmacokinetic properties, and therapeutic use in immunoregulatory disorders," *Drugs*, vol. 45, no. 6, pp. 953–1040, 1993.

[31] M. Nebbioso, G. Belcaro, C. Komaiha, C. Celani, and N. Pescosolido, "Keratoconjunctivitis by confocal microscopy after topical cyclosporine," *Panminerva Medica*, vol. 55, pp. 1–5, 2015.

[32] A. Lambiase, A. Leonardi, M. Sacchetti, V. Deligianni, S. Sposato, and S. Bonini, "Topical cyclosporine prevents seasonal recurrences of vernal keratoconjunctivitis in a randomized, double-masked, controlled 2-year study," *Journal of Allergy and Clinical Immunology*, vol. 128, no. 4, pp. 896-897, 2011.

[33] A. M. Zicari, A. Zicari, M. Nebbioso et al., "High-mobility group box-1 (HMGB-1) and serum soluble receptor for advanced glycation end products (sRAGE) in children affected by vernal keratoconjunctivitis," *Pediatric Allergy and Immunology*, vol. 25, no. 1, pp. 57–63, 2014.

Evaluation of Reliability and Validity of Three Common Dry Eye Questionnaires in Chinese

Fan Lu,[1] **Aizhu Tao** ⓘ**,**[1] **Yinu Hu,**[1] **Weiwei Tao,**[2] **and Ping Lu**[1]

[1]*School of Ophthalmology and Optometry, Wenzhou Medical University, Wenzhou, Zhejiang, China*
[2]*The First Affiliated Hospital of Wenzhou Medical University, Wenzhou, Zhejiang, China*

Correspondence should be addressed to Aizhu Tao; wztaz702@163.com

Academic Editor: Marta Sacchetti

Purpose. To investigate the psychometric properties of three commonly used dry eye questionnaires including McMonnies Questionnaire (MQ), the Ocular Surface Disease Index (OSDI), and the Salisbury Eye Evaluation Questionnaire (SEEQ) in Chinese. *Methods.* This prospective cross-sectional study was conducted at the Eye Hospital of Wenzhou Medical University. Ninety-eight participants completed three questionnaires in a random order. Ophthalmic examinations including tear break-up time, corneal fluorescein staining score, and Schirmer I test were performed. Reliability, validity, and accuracy were assessed for three questionnaires. *Results.* There were 35 mild-to-moderate dry eye patients, 14 severe dry eye patients, and 49 non-dry eye patients. The Cronbach α of MQ, OSDI, and SEEQ was 0.54, 0.74, and 0.76, respectively, and the intraclass correlation coefficients were 0.91, 0.90, and 0.94, respectively. There were significant differences ($P < 0.05$) in MQ and OSDI scores among different groups, but there were no statistically significant differences between the mild-to-moderate group and the severe group in terms of SEEQ scores. With cutoff values for abnormal MQ of 15, OSDI of 27.2, and SEED of 1, respectively, good dry eye diagnostic accuracies were obtained. *Conclusions.* The three questionnaires showed fair accuracy in the diagnosis of dry eye. The cutoff values of OSDI changed when applied to Chinese people.

1. Introduction

Dry eye is a kind of disease caused by abnormal tear quantity and quality or decreased stability of tear film due to abnormal tear dynamics, and it is accompanied by eye discomfort and/or tissue lesions characteristics of the eye [1]. Dry eye symptoms may be present in the absence of significant damage to the ocular surface, and one of the goals of dry eye treatment is to improve symptoms. Therefore, it is of great significance to evaluate the symptoms in the diagnosis and monitoring of the therapeutic efficacy of dry eye.

As early as 1986, McMonnies [2] pointed out that surveying a patient's medical history is of great significance for dry eye diagnosis and designed McMonnies dry eye questionnaire (McMonnies Questionnaire (MQ)). Since then, a series of dry eye questionnaires has been developed for epidemiological investigation and clinical study of dry eye [3, 4]. At present, the dry eye questionnaire used in clinical or scientific research in China is mainly based on the direct translation of foreign questionnaires. Three kinds of questionnaires have been used widely, including MQ, the Ocular Surface Disease Index (OSDI), and the Salisbury Eye Evaluation Questionnaire (SEEQ). These questionnaires differ in length and design, and there is a certain degree of blindness in the choice of questionnaire in clinical or scientific research. As the research object of these questionnaires is Western, when it is applied to the Chinese people, its reliability and validity will be changed, and the diagnostic value of dry eye will also need to be reevaluated. Therefore, in the present study, we compared the psychometric characteristics (reliability, validity, and accuracy) of the three common dry eye questionnaires, providing information for the further design and improvement of dry eye questionnaires.

2. Subjects and Methods

The study was approved by the human subjects' review board at the Eye Hospital of Wenzhou Medical University. Each subject signed a consent form and was treated in accordance with the principles of the Declaration of Helsinki. Ninety-eight subjects (46 females and 52 males, mean age: 33.4 ± 16.8 year, ranging from 18 to 76 years) were recruited from either students at Wenzhou Medical University or outpatients at the Affiliated Eye Hospital of Wenzhou Medical University. Patients with systemic or other ocular diseases were excluded from this study.

All subjects first completed the MQ, OSDI, and SEEQ in a random order and then had objective eye examinations according to the following order: tear film break-up time (TBUT), fluorescein corneal staining (FL), and Schirmer I test (SIT). Tear break-up time was defined as the interval between the last complete blink and the appearance of the first black spot. The mean value of 3 measurements of each eye was calculated. The cornea of each eye was divided into upper, middle, and lower parts during fluorescein staining score evaluation, with each part being graded from 0 to 3: no staining was defined as grade 0, tiny and scattered dyeing was grade 1, larger and diffuse staining was grade 3, staining between 1 and 3 was defined as 2, and the total score ranged from 0 to 9 points [5]. The length of wetting of filter strip in 5 minutes after surface anesthesia was measured and recorded as the Schirmer test value.

2-3 weeks after the first questionnaire survey, a survey of three dry questionnaires was derived via telephone interview. If subjects had dry eye intervention (such as the use of artificial tears, tears embolism, etc.) or ocular surgery or other eye diseases during the two surveys, the subjects were not included in the repeatability analysis.

The Japanese diagnostic criterion of dry eye was adopted in the present study [6]: (1) subjective symptoms of dry eye; (2) TBUT < 5 s or SIT < 5 mm/5 min; (3) ocular surface lesions: corneal fluorescein staining was greater than 3 points. If all criteria mentioned above were positive, the subject was diagnosed as dry eye. To evaluate the severity of dry eye, the following grade standard was adopted [7]: (1) at least three dry eye symptoms often occur; (2) corneal fluorescein staining was greater than 6; (3) TBUT < 5 s; (4) SIT < 5 mm/5 min. Any of the above being positive was recorded as 2 points, whereas negative results recorded as 1 point. The scores of 4 items were added together, and a total score of 4–6 points were identified as mild-to-moderate dry eye, whereas 7-8 points was identified as severe dry eye.

The SPSS Statistical Package Program 13.0 (SPSS, Cary, NC) was used for data processing; $P < 0.05$ was considered statistically significant. Data are presented as the mean ± standard deviations (SD). Reliability refers to the consistency of a measuring test. The internal consistency reliability of each questionnaire was evaluated by Cronbach's alpha coefficient; the test-retest reliability of each questionnaire was tested by the intraclass correlation coefficient (ICC). Validity refers to the degree to which a measurement corresponds accurately with reality. The construct validity of the questionnaire was evaluated with factor analysis, the concurrent validity of each

questionnaire was assessed by Spearman correlation analysis, and the discriminant validity of each questionnaire was evaluated by using the multiple comparison of rank sum test. Accuracy is the degree of closeness of a measurement to its actual value. The accuracy of each dry eye questionnaire for the diagnosis of dry eye was described by the area under the receiver operating characteristic curve (ROC). Based upon the normal MQ of 12.82 ± 5.21 [8], the minimum sample size to detect a 9.0 group difference with a 99% statistical power was 28 [9]. Similarly, based upon the normal OSDI of 9.6 ± 14.2 [7], the minimum sample size to detect a 20.0 group difference with a 99% statistical power was 40 [9]. Therefore, the 98 cases in this study were more than adequate.

3. Results

Ninety-eight subjects were recruited for this study: among these, 49 cases were diagnosed with dry eye (mild-to-moderate dry eye in 35 cases and severe dry eye in 14 cases). Another investigation was performed 2-3 weeks after the first survey: subjects who had either drug or surgical intervention for dry eye were removed, and 39 measurements were obtained for repeatability analysis. The average age of the dry eye group was 35.3 ± 18.1 years, the average age of the non-dry eye group was 31.4 ± 15.2 year, and there was no significant difference in age and gender between the two groups ($P = 0.564$ and 0.544, resp., χ^2 test). Dry eye questionnaire scores and clinical dry eye test results were statistically significantly different between the two groups ($P < 0.001$, Wilcoxon rank sum test, Table 1).

3.1. Reliability. The Cronbach's alpha coefficient of MQ was 0.54, and the average correlation coefficient of each item was 0.22, indicating that the internal consistency reliability of the questionnaire was low. The overall alpha reliability coefficient of OSDI was 0.74, and the alpha reliability coefficients of "eye symptoms," "visual function," and "environmental triggering factors" were 0.67, 0.71, and 0.86, respectively, indicating that the internal consistency reliability of the scale was relatively high. The overall alpha reliability coefficient of SEEQ was 0.76, and the average correlation coefficient of each item was 0.50, showing that the internal consistency was good.

The MQ scores of the two surveys were 10.2 ± 6.5 and 10.3 ± 6.3, the OSDI scores were 22.7 ± 13 and 22.5 ± 10.5, and the SEEQ scores were 0.6 ± 1 and 0.7 ± 0.9. Their ICC were 0.91 (95% confidence interval: 0.87–0.94), 0.90 (95% confidence interval: 0.85–0.94), and 0.94 (95% confidence interval: 0.90–0.96), respectively, showing that the test-retest reliability of the questionnaires was good.

3.2. Validity. The construct validity of the questionnaire was evaluated by factor analysis. The scores of each item in the questionnaire were rotated with the maximum variance, and the principal component analysis method was used for analysis. MQ and OSDI each identified 4 main common factors, and SEEQ identified 2 common factors (characteristic value was greater than 1). The factor loads of each

TABLE 1: Results of the questionnaires and clinical dry eye test in dry eye group ($n = 49$) and non-dry eye group ($n = 49$).

	Dry eye	Non-dry eye	P
MQ	16.4 ± 4.5	7.0 ± 4.6	<0.001
OSDI	35.8 ± 13.4	15.3 ± 9.9	<0.001
SEEQ	1.4 ± 0.9	0.1 ± 0.3	<0.001
TBUT (s)	3.2 ± 1.1	7.2 ± 3.3	<0.001
SIT (mm/5 min)	3.8 ± 2.2	7.9 ± 4.4	<0.001
FL	5.3 ± 2.2	0.4 ± 0.8	<0.001

MQ: McMonnies Questionnaire; OSDI: Ocular Surface Disease Index; SEEQ: Salisbury Eye Evaluation Questionnaire; TBUT: tear film break-up time; SIT: Schirmer I test; FL: fluorescein corneal staining.

item of the questionnaire were only on one factor and were in middle to high degree (>0.4, Tables 2–4), suggesting that the factors are independent of each other and the questionnaires have good construct validity.

Relationships between the questionnaires and the objective examination results of the dry eye group are shown in Table 5. We found that MQ and OSDI scores were positively correlated ($r = 0.597$, $P < 0.001$), the MQ score was positively correlated with the SEEQ score ($r = 0.381$, $P = 0.01$), and the OSDI score was positively correlated with the SEEQ score ($r = 0.400$, $P = 0.01$). Apart from the MQ score being negatively correlated with SIT values ($r = -0.309$, $P = 0.03$) and the SEEQ score being positively correlated with the corneal fluorescein staining ($r = 360$, $P = 0.01$), the questionnaire scores and other objective eye examination results were not correlated ($P > 0.05$).

There was significant difference in the MQ scores between the non-dry eye group and both the mild-to-moderate dry eye group and the severe dry eye group ($P < 0.001$, Table 6). Furthermore, the MQ score of the mild-to-moderate dry eye group was significantly different from that of the severe dry eye group ($P < 0.001$, Table 6). The OSDI total score and the dimension "visual function" were statistically significant among different groups ($P < 0.01$ for all comparisons, Table 6). There was statistical difference between the non-dry eye group and the mild-to-moderate dry eye group in the dimension "eye symptom" ($P < 0.001$, Table 6); there was no significant difference between the non-dry eye group and the mild-to-moderate dry eye group in the dimension "environmental trigger" ($P = 0.04$, $\alpha = 0.017$, according to $\alpha = 0.05$; the number of comparisons, Table 6); there was no statistically significant difference in the SEEQ score between the mild-to-moderate dry eye group and the severe dry eye group in the dimension of "eye symptoms"; and "environmental trigger" and SEEQ scores were not statistically different ($P > 0.02$, $\alpha = 0.017$ according to $\alpha = 0.05$; comparison of the number of times, Table 6), although the SEEQ scores among other groups were statistically significantly different ($P < 0.02$, $\alpha = 0.017$ according to $\alpha = 0.05$; comparison of the number of times, Table 6).

3.3. Accuracy. Using sensitivity as the longitudinal coordinate and 1-specificity as the horizontal coordinate, the ROC curves of MQ, OSDI, and SEEQ were constructed (Figure 1). The areas under the ROC curve were 0.92 ± 0.26,

0.89 ± 0.35, and 0.91 ± 0.33, respectively, showing that the values of the three questionnaires in the diagnosis of dry eye were high, especially for the MQ. The diagnosis threshold is determined when the sum of sensitivity and specificity is largest in this diagram. The diagnostic threshold value of MQ was 14.5 (as the questionnaire score is an integer, the actual diagnostic threshold value was 15); the OSDI diagnostic threshold was 27.2; and the diagnostic threshold value of SEEQ was 1. With the cutoff values mentioned above, the sensitivity and specificity of MQ, OSDI, and SEEQ for the diagnosis of dry eye were 75.5% and 93.9%, 75.5% and 87.8%, and 85.7% and 91.8%, respectively.

4. Discussions

Dry eye is a chronic, symptomatic ocular surface disease, with symptoms that differ in severity in different patients, and the irritation symptoms of dry eye cause adverse effects on the daily life of patients. However, the presence of a symptom is not always clear, especially when it is hidden, and patients may consider it as an inevitable result of visual symptoms (such as the general embodiment of ageing). The structured design of the questionnaire is helpful for finding these hidden symptoms. The International Dry Eye Workshop (2007) recommends that all clinical trials related to dry eye should include the use of a well-designed and effective questionnaire that evaluates subjective symptoms and visual function. Moreover, the questionnaire may be the best way to determine whether clinical treatment intervention is effective [10].

The importance of medical history in the diagnosis of dry eye was first proposed by McMonnies, who designed the MQ [2]. The total score of MQ is between 0 and 45, with patients whose total score ≥15 points being considered as dry eye [11]. MQ focuses on the risk factors for dry eye and can help to determine both the existence of dry eye and individuals who are exposed to the risk factors for dry eye. However, the recall period is not specified, symptoms that happened a long time ago may be overlaid with current symptoms. Meanwhile, as the symptoms and influencing factors are mixed in the answers, it is difficult to analyze the influencing factors after the diagnosis of dry eye. In the present study, we found that the alpha reliability coefficient of MQ was 0.54, indicating that the internal consistency reliability is low. As MQ covers a wide range of factors, it has a certain "heterogeneity"; this result can also be seen from factor analysis. Low internal consistency also suggests that, when using MQ either to compare two control groups or to conduct a longitudinal study, a large sample is needed. MQ has good reliability and construct validity. As some of the MQ's questions (such as age, gender, previous dry eye treatment, and medication history) did not change during the 2-3 weeks of our follow-up, this partly explained the observed ICC values. Assessment of the discriminant validity showed that MQ was effective at distinguishing the non-dry eye from the dry eye. Moreover, the level of score has a discriminant value for the severity of the dry eye. The higher the score, the more serious the degree of dry eye; these results were inconsistent with the results of Nichols et al. [12].

TABLE 2: Structural validity analysis of McMonnies dry eye questionnaire.

Question number	Common factor 1	Common factor 2	Common factor 3	Common factor 4
1	0.106	0.762	−0.013	−0.076
2	0.596	0.319	−0.322	0.359
3	0.840	0.188	0.024	−0.061
4	0.651	−0.172	0.142	0.117
5	0.387	−0.605	−0.146	0.144
6	0.067	−0.481	−0.567	−0.043
7	0.081	0.154	0.631	−0.242
8	0.190	0.499	0.051	0.047
9	0.138	0.111	0.656	0.390
10	0.193	−0.262	0.063	−0.703
11	0.249	−0.375	0.006	−0.624
12	0.685	0.063	0.338	−0.165

TABLE 3: Structural validity analysis of Ocular Surface Disease Index.

Dimension	Question number	Common factor 1	Common factor 2	Common factor 3	Common factor 4
1	1	0.664	−0.011	0.233	0.418
1	2	0.677	0.199	0.069	0.289
1	3	−0.045	0.040	−0.050	−0.855
2	4	−0.211	0.194	0.755	0.174
2	5	0.193	0.072	0.829	−0.147
2	6	−0.024	0.882	0.159	0.008
2	7	0.066	0.688	0.271	0.076
2	8	0.539	0.481	−0.247	−0.466
2	9	0.112	0.860	−0.075	−0.042
3	10	0.786	−0.105	0.059	−0.066
3	11	0.851	0.138	−0.118	−0.261
3	12	0.906	0.083	−0.114	−0.172

OSDI was designed by the Allergan research team [3]. The purpose of this questionnaire is to rapidly assess eye irritation symptoms associated with dry eye and the effects of these symptoms on visual function. Due to the subblock answer and the designated recall period of one week, patients can evaluate themselves each week. However, as the questionnaire does not involve dry eye-related factors (such as drug usage, etc.), it does not facilitate the patient's etiological therapy. We assume that the condition of the patient during the two repeated measurements is stable; however, in fact, the state of a typical dry eye patient is often volatile and inevitably affects the outcome of the retest. There were significant differences in the OSDI total score and the scores of "visual function" between the non-dry eye group and the dry eye group and between the mild-to-moderate dry eye group and the severe dry eye group. This showed that OSDI could not only identify non-dry eyes and dry eyes but also gauge the severity of dry eye. There was no significant difference between the scores of the mild-to-moderate dry eye group and the severe dry eye group in the dimensions of "eye symptoms" and "environmental trigger," indicating that simple eye symptoms and environmental factors have little value in judging the severity of dry eye; this differs from the results of Schiffman et al. [7]. This may be either because some severe dry eye symptoms in this experiment were tolerated or because relative corneal sensation decreased, accompanied by deterioration of the disease.

TABLE 4: Structural validity analysis of Salisbury Eye Evaluation Questionnaire.

Question number	Common factor 1	Common factor 2
1	−0.014	−0.900
2	0.364	0.780
3	0.578	0.205
4	0.640	0.538
5	0.860	−0.108
6	0.649	0.274

SEEQ was proposed by Schein et al. [4] and was originally designed for the epidemiological study of dry eye in old people. It involves 6 symptoms and signs of the eye. According to the frequency of occurrence, when at least one of the symptoms was frequent, the subject was considered as dry eye. As the questionnaire is simple and clear, the SEEQ is often used to study the epidemiology of dry eye in large populations; however, it misses dry eye patients with no obvious symptoms. The present study found that the alpha reliability coefficient of SEEQ was 0.76, showing that the internal consistency is good and the retest reliability and construct validity are all good. As regards discrimination validity, the results of the present study indicate that SEEQ can distinguish the non-dry eye from the dry eye, but it has no value in discriminating the severity of dry eye; the higher

TABLE 5: Relationships between questionnaires and the objective examination results of dry eye group.

	MQ	OSDI	SEEQ	TBUT	SIT	FL
MQ	—	0.597*	0.381*	−0.156	−0.309*	0.146
OSDI	—	—	0.400*	−0.246	−0.246	0.079
SEEQ	—	—	—	−0.192	−0.205	0.360*
TBUT	—	—	—	—	−0.104	−0.163
SIT	—	—	—	—	—	0.075

*There was a relationship between the two parameters ($P < 0.05$). MQ: McMonnies Questionnaire; OSDI: Ocular Surface Disease Index; SEEQ: Salisbury Eye Evaluation Questionnaire; TBUT: tear film break-up time; SIT: Schirmer I test; FL: fluorescein corneal staining.

TABLE 6: MQ, OSDI, and SEEQ evaluated according to the severity of dry eye.

	Non-dry eye ($n = 49$)	Mild-to-moderate dry eye ($n = 35$)	Severe dry eye ($n = 14$)
MQ	7.0 ± 4.6	15.2 ± 4.5	19.4 ± 2.7
OSDI	15.3 ± 9.9	32.2 ± 12.5	44.9 ± 11.7
Eye symptoms' dimension	10.9 ± 12.4	27.4 ± 18.4	39.3 ± 27.0
Visual function dimension	11.8 ± 11.0	20.2 ± 11.7	31.8 ± 7.8
Environmental trigger dimension	24.8 ± 19.1	36.4 ± 23.9	48.8 ± 18.4
SEEQ	0.1 ± 0.3	1.2 ± 0.8	1.9 ± 0.9

There was no statistically significant difference either between the non-dry eye group and the mild-to-moderate dry eye group in the dimension "environmental trigger" or between the mild to moderate dry eye group and severe dry eye group in the dimension of "eye symptoms," and "environmental trigger" and SEEQ scores were not statistically different. All other comparisons among different groups exhibited statistically significant differences. MQ: McMonnies Questionnaire; OSDI: Ocular Surface Disease Index; SEEQ: Salisbury Eye Evaluation Questionnaire.

the score, the higher the possibility of dry eye, but this does not mean that the degree of dry eye is more serious.

From the results of concurrent validity, the questionnaire scores were positively correlated with each other. However, the correlation in our study was not high, which suggests that the properties of some dry eye patients measured by OSDI were not reflected in the MQ questionnaire. Considering the different content and structure of the questionnaires, this correlation can be expected. In the present study, we found that the consistency of dry eye symptoms and clinical examination results were poor. This is similar to the results of previous studies on the correlation between dry eye symptoms and signs. Schein et al. [4] surveyed dry eye symptoms in 2,249 elderly people and found that the SIT value was not correlated with the frequency of symptoms; Nichols et al. [13] found that dryness and foreign body sensation of dry eye patients were not correlated with tear meniscus height, the phenol red thread, the SIT value, and corneal fluorescein staining. The lack of correlation between dry eye questionnaires and clinical examination may be due to the dry eye group containing different types of dry eye patients. When using a subtype of patients, the correlation was better [7]. There is a lack of correlation between self-reported symptoms and dry eye clinical examination, which is also a puzzling and difficult problem encountered in clinical dry eye treatment and research.

It is generally accepted that the MQ score is ≥15, and the SEEQ score is ≥1 for patients with dry eye [4, 11]. According to Schiffman et al. [7], the OSDI diagnostic threshold has been identified as 15. The diagnostic threshold of OSDI obtained in the present study differs from that of Western people, this may be due to differences in diagnostic criteria of dry eye, in addition to ethnic differences. As the three

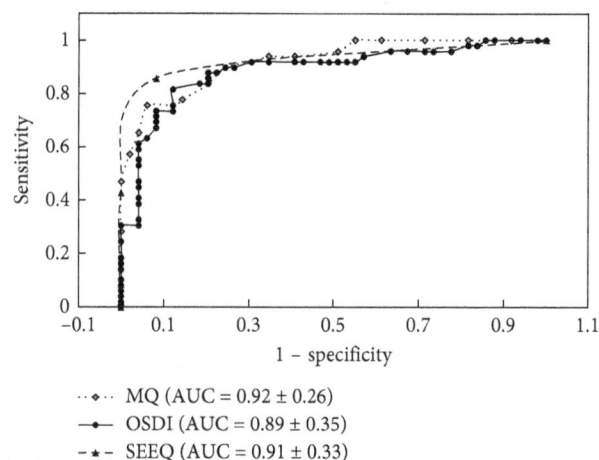

FIGURE 1: Receiver operating characteristic (ROC) curve of MQ, OSDI, and SEEQ. The area under the ROC curve (AUC) ranged from 0.89 to 0.92. MQ had the largest area, 0.92. When the cutoff value for abnormal MQ was 15, good diagnostic accuracy was obtained with 75.5% sensitivity and 93.9% specificity. MQ: McMonnies Questionnaire; OSDI: Ocular Surface Disease Index; SEEQ: Salisbury Eye Evaluation Questionnaire.

questionnaires were designed according to the Western cultural background and living environment, the threshold value of the diagnosis was changed when they were applied to the East. However, large sample population studies will be needed to confirm the specific threshold in future. Domestic dry eye researchers can combine the characteristics of dry eye questionnaires developed in foreign countries with Chinese people's habits and environment, thereby designing questionnaires that are more suitable for Chinese people. Future questionnaires may be focusing on developing electronic data system for assessing the effect of dry eye on quality of life and for self-monitoring.

In conclusion, the three questionnaires showed fair accuracy in the diagnosis of dry eye. The OSDI and the MQ scores were suitable for grading the severity of dry eye, and they were employed to screen individuals for the diagnosis of dry eye in the clinic. Furthermore, the OSDI has designated a recall period in the questionnaire and may be used to evaluate the effects of treatments. In contrast, the SEEQ did not prove suitable in discriminating between different levels of severity in dry eye patients. The SEEQ can be completed much more quickly than the OSDI and MQ, thus it may be the more convenient option for epidemiological studies. The cutoff values of OSDI changed when applied to Chinese people.

Conflicts of Interest

The authors declare that they have no conflicts of interest.

Authors' Contributions

Aizhu Tao, Yinu Hu, and Fan Lu designed the study; Aizhu Tao, Yinu Hu, Weiwei Tao, and Ping Lu performed data collection; Aizhu Tao, Weiwei Tao, and Ping Lu analyzed and interpreted the data; and Aizhu Tao, Yinu Hu, Weiwei Tao, Ping Lu, and Fan Lu were responsible for preparation, review, and approval of the manuscript.

Acknowledgments

This study was supported by the Medical Scientific Research Foundation of Zhejiang Province, China (2016KYB204), and the Development Program Project Grant from Wenzhou, China (Y20160149).

References

[1] M. A. Lemp, C. Baudouin, J. Baum et al., "The definition and classification of dry eye disease: report of the Definition and Classification Subcommittee of the International Dry Eye Workshop (2007)," *Ocular Surface*, vol. 5, no. 2, pp. 75–92, 2007.

[2] C. W. McMonnies, "Key questions in a dry eye history," *Journal of the American Optometric Association*, vol. 57, pp. 512–517, 1986.

[3] C. McAlinden, R. Gao, Q. Wang et al., "Rasch analysis of three dry eye questionnaires and correlates with objective clinical tests," *Ocular Surface*, vol. 15, no. 2, pp. 202–210, 2017.

[4] O. D. Schein, J. M. Tielsch, B. Munoz, K. Bandeen-Roche, and S. West, "Relationship between signs and symptoms of dry eye in the elderly. A population-based perspective," *Ophthalmology*, vol. 104, no. 9, pp. 1395–1401, 1997.

[5] O. P. van Bijsterveld, "Diagnostic tests in the Sicca syndrome," *Archives of Ophthalmology*, vol. 82, no. 1, pp. 10–14, 1969.

[6] Y. Mizuno, M. Yamada, Y. Miyake, and Dry Eye Survey Group of the National Hospital Organization of Japan, "Association between clinical diagnostic tests and health-related quality of life surveys in patients with dry eye syndrome," *Japanese Journal of Ophthalmology*, vol. 54, no. 4, pp. 259–265, 2010.

[7] R. M. Schiffman, M. D. Christianson, G. Jacobsen, J. D. Hirsch, and B. L. Reis, "Reliability and validity of the ocular surface disease index," *Archives of Ophthalmology*, vol. 118, no. 5, pp. 615–621, 2000.

[8] Y. Guo, R. Peng, K. Feng, and J. Hong, "Diagnostic performance of McMonnies questionnaire as a screening survey for dry eye: a multicenter analysis," *Journal of Ophthalmology*, vol. 2016, Article ID 6210853, 6 pages, 2016.

[9] E. Erdfelder, F. Faul, and A. Buchner, "GPOWER: a general power analysis program," *Behavior Research Methods Instruments and Computers*, vol. 28, no. 1, pp. 1–11, 1996.

[10] M. A. Lemp, "Report of the national eye institute/industry workshop on clinical trials in dry eyes," *CLAO Journal*, vol. 21, no. 4, pp. 221–232, 1995.

[11] C. W. McMonnies, A. Ho, and D. Wakefield, "Optimum dry eye classification using questionnaire responses," in *Advances in Experimental Medicine and Biology*, pp. 835–838, Springer, Boston, MA, USA, 1998.

[12] K. K. Nichols, J. J. Nichols, and G. L. Mitchell, "The reliability and validity of McMonnies dry eye index," *Cornea*, vol. 23, no. 4, pp. 365–371, 2004.

[13] K. K. Nichols, J. J. Nichols, and G. L. Mitchell, "The lack of association between signs and symptoms in patients with dry eye disease," *Cornea*, vol. 23, no. 8, pp. 762–770, 2004.

3

Efficacy Comparison of Intravitreal Anti-VEGF Therapy for Three Subtypes of Neovascular Age-Related Macular Degeneration

Jianqing Li (ID), Jiayi Xu, Yiyi Chen, Jiaju Zhang, Yihong Cao, and Peirong Lu (ID)

Department of Ophthalmology, The First Affiliated Hospital of Soochow University, 188 Shizi Street, Suzhou 215006, China

Correspondence should be addressed to Peirong Lu; lupeirong@suda.edu.cn

Academic Editor: Pierluigi Iacono

Purpose. Intravitreal antivascular endothelial growth factor (anti-VEGF) therapy has been widely used for the treatment of neovascularization (NV) secondary to age-related macular degeneration (AMD). This study aimed to compare the efficacy among different subtypes of neovascular age-related macular degeneration (nAMD). *Methods.* PubMed, Embase, and the Cochrane Library were searched for eligible studies. We performed meta-analysis using Review Manager 5.3 and Stata/SE 12.0. *Results.* A total of 24 studies met our inclusion criteria and were included in the systematic review. At 3 months, the mean logarithm of the minimum angle of resolution (logMAR) improvements were −0.09, −0.18, and −0.23 for type 1, 2, and 3, respectively, while the mean macular thickness (MT) changes were −104.83, −130.76, and −196.29 μm. At 12 months, the mean changes in Early Treatment of Diabetic Retinopathy Study (ETDRS) letters were 6.38, 8.12, and 9.37, while the MT decrease was 126.51, 126.52, and 139.85 μm, respectively. However, statistically significant difference was only found between type 1 and 3 in vision improvement, both in the short term ($p = 0.0002$) and long term ($p = 0.01$). *Conclusions.* The reactivity to VEGF inhibitors varied among different subtypes of nAMD. The efficacy of intravitreal anti-VEGF therapy in type 3 nAMD was statistically better than type 1 when considering vision improvement at 3 and 12 months. Thus, the lesion subtype is a predictor for the treatment outcome which can help guide prognosis.

1. Introduction

Age-related macular degeneration (AMD) is a progressive chronic disease of the central retina and a leading cause of vision loss worldwide [1] which basically has two types: exudative, neovascular, or wet AMD and nonexudative or dry AMD [2]. Neovascular age-related macular degeneration (nAMD), characterized by aberrant angiogenesis originating from the choroidal or, less frequently, the retinal circulation [3], is responsible for nearly 90% of the severe central visual acuity loss associated with AMD despite its lower incidence compared with the dry form [4].

The classification of nAMD was first developed in 1991 [5], which was based on fluorescein angiography (FA) and characterized lesion as "classic" or well-defined choroidal neovascularization (CNV) and "occult" or poorly defined CNV. A histologic classification proposed by Gass in 1994 [6] contained two different types: type 1 (located beneath the retinal pigment epithelium (RPE)) and type 2 (present beneath the sensory retina). Additional subtypes of nAMD, such as polypoidal choroidal vasculopathy (PCV) and retinal angiomatous proliferation (RAP), were further detailed with the development of optical coherence tomography (OCT). With advancements in imaging, a new anatomic classification based on FA and OCT was proposed [7], categorizing lesions as type 1 (sub-RPE), type 2 (subretinal), type 3 (intraretinal), or mixed neovascularization (NV). PCV was considered to be a special form of type 1 nAMD [7], while occult, classic, and RAP corresponded to type 1, 2, and 3, respectively, [8] in our meta-analysis.

Intravitreal antivascular endothelial growth factor (anti-VEGF) therapy has been identified to possess the potential to stabilize or even improve visual acuity in nAMD by clinical trials [9]. Several articles have studied the efficacy of anti-VEGF on different subtypes of nAMD [10–12]; however, there has been no meta-analysis focusing on the efficacy

TABLE 1: Baseline characteristics of the included studies.

First author (year)	Country	Subtype of nAMD	Sample size	Male (%)	Age (year)	Vision criteria for recruitment	Anti-VEGF use	Study design
Lai et al. (2007) [13]	China	Type 3	4	25.00	81.0±4.12	NA	Ranibizumab	Case report
Brown et al. (2009) [14]	America	Type 2	280	52.86	76.7±8.08	NA	Ranibizuma	RCT
Costagliola et al. (2010) [15]	Italy	Type 2	45	44.44	65.3±15	NA	Bevacizumab	RCT
Malgorzata and Stankiewicz (2011) [16]	Poland	Type 2	25	44.00	73.23±8.55	22–76 ETDRS letters	Ranibizumab	Clinical trial
Coscas et al. (2012) [17]	France	Type 2	29	34.48	76.3±10.9	20/400–20/40 by the ETDRS charts	Ranibizumab	RIS
Kramann et al. (2012) [18]	Germany	Type 3	26	30.77	77±8.25	NA	Ranibizumab	Retrospective case Series
Ying et al. (2013) [19]	America	Type 1, type 2, type 3	1105	38	79±8	20/25–20/320 on electronic VA testing	Ranibizumab or bevacizumab	RCT
Shin and Yu (2014) [20]	South Korea	Type 3	31	19.35	70.4±6.5	5–75 ETDRS letters (Snellen 20/32–20/800)	Ranibizumab	Clinical trial
Hata et al. (2015) [21]	Japan	Type 1 (PCV)	70	81.43	72.2±8.8	0.7 or less on a Landolt chart	Ranibizumab	RIS
Kano et al. (2015) [22]	Japan	Type 1	100	86	75.71±7.79	0.05 or better by the Japanese decimal VA chart	Ranibizumab or aflibercept	RIS
Park and Roh (2015) [23]	South Korea	Type 3	40	39.02	67.09±11.76	NA	Ranibizumab	RIS
Castro-Navarro et al. (2016) [24]	Spain	Type 3	7	14.29	79.42±7.14	<0.1 logMAR	Aflibercept	RIS
Chen et al. (2016) [25]	America	Type 1, type 3	36	36.11	80±8.0	19–73 ETDRS letters (Snellen 20/35–20/400)	Aflibercept	Clinical trial
Daniel et al. (2016) [26]	America	Type 3	126	30.95	81.7±7.30	20/25–20/320	Ranibizumab or bevacizumab	Clinical trial
Koizumi et al. (2016) [27]	Japan	Type 1 (PCV)	86	NA	NA	NA	Aflibercept	RIS
Lee et al. (2016) [28]	South Korea	Type 1, type 2	23	60.87	66.52±9.28	NA	Ranibizumab	RIS
Chevreaud et al. (2017) [29]	France	Type 1, PCV, type 2, type 3	109	33.03	76.9±8.3	NA	Ranibizumab	RIS
Kikushima et al. (2017) [30]	Japan	Type 1 (PCV)	69	83.9	72.9±7.9	Decimal BCVA≤1.2 in the Landolt chart	Aflibercept	RIS
Koh et al. (2017) [31]	Singapore	Type 1 (PCV)	154	75.3	68.2±9.0	78–24 ETDRS letters (Snellen 20/32–20/320)	Ranibizumab	RCT
Miere et al. (2017) [32]	Italy	Type 3	15	33.33	82.3±4.9	NA	Ranibizumab or bevacizumab	RIS
Saito et al. (2017) [33]	Japan	Type 1 (PCV)	20	90.00	72.2±6.4	NA	Aflibercept	Clinical trial
Gharbiya et al. (2018) [34]	Italy	Type 1, type 2, type 3	76	34.21	78.67±8.04	NA	Ranibizumab or aflibercept	Clinical trial
Matsumoto et al. (2018) [35]	Japan	Type 1 (half with PCV)	60	85.00	75.1±1.0	NA	Aflibercept	RIS
Mimura et al. (2018) [36]	Japan	Type 1 (PCV), type 3	58	65.52	73.08	NA	Aflibercept	RIS

†Data are mean±standard deviation or mean. ‡nAMD: neovascular age-related macular degeneration; anti-VEGF: antivascular endothelial growth factor; PCV: polypoidal choroidal vasculopathy; NA: not available; ETDRS: Early Treatment of Diabetic Retinopathy Study; RCT: randomized controlled trial; RIS: retrospective interventional study.

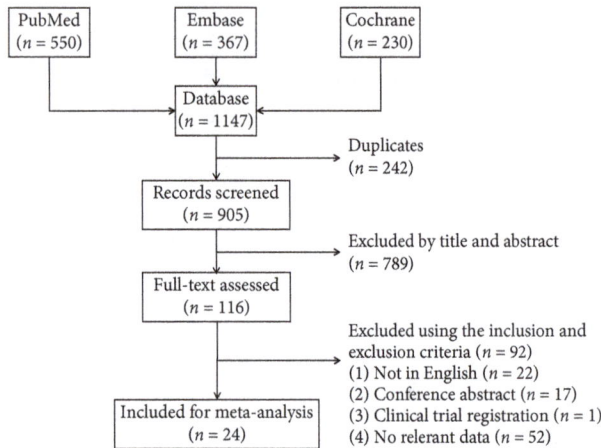

FIGURE 1: Flow diagram of the inclusion of studies in this meta-analysis.

comparison among all three types of nAMD. Therefore, we carried out a systematic review and meta-analysis in order to study the relationship between treatment efficacy and lesion subtype.

2. Materials and Methods

2.1. Search Strategy. Two independent reviewers (J. Li and J. Xu) performed a systematic search in PubMed, Embase, and the Cochrane Library on March 16, 2018, for articles focusing on the efficacy of intravitreal anti-VEGF on different subtypes of nAMD. The search strategy was [("nAMD" AND "subtype") AND "anti-VEGF"] using the MeSH or Emtree terms as well as free words. Here, "nAMD," "wet AMD," and "exudative AMD" were searched for "nAMD"; "Type 1," "PCV," "occult," "poorly-defined," "sub-RPE," "Type 2," "classic," "well-defined," "subretinal," "Type 3," "RAP," and "intraretinal" were for different subtypes of nAMD, while "pegaptanib," "bevacizumab," "ranibizumab," "aflibercept" and "conbercept" were searched for "anti-VEGF."

2.2. Selection Criteria. The eligibility criteria were as follows: (1) any subtype of nAMD, (2) treatment-naive nAMD, (3) anti-VEGF monotherapy, (4) efficacy measured by vision improvement or macular thickness (MT) changes, and (5) efficacy measured at 3 months or 12 months. Those studies which were not in English with no full text or irrelevant data were excluded. Any disagreements about the inclusion of an article for full review were resolved by a third researcher (P. Lu).

2.3. Assessment of Risk of Bias. "Risk of bias" of each included article was assessed using "risk of bias table," which was suitable for both randomized and nonrandomized studies, according to the Cochrane Handbook for Systematic Reviews of Interventions Version 5.1.

2.4. Data Extraction. The characteristics extracted from the eligible articles included the first author's name, publication

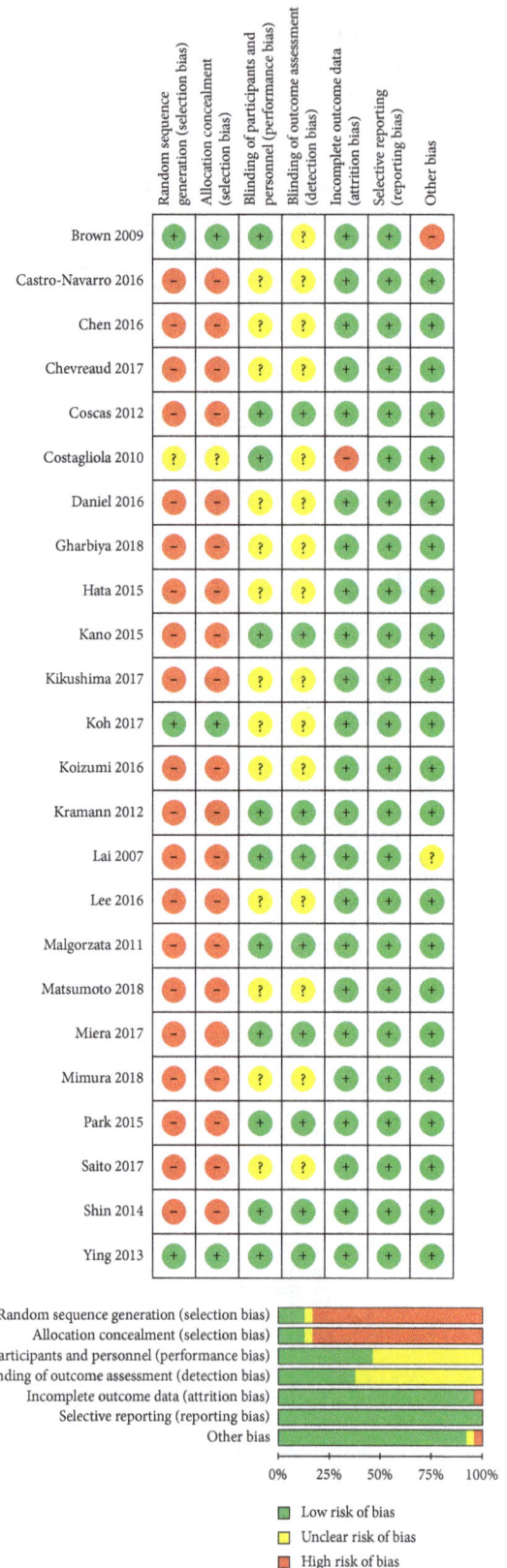

FIGURE 2: Risk of bias assessment of the included studies.

year, country where the study was conducted, subtype of nAMD, sample size, gender, mean age of the sample, vision criteria for recruitment, anti-VEGF use, and study design.

Study or subgroup	Mean difference	SE	Weight	Mean difference IV, random, 95% CI	Mean difference IV, random, 95% CI
1.1.1 Type 1					
Chevreaud et al. [29]	−0.0532	0.0301	11.2%	−0.05 (−0.11, 0.01)	
Kano et al. [22]	−0.0667	0.0154	13.9%	−0.07 (−0.10, −0.04)	
Kikushima et al. [30]	−0.11	0.0386	9.6%	−0.11 (−0.19, −0.03)	
Koizumi et al. [27]	−0.1	0.0318	10.9%	−0.10 (−0.16, −0.04)	
Lee et al. [28]	−0.07	0.0871	3.8%	−0.07 (−0.24, 0.10)	
Mimura et al. [36]	−0.12	0.0069	14.9%	−0.12 (−0.13, −0.11)	
Subtotal (95% CI)			64.2%	−0.09 (−0.12, −0.06)	

Heterogeneity: $\tau^2 = 0.00$; $\chi^2 = 13.79$, $df = 5$ ($P = 0.02$); $I^2 = 64\%$
Test for overall effect: $Z = 5.76$ ($P < 0.00001$)

1.1.2 Type 2					
Chevreaud et al. [29]	0.14	0.2041	0.9%	0.14 (−0.26, 0.54)	
Lee et al. [28]	−0.53	0.2306	0.7%	−0.53 (−0.98, −0.08)	
Malgorzata and Stankiewicz [16]	−0.19	0.054	7.1%	−0.19 (−0.30, −0.08)	
Subtotal (95% CI)			8.6%	−0.18 (−0.46, 0.10)	

Heterogeneity: $\tau^2 = 0.04$; $\chi^2 = 4.78$, $df = 2$ ($P = 0.09$); $I^2 = 58\%$
Test for overall effect: $Z = 1.29$ ($P = 0.20$)

1.1.3 Type 3					
Chevreaud et al. [29]	−0.26	0.2216	0.7%	−0.26 (−0.69, 0.17)	
Kramann et al. [18]	−0.22	0.0709	5.1%	−0.22 (−0.36, −0.08)	
Lai et al. [13]	−0.3	0.0431	8.8%	−0.30 (−0.38, −0.22)	
Mimura et al. [36]	−0.19	0.0228	12.6%	−0.19 (−0.23, −0.15)	
Subtotal (95% CI)			27.2%	−0.23 (−0.30, −0.16)	

Heterogeneity: $\tau^2 = 0.00$; $\chi^2 = 5.14$, $df = 3$ ($P = 0.16$); $I^2 = 42\%$
Test for overall effect: $Z = 6.81$ ($P < 0.00001$)

Total (95% CI)			100.0%	−0.14 (−0.17, −0.10)	

Heterogeneity: $\tau^2 = 0.00$; $\chi^2 = 53.33$, $df = 12$ ($P < 0.00001$); $I^2 = 77\%$
Test for overall effect: $Z = 6.94$ ($P < 0.00001$)
Test for subgroup differences: $\chi^2 = 14.22$, $df = 2$ ($P = 0.0008$); $I^2 = 85.9\%$

(a)

Study or subgroup	Mean difference	SE	Weight	Mean difference IV, random, 95% CI	Mean difference IV, random, 95% CI
2.1.1 Type 1					
Chevreaud et al. [29]	−162.8971	18.9396	7.9%	−162.90 (−200.02, −125.78)	
Gharbiya et al. [34]	−89	16.1658	8.0%	−89.00 (−120.68, −57.32)	
Hata et al. [21]	−123.4	22.328	7.7%	−123.40 (−167.16, −79.64)	
Kano et al. [22]	−59.32	11.6136	8.3%	−59.32 (−82.08, −36.56)	
Kikushima et al. [30]	−182	15.849	8.1%	−182.00 (−213.06, −150.94)	
Lee et al. [28]	−17.4	13.727	8.2%	−17.40 (−44.30, 9.50)	
Subtotal (95% CI)			48.1%	−104.83 (−156.93, −52.72)	

Heterogeneity: $\tau^2 = 3961.15$; $\chi^2 = 85.69$, $df = 5$ ($P = 0.00001$); $I^2 = 94\%$
Test for overall effect: $Z = 3.94$ ($P < 0.0001$)

2.1.2 Type 2					
Chevreaud et al. [29]	−135	101.5364	2.6%	−135.00 (−334.01, 64.01)	
Gharbiya et al. [34]	−79.5	24.6667	7.5%	−79.50 (−127.85, −31.15)	
Lee et al. [28]	−185.78	53.682	5.2%	−185.78 (−290.99, −80.57)	
Malgorzata and Stankiewicz [16]	−150.32	13.0154	8.2%	−150.32 (−175.83, −124.81)	
Subtotal (95% CI)			23.5%	−130.76 (−181.07, −80.45)	

Heterogeneity: $\tau^2 = 1315.03$; $\chi^2 = 7.31$, $df = 3$ ($P = 0.06$); $I^2 = 59\%$
Test for overall effect: $Z = 5.09$ ($P = 0.00001$)

2.1.3 Type 3					
Chevreaud et al. [29]	−303.3	56.7403	5.0%	−303.30 (−414.51, −192.09)	
Gharbiya et al. [34]	−110.1	26.1171	7.4%	−110.10 (−161.29, −58.91)	
Kramann et al. [18]	−130	14.9473	8.1%	−130.00 (−159.30, −100.70)	
Lai et al. [13]	−269	19.6373	7.8%	−269.00 (−307.49, −230.51)	
Subtotal (95% CI)			28.4%	−196.29 (−285.05, −107.53)	

Heterogeneity: $\tau^2 = 7229.58$; $\chi^2 = 43.25$, $df = 3$ ($P = 0.00001$); $I^2 = 93\%$
Test for overall effect: $Z = 4.33$ ($P < 0.0001$)

Total (95% CI)			100.0%	−136.95 (−175.62, −98.27)	

Heterogeneity: $\tau^2 = 4578.10$; $\chi^2 = 185.15$, $df = 13$ ($P < 0.00001$); $I^2 = 93\%$
Test for overall effect: $Z = 6.94$ ($P < 0.00001$)
Test for subgroup differences: $\chi^2 = 3.04$, $df = 2$ ($P = 0.22$); $I^2 = 34.2\%$

(b)

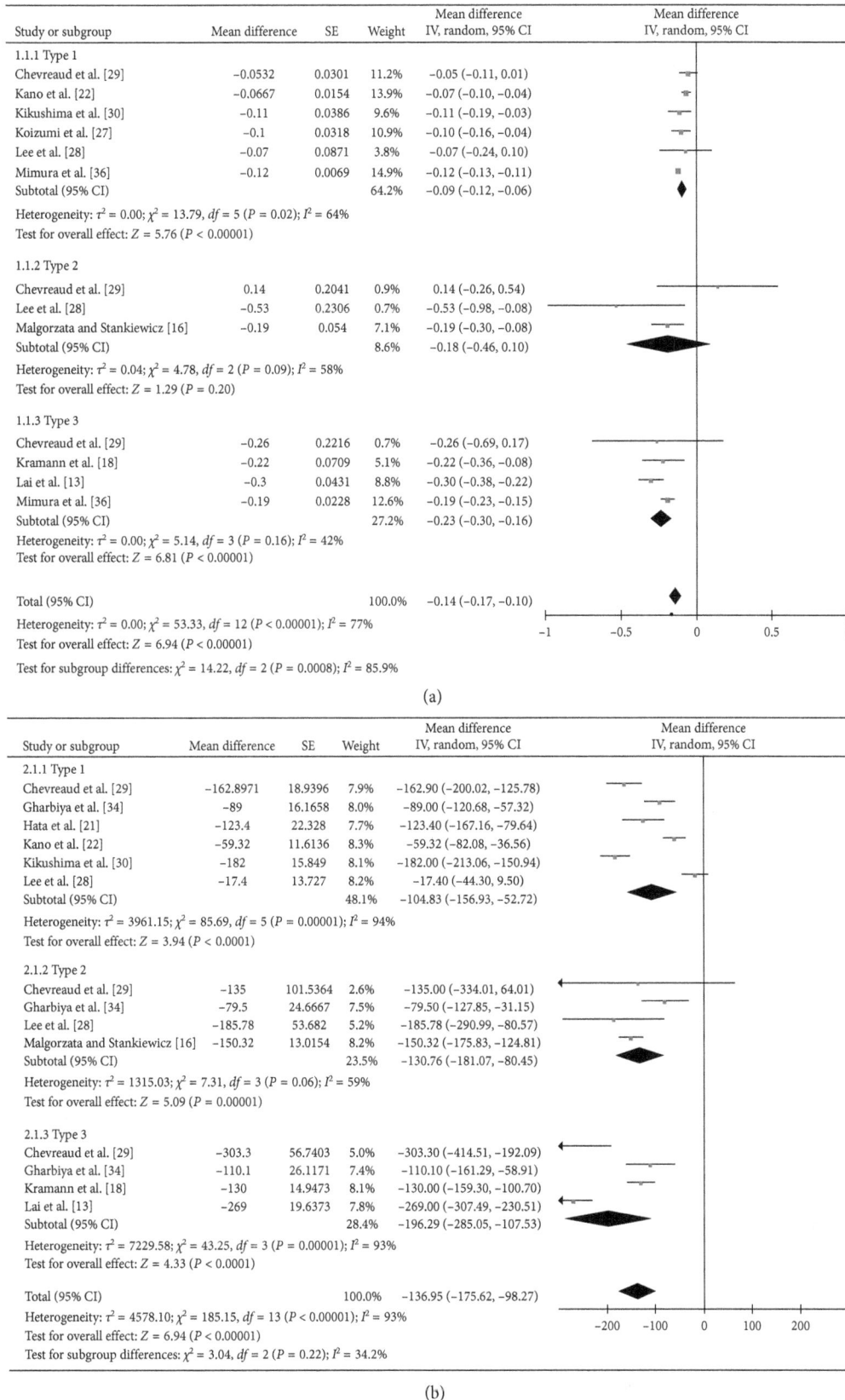

FIGURE 3: The short-term (3 months) efficacy comparison of antivascular endothelial growth factor (anti-VEGF) therapy for three subtypes of neovascular age-related macular degeneration (nAMD). (a) Vision improvement of the three types of nAMD, measured by logarithm of the minimum angle of resolution (logMAR), were −0.09 (95% confidence interval (CI): −0.12, −0.06), −0.18 (95% CI: −0.46, 0.10), and −0.23 (95% CI: −0.30, −0.16). (b) Macular thickness decreases were −104.83 (95% CI: −156.93, −52.72), −130.76 (95% CI: −181.07, −80.45), and −196.29 (95% CI: −285.05, −107.53) μm, respectively.

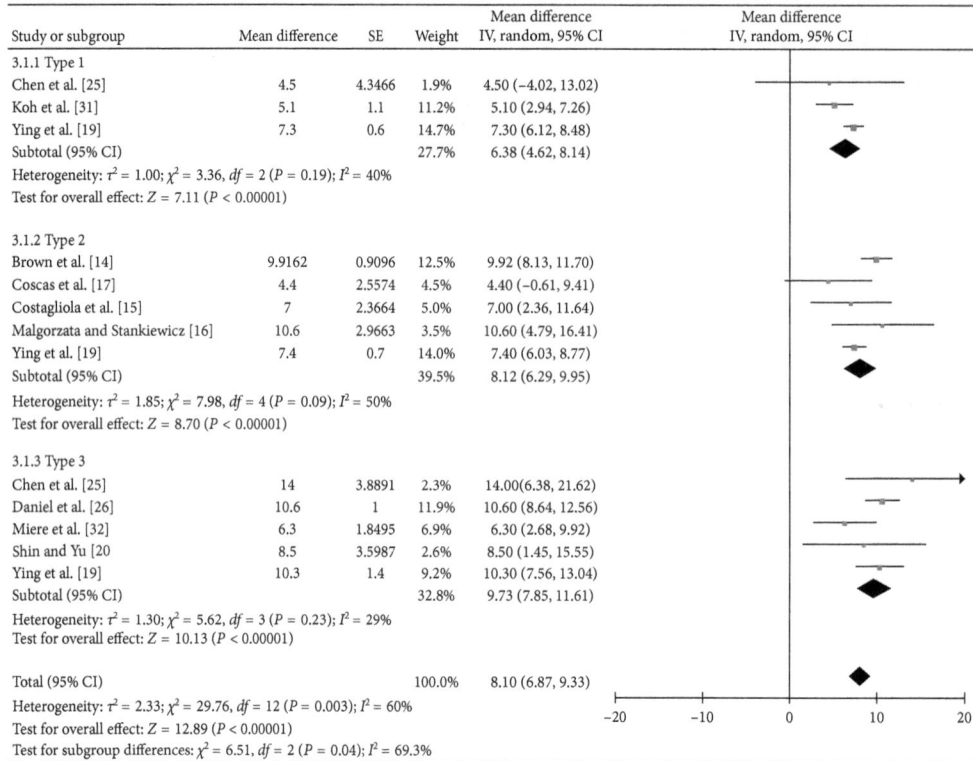

(a)

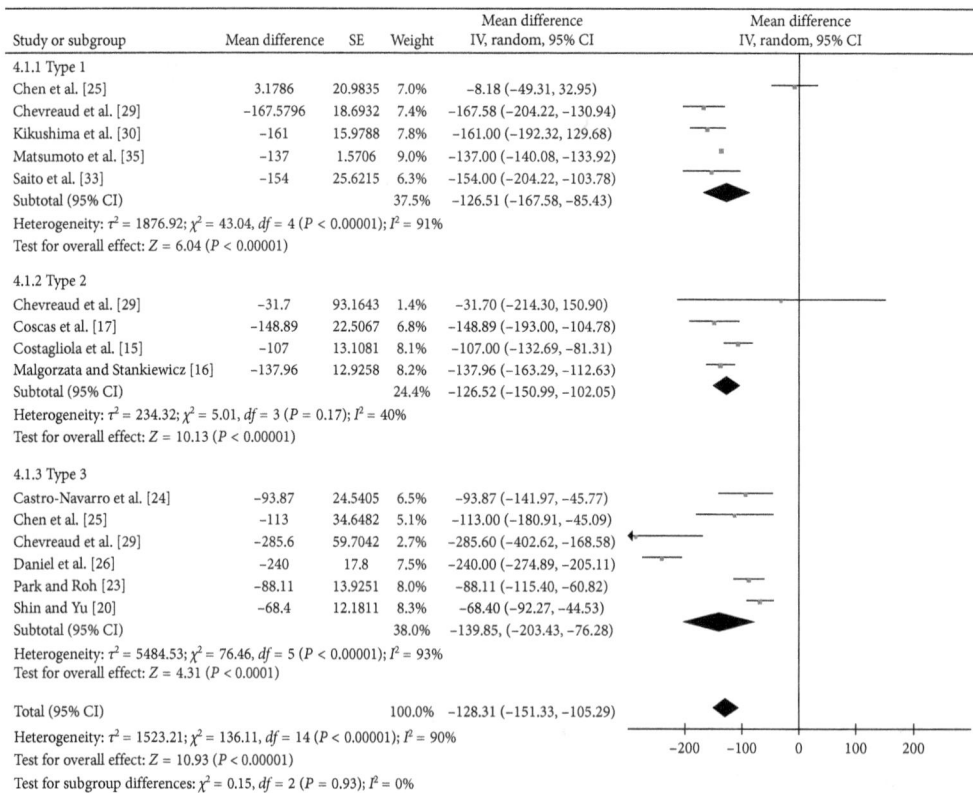

(b)

FIGURE 4: The long-term (12 months) efficacy comparison among three subtypes of neovascular age-related macular degeneration (nAMD) was presented. (a) Vision improvement, evaluated by Early Treatment of Diabetic Retinopathy Study (ETDRS) letters, were 6.38 (95% CI: 4.62, 8.14), 8.12 (95% CI: 6.29, 9.95), and 9.73 (95% CI: 7.85, 11.61) for the three types of nAMD. (b) Macular thickness changes were −126.51 (95% CI: −167.58, −85.43), −126.52 (95% CI: −150.99, −102.05), and −139.85 (95% CI: −203.43, −76.28) μm, respectively.

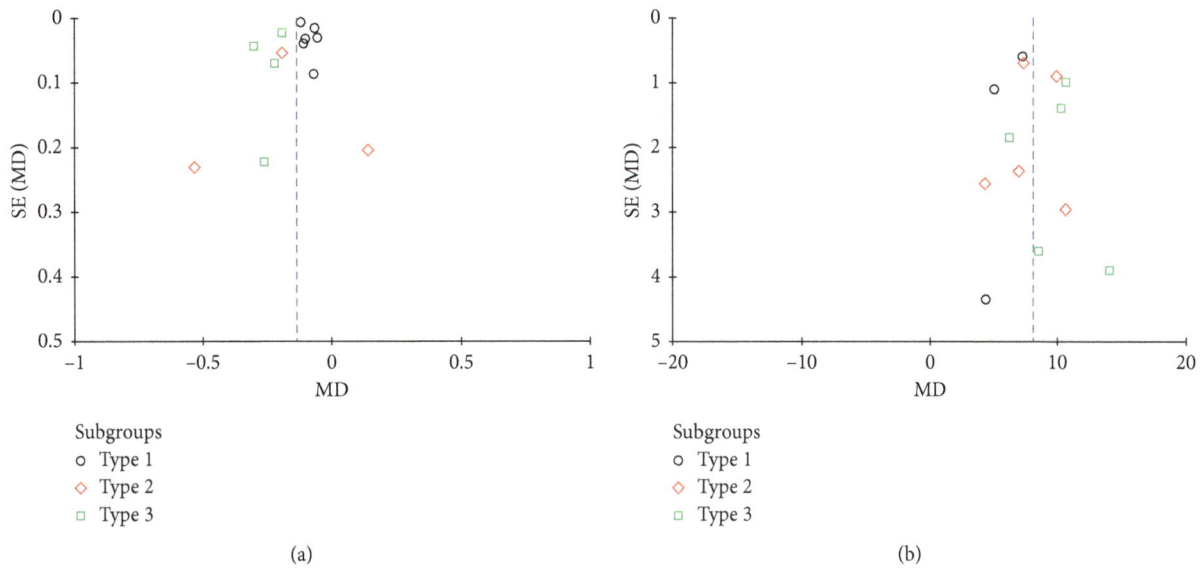

FIGURE 5: Funnel plots for short-term (a) and long-term (b) vision improvement comparison.

Besides, PCV was marked in the column of subtype of nAMD in Table 1 since it was a variant of type 1 nAMD.

The main outcome of this meta-analysis was efficacy comparison of intravitreal anti-VEGF therapy for three subtypes of nAMD. The efficacy was measured by vision improvement or macular thickness (MT) changes at 3 or 12 months; therefore, these data were extracted for further analysis. Since meta-analysis was a second source, the relevant data were extracted either directly from the article or by extrapolation. In this study, no authors were contacted for the raw data of each patient, thus we could not adjust some different factors such as visual acuity at baseline.

2.5. Statistical Analysis. All the statistical analyses in our study were completed using Review Manager (RevMan) version 5.3 (The Nordic Cochrane Centre, Copenhagen, Denmark) and Stata version 12.0 (StataCorp, Texas, America). The effect value in this meta-analysis was the mean difference (MD). Before the analysis, the study heterogeneity was tested using both the I-squared and chi-squared test statistics. An $I^2 \geq 50\%$ and/or a Q-statistic of $p < 0.05$ was evidence supporting the presence of heterogeneity, in which the random-effects modeling method was needed. Otherwise, the fixed-effects modeling method was applied. In addition, publication bias and sensitivity analysis were conducted to study the relevant bias as well as stability and reliability of the outcomes.

3. Results

3.1. Description of Studies. A total of 1147 articles were identified, and their records were included in EndNote X8 (Clarivate Analytics, Philadelphia, PA, US). After removing 242 duplicates, the remaining 905 articles were screened based on the titles and abstracts by two reviewers according to our inclusion criteria. Any disagreements about the inclusion of an article for full review were resolved by the third researcher. Full-text assessment was conducted on the rest of the 116 articles. Finally, 24 articles [13–36] were included in this meta-analysis. The article searches and selection process is summarized in Figure 1.

3.2. Study Quality and Characteristics. "Risk of bias" of these studies was assessed by "risk of bias table," and the outcome is summarized in Figure 2. The selection bias, which contained random sequence generation and allocation concealment, was mainly of high risk, predominantly due to those nonrandomized studies. Although blinding of performance and detection was not performed in most of the included studies, the outcome was not likely to be influenced by lack of blinding or there was insufficient information to permit judgement of "Low risk" or "High risk."

Among the included studies, 4 were randomized controlled trials (RCT), 12 were retrospective interventional studies (RIS), 6 were clinical trials, and the left 2 were case reports. Altogether, 2594 patients were involved in this review. The demographic characteristics of the studies were summarized in Table 1.

3.3. Critical Appraisal Tool

3.3.1. Short-Term Outcome. Figure 3 illustrated the short-term (3 months) efficacy comparison. In Figure 3(a), vision improvements of the three types of nAMD, measured by logarithm of the minimum angle of resolution (logMAR), were −0.09 (95% confidence interval (CI): −0.12, −0.06), −0.18 (95% CI: −0.46, 0.10), and −0.23 (95% CI: −0.30, −0.16). While MT changes, displayed in Figure 3(b), were −104.83 (95% CI: −156.93, −52.72), −130.76 (95% CI: −181.07, −80.45), and −196.29 (95% CI: −285.05, −107.53) μm, respectively. It was obvious that the efficacy varied among different subtypes of nAMD; however, the subtype difference was only statistically significant between type 1 and type 3 in vision improvement ($p = 0.0002$).

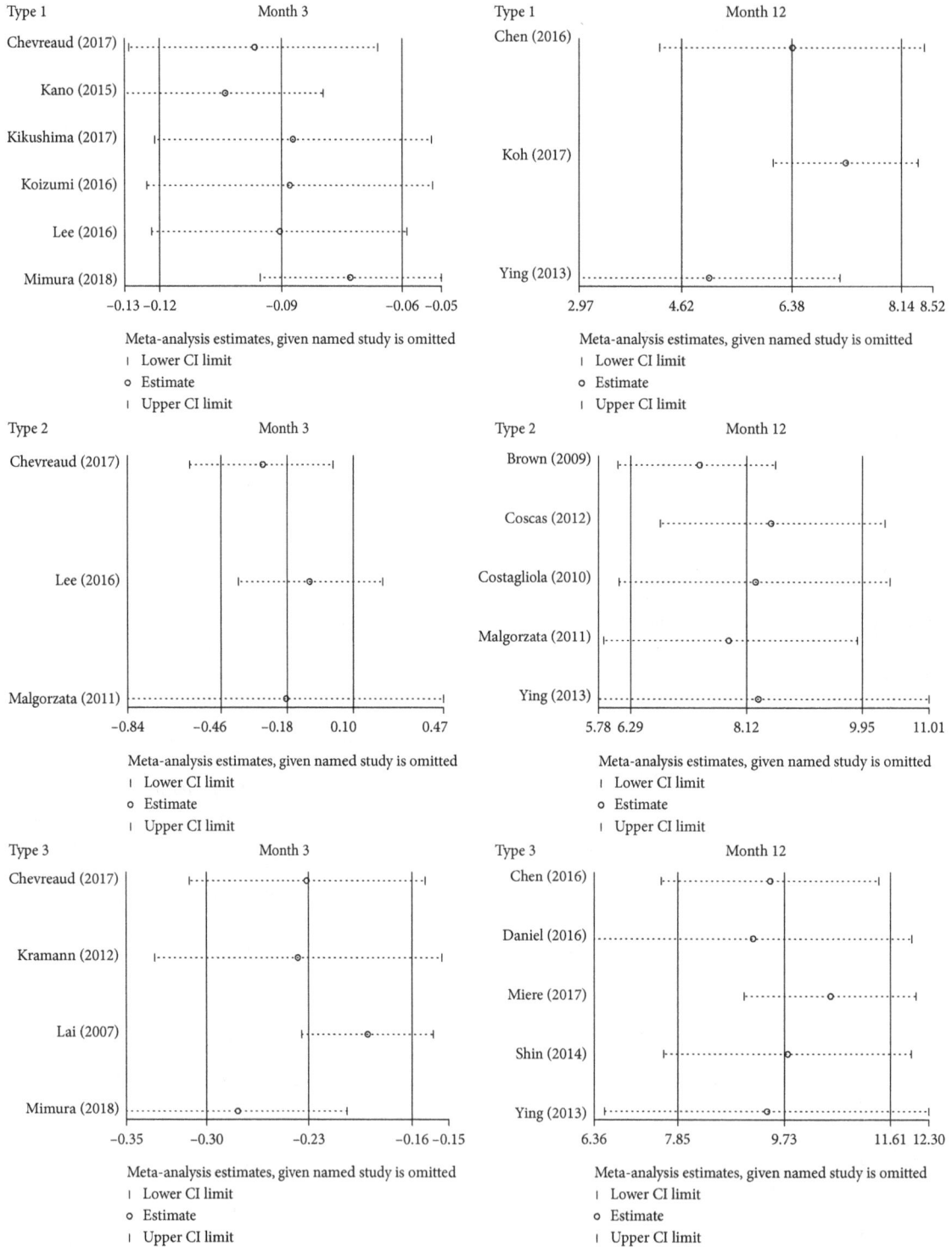

FIGURE 6: Sensitivity analysis on the outcome of vision improvement at 3 and 12 months.

3.3.2. Long-Term Outcome. The long-term (12 months) efficacy comparison was presented in Figure 4. Vision improvements, evaluated by Early Treatment of Diabetic Retinopathy Study (ETDRS) letters, were 6.38 (95% CI: 4.62, 8.14), 8.12 (95% CI: 6.29, 9.95), and 9.73 (95% CI: 7.85, 11, 61) for the three types of nAMD. In Figure 4(b), MT changes were −126.51 (95% CI: −167.58, −85.43), −126.52 (95% CI: −150.99, −102.05), and −139.85 (95% CI: −203.43, −76.28) μm,

respectively. Although the efficacy differed in the three types of nAMD, the statistically significant subtype difference still only existed between type 1 and type 3 in vision improvement ($p < 0.0001$).

3.4. Publication Bias. Funnel plots for short-term and long-term vision improvement comparison are shown in Figure 5.

The two plots were both relatively symmetrical, which indicated little evidence of publication bias.

3.5. Sensitivity Analysis. The impact of individual data was examined for sensitivity analysis, which was conducted on the outcome of vision improvement at 3 and 12 months (Figure 6). When omitting each study, we found no obvious changes to the results, thus drawing a conclusion that our results on vision efficacy were stable and reliable.

4. Discussion

To our knowledge, this was the first meta-analysis quantitatively comparing treatment efficacy of intravitreal anti-VEGF therapy for three subtypes of nAMD. A total of 24 articles were included in our systematic review. In order to assess the efficacy, the relevant data about vision improvement and MT changes at 3 months or 12 months were extracted for further pooled analysis. We found that although the efficacy of type 2 nAMD was superior to type 1 and inferior to type 3, statistically significant difference was only found between type 1 and 3 in vision improvement, both during the short term ($p = 0.0002$) and long term ($p = 0.01$). We could draw a conclusion that the reactivity to VEGF inhibitors varied among different subtypes of nAMD. Thus, the lesion subtype could be considered as a predictor for the treatment outcome.

There are several potential explanations for our results. First of all, the three types of nAMD are characterized with different locations of NV: sub-RPE, subretina, and intraretina. The closer to the retinal photoreceptors, the earlier and more severe the clinical symptoms of nAMD appear. Therefore, the three subtypes suffer from different durations and various severities. Another theory is anti-VEGF resistance, which means that tissues treated with anti-VEGF may develop resistance to hypoxia and become less dependent on angiogenesis or develop more mature vessels through remodeling, which is less responsive to anti-angiogenic therapy [37]. Patients with type 1 nAMD tend to agonize over longer duration, thus are more likely to develop anti-VEGF resistance. Therefore, treatment efficacy for type 1 is inferior to type 2 and 3.

So far, the three types of nAMD have been classified based on the location of abnormal vessels using fluorescence angiography (FA) and optical coherence tomography (OCT). Nevertheless, OCTA (and a possible OCTA classification) may offer additional information on treatment-response and anti-VEGF resistance by providing morphological information and quantitative measures (area, vascular density, fractal dimension, etc.), but that the clinical relevance of such findings is still debated [32, 38, 39].

Some limitations did exist in our systematic review. Firstly, this meta-analysis consisted mostly of nonrandomized studies which were more likely to be influenced by various kinds of biases. Hence, it was not surprising that almost all of them were at relatively high risk when we assessed the risk of bias as shown in Figure 2. However, there has been no way to control these biases and no method to assess their impact on the outcome so far. Secondly, heterogeneity was statistically significant across several results (Figures 3 and 4). One possible explanation was that nonrandomized studies were more likely to introduce heterogeneity due to confounding factors and all kinds of biases. Moreover, no authors were contacted for primary statistics. The relevant data were extracted either directly from the article or by extrapolation, thus we could not adjust some different factors at baseline. For example, of the 24 included studies, only 11 were involved with vision criteria for enrollment, and these criteria were various. However, we had no way to adjust visual acuity at baseline because of lacking individual patient data. Nevertheless, this problem might be a common limitation of meta-analysis.

5. Conclusion

In summary, we believe that this meta-analysis, comparing treatment efficacy among different types of nAMD, is of great significance to clinical practice. The results indicate that lesion subtype is a predictor for the treatment outcome which could help guide prognosis.

Conflicts of Interest

The authors declare that they have no conflicts of interest.

Authors' Contributions

Jianqing Li and Peirong Lu designed the study and wrote the paper; Jianqing Li and Jiayi Xu searched the literature; Jianqing Li, Yiyi Chen, Jiaju Zhang, and Yihong Cao extracted and analyzed the data; Jianqing Li and Peirong Lu contributed to the improvement of the manuscript. All authors approved the submitted and final version.

Acknowledgments

This work was supported by the National Natural Science Foundation of China (NSFC No. 81671641), Jiangsu Provincial Medical Innovation Team (No. CXTDA2017039), Jiangsu Provincial Natural Science Foundation (No. BK20151208), and the Soochow Scholar Project of Soochow University (No. R5122001).

References

[1] L. S. Lim, P. Mitchell, J. M. Seddon, F. G. Holz, and T. Y. Wong, "Age-related macular degeneration," *The Lancet*, vol. 379, no. 9827, pp. 1728–1738, 2012.

[2] I. Bhutto and G. Lutty, "Understanding age-related macular degeneration (AMD): relationships between the photoreceptor/retinal pigment epithelium/Bruch's membrane/choriocapillaris complex," *Molecular Aspects of Medicine*, vol. 33, no. 4, pp. 295–317, 2012.

[3] J. D. Gass, A. Agarwal, A. M. Lavina, and K. A. Tawansy, "Focal inner retinal hemorrhages in patients with drusen: an early sign of occult choroidal neovascularization and chorioretinal anastomosis," *Retina*, vol. 23, no. 6, pp. 741–751, 2003.

[4] American Academy of Ophthalmology Retina/Vitreous Panel, *Preferred Practice Pattern®Guidelines. Age-Related Macular Degeneration*, American Academy of Ophthalmology, San Francisco, CA, USA, 2015, http://www.aao.org/ppp.

[5] Macular Photocoagulation Study Group, "Laser photocoagulation of subfoveal neovascular lesions in age-related macular degeneration. Results of a randomized clinical trial," *Archives of Ophthalmology*, vol. 109, no. 9, pp. 1220–1231, 1991.

[6] J. D. Gass, "Biomicroscopic and histopathologic considerations regarding the feasibility of surgical excision of subfoveal neovascular membranes," *American Journal of Ophthalmology*, vol. 118, no. 3, pp. 285–298, 1994.

[7] K. B. Freund, S. A. Zweifel, and M. Engelbert, "Do we need a new classification for choroidal neovascularization in age-related macular degeneration?," *Retina*, vol. 30, no. 9, pp. 1333–1349, 2010.

[8] J. J. Jung, C. Y. Chen, S. Mrejen et al., "The incidence of neovascular subtypes in newly diagnosed neovascular age-related macular degeneration," *American Journal of Ophthalmology*, vol. 158, no. 4, pp. 769–779.e2, 2014.

[9] H. Mehta, A. Tufail, V. Daien et al., "Real-world outcomes in patients with neovascular age-related macular degeneration treated with intravitreal vascular endothelial growth factor inhibitors," *Progress in Retinal and Eye Research*, vol. 64, pp. 127–146, 2018.

[10] H. Koizumi, M. Kano, A. Yamamoto et al., "Short-term changes in choroidal thickness after aflibercept therapy for neovascular age-related macular degeneration," *American Journal of Ophthalmology*, vol. 159, no. 4, pp. 627–633, 2015.

[11] B. Chae, J. J. Jung, S. Mrejen et al., "Baseline predictors for good versus poor visual outcomes in the treatment of neovascular age-related macular degeneration with intravitreal anti-VEGF therapy," *Investigative Opthalmology & Visual Science*, vol. 56, no. 9, pp. 5040–5047, 2015.

[12] K. Hufendiek, K. Hufendiek, G. Panagakis, H. Helbig, and M. A. Gamulescu, "Visual and morphological outcomes of bevacizumab (Avastin®) versus ranibizumab (Lucentis®) treatment for retinal angiomatous proliferation," *International Ophthalmology*, vol. 32, no. 3, pp. 259–268, 2012.

[13] T. Y. Lai, W. M. Chan, D. T. Liu, and D. S. Lam, "Ranibizumab for retinal angiomatous proliferation in neovascular age-related macular degeneration," *Graefe's Archive for Clinical and Experimental Ophthalmology*, vol. 245, no. 12, pp. 1877–1880, 2007.

[14] D. M. Brown, M. Michels, P. K. Kaiser et al., "Ranibizumab versus verteporfin photodynamic therapy for neovascular age-related macular degeneration: two-year results of the ANCHOR study," *Ophthalmology*, vol. 116, no. 1, pp. 57–65.e5, 2009.

[15] C. Costagliola, M. R. Romano, M. Rinaldi et al., "Low fluence rate photodynamic therapy combined with intravitreal bevacizumab for neovascular age-related macular degeneration," *British Journal of Ophthalmology*, vol. 94, no. 2, pp. 180–184, 2010.

[16] F. Małgorzata and A. Stankiewicz, "Effectiveness of ranibizumab intravitreal injections for exudative age-related macular degeneration treatment: 12-month outcomes," *Medical Science Monitor*, vol. 17, no. 9, pp. CR485–CR490, 2011.

[17] F. Coscas, G. Querques, R. Forte, C. Terrada, G. Coscas, and E. H. Souied, "Combined fluorescein angiography and spectral-domain optical coherence tomography imaging of classic choroidal neovascularization secondary to age-related macular degeneration before and after intravitreal ranibizumab injections," *Retina*, vol. 32, no. 6, pp. 1069–1076, 2012.

[18] C. A. Kramann, K. Schöpfer, K. Lorenz, I. Zwiener, B. M. Stoffelns, and N. Pfeiffer, "Intravitreal ranibizumab treatment of retinal angiomatous proliferation," *Acta Ophthalmologica*, vol. 90, no. 5, pp. 487–491, 2012.

[19] G. S. Ying, J. Huang, M. G. Maguire et al., "Baseline predictors for one-year visual outcomes with ranibizumab or bevacizumab for neovascular age-related macular degeneration," *Ophthalmology*, vol. 120, no. 1, pp. 122–129, 2013.

[20] J. Y. Shin and H. G. Yu, "Optical coherence tomography-based ranibizumab monotherapy for retinal angiomatous proliferation in Korean patients," *Retina*, vol. 34, no. 12, pp. 2359–2366, 2014.

[21] M. Hata, A. Tsujikawa, M. Miyake et al., "Two-year visual outcome of ranibizumab in typical neovascular age-related macular degeneration and polypoidal choroidal vasculopathy," *Graefe's Archive for Clinical and Experimental Ophthalmology*, vol. 253, no. 2, pp. 221–227, 2015.

[22] M. Kano, T. Sekiryu, Y. Sugano et al., "Foveal structure during the induction phase of anti-vascular endothelial growth factor therapy for occult choroidal neovascularization in age-related macular degeneration," *Clinical Ophthalmology*, vol. 9, pp. 2049–2056, 2015.

[23] Y. G. Park and Y. J. Roh, "One year results of intravitreal ranibizumab monotherapy for retinal angiomatous proliferation: a comparative analysis based on disease stages," *BMC Ophthalmology*, vol. 15, no. 1, p. 182, 2015.

[24] V. Castro-Navarro, E. Cervera-Taulet, J. Montero-Hernández, and C. Navarro-Palop, "One-year outcomes of the treat-and-extend approach with aflibercept in age-related macular degeneration: effects on typical choroidal neovascularization and retinal angiomatous proliferation," *Ophthalmologica*, vol. 236, no. 4, pp. 215–222, 2016.

[25] X. Chen, M. Al-Sheikh, C. K. Chan et al., "Type 1 versus type 3 neovascularization pigment epithelial detachments associated with age-related macular degeneration after anti-vascular endothelial growth factor therapy: a prospective Study," *Retina*, vol. 36, no. 1, pp. S50–S64, 2016.

[26] E. Daniel, J. Shaffer, G. S. Ying et al., "Outcomes in eyes with retinal angiomatous proliferation in the comparison of age-related macular degeneration treatments trials (CATT)," *Ophthalmology*, vol. 123, no. 3, pp. 609–616, 2016.

[27] H. Koizumi, M. Kano, A. Yamamoto et al., "Subfoveal choroidal thickness during aflibercept therapy for neovascular age-related macular degeneration: twelve-month results," *Ophthalmology*, vol. 123, no. 3, pp. 617–624, 2016.

[28] J. Y. Lee, H. Chung, and H. C. Kim, "Changes in fundus autofluorescence after anti-vascular endothelial growth factor according to the type of choroidal neovascularization in age-related macular degeneration," *Korean Journal of Ophthalmology*, vol. 30, no. 1, pp. 17–24, 2016.

[29] O. Chevreaud, H. Oubraham, S. Y. Cohen et al., "Ranibizumab for vascularized pigment epithelial detachment: 1-year anatomic and functional results," *Graefe's Archive for Clinical and Experimental Ophthalmology*, vol. 255, no. 4, pp. 743–751, 2017.

[30] W. Kikushima, Y. Sakurada, S. Yoneyama et al., "Incidence and risk factors of retreatment after three-monthly aflibercept therapy for exudative age-related macular degeneration," *Scientific Reports*, vol. 7, no. 1, p. 44020, 2017.

[31] A. Koh, T. Y. Y. Lai, K. Takahashi et al., "Efficacy and safety of ranibizumab with or without verteporfin photodynamic therapy for polypoidal choroidal vasculopathy: a randomized

clinical trial," *JAMA Ophthalmology*, vol. 135, no. 11, pp. 1206–1213, 2017.

[32] A. Miere, G. Querques, O. Semoun et al., "Optical coherence tomography angiography changes in early type 3 neo-vascularization after anti-vascular endothelial growth factor treatment," *Retina*, vol. 37, no. 10, pp. 1873–1879, 2017.

[33] M. Saito, M. Kano, K. Itagaki, and T. Sekiryu, "Efficacy of intravitreal aflibercept in Japanese patients with exudative age-related macular degeneration," *Japanese Journal of Ophthalmology*, vol. 61, no. 1, pp. 74–83, 2017.

[34] M. Gharbiya, R. Giustolisi, J. Marchiori et al., "Comparison of short-term choroidal thickness and retinal morphological changes after intravitreal anti-VEGF therapy with ranibizu-mab or aflibercept in treatment-naive eyes," *Current Eye Research*, vol. 43, no. 3, pp. 391–396, 2018.

[35] H. Matsumoto, T. Hiroe, M. Morimoto, K. Mimura, A. Ito, and H. Akiyama, "Efficacy of treat-and-extend regimen with aflibercept for pachychoroid neovasculopathy and type 1 neovascular age-related macular degeneration," *Japanese Journal of Ophthalmology*, vol. 62, no. 2, pp. 144–150, 2018.

[36] K. Mimura, H. Matsumoto, M. Morimoto, and H. Akiyama, "Development of age-related macular degeneration (AMD) in the fellow eye of patients with AMD treated by treat-and-extend intravitreal therapy with aflibercept," *Oph-thalmologica*, vol. 239, no. 2-3, pp. 121–127, 2018.

[37] S. Yang, J. Zhao, and X. Sun, "Resistance to anti-VEGF therapy in neovascular age-related macular degeneration: a comprehensive review," *Drug Design, Development and Therapy*, vol. 10, pp. 1857–1867, 2016.

[38] D. Xu, J. P. Dávila, M. Rahimi et al., "Long-term progression of type 1 neovascularization in age-related macular degen-eration using optical coherence tomography angiography," *American Journal of Ophthalmology*, vol. 187, pp. 10–20, 2018.

[39] A. Carnevali, M. V. Cicinelli, V. Capuano et al., "Optical coherence tomography angiography: a useful tool for diag-nosis of treatment-naïve quiescent choroidal neovasculari-zation," *American Journal of Ophthalmology*, vol. 169, pp. 189–198, 2016.

4

Deep Neural Network-Based Method for Detecting Central Retinal Vein Occlusion using Ultrawide-Field Fundus Ophthalmoscopy

Daisuke Nagasato ⓘ,[1] **Hitoshi Tabuchi,**[1] **Hideharu Ohsugi,**[1] **Hiroki Masumoto,**[1] **Hiroki Enno,**[2] **Naofumi Ishitobi,**[1] **Tomoaki Sonobe,**[1] **Masahiro Kameoka,**[1] **Masanori Niki,**[3] **Ken Hayashi,**[4] **and Yoshinori Mitamura** ⓘ[3]

[1]*Department of Ophthalmology, Tsukazaki Hospital, Himeji, Japan*
[2]*Rist Inc., Tokyo, Japan*
[3]*Department of Ophthalmology, Institute of Biomedical Sciences, Tokushima University Graduate School, Tokushima, Japan*
[4]*Hayashi Eye Hospital, Fukuoka, Japan*

Correspondence should be addressed to Daisuke Nagasato; d.nagasato@tsukazaki-eye.net

Academic Editor: Elad Moisseiev

The aim of this study is to assess the performance of two machine-learning technologies, namely, deep learning (DL) and support vector machine (SVM) algorithms, for detecting central retinal vein occlusion (CRVO) in ultrawide-field fundus images. Images from 125 CRVO patients ($n = 125$ images) and 202 non-CRVO normal subjects ($n = 238$ images) were included in this study. Training to construct the DL model using deep convolutional neural network algorithms was provided using ultrawide-field fundus images. The SVM uses scikit-learn library with a radial basis function kernel. The diagnostic abilities of DL and the SVM were compared by assessing their sensitivity, specificity, and area under the curve (AUC) of the receiver operating characteristic curve for CRVO. For diagnosing CRVO, the DL model had a sensitivity of 98.4% (95% confidence interval (CI), 94.3–99.8%) and a specificity of 97.9% (95% CI, 94.6–99.1%) with an AUC of 0.989 (95% CI, 0.980–0.999). In contrast, the SVM model had a sensitivity of 84.0% (95% CI, 76.3–89.3%) and a specificity of 87.5% (95% CI, 82.7–91.1%) with an AUC of 0.895 (95% CI, 0.859–0.931). Thus, the DL model outperformed the SVM model in all indices assessed ($P < 0.001$ for all). Our data suggest that a DL model derived using ultrawide-field fundus images could distinguish between normal and CRVO images with a high level of accuracy and that automatic CRVO detection in ultrawide-field fundus ophthalmoscopy is possible. This proposed DL-based model can also be used in ultrawide-field fundus ophthalmoscopy to accurately diagnose CRVO and improve medical care in remote locations where it is difficult for patients to attend an ophthalmic medical center.

1. Introduction

Central retinal vein occlusion (CRVO) is a vascular disease of the eye and a known cause of significant visual morbidity, including sudden blindness [1]. Pathogenesis of CRVO is believed to follow the principles of Virchow's triad of thrombogenesis, namely, vessel damage, stasis, and hypercoagulability [2]. In CRVO, the fundus may show retinal hemorrhages, dilated tortuous retinal veins, cotton-wool spots, optic edema, and macular edema (ME); ME is the most important cause of visual impairment in CRVO [3].

Intravitreous injections of antivascular endothelial growth factor (VEGF) agents have been shown to significantly improve visual acuity in eyes with CRVO-associated ME [4]. However, any delay in treatment with anti-VEGF agents results in poor functional improvement, and it is difficult to subsequently achieve satisfactory improvement in vision [5–7].

Thus, it is important to treat CRVO patients in an ophthalmic specialty center immediately after the onset to preserve visual function. However, establishing a large number of such centers is impractical because of rising public healthcare costs, a problem that is burdening several nations worldwide [8].

Recent remarkable advances in medical equipment include the ultrawide-field scanning laser ophthalmoscope, the Optos 200T× (Optos PLC, Dunfermline, United Kingdom). The Optos can easily and noninvasively provide wide-field fundus images (Figure 1) without mydriatic agent use, and it has been used for diagnosing or monitoring multiple conditions and for treatment evaluation in peripheral retinal and vascular pathology [9]. Importantly, if pupillary block and elevated intraocular pressure associated with dilation can be avoided, a trained non-medical personnel can safely capture images to use them in telemedicine applications, especially in areas without ophthalmologists.

Image processing approaches using two machine-learning algorithms, namely, deep learning (DL) and support vector machines (SVMs), have retained investigator attention for years because of their extremely high-performance levels; in fact, increasing number of studies have assessed their applications in medical imaging [10–14]. Nonetheless, in ophthalmology, the use of image processing technology that uses DL algorithms and SVM models to analyze medical images has been previously reported [13, 15, 16]. However, to the best of our knowledge, no study has evaluated the possibility of automated CRVO diagnosis using Optos images and machine-learning technology. Therefore, in this study, we assessed the ability of a DL model to detect CRVO using Optos images and compared the results between DL- and SVM-based algorithms.

2. Materials and Methods

2.1. Image Dataset. Optos images of patients with acute CRVO and those without fundus diseases were extracted from the clinical database of the ophthalmology departments of the Tsukazaki Hospital, Tokushima University Hospital, and Hayashi Eye Hospital. These images were reviewed by a retinal specialist and stored in an analytical database. Of the 363 fundus images selected, 125 were from CRVO patients and 238 were from non-CRVO healthy subjects.

We used K-fold cross validation in this study, and it has been described in detail elsewhere [17, 18]. Briefly, image data were divided into K groups, and $(K - 1)$ groups were used as training data, whereas one data group was used for validation. This process was repeated K times until each of the K groups became a validation dataset. The number of groups (K) was calculated using Sturges' formula ($K = 1 + \log_2 N$). Sturges' formula is used to decide the number of classes in the histogram [19, 20]. Thus, in this study, we categorized the data into nine groups.

Images in the training dataset were augmented by adjusting for brightness, gamma correction, histogram equalization, noise addition, and inversion so that the amount of training data increased by 18-fold. The deep convolutional neural network (DNN) model, as detailed below, was created and was trained using preprocessed image data.

This study was conducted in compliance with the principles of the Declaration of Helsinki and was approved by the ethics committees of Tsukazaki Hospital, Tokushima University Hospital, and Hayashi Eye Hospital.

2.2. Deep Learning Model and Training. A DNN model called the Visual Geometry Group-16 (VGG-16) [21] was used in the present study, and its schematic is shown in Figure 2. This type of DNN is configured to automatically learn local features of images and generate a classification model [22–24]. The aspect ratio of the original Optos images was $3,900 \times 3,072$ pixels; however, for analysis, we changed the aspect ratio of all input images and resized them to 256×192 pixels. As the RGB input of images had a range of 0–255, it was first normalized to a range of 0–1 by dividing it by 255.

The VGG-16 model comprises five blocks and three fully connected layers. Each block includes convolutional layers followed by a max-pooling layer with decreasing position sensitivity but greater generic recognition [25]. Flattening of the output from block 5 results in only two fully connected layers. The first layer removes spatial information from the extracted feature vectors, and the second layer is a classification layer that uses feature vectors from target images acquired in previous layers in combination with the softmax function for binary classification. To improve generalization performance, dropout processing was performed such that masking was achieved with a probability of 25% in the first fully connected layer.

Fine tuning was used to increase the learning speed and achieve higher performance with lower quantitates of data [26, 27]. We used the following parameters from ImageNet: blocks 1 to 4 were fixed, whereas block 5 and the fully connected layers were trained.

The weights of block 5 and the fully connected layers were updated using the optimization momentum stochastic gradient descent algorithm (learning coefficient = 0.0005, inertial term = 0.9) [28, 29]. Of the 40 DL models obtained in 40 learning cycles, the one with the highest rate of correct answers for the test data was selected as the DL model to be evaluated in this study. For this purpose, Keras (https://keras.io/ja/) was run on TensorFlow (https://www.tensorflow.org/) written in Python and was used to build and evaluate the model. We trained the model using the CPU of Core (TM) i7-8700K by Intel and the GPU of GeForce GTX 1080 Ti by NVIDIA.

2.3. Support Vector Machine Model. We used the soft-margin SVM implemented in the scikit-learn library using the radial basis function kernel [30]. We reduced all images to 60 dimensions as this was the number of dimensions that was found to provide the highest correct answer rate for the test data; for this, we tested 10–70 dimensions in steps of 10. The optimal values for cost parameter "C" of the SVM algorithm and parameter "γ" of the radial basis function were determined by grid search using quadrant cross validation, and the combination with the highest average correct answer rate was selected. The parameter values tested for C were 1, 10, 100, and 1000 and those for γ were 0.0001, 0.001, 0.01,

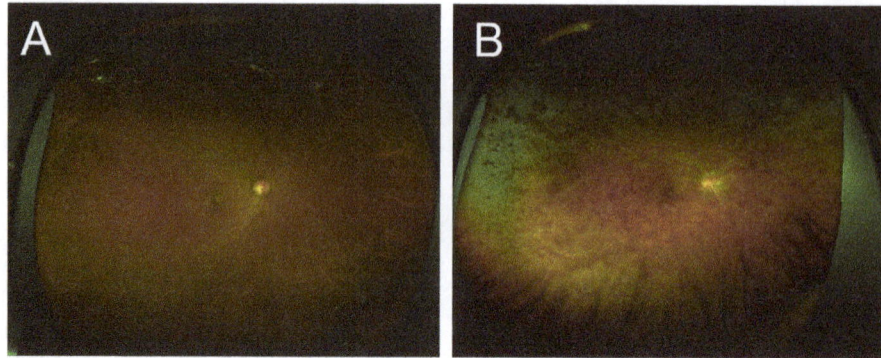

FIGURE 1: Representative fundus images obtained using ultrawide-field scanning laser ophthalmoscopy. Ultrawide-field fundus images of the right eye without central retinal vein occlusion (CRVO) (A) and with CRVO (B).

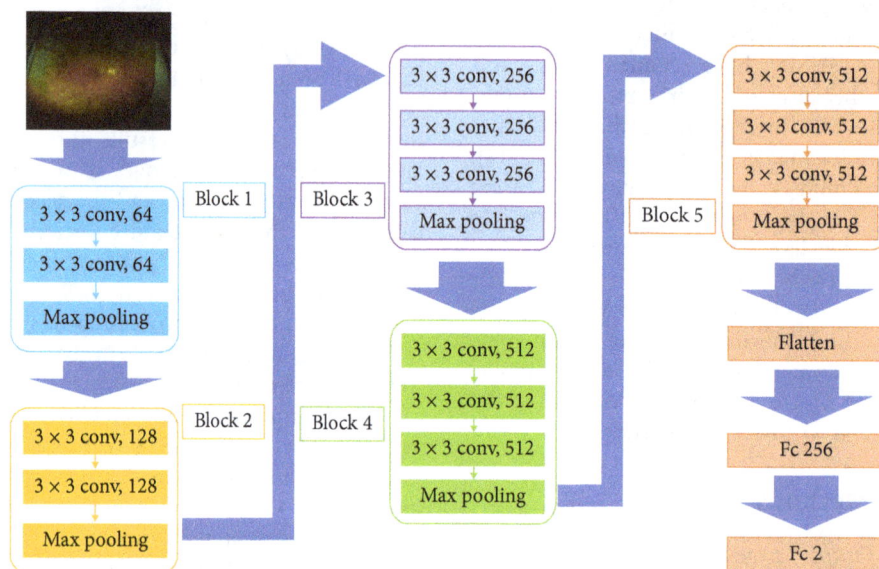

FIGURE 2: Overall architecture of Visual Geometry Group-16 model. Visual Geometry Group-16 (VGG-16) comprises five blocks and three fully connected layers. Each block includes convolutional layers followed by a max-pooling layer. Flattening of the output matrix after block 5 resulted in two fully connected layers for binary classification. The deep convolutional neural network used ImageNet parameters; the weights of blocks 1–4 were fixed, whereas the weights of block 5 and the fully connected layers were adjusted.

0.1, and 1. The final learning model was generated using the optimized parameter values of $C = 10$ and $\gamma = 0.0001$.

2.4. Outcomes. Receiver operating characteristic (ROC) curves for CRVO were created on the basis of the ability of the DL and SVM models to distinguish between CRVO and non-CRVO images, and the models were compared using area under the curve (AUC), sensitivity, and specificity values.

2.5. Heat Map. A heat map of the DNN focus site was created and classified using gradient-weighted class activation mapping [21]. Next, composite images were created by overlaying heat maps of the DNN focus site on the corresponding CRVO and non-CRVO images. The third convolution layer in block 3 was defined as the target layer, and the rectified linear unit was used as the backprop

modifier. This process was performed using Python Keras-vis (https://raghakot.github.io/keras-vis/).

2.6. Statistical Analysis. Patient demographic data such as age were compared using Student's *t*-test, whereas Fisher's exact test was used for comparing the gender ratio and the ratio of the right to left eye images.

The 95% confidence interval (CI) of AUC was obtained as follows. Images judged to exceed a threshold were defined as positive for CRVO, and the ROC curve was created. We created nine such models and nine ROC curves. For determining AUC, the 95% CI was obtained by assuming normal distribution and using the average and standard deviation of the nine ROC curves. For estimating sensitivity and specificity, optimal cutoff values, which are the points closest to the point at which both sensitivity and specificity are 100% in each ROC curve, were used [26]. The sensitivity and specificity at the optimal cutoff value were calculated using the Youden index [31]. The ROC curve was calculated using scikit-learn, and CIs for sensitivity and specificity were determined using SciPy. The paired t-test was used to compare AUCs between the DL and the SVM models.

3. Results

We used 125 CRVO images from 125 patients (mean age, 67.8 ± 13.9 years; 67 men and 58 women; 61 left fundus and 64 right fundus images) and 238 non-CRVO images from 202 subjects (mean age, 68.6 ± 7.9 years; 104 men and 98 women; 122 left fundus and 116 right fundus images) in this analysis. No significant differences were detected between these two groups with respect to age, gender ratio, and left-right eye image ratio (Table 1).

The DL model's sensitivity for diagnosing CRVO was 98.4% (95% CI, 94.3–99.8%), its specificity was 97.9% (95% CI, 94.6–99.1%), and the AUC was 0.989 (95% CI, 0.980–0.999); in contrast, sensitivity of the SVM model was 84.0% (95% CI, 76.3–89.3%), its specificity was 87.5% (95% CI, 82.7–91.1%), and the AUC was 0.895 (95% CI, 0.859–0.931). In ROC curves, AUC of the DL model was significantly higher than that of the SVM model ($P < 0.001$) (Figure 3).

A composite image, comprising the fundal image superimposed with its corresponding heat map, was created by the DNN, and these images showed that DNNs could accurately identify crucial areas in the fundal images; a representative composite image is presented in Figure 4. Blue was used to indicate the strength of DNN-based identification, and an increase in color intensity was observed in areas with retinal hemorrhage and at the focus points. Thus, in non-CRVO images, the heat map showed that focal points accumulated around the optic disc, whereas in CRVO images, focal points accumulated around the optic disc and around retinal hemorrhages. These results imply that DNNs may be able to distinguish between CRVO eyes and normal eyes by identifying and highlighting retinal hemorrhages.

4. Discussion

The fundamental aim of this study was to explore the possibility of early detection of CRVO from Optos fundus photographs using DL-based algorithms. If screening for CRVO is possible noninvasively and without the use of mydriatic agents, this approach would be medically viable. Currently, it is unreasonable to expect ophthalmologists to interpret all Optos-acquired fundus images because of associated medical resource costs. Therefore, a DL model that can accurately diagnose conditions based on ultrawide-field fundus ophthalmoscopy images without the need for human input can be used to screen and diagnose a very large number of patients at a very low cost.

Here, we have used DL technology to identify Optos images that show presence of CRVO. Our results show that the DL model has higher sensitivity, specificity, and AUC values than the SVM model for detecting CRVO in Optos-derived fundus photographs.

TABLE 1: Patient demographics.

	CRVO	Non-CRVO	p value
Number of images (patients)	125 (125)	238 (202)	—
Age (yrs)	67.8 ± 13.9	68.6 ± 7.9	0.489 (Student's t-test)
Sex, female	58 (46.4%)	98 (48.5%)	0.734 (Fisher's exact test)
Left fundus	61 (48.8%)	122 (51.3%)	0.660 (Fisher's exact test)

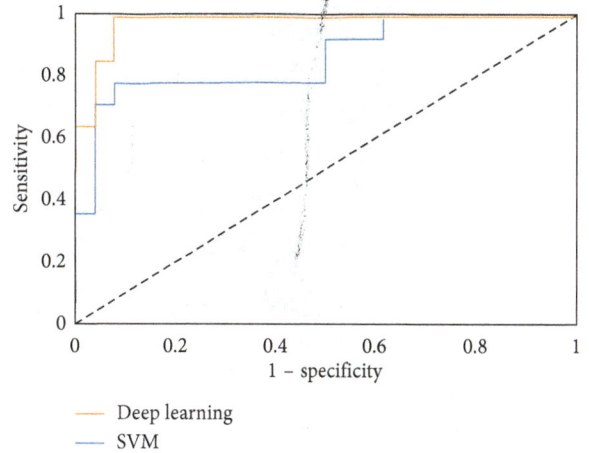

FIGURE 3: Receiver operating characteristic (ROC) curve for central retinal vein occlusion.

Further, using heat maps, we show that DNN could accurately identify an area around the optic disc in the non-CRVO images, whereas in CRVO images, it focused on the area around the optic disc and could highlight retinal hemorrhages. This result implies that the proposed DNN model may be able to identify CRVO by focusing on areas with suspected retinal hemorrhages. It is known that DL algorithm-based models can automatically learn local feature values of images and generate classification models [22, 26, 29, 31]. Additionally, DL includes several layers for the identification of local features of complicated differences, which can subsequently be combined [29].

In recent years, a number of studies have addressed that CNN hugely outperforms classic ML algorithms in image classification tasks [16, 32–34]. Recently, Wang et al. have reported that the performance of the DL model was not significantly different from that of the best classical methods, including SVM and human physicians, when classifying mediastinal lymph node metastasis in nonsmall cell lung cancer using positron emission tomography/computed tomography images [35]. This could be because image information necessary for classification was lost during image convolution in DL. In contrast, we found that the performance of the DL model was better than that of the SVM model in accurately diagnosing CRVO using Optos images. As most cases of CRVO need early intervention, patients diagnosed with CRVO using this method can immediately consult retinal specialists and receive necessary advanced

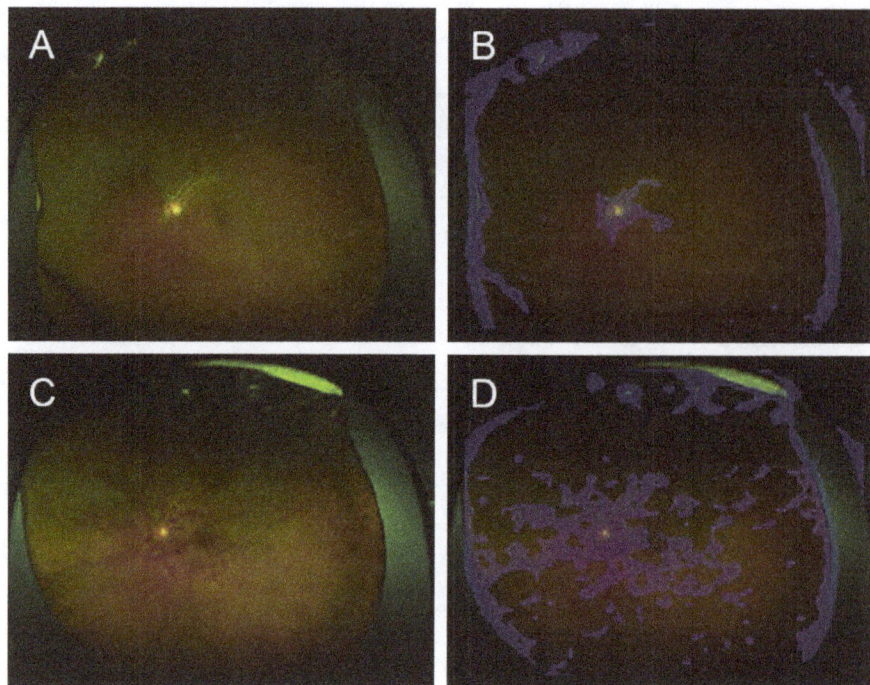

FIGURE 4: Representative ultrawide-field fundus images and corresponding heat maps. The ultrawide-field fundus image without central retinal vein occlusion (CRVO) (A), and its corresponding superimposed heat map (B); with CRVO (C), and its corresponding superimposed heat map (D). In the image without CRVO (A), the deep convolution neural network focused on the optic disc (blue), whereas in the image with CRVO (B), the model focused on the optic disc and on the retinal hemorrhages (blue) (D).

treatment at an ophthalmic medical center. The Optos-based telemedicine technology being proposed here could significantly help us in preserving good visual function in CRVO patients living in areas with inadequate ophthalmic care and could potentially be used to cover large areas without adequate care facilities.

Despite the above, our study has a few limitations. First, we have only compared images of normal retinas with CRVO retinas and did not include images of other retinal diseases. Based on the image examples presented in this study, it may be expected that a CNN algorithm should easily be able to classify between the two types of images. To use this model under clinical conditions, further development and testing to ensure accurate identification of multiple conditions other than CRVO would be essential. Additionally, clarity of the eye may decrease in patients with mature cataract or severe vitreous hemorrhage, and in such cases, analysis of images captured using Optos may be difficult. Thus, future studies should extensively evaluate the performance and versatility of DL using larger samples and with images of other fundus diseases.

5. Conclusions

In conclusion, the DL model performed better than the SVM model in terms of its ability to distinguish between CRVO and normal eyes using ultrawide-field fundus ophthalmoscopic images. This technology has significant potential clinical usefulness as it can be combined with telemedicine to reach large areas where no specialist care is available.

Conflicts of Interest

The authors declare that there are no conflicts of interest regarding the publication of this paper.

Acknowledgments

We thank Masayuki Miki and orthoptists at Tsukazaki Hospital for their support in data collection.

References

[1] J. W. Yau, P. Lee, T. Y. Wong, J. Best, and A. Jenkins, "Retinal vein occlusion: an approach to diagnosis, systemic risk factors and management," *Internal Medicine Journal*, vol. 38, no. 12, pp. 904–910, 2008.

[2] S. Rogers, R. L. McIntosh, N. Cheung et al., "The prevalence of retinal vein occlusion: pooled data from population studies from the United States, Europe, Asia, and Australia," *Ophthalmology*, vol. 117, no. 2, pp. 313–319, 2010.

[3] S. S. Hayreh and M. B. Zimmerman, "Fundus changes in central retinal vein occlusion," *Retina*, vol. 35, no. 1, pp. 29–42, 2015.

[4] S. Yeh, S. J. Kim, A. C. Ho et al., "Therapies for macular edema associated with central retinal vein occlusion: a report by the

American Academy of Ophthalmology," *Ophthalmology*, vol. 122, no. 4, pp. 769–778, 2015.

[5] P. A. Campochiaro, D. M. Brown, C. C. Awh et al., "Sustained benefits from ranibizumab for macular edema following central retinal vein occlusion: twelve-month outcomes of a phase III study," *Ophthalmology*, vol. 118, no. 10, pp. 2041–2049, 2011.

[6] D. M. Brown, J. S. Heier, W. L. Clark et al., "Intravitreal aflibercept injection for macular edema secondary to central retinal vein occlusion: 1-year results from the phase 3 COPERNICUS study," *American Journal of Ophthalmology*, vol. 155, no. 3, pp. 429–437, 2013.

[7] J. F. Korobelnik, F. G. Holz, J. Roider et al., "Intravitreal aflibercept injection for macular edema resulting from central retinal vein occlusion: one-year results of the phase 3 GALILEO study," *Ophthalmology*, vol. 121, no. 1, pp. 202–208, 2014.

[8] M. Mrsnik, *Global Aging 2013: Rising to the Challenge*, Standard & Poor's Rating Services, 2013, https://www.nact.org/resources/2013_NACT_Global_Aging.pdf.

[9] A. Nagiel, R. A. Lalane, S. R. Sadda, and S. D. Schwarttz, "Ultra-wide field fundus imaging: a review of clinical applications and future trends," *Retina*, vol. 36, no. 4, pp. 660–678, 2016.

[10] Y. LeCun, Y. Bengio, and G. Hinton, "Deep learning," *Nature*, vol. 521, no. 7553, pp. 436–444, 2015.

[11] S. Liu, S. Liu, W. Cai et al., "Multimodal neuroimaging feature learning for multiclass diagnosis of Alzheimer's disease," *IEEE Transactions on Biomedical Engineering*, vol. 62, no. 4, pp. 1132–1140, 2015.

[12] G. Litjens, C. I. Sánchez, N. Timofeeva et al., "Deep learning as a tool for increased accuracy and efficiency of histopathological diagnosis," *Scientific Reports*, vol. 6, no. 1, article 26286, 2016.

[13] V. Gulshan, L. Peng, M. Coram et al., "Development and validation of a deep learning algorithm for detection of diabetic retinopathy in retinal fundus photographs," *JAMA*, vol. 316, no. 22, pp. 2402–2410, 2016.

[14] W. H. Pinaya, A. Gadelha, O. M. Doyle et al., "Using deep belief network modelling to characterize differences in brain morphometry in schizophrenia," *Scientific Reports*, vol. 6, no. 1, article 38897, 2016.

[15] R. Gargeya and T. Leng, "Automated identification of diabetic retinopathy using deep learning," *Ophthalmology*, vol. 124, no. 7, pp. 962–969, 2017.

[16] H. Ohsugi, H. Tabuchi, H. Enno, and N. Ishitobi, "Accuracy of deep learning, a machine-learning technology, using ultra-wide-field fundus ophthalmoscopy for detecting rhegmatogenous retinal detachment," *Scientific Reports*, vol. 7, no. 1, p. 9425, 2017.

[17] F. Mosteller and J. W. Tukey, "Data analysis, including statistics," in *Handbook of Social Psychology, Research Methods*, G. Lindzey and E. Aronson, Eds., Vol. 2, Addison-Wesley, Reading, MA, USA, 1968.

[18] R. Kohavi, "A study of cross-validation and bootstrap for accuracy estimation and model selection," in *Proceedings of International Joint Conference on Artificial Intelligence (IJCAI)*, pp. 1137–1145, Stanford University, Stanford, CA, USA, 1995.

[19] D. M. Maslove, T. Podchiyska, and H. J. Lowe, "Discretization of continuous features in clinical datasets," *Journal of the American Medical Informatics Association*, vol. 20, no. 3, pp. 544–553, 2013.

[20] H. A. Sturges, "The choice of a class interval," *Journal of the American Statistical Association*, vol. 21, no. 153, pp. 65-66, 1926.

[21] A. K. Akobeng, "Understanding diagnostic tests 3: receiver operating characteristic curves," *Acta Paediatrica*, vol. 96, no. 5, pp. 644–647, 2007.

[22] J. Deng, W. Dong, R. Socher, L. J. Li, K. Li, and L. Fei-Fei, "Imagenet: a large-scale hierarchical image database," in *Proceedings of IEEE Conference on Computer Vision and Pattern Recognition*, pp. 248–255, 2009.

[23] O. Russakovsky, J. Deng, H. Su et al., "Imagenet large scale visual recognition challenge," *International Journal of Computer Vision*, vol. 115, no. 3, pp. 211–252, 2015.

[24] C. Y. Lee, S. Xie, P. Gallagher, Z. Zhang, and Z. Tu, "Deeply-supervised nets," in *Proceedings of 18th International Conference on Artificial Intelligence and Statistics AISTATS*, vol. 2, San Diego, CA, USA, 2015.

[25] D. Scherer, M. Andreas, and B. Sven, "Evaluation of pooling operations in convolutional architectures for object recognition," in *Proceedings of 20th International Artificial Neural Networks–ICANN*, pp. 92–101, Thessaloniki, Greece, 2010.

[26] J. Redmon, S. Divvala, R. Girshick, and F. Farhadi, "You only look once: unified, real-time object detection," arXivpreprint arXiv; 1506.02640, 2015.

[27] P. Agrawal, R. Girshick, and J. Malik, "Analyzing the performance of multilayer neural networks for object recognition," in *Proceedings of European Conference on Computer Vision*, pp. 329–344, Zurich, Switzerland, 2014.

[28] N. Qian, "On the momentum term in gradient descent learning algorithms," *Neural Networks*, vol. 12, no. 1, pp. 145–151, 1999.

[29] Y. Nesterov, "A method for unconstrained convex minimization problem with the rate of convergence O $(1/k^2)$," *Doklady AN USSR*, vol. 269, pp. 543–547, 1983.

[30] R. G. Brereton and G. R. Lloyd, "Support vector machines for classification and regression," *Analyst*, vol. 135, no. 2, pp. 230–267, 2010.

[31] E. F. Schisterman, D. Faraggi, B. Reiser, and J. Hu, "Youden Index and the optimal threshold for markers with mass at zero," *Statistics in Medicine*, vol. 27, no. 2, pp. 297–315, 2008.

[32] C. Quan, L. Hua, X. Sun, and W. Bai, "Multichannel convolutional neural network for biological relation extraction," *BioMed Research International*, vol. 2016, Article ID 1850404, 10 pages, 2016.

[33] S. B. Seong, C. Pae, and H. J. Park, "Geometric convolutional neural network for analyzing surface-based neuroimaging data," *Frontiers in Neuroinformatics*, vol. 12, p. 42, 2018.

[34] T. Maruyama, N. Hayashi, Y. Sato et al., "Comparison of medical image classification accuracy among three machine learning methods," *Journal of X-Ray Science and Technology*, pp. 1–9, 2018.

[35] H. Wang, Z. Zhou, Y. Li et al., "Comparison of machine learning methods for classifying mediastinal lymph node metastasis of non-small cell lung cancer from 18F-FDG PET/CT images," *EJNMMI Research*, vol. 7, no. 1, p. 11, 2017.

5

Early Changes in Visual Quality and Corneal Structure after DMEK: Does DMEK Approach Optical Quality of a Healthy Cornea?

Maria Satue ⓘ,[1,2] Miriam Idoipe,[1,2] Alicia Gavin,[2] Maria Romero-Sanz,[2] Vasilios S. Liarakos,[3] Antonio Mateo,[1,2] Elena Garcia-Martin ⓘ,[1,2] Alejandro Blasco-Martinez,[1,2] and Antonio Sanchez-Perez[1,2]

[1]IIS-Aragon, Aragon Institute for Health Research (IIS Aragón), Zaragoza, Spain
[2]Ophthalmology Department, Miguel Servet University Hospital, Zaragoza, Spain
[3]Ophthalmology Department, Naval Hospital, Athens, Greece

Correspondence should be addressed to Maria Satue; mariasatue@gmail.com

Academic Editor: Naoki Okumura

Purpose. To evaluate early changes in visual function and visual quality parameters after Descemet membrane endothelial keratoplasty (DMEK) and to compare the outcomes with healthy controls. *Methods.* Thirteen patients who underwent DMEK and 14 controls were evaluated. All subjects underwent visual function evaluation, including visual acuity under photopic and mesopic lighting conditions and contrast sensitivity (CSV) tests CSV 1000 and Pelli-Robson. Corneal parameters were assessed with Oculus Pentacam. Corneal mean keratometry (Km), corneal densitometry values, and low and high order aberrations (LOA and HOA) were recorded. In DMEK patients, all tests were performed before surgery and 1 and 6 months after surgery. *Results.* In patients who underwent DMEK, photopic visual acuity improved from 0.59 to 0.31 at 1 month ($p = 0.013$) and 0.13 at 6 months ($p = 0.008$); mesopic visual acuity and all contrast sensitivity values (both CSV and Pelli-Robson test) improved significantly in the first month ($p < 0.005$). A significant decrease was observed in corneal density in the 0–2 mm ring (from 43.83 to 35.60, $p = 0.043$) and mean posterior Km (from −5.84 to −6.80, $p = 0.005$) in the first month. Corneal HOAs and all corneal densities improved at 6 months after DMEK ($p < 0.05$). All visual function parameters and corneal aberrations remained lower and higher, respectively, compared with healthy controls ($p < 0.05$). Corneal densities were comparable with controls at 6 months after DMEK ($p > 0.05$). *Conclusions.* Patients undergoing DMEK present visual function improvement and a decrease in corneal density at 1 month after surgery. Decrease in corneal posterior HOAs can be observed at 6 months. However, visual function outcomes and corneal aberrations remained worse compared with healthy controls.

1. Introduction

In the last decade, selective replacement of the diseased endothelium with a donor endothelial graft has superseded traditional full-thickness penetrating keratoplasty [1], in the treatment of endothelial disorders such as Fuchs endothelial dystrophy and pseudophakic bullous keratopathy. Benefits of endothelial keratoplasty (EK) over penetrating keratoplasty include superior biomechanical integrity, faster visual recovery with better uncorrected visual acuity, and a more predictable refractive outcome with less induced astigmatism [2–4].

It has been well established that Descemet membrane endothelial keratoplasty (DMEK) produces better visual outcomes than other EK techniques. Theories explaining this improvement in visual results include a more regular posterior graft surface with greater thickness uniformity [5–7], thinner grafts with a better match in curvature, improved parallelism between the graft and recipient, and improved optical compensation by the posterior cornea [8]. These advantageous structural results might be explained by the transplantation of only an isolated Descemet membrane and its endothelium in DMEK, apparently resulting in near-normal anatomic corneal restoration. Thus, it has been suggested that a transplanted DMEK cornea may approach the optical quality of a healthy cornea [9].

Corneal aberrations after DMEK have been previously studied [9, 10]. However, research on visual function (which overall provide more accurate information on the patient's visual performance than high contrast visual acuity) and other corneal parameters such as corneal light scatter after DMEK is scarce, and surgery outcomes are mostly compared with other keratoplasty techniques rather than healthy controls. The purpose of the present study was to provide further and complete information on early changes in visual function and corneal parameters after DMEK and to compare visual and structural outcomes with healthy controls. This is the first longitudinal follow-up study in DMEK patients including all these visual function tests and densitometry analysis.

2. Methods

Thirteen patients who underwent DMEK surgery and 14 healthy controls were included in the study. All procedures adhered to the tenets of the Declaration of Helsinki, and all participants provided informed consent to participate in the study. The protocol and informed consent were approved by the local ethics committee for scientific research in Aragón (Comité Ético de Investigaciones Científicas de Aragón-CEICA, PI16/0010).

Pseudophakic patients with different stages of corneal edema secondary to endothelial disease (FED/BK) were selected for the study. The reason to include only pseudophakic patients was to avoid any alterations in the visual quality measurements caused by lens opacifications (cataract of any kind). DMEK surgery was programmed in all cases. The Descemet endothelial grafts were harvested from 13 donor corneoscleral buttons using the standardized "no touch" technique for endothelial graft preparation [11]. All DMEK procedures were carried out following the standardized "no touch" technique. To summarize, a descemetorhexis was performed up to 1 mm from the limbus under air. An anterior chamber maintainer (Centurion Vision System, Alcon laboratories Inc.) with continuous air infusion was used to fill the anterior chamber with air during descemetorhexis. The donor Descemet endothelial roll was inserted into the anterior chamber of the patient with a glass injector after staining with 0.06% trypan blue. The graft was oriented with the donor DM facing the recipient posterior stroma and attached onto the recipient posterior stroma with air. The anterior chamber was pressurized with air for 60 to 80 minutes, followed by an air-fluid exchange leaving a 50% air bubble.

Patients who experienced intraoperative and/or post-operative complications were excluded from the study. Complications were defined as any event that could potentially affect visual quality measurements: significant graft detachment or any detachment causing corneal edema (even if edema was not affecting the visual axis), the use of corneal sutures, paralytic mydriasis caused by ischaemia during the anterior chamber pressurization, the presence of significant amount of pigment on the intraocular lens, and delayed epithelial wound healing (more than 3 weeks). Other exclusion criteria were the presence of significant refractive errors prior to DMEK surgery (>5 diopters of spherical equivalent refraction or 3 diopters of astigmatism); axial length >26 mm or <22 mm; intraocular pressure ≥21 mmHg; media opacifications such as corneal fibrosis, cataract, or vitreous opacifications; concomitant ocular diseases, including history of glaucoma or retinal pathology; and systemic conditions that could affect the visual system. All controls included in the study were pseudophakic (uncomplicated surgery) and had no history nor evidence of ocular or neurologic disease of any nature; their best-corrected visual acuity (BCVA) was >20/30 based on the Snellen scale. Only one eye per subject was randomly selected in the control group and included. From a total of 20 consecutive patients planned for DMEK, 7 patients were excluded (2 due to significant detachment that produced corneal edema for longer than a month; 2 patients were excluded due to corneal epithelial ulcers with delayed healing; 1 due to iris ischaemia, 1 due to superficial corneal fibrosis, and 1 due to fibrotic maculopathy), and their data (preoperative and postoperative) were withdrawn from the final statistical analysis.

All patients underwent visual function and visual quality evaluation before surgery (from 1 week to a maximum of 2 months prior the intervention) and at one and six months after the DMEK procedure. Controls were evaluated in one visit, at least 6 months after cataract surgery. Visual function was assessed in all participants by evaluating BCVA using an Early Treatment Diabetic Retinopathy Study (ETDRS) chart and contrast sensitivity vision (CSV) using the Pelli-Robson and CSV-1000E tests. Structural corneal parameters were evaluated with the Pentacam® system (OCULUS, Wetzlar, Germany).

LogMAR visual acuity (VA) was assessed under monocular vision with best spectacle correction, in two different controlled lighting conditions: photopic ($85 \, cd/m^2$) and mesopic ($3 \, cd/m^2$). Contrast sensitivity provides more complete information about visual function than does visual acuity tests. CSV was evaluated in our patients using the Pelli-Robson chart and the CSV-1000E test. The Pelli-Robson chart comprises horizontal lines of capital letters organized into groups of three (triplets) with two triplets per line. The contrast decreases from one triplet to the next, even within each line. All patients were evaluated under monocular vision at a distance of 1 meter from the chart and under controlled photopic conditions ($85 \, cd/m^2$). The score corresponding to the last triplet of letters seen by the patient was recorded. The CSV-1000E instrument is used worldwide for standardized CSV and glare testing. All patients were evaluated at a distance of 2.5 meters from the chart under monocular vision at 4 different spatial frequencies (3, 6, 12, and 18 cycles per degree (cpd)), under 3 different lighting conditions: photopic ($85 \, cd/m^2$), mesopic ($3 \, cd/m^2$), and mesopic with glare ($3 \, cd/m^2 + 90/100$). The chart comprises four rows with 17 circular patches each. The patches present a grating that decreases in contrast moving from left to right across the row. The patient indicates whether the grating appears in the top patch or the bottom patch for each column. Each contrast value for each spatial frequency was transformed into a logarithmic scale according to standardized values.

Corneal quality parameters were evaluated using the Pentacam® system (OCULUS, Wetzlar, Germany). This device uses a rotational Scheimpflug camera that produces high-resolution three-dimensional images of the anterior pole of the eye. It provides different corneal maps (curvature, refraction, elevation, and pachymetric maps) and calculates numerical parameters of keratometry. Additionally, the software calculates corneal densitometry (backscattered light) in 3 different fixed corneal layers (anterior layer (anterior 120 mm), central layer, and posterior layer (posterior 60 mm)), as well as in fixed corneal concentric rings around the apex (central 0–2 mm, 2–6 mm, 6–10 mm, and 10–12 mm) [12].

For this study, central, anterior, and posterior corneal densitometry (0–2 mm zone and total); mean keratometry (Km); and the root mean square values (RMS) for total, low-order, and high-order aberrations (LOA and HOA, respectively) were calculated for anterior and posterior cornea and recorded. LOA include the second-order Zernike polynomials which represent the conventional aberrations defocus (myopia, hyperopia, and astigmatism). These aberrations represent 85% of total aberrations in the eye. HOA describe Zernike aberrations above second-order: third-order Zernike terms are coma and trefoil; fourth-order Zernike terms include spherical aberration. Higher-order aberrations make up about 15% of the overall number of aberrations in an eye and cannot be corrected by any means of present technology. Central corneal thickness and endothelial cell density at 6 months were also measured in our patients.

All data analyses were performed using SPSS software version 20.0 (SPSS Inc., Chicago, IL). To monitor the progression of corneal changes after DMEK, visual function and visual quality parameters were compared within the patients groups: preoperative data were compared with data obtained at one month after surgery, and the latter were compared with measurements obtained at 6 months after DMEK. To evaluate the differences between corneas which underwent DMEK surgery and healthy corneas, parameters obtained at 6 months after DMEK in patients were compared with measurements obtained in controls. Due to the nonparametric distribution of the data, comparisons between the different groups were calculated using the Mann–Whitney U test. A correlation analysis between visual function and topographic parameters was performed using Spearman's Rho test. A level of significance was considered at $p < 0.05$. To avoid a high false-positive rate, the Bonferroni correction for multiple tests was calculated, and the corrected p values were added to the previously calculated data.

3. Results

A total of 13 eyes in 13 different patients who underwent DMEK surgery and 14 eyes of 14 healthy controls were included in the study. Mean age in the patients group was 69.45 ± 7.51 years and in the control group was 72.62 ± 9.38 years ($p = 0.296$). Mean axial length was 23.58 ± 1.74 mm in the DMEK group and 23.47 ± 1.25 mm in the control group ($p = 0.722$). Anterior and posterior keratometric values were similar between both groups ($p = 0.841$ and $p = 0.080$, respectively). The indication for DMEK was Fuchs endothelial dystrophy ($n = 8$), bullous keratopathy ($n = 2$), or both ($n = 3$). At 6 months postoperative, mean central corneal thickness in patients was 507 ± 36 microns, and mean endothelial cell density was 912 ± 326 cells/mm^2.

3.1. Improvement of Visual and Corneal Parameters after DMEK. Patients who underwent DMEK experienced a significant improvement in all visual function parameters at one month after surgery (Table 1). After the first postoperative month, all parameters continued to improve. However, only photopic BCVA (0.31 ± 0.19 at 1 month vs 0.13 ± 0.09 at 6 months, $p = 0.008$), CSV at 6 cpd under mesopic conditions + glare (1.06 ± 0.58 at 1 month vs 1.46 ± 0.33 at 6 months, $p = 0.034$), and CSV as measured with the Pelli-Robson chart (1.29 ± 0.18 at 1 month vs 1.48 ± 0.14 at 6 months, $p = 0.006$) improved significantly at 6 months (Table 1).

A significant decrease of the 0–2 mm density both in the anterior (43.83 ± 10.50 preoperative vs 35.60 ± 12.16 at 1 month postoperative, $p = 0.045$) and posterior cornea (27.70 ± 4.20 vs 22.07 ± 7.45, $p = 0.006$) was observed at one month after DMEK. A significant improvement of the posterior Km was also observed at 1 month after surgery (-5.84 ± 0.23 preoperative vs -6.80 ± 0.67 at 1 month postoperative, $p = 0.005$). Total corneal densities and posterior aberrations (LOA and total) also improved compared with preoperative levels without reaching significance. Posterior HOA did not change within the first month. A significant increase in the anterior corneal aberrations was observed at 1 month after DMEK (RMS LOA, 3.36 ± 1.23 preoperative vs 4.73 ± 1.67 at 1 month, $p = 0.026$; RMS total aberrations, 3.60 ± 1.28 vs 5.04 ± 1.77, $p = 0.022$) (Table 2).

Central corneal density (33.60 ± 13.87 at 1 month vs 24.32 ± 2.92 at 6 months, $p = 0.006$), all anterior corneal densities (0–2, 35.60 ± 12.16 vs 25.21 ± 5.40, $p = 0.035$; total, 38.40 ± 10.03 vs 29.25 ± 6.52 $p = 0.029$), posterior 0–2 mm density (22.07 ± 7.45 vs 17.60 ± 2.83, $p = 0.010$), and all posterior aberrations continued to decrease significantly at 6 months (RMS HOA, 0.69 ± 0.26 vs 0.47 ± 0.13, $p = 0.015$; RMS LOA, 1.54 ± 0.56 vs 1.04 ± 0.29, $p = 0.020$; RMS total 1.71 ± 0.57 vs 1.15 ± 0.29, $p = 0.015$). Anterior corneal aberrations decreased at 6 months compared with 1 month after surgery. However, the differences did not reach significance levels (Table 2).

A representative case of preoperative-postoperative changes after DMEK can be seen in Figure 1.

3.2. Comparison between DMEK Corneas and Healthy Corneas. Compared with healthy subjects, patients who underwent DMEK presented worse visual function at 6 months after DMEK, in all parameters except the CSV at 3

TABLE 1: Visual function parameters in patients undergoing DMEK as measured preoperative and at 1 month and at 6 months postoperative.

Functional parameter	Preoperative	1 month postoperative	P (preoperative vs 1 month postoperative)	6 month postoperative	P (1 month vs 6 months postoperative)
Visual Acuity					
VA ETDRS photopic	0.59 (0.33)	0.31 (0.19)	**0.013**	0.13 (0.09)	**0.008**
VA ETDRS mesopic	0.75 (0.25)	0.50 (0.22)	**0.012**	0.36 (0.15)	0.130
Contrast sensitivity					
CSV 3cpd	0.46 (0.52)	1.06 (0.61)	**0.005**	1.49 (0.45)	0.077
CSV 6cpd	0.23 (0.52)	1.17 (0.65)	**<0.001***	1.33 (0.47)	0.363
CSV12cpd	0.21 (0.41)	0.58 (0.50)	**0.031**	0.80 (0.46)	0.217
CSV18cpd	0.08 (0.18)	0.29 (0.31)	**0.015**	0.45 (0.46)	0.264
CSV-M 3cpd	0.44 (0.48)	1.20 (0.48)	**0.001***	1.52 (0.28)	0.056
CSV-M 6cpd	0.19 (0.44)	1.19 (0.55)	**<0.001***	1.26 (0.66)	0.401
CSV-M 12cpd	0.13 (0.31)	0.71 (0.67)	**0.004**	0.76 (0.56)	0.741
CSV-M 18cpd	0.07 (0.18)	0.23 (0.30)	**0.022**	0.34 (0.28)	0.350
CSV-MG 3cpd	0.21 (0.45)	1.06 (0.58)	**0.001***	1.46 (0.33)	**0.034**
CSV-MG 6cpd	0.12 (0.35)	0.83 (0.57)	**<0.001***	0.84 (0.64)	0.867
CSV-MG 12cpd	0.04 (0.15)	0.43 (0.39)	**0.001***	0.59 (0.56)	0.434
CSV-MG 18cpd	0.05 (0.35)	0.27 (0.33)	**0.002***	0.34 (0.28)	0.755
Pelli-Robson	1.00 (0.29)	1.29 (0.18)	**0.005**	1.48 (0.14)	**0.006**

P values correspond to comparisons preoperative versus 1 month and 1 month versus 6 months. Bold letters indicate *p* < 0.05. Asterisks mark Bonferroni values less than 0.003. DMEK, Descemet membrane endothelial keratoplasty; VA, visual acuity; ETDRS, Early Treatment Diabetic Retinopathy Study; CSV, contrast sensitivity vision; cpd, cycles per degree.

TABLE 2: Visual quality parameters as obtained with Oculus Pentacam of corneas undergoing Descemet membrane endothelial keratoplasty (DMEK) measured preoperative and at 1 month and at 6 months postoperative.

Quality parameter	Preoperative	1 month postoperative	P (preoperative vs 1 month postoperative)	6 months postoperative	P (1 month vs 6 months postoperative)
Anterior cornea					
Central density	39.81 (10.99)	33.60 (13.87)	0.069	24.32 (2.92)	**0.006***
0–2 mm density	43.83 (10.50)	35.60 (12.16)	**0.045**	25.21 (5.40)	**0.035**
Total density	41.06 (10.43)	38.40 (10.03)	0.489	29.25 (6.52)	**0.029**
Km	43.83 (2.03)	43.13 (1.86)	0.281	42.85 (1.50)	0.607
RMS HOA (μm)	1.19 (0.52)	1.66 (0.79)	0.249	1.50 (1.11)	0.317
RMS LOA (μm)	3.36 (1.23)	4.73 (1.67)	**0.026**	3.86 (2.24)	0.427
RMS total (μm)	3.60 (1.28)	5.04 (1.77)	**0.022**	4.39 (2.23)	0.522
Posterior cornea					
0–2 mm density	27.70 (4.20)	22.07 (7.45)	**0.006***	17.60 (2.83)	**0.010**
Total density	29.06 (4.56)	26.26 (5.44)	0.214	23.38 (3.52)	0.128
Km	−5.84 (0.23)	−6.80 (0.67)	**0.005***	−6.52 (0.39)	0.217
RMS HOA (μm)	0.69 (0.34)	0.69 (0.26)	0.828	0.47 (0.13)	**0.015**
RMS LOA (μm)	1.71 (1.08)	1.54 (0.56)	0.870	1.04 (0.29)	**0.020**
RMS total (μm)	1.86 (1.11)	1.71 (0.57)	0.703	1.15 (0.29)	**0.015**

Bold letters indicate *p* < 0.05. Asterisk marks Bonferroni values <0.007. DMEK, Descemet membrane endothelial keratoplasty; Km, mean keratometry; RMS, root mean square; HOA, high-order aberrations; LOA, low-order aberrations; μm, microns.

cpd (photopic, *p* = 0.676; mesopic, *p* = 0.064 and mesopic + glare, *p* = 0.786) (Table 3).

No significant differences were observed between DMEK corneas at 6 months after surgery and healthy corneas in the central, anterior, and posterior corneal densitometry and in the anterior and posterior Km values (*p* > 0.05) (Table 4). Anterior (HOA, 1.50 ± 1.11 in patients vs 0.76 ± 0.21 in controls, *p* = 0.021 and total 4.39 ± 2.23 vs 2.54 ± 0.74, *p* = 0.014) and posterior (HOA, 0.47 ± 0.13 in patients vs 0.25 ± 0.10 in controls, *p* < 0.001; LOA, 1.04 ± 0.29 vs 0.67 ± 0.33, *p* = 0.005 and total, 1.15 ± 0.29 vs 0.72 ± 0.34, *p* = 0.002) aberrations remained higher in the group of DMEK patients compared with healthy controls (Table 4).

The correlation analysis did not reveal any significant association between visual function parameters and topographical changes in DMEK patients. An additional analysis was performed over a selected group of 8 patients who presented better visual results (BCVA≤0.1), and anterior and posterior HOAs were compared with controls. Patients with good visual outcomes 6 months after DMEK presented higher posterior HOAs compared with controls (0.62 ± 0.30 in DMEK vs 0.26 ± 0.11 in controls, *p* = 0.001). However, though higher, no significant differences were observed in anterior HOAs between both groups (1.49 ± 0.70 in DMEK vs 0.78 ± 0.22 in controls, *p* = 0.065).

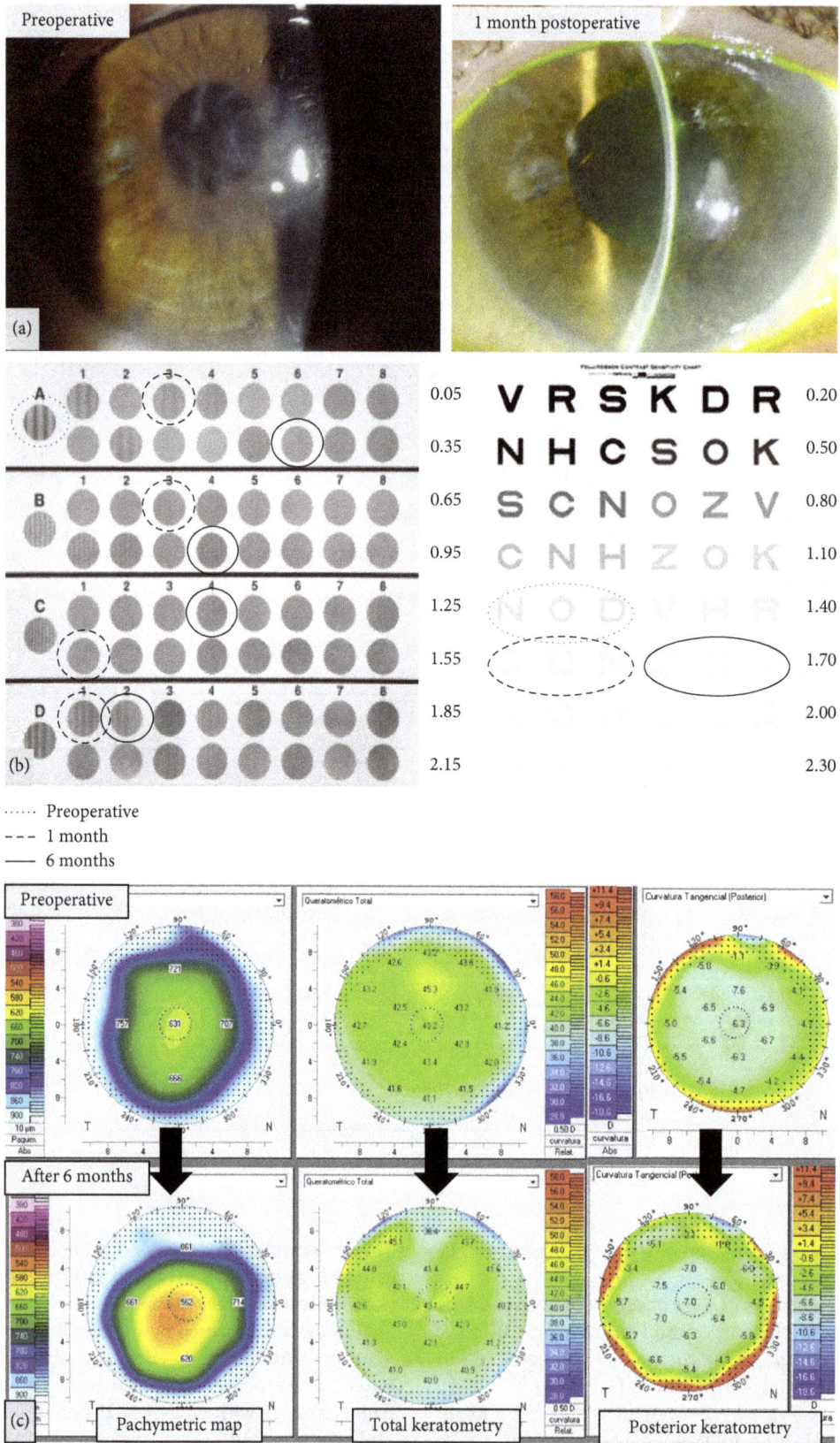

FIGURE 1: Representative case of a patient included in the study, who underwent DMEK. (a) Preoperative (left) and 1 month postoperative (right) slitlamp image of the right eye of a 62-year-old female patient who underwent DMEK. (b) Contrast sensitivity results: left, CSV 1000 test results marked with discontinuous-continuous circled lines (see legend in the figure); in frequencies B, C, and D, no preoperative circle was marked since the patient could not even identify the first image; right, Pelli-Robson results at preoperative and 1 month and 6 months postoperative. (c) Topographic changes preoperative and at 6 months postoperative: left, corneal thickness map; center, keratometric map of the frontal cornea; right, keratometric map of the posterior cornea.

TABLE 3: Visual function parameters in patients undergoing Descemet membrane endothelial keratoplasty (DMEK) at 6 months postoperative compared with healthy corneas.

Functional parameter	DMEK	Controls	p
Visual Acuity			
VA ETDRS photopic	0.13	−0.15	**0.002***
VA ETDRS mesopic	0.36	0.23	**0.044**
Contrast sensitivity			
CSV 3cpd	1.49	1.62	0.676
CSV 6cpd	1.33	1.79	**<0.001***
CSV 12cpd	0.80	1.39	**0.006**
CSV 18cpd	0.45	0.95	**0.006**
CSV-M 3cpd	1.52	1.72	0.064
CSV-M 6cpd	1.26	1.81	**0.005**
CSV-M 12cpd	0.76	1.46	**0.001***
CSV-M 18cpd	0.34	0.94	**<0.001***
CSV-MG 3cpd	1.46	1.61	0.786
CSV-MG 6cpd	0.84	1.63	**0.001***
CSV-MG 12cpd	0.59	1.33	**0.001***
CSV-MG 18cpd	0.39	1.10	**0.002***
Pelli-Robson	1.48	1.71	**0.002***

Bold letters indicate $p < 0.05$. Asterisks mark Bonferroni values less than 0.003. DMEK, Descemet membrane endothelial keratoplasty; VA, visual acuity; ETDRS, Early Treatment Diabetic Retinopathy Study; CSV, contrast sensitivity vision; cpd, cycles per degree.

TABLE 4: Visual quality parameters as obtained with Oculus Pentacam of corneas undergoing Descemet membrane endothelial keratoplasty (DMEK) at six months after surgery compared with healthy controls.

Quality parameter	DMEK	Controls	p
Anterior cornea			
Central density	24.32 (2.92)	23.84 (9.87)	0.099
0–2 mm density	25.21 (5.40)	29.83 (9.30)	0.275
Total density	29.25 (6.52)	36.35 (9.54)	0.052
Km	42.85 (1.50)	44.15 (1.77)	0.058
RMS HOA (μm)	1.50 (1.11)	0.76 (0.21)	**0.021**
RMS LOA (μm)	3.86 (2.24)	2.42 (0.73)	0.069
RMS total (μm)	4.39 (2.23)	2.54 (0.74)	**0.014**
Posterior cornea			
0–2 mm density	17.60 (2.83)	18.46 (6.51)	0.734
Total density	23.38 (3.52)	26.72 (6.33)	0.234
Km	−6.52 (0.39)	−6.36 (0.24)	0.292
RMS HOA (μm)	0.47 (0.13)	0.25 (0.10)	**<0.001**
RMS LOA (μm)	1.04 (0.29)	0.67 (0.33)	**0.005**
RMS total (μm)	1.15 (0.29)	0.72 (0.34)	**0.002**

Central density has been included in the anterior corneal measurements group. Bold letters indicate $p < 0.05$. DMEK, Descemet membrane endothelial keratoplasty; Km, mean keratometry; RMS, root mean square; HOA, high-order aberrations; LOA, low-order aberrations; μm, microns.

3.3. Discussion. In the present study, we evaluated early visual rehabilitation and progressive corneal changes in 13 eyes which underwent DMEK surgery and compared them with a group of healthy subjects. Research on visual and corneal changes after DMEK typically focused on the outcomes at six months postoperative [9, 10, 13]. Despite published studies by the Melles team on early outcomes after DMEK, these results refer mainly to BCVA in photopic conditions [14, 15]. Measuring BCVA and contrast

sensitivity in different lighting conditions may provide more accurate information about the visual system and the patient's possible performance in everyday situations (such as driving and reading) [16, 17]. Our patients' visual function (photopic and mesopic BCVA and CSV) improved dramatically after surgery, and most of the measured parameters stabilized at 1 month after the procedure. BCVA in photopic conditions additionally improved significantly at 6 months. Improvement in light scattering (both anterior and posterior) and posterior mean keratometry was observed in the first month. However, posterior HOA did not decrease until six months after surgery. Anterior HOAs did not change after DMEK in our patients.

Despite the observed changes and early improvement after DMEK, visual function at 6 months was worse than that in controls (except CSV in the 3 cpd frequency), and corneal HOA remained higher in patients than in healthy controls. These results support previous studies in which contrast sensitivity and posterior aberrations in eyes undergoing DMEK did not reach the same levels as controls [9, 13]. Garrido et al. demonstrated that CSV (as measured with the Pelli-Robson test) in pseudophakic patients undergoing DMEK remained worse than CSV in phakic healthy controls. Additionally, CSV 1000 test was used by Garrido et al. to assess CSV after DMEK and compare the results with other keratoplasty techniques [18]. DMEK demonstrated to preserve better CSV at 12 and 18 cpd compared with other procedures. However, these outcomes were never compared with a healthy population. Despite the numerous published articles on DMEK visual outcomes, we could not find any study performing a complete evaluation of visual function parameters (that is, measuring BCVA and CSV at different spatial frequencies and lighting situations) in DMEK patients compared with healthy controls. The present study provides not only a complete analysis of visual function changes after DMEK but also compares visual outcomes with a healthy population in similar circumstances.

Previous research by Van Dijk et al demonstrated that DMEK corneas presented a significant decrease in posterior HOA at six months after surgery, but as it was also observed in our patients, these aberrations remained higher compared with controls [9]. Rudolph et al. demonstrated that DMEK corneas presented higher HOA in the posterior 4 mm of the cornea compared to healthy eyes [10]. However, they failed to detect changes in anterior HOA and LOA, whereas van Dijk et al. found higher anterior HOA in their patients compared with controls [9]. Increased anterior and posterior HOAs were also observed recently in the 6 mm central cornea, in DMEK patients compared with controls [19]. Our patients did not experience any significant changes in anterior HAO; however, anterior LOA increased significantly in the first month, contrary to that observed by van Dijk et al. and Rudolph et al. [9, 10]. HOAs have been correlated to visual acuity after EK and PKP due to the degradation by HOAs of the small-angle domain of the retinal point-spread function [7, 19]. Posterior corneal HOAs increased after EK compared with healthy controls [19–23], and it has been suggested that the posterior corneal surface is the source of increased whole-eye HOAs after Descemet stripping endothelial keratoplasty (DSEK) compared with normal eyes [21, 24]. Posterior HOAs have been linked to BCVA after EK [19]; however, several studies have failed to find an association between posterior corneal HOAs and postoperative BCVA [9, 23, 25, 26], leading some authors to suggest that changes in the posterior cornea should not affect visual acuity [21, 27]. Anterior HOAs have been found to be higher after DSAEK than in normal corneas [28], and a significant correlation has been demonstrated between anterior corneal HOAs and postoperative BCVA [10, 22, 23]. Since EK itself causes minimal disruption of the anterior corneal surface, it is reasonable to suggest that other sources (that is, other than the surgical technique) of increased HOAs must exist in these patients, such as factors related to the underlying disease. In our patients, anterior HOAs after DMEK remained higher than in controls, and a significant increase in anterior LOAs was observed in the first month, whereas visual function and corneal densities improved. These observed changes might be due to preexistent chronic stromal edema, degeneration of keratocytes, and collagen reorganization after DMEK. Additionally, when our patients with better visual outcomes were analysed separately, no differences in anterior HOAs were observed compared with controls. This might also suggest that anterior HOAs play a more important role concerning BCVA results in these patients than do posterior HOAs. These results should still be analysed with caution due to the small sample size and the limitation to the statistical calculations.

Though corneal aberrations have been widely studied after EK, literature on light scattering after DMEK is scarce. We could only find one published study in which corneal density after DMEK was analysed and compared with healthy corneas [9]. In their study, Van Dijk et al. found a strong significant correlation between anterior corneal haze and postoperative BCVA.

It has been argued that light scatter alone cannot affect high-contrast visual acuity [6, 29]. However, increased light scatter may reduce visual quality after EK [29–31], and this is more evident in everyday low-contrast situations [21]. The anterior recipient cornea has been proved to be the main source of haze after other EK techniques such as DSEK and deep lamellar endothelial keratoplasty [6, 29]. Changes associated with this stromal haze seem to be independent of preoperative edema or fibrosis [32]. In our patients, corneal 0–2 mm anterior and posterior densities decreased significantly in the first month after DMEK. These early changes in light scattering had not been documented before since most DMEK studies evaluate their outcomes at 6 months after the procedure. All densities in our patients improved at 6 months after surgery reaching similar light scattering levels to healthy corneas. However, visual function outcomes remained worse than controls, suggesting that other factors such as anterior and posterior HOAs may be limiting postoperative visual quality outcomes in our patients. Our results differ from previous observations on light scattering after DMEK, where corneal densities at 6 months postoperative remained higher than those in healthy corneas. More studies evaluating changes in corneal density after DMEK are needed to corroborate our findings.

The most important limitation to our study is the small sample size, which may be limiting the statistical findings. We believe that correlations between visual results and corneal parameters were not observed in our study due to the small sample size, and further studies analysing visual function with a larger number of patients are needed to establish a correlation between BCVA and CSV and topographic changes in these patients. Given the large samples included in other studies (especially those from the Melles group), our study should be interpreted with caution when compared with other similar research studies, and factors responsible for visual function outcomes in our patients cannot be taken further from speculation.

4. Conclusions

Patients undergoing DMEK present visual function improvement and a decrease in anterior and posterior corneal density at 1 month after the procedure. A further decrease in corneal posterior HOAs was observed at 6 months. Despite this remarkable improvement, visual function outcomes remained worse compared with healthy corneas. Corneal parameters such as mean keratometry and corneal density were comparable to controls; however, HOAs remained higher in DMEK patients at 6 months after surgery. Similar studies with a larger simple size are needed in order to establish a possible correlation between visual function outcomes and corneal parameters after DMEK.

Conflicts of Interest

The authors declare that they have no conflicts of interest.

Acknowledgments

This work was supported by MAT2017-83858-C2-2 MINECO/AEI/FEDER, UE.

References

[1] S. V. Patel, "Keratoplasty for endothelial dysfunction," *Ophthalmology*, vol. 114, no. 4, pp. 627-628, 2007.

[2] I. Bahar, I. Kaiserman, P. McAllum, A. Slomovic, and D. Rootman, "Comparison of posterior lamellar keratoplasty techniques to penetrating keratoplasty," *Ophthalmology*, vol. 115, no. 9, pp. 1525–1533, 2008.

[3] J. Hjortdal and N. Ehlers, "Descemet's stripping automated endothelial keratoplasty and penetrating keratoplasty for Fuchs' endothelial dystrophy," *Acta Ophthalmologica*, vol. 87, no. 3, pp. 310–314, 2009.

[4] T. Tourtas, K. Laaser, B. O. Bachmann, C. Cursiefen, and F. E. Kruse, "Descemet membrane endothelial keratoplasty versus Descemet stripping automated endothelial keratoplasty," *American Journal of Ophthalmology*, vol. 153, no. 6, pp. 1082–1090, 2012.

[5] M. Dirisamer, J. Parker, M. Naveiras et al., "Identifying causes for poor visual outcome after DSEK/DSAEK following secondary DMEK in the same eye," *Acta Ophthalmologica*, vol. 91, no. 2, pp. 131–139, 2013.

[6] J. W. McLaren and S. V. Patel, "Modeling the effect of forward scatter and aberrations on visual acuity after endothelial keratoplasty," *Investigative Opthalmology & Visual Science*, vol. 53, no. 9, pp. 5545–5551, 2012.

[7] L. S. Seery, C. B. Nau, J. W. McLaren, K. H. Baratz, and S. V. Patel, "Graft thickness, graft folds, and aberrations after Descemet stripping endothelial keratoplasty for Fuchs dystrophy," *American Journal of Ophthalmology*, vol. 152, no. 6, pp. 910–916, 2011.

[8] T. Yamaguchi, K. Ohnuma, D. Tomida et al., "The contribution of the posterior surface to the corneal aberrations in eyes after keratoplasty," *Investigative Opthalmology & Visual Science*, vol. 52, no. 9, pp. 6222–6229, 2011.

[9] K. van Dijk, K. Droutsas, J. Hou, S. Sangsari, V. S. Liarakos, and G. R. Melles, "Optical quality of the cornea after Descemet membrane endothelial keratoplasty," *American Journal of Ophthalmology*, vol. 158, no. 1, pp. 71–79, 2014.

[10] M. Rudolph, K. Laaser, B. O. Bachmann, C. Cursiefen, D. Epstein, and F. E. Kruse, "Corneal higher-order aberrations after Descemet's membrane endothelial keratoplasty," *Ophthalmology*, vol. 119, no. 3, pp. 528–535, 2012.

[11] E. A. Groeneveld-van Beek, J. T. Lie, J. van der Wees, M. Bruinsma, and G. R. J. Melles, "Standardized 'no-touch' donor tissue preparation for DALK and DMEK: harvesting undamaged anterior and posterior transplants from the same donor cornea," *Acta Ophthalmologica*, vol. 91, no. 2, pp. 145–150, 2013.

[12] Oculus Optikgeräte GmbH, *Oculus Pentacam Instruction Manual. Measurement and Evaluation System for the Anterior Segment of the Eye*, Oculus Optikgeräte, Wetzlar, Germany, 2018.

[13] J. Cabrerizo, E. Livny, F. U. Musa, P. Leeuwenburgh, K. van Dijk, and G. R. Melles, "Changes in color vision and contrast sensitivity after descemet membrane endothelial keratoplasty for fuchs endothelial dystrophy," *Cornea*, vol. 33, no. 10, pp. 1010–1015, 2014.

[14] M. Satué, M. Rodríguez-Calvo-de-Mora, M. Naveiras, J. Cabrerizo, I. Dapena, and G. R. Melles, "Standardization of the Descemet membrane endothelial keratoplasty technique: outcomes of the first 450 consecutive cases," *Archivos de la Sociedad Española de Oftalmología*, vol. 90, no. 8, pp. 356–364, 2015.

[15] M. Rodríguez-Calvo-de-Mora, R. Quilendrino, L. Ham et al., "Clinical outcome of 500 consecutive cases undergoing Descemet's membrane endothelial keratoplasty," *Ophthalmology*, vol. 122, no. 3, pp. 464–470, 2015.

[16] S. J. Leat and G. C. Woo, "The validity of current clinical tests of contrast sensitivity and their ability to predict reading speed in low vision," *Eye*, vol. 11, no. 6, pp. 893–899, 1997.

[17] J. M. Wood, "Age and visual impairment decrease driving performance as measured on a closed-road circuit," *Human Factors*, vol. 44, no. 3, pp. 482–494, 2002.

[18] C. Garrido, G. Cardona, J. L. Güell, and J. Pujol, "Visual outcome of penetrating keratoplasty, deep anterior lamellar keratoplasty and Descemet membrane endothelial keratoplasty," Journal of Optometry, pii: S1888-4296(17)30069-9, 2017.

[19] T. Hayashi, T. Yamaguchi, K. Yuda, N. Kato, Y. Satake, and J. Shimazaki, "Topographic characteristics after Descemet's membrane endothelial keratoplasty and Descemet's stripping automated endothelial keratoplasty," *PLoS One*, vol. 12, no. 11, Article ID e0188832, 2017.

[20] W. Chamberlain, N. Omid, A. Lin et al., "Comparison of corneal surface higher-order aberrations after endotelial keratoplasty, femtosecond laser-assisted keratoplasty, and conventional penetrating keratoplasty," *Cornea*, vol. 31, pp. 6–13, 2011.

[21] H. B. Hindman, K. R. Huxlin, S. M. Pantanelli et al., "Post-DSAEK optical changes: a comprehensive prospective analysis on the role of ocular wavefront aberrations, haze and corneal thickness," *Cornea*, vol. 32, no. 12, pp. 1567–1577, 2013.

[22] O. Muftuoglu, P. Prasher, R. W. Bowman, J. P. McCulley, and V. Vinod Mootha, "Corneal higherorder aberrations after Descemet's stripping automated endothelial keratoplasty," *Ophthalmology*, vol. 117, no. 5, pp. 878–884, 2010.

[23] T Yamaguchi, K Negishi, K Yamaguchi et al., "Effect of anterior and posterior corneal surface irregularity on vision after Descemet-stripping endothelial keratoplasty," *Journal of Cataract & Refractive Surgery*, vol. 35, no. 4, pp. 688–694, 2009.

[24] S. V. Patel, J. W. McLaren, D. O. Hodge, and K. H. Baratz, "Scattered light and visual function in a randomized trial of deep lamellar endothelial keratoplasty and penetrating keratoplasty," *American Journal of Ophthalmology*, vol. 145, no. 1, pp. 97–105, 2008.

[25] N. Morishige, N. Yamada, S. Teranishi, T.-i Chikama, T. Nishida, and A. Takahara, "Detection of subepithelial fibrosis associated with corneal stromal edema by second harmonic generation imaging microscopy," *Investigative Opthalmology & Visual Science*, vol. 50, no. 7, pp. 3145–3150, 2009.

[26] S. Koh, N. Maeda, T. Nakagawa, and K. Nishida, "Quality of vision in eyes after selective lamellar keratoplasty," *Cornea*, vol. 31, no. 1, pp. S45–S49, 2012.

[27] T. Yamaguchi, K. Negishi, K. Yamaguchi et al., "Comparison of anterior and posterior corneal surface irregularity in Descemet stripping automated endothelial keratoplasty and penetrating keratoplasty," *Cornea*, vol. 29, no. 10, pp. 1086–1090, 2010.

[28] S. Koh, N. Maeda, T. Nakagawa et al., "Characteristic higherorder aberrations of the anterior and posterior corneal surfaces in 3 corneal transplantation techniques," *American Journal of Ophthalmology*, vol. 153, no. 2, pp. 284–290, 2012.

[29] S. V. Patel and J. W. McLaren, "In vivo confocal microscopy of Fuchs endothelial dystrophy before and after endothelial keratoplasty," *JAMA Ophthalmology*, vol. 131, no. 5, pp. 611–618, 2013.

[30] S. V. Patel, K. H. Baratz, L. J. Maguire, D. O. Hodge, and J. W. McLaren, "Anterior corneal aberrations after Descemet's stripping endothelial keratoplasty for Fuchs' endothelial dystrophy," *Ophthalmology*, vol. 119, no. 8, pp. 1522–1529, 2012.

[31] I. J. Van der Meulen, S. V. Patel, R. Lapid-Gortzak et al., "Quality of vision in patients with Fuchs endothelial dystrophy and after Descemet stripping endothelial keratoplasty," *Archives of Ophthalmology*, vol. 129, no. 12, pp. 1537–1542, 2011.

[32] S. V. Patel, K. H. Baratz, D. O. Hodge, L. J. Maguire, and J. W. McLaren, "The effect of corneal light scatter on vision after Descemet stripping with endothelial keratoplasty," *Archives of Ophthalmology*, vol. 127, no. 2, pp. 153–160, 2009.

6

Association between Visual Acuity and Retinal Layer Metrics in Diabetics with and without Macular Edema

LakshmiPriya Rangaraju ⓘ,[1] Xuejuan Jiang,[2] J. Jason McAnany ⓘ,[1] Michael R. Tan,[1] Justin Wanek ⓘ,[1] Norman P. Blair,[1] Jennifer I. Lim,[1] and Mahnaz Shahidi ⓘ[2]

[1]Department of Ophthalmology and Visual Sciences, University of Illinois at Chicago, Chicago, IL, USA
[2]Department of Ophthalmology, University of Southern California, Los Angeles, CA, USA

Correspondence should be addressed to Mahnaz Shahidi; mshahidi@usc.edu

Academic Editor: Alejandro Cerviño

Purpose. Diabetes is known to cause alterations in retinal microvasculature and tissue that progressively lead to visual impairment. Optical coherence tomography (OCT) is useful for assessment of total retinal thickening due to diabetic macular edema (DME). In the current study, we determined associations between visual acuity (VA) and retinal layer thickness, reflectance, and interface disruption derived from enface OCT images in subjects with and without DME. *Materials and Methods.* Best corrected VA was measured and high-density OCT volume scans were acquired in 149 diabetic subjects. A previously established image segmentation method identified retinal layer interfaces and locations of visually indiscernible (disrupted) interfaces. Enface thickness maps and reflectance images of the nerve fiber layer (NFL), combined ganglion cell and inner plexiform layer (GCLIPL), inner nuclear layer (INL), outer plexiform layer (OPL), outer nuclear layer (ONL), photoreceptor outer segment layer (OSL), and retinal pigment epithelium (RPE) were generated in the central macular subfield. The associations among VA and retinal layer metrics were determined by multivariate linear regressions after adjusting for covariates (age, sex, race, HbA1c, diabetes type, and duration) and correcting for multiple comparisons. *Results.* In DME subjects, increased GCLIPL and OPL thickness and decreased OSL thickness were associated with reduced VA. Furthermore, increased NFL reflectance and decreased OSL reflectance were associated with reduced VA. Additionally, increased areas of INL and ONL interface disruptions were associated with reduced VA. In subjects without DME, increased INL thickness was associated with reduced VA, whereas in subjects without DME but with previous antivascular endothelium growth factor treatment, thickening of OPL was associated with reduced VA. *Conclusions.* Alterations in retinal layer thickness and reflectance metrics derived from enface OCT images were associated with reduced VA with and without presence of DME, suggestive of their potential for monitoring development, progression, and treatment of DME.

1. Introduction

Diabetes is known to cause alterations in retinal microvasculature and tissue that progressively lead to visual impairment. Indeed, diabetic retinopathy (DR) is the leading cause of vision loss in working-age adults [1]. One consequence of DR is the development of diabetic macular edema (DME) due to the accumulation of fluid within the central retinal tissue, which is a major contributor towards vision loss [2]. Reduction in visual acuity (VA) with progression of DR based on fundus photography in individuals with DME

has been established [3]. Optical coherence tomography (OCT) is currently the standard of clinical care for detecting abnormalities in retinal structure and quantifying the extent of retinal thickening due to DME [4]. Furthermore, high-resolution OCT can also quantify subtle retinal thickening not discernible on clinical examination in individuals with mild DME [5]. Additionally, previous studies have shown methods for 3D OCT imaging [6] and repeatable retinal layer thickness measurements in healthy and multiple sclerosis patients using commercially available OCT instruments (Cirrus HD-OCT and Spectralis SD-OCT) [7].

Although the total retinal thickness in the central subfield has been shown to be correlated with VA, the association was weaker than that of individual retinal layers [7, 8]. Specifically, thinning of the nerve fiber layer (NFL) in individuals with minimal or no DR and thickening of the inner nuclear layer (INL) and outer plexiform layer (OPL) in individuals with DME have been reported [9–15]. In addition to these changes, reduced VA has been correlated with thinning of the ganglion cell layer + inner plexiform layer (GCLIPL) and the photoreceptor outer segment layer (OSL) in subjects with and without DME [16, 17].

In addition to retinal thickness, alterations in retinal layer reflectance and interface have also been reported in DR. Specifically, in subjects with DME, reductions in photoreceptor outer segment length and disruptions of photoreceptor inner/outer segment junctions have been related to reduced VA [18, 19]. Additionally, inner retinal layer interface disruptions (visually indiscernible layer interfaces) and discontinuities in the inner segment/outer segment junction and in the external limiting membrane were associated with reduced VA [20–23]. However, most previous studies have examined retinal layer thickness, reflectance, and interface disruption from single OCT B-scans which limits localization of the spatial extent of retinal abnormalities. To better understand the spatial characteristics of retinal pathology, a method of retinal layer segmentation that generates three-dimensional outer retinal topography and reflectivity maps has been developed [24]. Although this approach provides more information than that obtained from single B-scans, the algorithms were based on images obtained using a spectral domain OCT prototype instrument. Using a commercially available OCT instrument, we have previously reported and validated methods for generating enface thickness maps and reflectance images of individual retinal layers from a high-density raster of OCT B-scan images and demonstrated alterations at different stages of DR [25–27]. In the current study, we identified individual retinal layers with thickness, reflectance, and interface disruption associated with VA in groups of DR subjects with and without DME.

2. Methods

2.1. Subjects. The research study was approved by an Institutional Review Board at the University of Illinois at Chicago and followed the tenets of the Declaration of Helsinki. Prior to enrollment, the study was explained to the subjects and informed consent was obtained. A total of 149 diabetic subjects participated in the study. All subjects underwent clinical examination by retinal specialists. Exclusion criteria were refractive error greater than 6 diopters of myopia, clinical diagnosis of glaucoma, age-related macular degeneration, retinal vascular occlusions or other conditions that could alter the anatomic integrity of the retina, history of intraocular surgery, cataract surgery performed less than 4 months prior to imaging, lens nuclear sclerosis score greater than 2+, or posterior subcapsular cataract concurrent with VA less than 20/20. One eye per subject was selected based on the exclusion criteria. If both

eyes qualified, the eye with better image quality was included. Based on clinical examination by retina specialists, subjects' eyes were classified as no DR (NDR; $N = 51$), nonproliferative DR (NPDR; $N = 59$), or proliferative DR (PDR; $N = 39$). The subjects were categorized into two subgroups, DME and no-DME, based on central subfield thickness (CST) being greater than $320\,\mu m$ (males) and $304\,\mu m$ (females) [28]. Twenty-eight subjects (NDR = 2; NPDR = 16; PDR = 10) had DME and 121 did not have DME at the time of imaging. Twenty-one of the 28 DME and 25 of the 121 no-DME subjects had previously received anti-VEGF therapy. Best-corrected VA was measured at a 4-meter distance using a retro-illuminated Early Treatment Diabetic Retinopathy Study (ETDRS) chart by an ophthalmic technician who was trained in the ETDRS protocol.

2.2. Image Acquisition. Spectral domain OCT (SDOCT) imaging of a retinal area of $20° \times 15°$ centered on the fovea was performed using a commercially available instrument (Spectralis; Heidelberg Engineering, Heidelberg, Germany). A high-density SDOCT raster volume scan was generated from 73 raster horizontal B-scans (9 averaged frames) with a vertical spacing of $62\,\mu m$. Each B-scan consisted of 1024 A-scans and had a depth resolution of $3.9\,\mu m$.

2.3. Image Analysis. SDOCT B-scans were analyzed using our previously described automated image segmentation software based on graph theory and dynamic programming [25]. In brief, a graph was generated for all SDOCT B-scans with edge weights designated according to vertical gradients in the images. A horizontal path through the graph that minimized the total sum of the weights was found using Dijkstra's algorithm and defined a line separating two retinal cell layers. Figure 1 displays eight retinal interfaces that were detected: (1) vitreous and NFL, (2) NFL and GCLIPL, (3) GCLIPL and INL, (4) INL and OPL, (5) OPL and outer nuclear layer (ONL), (6) ONL and OSL, (7) OSL and retinal pigment epithelium (RPE), and (8) RPE and choroid. Following our previously reported method, an operator was able to review the automated interface detection results by scrolling through all SDOCT B-scans. If necessary, errors were corrected by manually selecting the segmentation line that required adjustment and drawing a revised line corresponding to the visualized cell-layer interface. The program then regenerated an automated line by restricting the graph search area to a small vertical image region around the manually drawn line and recalculating the minimum graph cut solution, as previously described [25]. Locations of retinal layer interfaces that were not visually discernible (disruptions) due to gross abnormalities in retinal cell layer architecture were manually selected by the operator. The automated image segmentation method was previously validated [25] by demonstrating a high correlation with data provided by commercial instruments and also showing a decrease in retinal thickness with increased age, consistent with previous reports. Additionally, the average error rate obtained by the automated segmentation method was shown to be 7% in NPDR subjects [25].

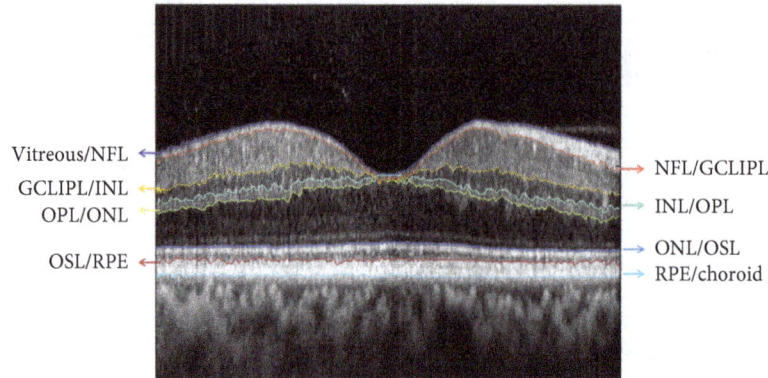

FIGURE 1: Example of an OCT B-scan in a DR subject without DME, representing the eight segmented retinal layer interfaces.

Enface thickness maps and reflectance images were generated for each of 7 retinal layers (NFL, GCLIPL, INL, OPL, ONL, OSL, and RPE) based on segmentation of the 8 retinal interfaces in the SDOCT B-scans. Regions containing retinal layer interface disruption were not assigned thickness or reflectance values. Retinal layer metrics of thickness, reflectance, and areas of interface disruption were evaluated in the ETDRS central subfield (1 mm diameter) [29]. Mean thickness metrics were calculated for each layer (NFL_T, $GCLIPL_T$, INL_T, OPL_T, ONL_T, and OSL_T). Reflectance ratio metrics were also calculated in the central subfield for each layer (NFL_R, $GCLIPL_R$, INL_R, OPL_R, ONL_R, and OSL_R) as the mean intensity of each layer divided by the mean intensity of the RPE ($layer_{Intensity}/RPE_{Intensity}$).

Percent areas of layer interface disruption relative to the total central ETDRS subfield area (NFL_d, INL_d, ONL_d, and RPE_d) were calculated. NFL_d was calculated based on the interface disruption of both vitreous/NFL and NFL/GCLIPL interfaces relative to the total central subfield area. Similarly, INL_d was calculated based on disruptions of both GCLIPL/INL and INL/OPL interfaces; ONL_d was calculated based on disruptions of both OPL/ONL and ONL/OSL interfaces; RPE_d was calculated based on disruptions of both OSL/RPE and RPE/choroid interfaces.

2.4. Statistical Analysis. Associations of retinal layer thickness, reflectance, and percent area of interface disruptions were determined by multivariate general linear models, adjusting for age, sex, race, diabetes type, diabetes duration, and HbA1C level. Diagnostics of model assumptions were performed on all models and residuals for VA followed a normal distribution. Potential influential data points were also identified; sensitivity analyses excluding those data points were performed and the regression results were not changed materially. With a sample size of 28, the statistical power for multivariate linear regression (with 7 variables) was 80% to detect a partial correlation of 0.56 or greater, and with a sample size of 121, the power was 80% to detect a partial correlation of 0.26 or greater. For the associations between VA and retinal layer interface disruptions, Kruskal–Wallis tests were also performed and results were similar to those obtained by analysis of variance. All statistical tests were conducted using SAS 9.4 (SAS Institute

Inc., Cary, NC). All P-values were from two-sided tests. For the associations between VA and layer-specific measurements, significance was accepted at $P < 0.008$ to account for multiple comparisons using Bonferroni correction.

3. Results

Demographic details and ocular characteristics of subjects are presented in Table 1. Mean CST in all subjects was $283 \pm 56 \, \mu m$ ($N = 149$). As expected, CST was greater in subjects with DME ($371 \pm 70 \, \mu m$; $N = 28$), compared with subjects without DME ($263 \pm 23 \, \mu m$; $N = 121$) ($P < 0.001$). Log MAR VA of all subjects was 0.04 ± 0.13. Subjects with DME had worse VA (0.14 ± 0.16 log MAR), compared with subjects with no DME (0.02 ± 0.11 log MAR) ($P < 0.001$). Examples of enface retinal layer thickness maps and reflectance images (not normalized to RPE reflectance) in a DR subject with DME are displayed in Figure 2. On average, ONL and NFL have the largest and smallest thickness, respectively. Due to the foveal depression, GCLIPL has minimal thickness in the center of the fovea. The ONL and OSL have the lowest and highest reflectance, respectively. Regions of retinal layer interface disruptions are represented by black and yellow on the thickness and reflectance layer maps, respectively.

3.1. Retinal Layer Thickness. Mean retinal layer thickness and regression coefficients obtained in DME subjects after adjusting for age, sex, race, diabetes type, diabetes duration, and HbA1c are listed in Table 2. Increased $GCLIPL_T$ and OPL_T (coefficients ≥ 0.03 log MAR/10 micron) and decreased OSL_T (coefficient $= -0.117$ log MAR/10 micron) were associated with reduced VA ($P < 0.008$). That is, each 10 micron increase in $GCLIPL_T$ and OPL_T resulted in an approximate 1 or 2 letter loss of VA, whereas each 10 micron decrease in OSL_T resulted in approximately 5 letters of VA loss. Mean retinal layer thickness and regression coefficients obtained in no-DME subjects after adjusting for age, sex, race, diabetes type, diabetes duration, and HbA1c are listed in Table 3. Increased INL_T was associated with reduced VA (coefficient $= 0.048$ log MAR/10 micron). Mean retinal layer thickness and regression coefficients obtained in no-DME subjects with a history of anti-VEGF treatment after adjusting for age, sex, race, diabetes type, diabetes duration,

TABLE 1: Study population and ocular characteristics.

	Total sample size = 149
Population characteristics	
Age, mean (SD), years	56.0 (11.8)
Female sex, number (%)	87 (58.4%)
Race/ethnicity, number (%)	
White	25 (16.8%)
African American	77 (51.7%)
Hispanic or Latino	42 (28.2%)
Asian	5 (3.4%)
DM type, number (%)	
1	12 (8.1%)
2	137 (91.9%)
DM duration, mean (SD), years	16.3 (10.1)
Glycated hemoglobin level, mean (SD), %	7.9 (1.7)
Ocular characteristics	
Study eye, number (%)	
Right	96 (64%)
Left	53 (36%)
Spherical equivalent refractive error, mean (SD), D	−0.66 (1.74)
Visual acuity, mean (SD), log MAR units	0.04 (0.13)
Diabetic retinopathy stage, number (%)	
No DR	51 (34%)
NPDR	59 (40%)
PDR	39 (27%)
Presence of DME, number (%)	28 (18.8%)
Central subfield thickness, mean (SD), μm	283 (56)

DM = diabetes mellitus; DR = diabetic retinopathy; PDR = proliferative diabetic retinopathy; NPDR = nonproliferative diabetic retinopathy; DME = diabetic macular edema; SD = standard deviation.

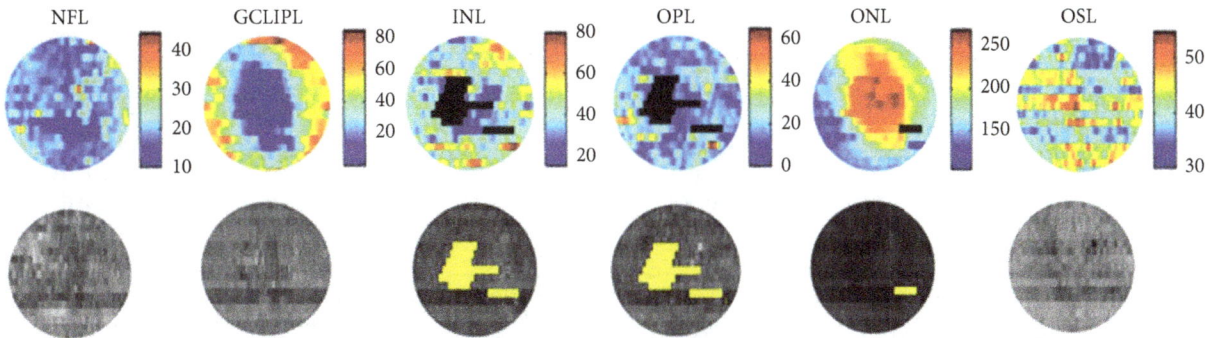

FIGURE 2: Enface thickness maps and reflectance images in a DR subject with DME. Top (left to right): ETDRS central subfield thickness maps of NFL, GCLIPL, INL, OPL, ONL, OSL, and RPE retinal layers. Bottom (left to right): reflectance images of NFL, GCLIPL, INL, OPL, ONL, OSL, and RPE retinal layers. Regions of retinal layer interface disruptions are represented by black and yellow on retinal layer thickness and reflectance maps, respectively. In these regions of disrupted interfaces, thickness and reflectance values were not assigned.

and HbA1c are listed in Table 4. Increased OPL_T was associated with reduced VA (coefficient = 0.061 log MAR/10 micron).

3.2. Retinal Layer Reflectance.

Mean retinal layer reflectance and regression coefficients obtained in DME subjects after adjusting for age, sex, race, diabetes type, diabetes duration, and HbA1c are listed in Table 2. Increased NFL_R (coefficient = 0.077 log MAR/0.1 reflectance ratio) and decreased OSL_R (coefficient = −0.069 log MAR/0.1 reflectance ratio) were associated with reduced VA ($P < 0.008$). Mean retinal layer reflectance and regression coefficients obtained in no-DME subjects after adjusting for age, sex, race, diabetes type,

diabetes duration, and HbA1c are listed in Table 3. Retinal layer reflectance changes were not associated with reduced VA. Similarly, in no-DME subjects with a history of anti-VEGF treatment, there was no significant association between retinal layer reflectance and VA (Table 4).

3.3. Retinal Interface Disruption.

Both increased INL_d and ONL_d were associated with worse VA after adjusting for age, sex, race, diabetes type, diabetes duration, and HbA1c ($P < 0.008$). The mean VA values for subjects with 0%, <10%, and ≥10% INL_d were 0.02 ± 0.12 ($N = 124$), 0.09 ± 0.13 ($N = 13$), and 0.18 ± 0.14 ($N = 12$) log MAR, respectively ($P < 0.01$). The mean VA values in subjects with 0%, <10%,

TABLE 2: Multivariate associations of retinal layer thickness and reflectance ratio with logMAR visual acuity based on data from DME subjects ($N = 28$).

Metrics	Thickness (microns), mean ± SD	Regression coefficient (95% CI) [1]
NFL_T	21 ± 6	0.074 (−0.020, 0.167)
$GCLIPL_T$	43 ± 26	0.030 (0.013, 0.048)**
INL_T	55 ± 57	0.014 (0.003, 0.024)
OPL_T	24 ± 8	0.101 (0.043, 0.160)**
ONL_T	159 ± 57	−0.007 (−0.018, 0.003)
OSL_T	42 ± 9	−0.117 (−0.165, −0.069)**
Metrics	Reflectance ratio, mean ± SD	Regression coefficient (95% CI) [1]
NFL_R	0.63 ± 0.12	0.077 (0.040, 0.114)**
$GCLIPL_R$	0.65 ± 0.07	0.085 (−0.003, 0.173)
INL_R	0.49 ± 0.08	−0.028 (−0.123, 0.068)
OPL_R	0.53 ± 0.08	0.057 (−0.035, 0.150)
ONL_R	0.35 ± 0.04	0.012 (−0.130, 0.154)
OSL_R	0.76 ± 0.11	−0.069 (−0.117, −0.021)**

** $P \leq 0.008$. [1] Regression coefficients represent logMAR change with 10 micron increase in thickness or 0.1 increase in reflectance ratio, after adjusting for age, sex, race, diabetes type, diabetes duration, and HbA1c. NFL = nerve fiber layer; GCLIPL = ganglion cell layer + inner plexiform layer; INL = inner nuclear layer; OPL = outer plexiform layer; ONL = outer nuclear layer; OSL = photoreceptor outer segment layer; RPE = retinal pigment epithelium. Suffix T = thickness; suffix R = reflectance ratio.

TABLE 3: Multivariate associations of retinal layer thickness and reflectance ratio with logMAR visual acuity based on data from subjects without DME ($N = 121$).

Metrics	Thickness (microns), mean ± SD	Regression coefficient (95% CI) [1]
NFL_T	18 ± 13	0.004 (−0.060, 0.068)
$GCLIPL_T$	28 ± 12	−0.003 (−0.021, 0.016)
INL_T	21 ± 8	0.048 (0.023, 0.073)**
OPL_T	21 ± 8	0.029 (0.001, 0.056)
ONL_T	114 ± 22	−0.002 (−0.012, 0.007)
OSL_T	44 ± 7	−0.008 (−0.036, 0.019)
Metrics	Reflectance ratio, mean ± SD	Regression coefficient (95% CI) [1]
NFL_R	0.54 ± 0.07	0.029 (0, 0.057)
$GCLIPL_R$	0.61 ± 0.07	0.021 (−0.010, 0.052)
INL_R	0.50 ± 0.06	0.010 (−0.025, 0.044)
OPL_R	0.52 ± 0.06	0.009 (−0.026, 0.045)
ONL_R	0.37 ± 0.05	0.043 (0.001, 0.085)
OSL_R	0.81 ± 0.07	−0.007 (−0.037, 0.023)

** $P \leq 0.008$. [1] Regression coefficients represent logMAR change with 10 micron increase in thickness or 0.1 increase in reflectance ratio, after adjusting for age, sex, race, diabetes type, diabetes duration, and HbA1c. NFL = nerve fiber layer; GCLIPL = ganglion cell layer + inner plexiform layer; INL = inner nuclear layer; OPL = outer plexiform layer; ONL = outer nuclear layer; OSL = photoreceptor outer segment layer; RPE = retinal pigment epithelium. Suffix T = thickness; suffix R = reflectance ratio.

and ≥10% ONL_d were 0.02 ± 0.12 ($N = 125$), 0.11 ± 0.15 ($N = 11$), and 0.16 ± 0.14 ($N = 13$) log MAR, respectively ($P < 0.01$). When the analyses were conducted separately for DME and no-DME subjects, there was no significant association between VA and INL_d or ONL_d ($P > 0.05$).

4. Discussion

In the current study, we determined associations between VA and retinal layer thickness and reflectance in DR subjects with and without DME. In DME subjects, GCLIPL and OPL thickening and OSL thinning, as well as hyper-reflectance of the NFL and hypo-reflectance of the OSL, were associated with reduced VA. Moreover, VA was reduced in regions of disrupted retinal interfaces bordering the INL and ONL.

Interestingly, in subjects without DME, thickening of the INL was associated with reduced VA, whereas in the subset of these subjects who had previous anti-VEGF treatment, thickening of OPL was associated with reduced VA.

In DME subjects, increased $GCLIPL_T$ and OPL_T were associated with decreased VA. The relationship between increased OPL_T and decreased VA is consistent with previous studies, which reported a correlation between increased edema and reduced VA [20]. Our findings are also consistent with other reports of the presence of cystoid spaces or increased OPL thickness, although the relation to VA was not reported in these studies [9, 11]. Decreased OSL_T was associated with reduced VA, consistent with the findings of a previous study [18]. This change in OSL_T suggests that photoreceptor degeneration, possibly secondary to macular

TABLE 4: Multivariate associations of retinal layer thickness and reflectance ratio with logMAR visual acuity based on data from subjects without DME but with a history of anti-VEGF treatment ($N = 25$).

Metrics	Thickness (microns), mean $\pm$ SD	Regression coefficient (95% CI) [1]
NFL_T	18 ± 3	$0.132 \ (-0.054, 0.318)$
$GCLIPL_T$	29 ± 11	$0.012 \ (-0.034, 0.057)$
INL_T	28 ± 10	$0.046 \ (0.007, 0.086)$
OPL_T	21 ± 12	$0.061 \ (0.028, 0.093)^{**}$
ONL_T	117 ± 39	$-0.009 \ (-0.02, 0.002)$
OSL_T	41 ± 8	$-0.021 \ (-0.078, 0.036)$
Metrics	Reflectance ratio, mean $\pm$ SD	Regression coefficient (95% CI) [1]
NFL_R	0.55 ± 0.09	$0.031 \ (-0.037, 0.098)$
$GCLIPL_R$	0.61 ± 0.08	$0.017 \ (-0.056, 0.09)$
INL_R	0.49 ± 0.07	$-0.002 \ (-0.079, 0.076)$
OPL_R	0.51 ± 0.07	$-0.014 \ (-0.09, 0.061)$
ONL_R	0.38 ± 0.06	$0.01 \ (-0.068, 0.088)$
OSL_R	0.79 ± 0.07	$0.003 \ (-0.079, 0.085)$

$^{**}P \leq 0.008$. [1]Regression coefficients represent logMAR change with 10 micron increase in thickness or 0.1 increase in reflectance ratio, after adjusting for age, sex, race, diabetes type, diabetes duration, and HbA1c. NFL = nerve fiber layer; GCLIPL = ganglion cell layer + inner plexiform layer; INL = inner nuclear layer; OPL = outer plexiform layer; ONL = outer nuclear layer; OSL = photoreceptor outer segment layer; RPE = retinal pigment epithelium. Suffix T = thickness; suffix R = reflectance ratio.

edema, may contribute to vision loss. Further studies are needed to confirm our findings, given the limited number of DME subjects in this study, and to determine whether treatment based on thickening of specific retinal layers can potentially improve visual outcomes.

In subjects without DME, increased INL_T was associated with reduced VA. This finding suggests that thickening of the INL can occur and perhaps precede the development of DME. Of note, the regression coefficient for the association between INL_T and VA in no-DME subjects with a history of anti-VEGF treatment was similar to the value in subjects without DME, though it did not reach statistical significance after adjusting for multiple comparisons, possibly due to the smaller sample size. Interestingly, in no-DME subjects with a history of anti-VEGF treatment, thickening of OPL was associated with reduced VA, similar to the finding in DME subjects. Future longitudinal studies are needed to investigate thickness alterations in this retinal layer as an early indicator for recurrent DME or as a marker for the adequacy of DME treatment.

The current study demonstrated associations between changes in retinal layer reflectance and reduced VA. In the DME subjects, decreased OSL_R and increased NFL_R were associated with reduced VA. The association of OSL_R and VA is consistent with a previous study that reported reduced reflectance of the photoreceptor layer when cystoid spaces were present in the OPL [30] and other studies that showed a correlation between the continuity of the photoreceptor inner and outer segment (ellipsoid) and VA [7, 19–21, 31, 32]. However, these previous studies evaluated the inner and outer segment junction visibility based on a single B-scan or a low-density raster of B-scans. In the current study, enface reflectance images of the OSL were obtained from high-density OCT B-scans, thereby providing a more accurate localization of the spatial extent of reduced OSL reflectance. To our knowledge, an association between increased NFL_R and reduced VA has not been previously reported.

Several previous studies have reported methods for segmentation of different retinal layers in DR [33–39]. The accuracy of automated segmentation of retinal layers in healthy and DR subjects relies on the presence of distinct interfaces between layers. However, in DME subjects who have severe pathology, these interfaces cannot be clearly identified, even by expert human evaluation. The method presented in the current study allowed quantitative measurement of areas in which retinal layer interfaces were visually indiscernible due to pathologies and macular edema, thus providing a useful metric for assessing retinal integrity. The finding of an association between reduced VA and disrupted INL and ONL interfaces is consistent with previous studies that reported a correlation between combined inner retinal interface disruptions (NFL/GCLIPL, GCLIPL/INL/OPL, and OPL/ONL) and VA, although they did not evaluate disruptions in other layer interfaces (ONL/OSL and OSL/RPE) [22, 23].

5. Conclusion

Quantitative assessment of retinal layer integrity by enface OCT imaging may be clinically relevant for monitoring the progression of pathologies due to disease or their resolution following treatment. Concurrent assessment of thickness, reflectance, and interface disruption of individual retinal layers by enface OCT imaging provides a comprehensive approach for identifying anatomic outcomes that may be useful for monitoring development, progression, and treatment efficacy of DME.

Conflicts of Interest

The authors declare that they have no conflicts of interest.

Acknowledgments

This work was supported by the NIH grants DK010439 (MS), EY001792 (UIC Core), and EY026004 (JM), a Senior Scientific Investigator Award (MS), a Dolly Green Special Scholar Award (JM), and an unrestricted departmental grant from Research to Prevent Blindness.

References

[1] S. Wild, A. Green, R. Sicree, and H. King, "Global prevalence of diabetes: estimates for the year 2000 and projections for 2030," *Diabetes Care*, vol. 27, no. 5, pp. 1047–1053, 2004.

[2] R. Lee, T. Y. Wong, and C. Sabanayagam, "Epidemiology of diabetic retinopathy, diabetic macular edema and related vision loss," *Eye and Vision*, vol. 2, no. 1, p. 17, 2015.

[3] B. Bengtsson, A. Heijl, and E. Agardh, "Visual fields correlate better than visual acuity to severity of diabetic retinopathy," *Diabetologia*, vol. 48, no. 12, pp. 2494–2500, 2005.

[4] L. M. Sakata, J. Deleon-Ortega, V. Sakata, and C. A. Girkin, "Optical coherence tomography of the retina and optic nerve- a review," *Clinical & Experimental Ophthalmology*, vol. 37, no. 1, pp. 90–99, 2009.

[5] J. C Brown, S. D. Solomon, S. B. Bressler, A. P. Schachat, C. DiBernardo, and N. M. Bressler, "Detection of diabetic foveal edema: contact lens biomicroscopy compared with optical coherence tomography," *Archives of Ophthalmology*, vol. 122, no. 3, pp. 330–335, 2004.

[6] C. Hitzenberger, P. Trost, P. W. Lo, and Q. Zhou, "Three-dimensional imaging of the human retina by high-speed optical coherence tomography," *Optics Express*, vol. 11, no. 21, pp. 2753–2761, 2003.

[7] T. Otani, Y. Yamaguchi, and S. Kishi, "Correlation between visual acuity and foveal microstructural changes in diabetic macular edema," *Retina*, vol. 30, no. 5, pp. 774–780, 2010.

[8] D. J. Browning, A. R. Glassman, L. P. Aiello et al., "Relationship between optical coherence tomography-measured central retinal thickness and visual acuity in diabetic macular edema," *Ophthalmology*, vol. 114, no. 3, pp. 525–536, 2007.

[9] F. Bandello, A. N. Tejerina, S. Vujosevic et al., "Retinal layer location of increased retinal thickness in eyes with subclinical and clinical macular edema in diabetes type 2," *Ophthalmic Research*, vol. 54, no. 3, pp. 112–117, 2015.

[10] J. Chhablani, A. Sharma, A. Goud et al., "Neurodegeneration in type 2 diabetes: evidence from spectral-domain optical coherence tomography," *Investigative Ophthalmology & Visual Science*, vol. 56, no. 11, pp. 6333–6338, 2015.

[11] T. Murakami and N. Yoshimura, "Structural changes in individual retinal layers in diabetic macular edema," *Journal of Diabetes Research*, vol. 2013, Article ID 920713, 11 pages, 2013.

[12] P. H. Peng, H. S. Lin, and S. Lin, "Nerve fibre layer thinning in patients with preclinical retinopathy," *Canadian Journal of Ophthalmology*, vol. 44, no. 4, pp. 417–422, 2009.

[13] H. W. Van Dijk, F. D. Verbraak, P. H. Kok et al., "Early neurodegeneration in the retina of type 2 diabetic patients," *Investigative Opthalmology & Visual Science*, vol. 53, no. 6, pp. 2715–2719, 2012.

[14] A. Verma, R. Raman, K. Vaitheeswaran et al., "Does neuronal damage precede vascular damage in subjects with type 2 diabetes mellitus and having no clinical diabetic retinopathy?," *Ophthalmic Research*, vol. 47, no. 4, pp. 202–207, 2012.

[15] S. Vujosevic and E. Midena, "Retinal layers changes in human preclinical and early clinical diabetic retinopathy support early retinal neuronal and Muller cells alterations," *Journal of Diabetes Research*, vol. 2013, Article ID 905058, 8 pages, 2013.

[16] T. Alasil, P. A. Keane, J. F. Updike et al., "Relationship between optical coherence tomography retinal parameters and visual acuity in diabetic macular edema," *Ophthalmology*, vol. 117, no. 12, pp. 2379–2386, 2010.

[17] S. Bonnin, R. Tadayoni, A. Erginay, P. Massin, and B. Dupas, "Correlation between ganglion cell layer thinning and poor visual function after resolution of diabetic macular edema," *Investigative Ophthalmology & Visual Science*, vol. 56, no. 2, pp. 978–982, 2015.

[18] F. Forooghian, P. F. Stetson, S. A. Meyer et al., "Relationship between photoreceptor outer segment length and visual acuity in diabetic macular edema," *Retina*, vol. 30, no. 1, pp. 63–70, 2010.

[19] A. S. Maheshwary, S. F. Oster, R. M. Yuson, L. Cheng, F. Mojana, and W. R. Freeman, "The association between percent disruption of the photoreceptor inner segment-outer segment junction and visual acuity in diabetic macular edema," *American Journal of Ophthalmology*, vol. 150, no. 1, pp. 63.e61–67.e61, 2010.

[20] T. Murakami, K. Nishijima, A. Sakamoto, M. Ota, T. Horii, and N. Yoshimura, "Association of pathomorphology, photoreceptor status, and retinal thickness with visual acuity in diabetic retinopathy," *American Journal of Ophthalmology*, vol. 151, no. 2, pp. 310–317, 2011.

[21] H. J. Shin, S. H. Lee, H. Chung, and H. C. Kim, "Association between photoreceptor integrity and visual outcome in diabetic macular edema," *Graefe's Archive for Clinical and Experimental Ophthalmology*, vol. 250, no. 1, pp. 61–70, 2012.

[22] J. K. Sun, M. M. Lin, J. Lammer et al., "Disorganization of the retinal inner layers as a predictor of visual acuity in eyes with center-involved diabetic macular edema," *JAMA Ophthalmology*, vol. 132, no. 11, pp. 1309–1316, 2014.

[23] J. K. Sun, S. H. Radwan, A. Z. Soliman et al., "Neural retinal disorganization as a robust marker of visual acuity in current and resolved diabetic macular edema," *Diabetes*, vol. 64, no. 7, pp. 2560–2570, 2015.

[24] M. Wojtkowski, B. L. Sikorski, I. Gorczynska et al., "Comparison of reflectivity maps and outer retinal topography in retinal disease by 3-D Fourier domain optical coherence tomography," *Optics Express*, vol. 17, no. 5, pp. 4189–4207, 2009.

[25] J. Wanek, N. P. Blair, F. Y. Chau, Y. I. Lim, Y. I. Leiderman, and M. Shahidi, "Alterations in retinal layer thickness and reflectance at different stages of diabetic retinopathy by enface optical coherence tomography," *Investigative Ophthalmology & Visual Science*, vol. 57, no. 9, pp. OCT341–OCT347, 2016.

[26] F. Mohammad, J. Wanek, R. Zelkha, J. I. Lim, J. Chen, and M. Shahidi, "A method for en face OCT imaging of subretinal fluid in age-related macular degeneration," *Journal of Ophthalmology*, vol. 2014, Article ID 720243, 6 pages, 2014.

[27] J. Wanek, R. Zelkha, J. I. Lim, and M. Shahidi, "Feasibility of a method for en face imaging of photoreceptor cell integrity," *American Journal of Ophthalmology*, vol. 152, no. 5, pp. 807.e1–814.e1, 2011.

[28] K. V. Chalam, S. B. Bressler, A. R. Edwards et al., "Retinal thickness in people with diabetes and minimal or no diabetic retinopathy: Heidelberg Spectralis optical coherence tomography," *Investigative Ophthalmology & Visual Science*, vol. 53, no. 3, pp. 8154–8161, 2012.

[29] ETDRS Research Group, "Early Treatment Diabetic Retinopathy Study design and baseline patient characteristics.

ETDRS report number 7," *Ophthalmology*, vol. 98, no. 5, pp. 741–756, 1991.

[30] T. Murakami, K. Nishijima, T. Akagi et al., "Optical coherence tomographic reflectivity of photoreceptors beneath cystoid spaces in diabetic macular edema," *Investigative Ophthalmology & Visual Science*, vol. 53, no. 3, pp. 1506–1511, 2012.

[31] A. Sakamoto, K. Nishijima, M. Kita, H. Oh, A. Tsujikawa, and N. Yoshimura, "Association between foveal photoreceptor status and visual acuity after resolution of diabetic macular edema by pars plana vitrectomy," *Graefe's Archive for Clinical and Experimental Ophthalmology*, vol. 247, no. 10, pp. 1325–1330, 2009.

[32] Y. Shen, K. Liu, and X. Xu, "Correlation between visual function and photoreceptor integrity in diabetic macular edema: spectral-domain optical coherence tomography," *Current Eye Research*, vol. 41, no. 3, pp. 391–399, 2016.

[33] F. Mohammad, R. Ansari, J. Wanek, A. Francis, and M. Shahidi, "Feasibility of level-set analysis of enface OCT retinal images in diabetic retinopathy," *Biomedical Optics Express*, vol. 6, no. 5, pp. 1904–1918, 2015.

[34] Y. Huang, R. P. Danis, J. W. Pak et al., "Development of a semi-automatic segmentation method for retinal OCT images tested in patients with diabetic macular edema," *PLoS One*, vol. 8, no. 12, Article ID e82922, 2013.

[35] M. K. Garvin, M. D. Abramoff, X. Wu, S. R. Russell, T. L. Burns, and M. Sonka, "Automated 3-D intraretinal layer segmentation of macular spectral-domain optical coherence tomography images," *IEEE Transactions on Medical Imaging*, vol. 28, no. 9, pp. 1436–1447, 2009.

[36] K. A. Vermeer, J. Van Der Schoot, H. G. Lemij, and J. F. De Boer, "Automated segmentation by pixel classification of retinal layers in ophthalmic OCT images," *Biomedical Optics Express*, vol. 2, no. 6, pp. 1743–1756, 2011.

[37] S. J. Chiu, M. J. Allingham, P. S. Mettu, S. W. Cousins, J. A. Izatt, and S. Farsiu, "Kernel regression based segmentation of optical coherence tomography images with diabetic macular edema," *Biomedical Optics Express*, vol. 6, no. 4, pp. 1172–1194, 2015.

[38] S. J. Chiu, X. T. Li, P. Nicholas, C. A. Toth, J. A. Izatt, and S. Farsiu, "Automatic segmentation of seven retinal layers in SDOCT images congruent with expert manual segmentation," *Optics Express*, vol. 18, no. 18, pp. 19413–19428, 2010.

[39] S. J. Chiu, C. A. Toth, C. Bowes Rickman, J. A. Izatt, and S. Farsiu, "Automatic segmentation of closed-contour features in ophthalmic images using graph theory and dynamic programming," *Biomedical Optics Express*, vol. 3, no. 5, pp. 1127–1140, 2012.

7

Corneal Epithelial Damage and Impaired Tear Functions in Patients with Inflamed Pinguecula

Erkut Küçük ⓘ,[1] Uğur Yılmaz,[2] and Kürsad Ramazan Zor[1]

[1]*Ophthalmology Department, Niğde Ömer Halisdemir University, Faculty of Medicine, 51240 Niğde, Turkey*
[2]*Ophthalmology Department, Pamukkale University Faculty of Medicine, 20160 Denizli, Turkey*

Correspondence should be addressed to Erkut Küçük; erkutkucuk@yahoo.com

Academic Editor: Jesús Pintor

Purpose. In this study, we evaluated corneal epithelial integrity and tear film parameters in patients with inflamed pinguecula and compared these findings with their fellow eyes and with healthy controls. *Methods.* We evaluated the fluorescein staining properties and performed the tear break-up time (TBUT) test and Schirmer 2 test (ST2) measurements of 32 patients who had symptomatic unilateral inflamed pinguecula and compared the results with their fellow eyes and also with an age- and sex-matched control group. *Results.* Twenty-three eyes (72%) in the inflamed pinguecula group and 1 eye (3.1%) in the fellow eyes group had punctate epithelial staining (PES) or epithelial defect on the nasal cornea ($p < 0.001$). There was no PES or epithelial defect in the control group. Eyes with inflamed pinguecula ($n = 32$) had lower TBUT and ST2 values compared to the control group ($n = 32$) ($p < 0.001$ for both). Fellow eyes ($n = 32$) also had lower TBUT and ST2 values compared to the control group ($p = 0.003$ for both). There was no difference in the TBUT and ST2 results between the eyes with inflamed pinguecula and fellow eyes ($p = 0.286$ and $p = 0.951$, respectively). *Conclusion.* A high percentage of eyes with inflamed pinguecula had nasal corneal epithelial staining or epithelial defect. We also found lower TBUT and ST2 results in eyes with inflamed pinguecula and the fellow eyes compared to the control group. These findings may be important in pathogenesis of pinguecula and pterygium and also in uncovering their relation.

1. Introduction

Pinguecula is a yellowish elevated mass commonly located on the nasal bulbar conjunctiva close to the limbus [1]. Its prevalence increases with age, and ultraviolet radiation (UVR) is a risk factor in its pathogenesis [2, 3]. Male gender and diabetes mellitus are also reported risk factors [4]. Histological studies reported abnormal differentiation and squamous metaplasia of the conjunctival epithelium, exaggeration and distortion in the production of elastic fibers, and abnormality of their organization in the subepithelial connective tissue [5–7]. It was reported that 22.5% to 70.1% of the population has pinguecula [4, 8]. This heterogeneity in the prevalence may be due to differences in age, geographic location, and ethnicity of participants. Pinguecula may be inflamed, causing hyperemia, pain, and foreign body sensation.

Pterygium is a triangular growth of conjunctival fibrovascular tissue onto the cornea, usually located at the nasal

cornea. Its prevalence is lower than that of pinguecula. It can cause decreased visual acuity, irritation, and pain due to inflammation and cosmetic problems. Although surgery is effective in its treatment, the risk of recurrence is still an important problem. Ultraviolet radiation (UVR) is thought to be a factor in the development of both pinguecula and pterygium. It is hypothesized that UVR causes conjunctival degeneration and the formation of pinguecula. With increased exposure, corneal epithelial and stem cells may be affected and lead to the formation of pterygium [9, 10]. But it is still unknown if pinguecula is a precursor of pterygium or if so, what causes its progress to pterygium.

Several studies reported abnormalities of tear function tests in pinguecula patients [2, 11]. The abnormality of the tear film and mechanical trauma may cause inflammation of pinguecula [12]. Inflamed pinguecula has attracted little attention in the ophthalmic community. In this study, we investigated the fluorescein staining properties and tear film parameters in patients with inflamed pinguecula. We also discussed the role of these parameters in the possible evolution of the inflamed pinguecula to pterygium.

2. Materials and Methods

This controlled multicenter study was performed in the Ophthalmology Department of Niğde Ömer Halisdemir University (Niğde, Turkey) and Ophthalmology Department of Pamukkale University Hospital (Denizli, Turkey). Both cities are located at the same latitude (38°), and they have the same distance from the equator. Denizli is located approximately 124 km from the Aegean Sea, and Niğde is located 130 km from the Mediterranean Sea. Although regional differences can exist, these two cities show similar climatic characteristics. Thirty-two consecutive patients who applied to these clinics between July 2017 and September 2017 and had symptomatic unilateral inflamed pinguecula were included. Twelve of these patients were from Pamukkale University Hospital and 20 from Niğde Ömer Halisdemir University Ophthalmology Department. Symptomatic inflamed pinguecula was described as a combination of vascular congestion and hyperemia of the pinguecula and adjacent conjunctiva in biomicroscopic examination together with patients' description of a recent increase in ocular redness and one or more of the following symptoms: photophobia, pain, foreign-body sensation, discomfort, and tearing. Two independent experienced ophthalmologists (EK and UY) diagnosed the patients for inclusion criteria. A control group ($n = 32$) was formed from age-matched individuals that did not have any ophthalmic disease other than refractive problems. Subjects who had corneal pathologies, allergic conditions, previous corneal and/or conjunctival surgery, meibomian gland dysfunction, active ocular infection, and contact lens users were excluded. All participants underwent complete ophthalmologic examination. To ensure reproductivity, all patients diagnosed with inflamed pinguecula were reexamined, and tests of the tear function were performed on the following day in the morning in the ophthalmologists' dimly lit examination room. Corneal staining properties were evaluated using fluorescein sodium solution 2% (Fluorescite®; Alcon Laboratories, Inc., Fort Worth, Texas 76134, USA). For TBUT test measurements, a drop of 2% fluorescein solution was applied to the lateral inferior fornix. The patient was asked to blink several times for uniform distribution of fluorescein and then instructed to look ahead without blinking. The time from the last blink to the appearance of the first dry spot on the cornea was recorded using the cobalt blue filter of the biomicroscope and a stopwatch. Three consecutive measurements were made, and the mean of measurements was recorded. Thirty minutes later, in the dimly lit examining room, a topical anesthetic agent proparacaine hydrochloride 0.5% drop (Alcaine®; Alcon, Fort Worth, TX) was applied to the inferior fornix, and three minutes later, a standard Schirmer test filter strip (Bio Schirmer®; Bio-Tech Vision Care, Ahmedabad, Gujarat, India) was inserted into the lateral inferior fornix at the junction of the middle and lateral thirds of the lower eyelid, taking care not to touch cornea. The patient was asked to keep eyes open and blink as necessary. After five minutes, the filter strip was removed and wetting was recorded. This study was performed according to the tenets of Declaration of Helsinki, and the study received approval from Pamukkale University Ethics Committee. Written informed consent and verbal informed consent were taken from patients and controls.

Statistical analysis was performed using SPSS version 20.0 (IBM Corporation, Armonk, NY). Test results were expressed as mean ± standard deviation (SD). The distribution of the variables was tested using the Kolmogorov–Smirnov test. The chi-square test was used to compare groups for gender and nasal corneal epithelial staining. Independent-samples T test was used to compare the groups for age. For BUT and ST2 values, the Kruskal–Wallis one-way test was used to test the difference among groups and Mann–Whitney U test was used to compare groups. In all analyses, p values <0.05 were considered as statistically significant.

3. Results

There was no significant difference in age and gender between inflamed pinguecula and control groups ($p = 0.862$ and $p = 0.794$, respectively) (Table 1). Thirty-two eyes of 32 patients had inflamed pinguecula. All inflamed pingueculae were on the nasal conjunctiva (Figure 1). There were pinguecula in 13 (40 %) and pterygium in 3 (9%) of the fellow eyes ($n = 32$). There was no pinguecula or pterygium in the control group.

Twenty-three eyes (72%) had punctate epithelial staining (PES) or epithelial defect on the nasal cornea in eyes with inflamed pinguecula (Figures 2(a) and 2(b)). There was one eye (3.1%) with corneal PES in the fellow eyes group. The difference was statistically significant ($p < 0.001$). There was no corneal PES or epithelial defect in the control group.

The mean values of TBUT tests of eyes with inflamed pinguecula, fellow eyes, and control eyes were 8.1 ± 3.9 s, 9.3 ± 4.3 s, and 13.5 ± 4.9 s, respectively (Table 2). The eyes with inflamed pinguecula had significantly lower TBUT values compared to the control group ($p < 0.001$). Fellow eyes also had lower TBUT values than the control group ($p = 0.003$). There was no significant difference in the TBUT results between eyes with inflamed pinguecula and fellow eyes ($p = 0.286$). The mean values of ST2 results of eyes with inflamed pinguecula, fellow eyes, and control eyes were 11.6 ± 5.1 s, 11.6 ± 5.3 s, and 17.6 ± 7.8 s, respectively. The eyes with inflamed pinguecula had significantly lower ST2 values compared to the control group ($p < 0.001$). Fellow eyes also had lower ST2 values than the control group ($p = 0.003$). There was no significant difference in the ST2 results between the eyes with inflamed pinguecula and fellow eyes ($p = 0.951$).

4. Discussion

Pinguecula is a common disease of the conjunctiva whose exact etiology is unknown. UVR is reported to be an important factor [2, 3]. Fluorescein is a diagnostic dye commonly used in ophthalmic practice. Although the underlying cellular mechanism of corneal staining is incompletely understood, fluorescein staining of the ocular surface is a common diagnostic feature of ocular diseases, and it is

TABLE 1: Demographic characteristics of groups.

	Inflamed pinguecula group ($n = 32$)	Control group ($n = 32$)	p
Age (years) (mean ± SD)	32.78 ± 10.35	32.31 ± 11.07	**0.862[a]**
Sex Female, n (%)	21 (65.6%)	20 (62.5%)	**0.794[b]**
Male, n (%)	11 (34.4%)	12 (37.5%)	

[a]Independent-samples T test; [b]chi-square test; p value <0.05 is statistically significant.

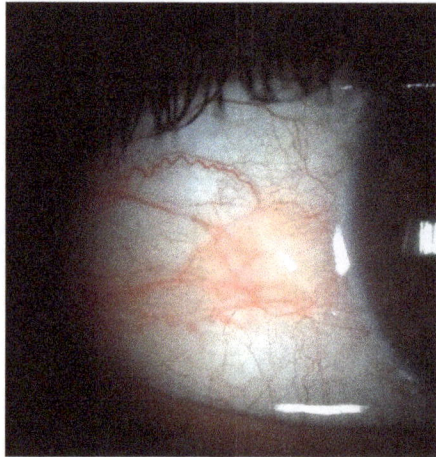

FIGURE 1: An inflamed pinguecula.

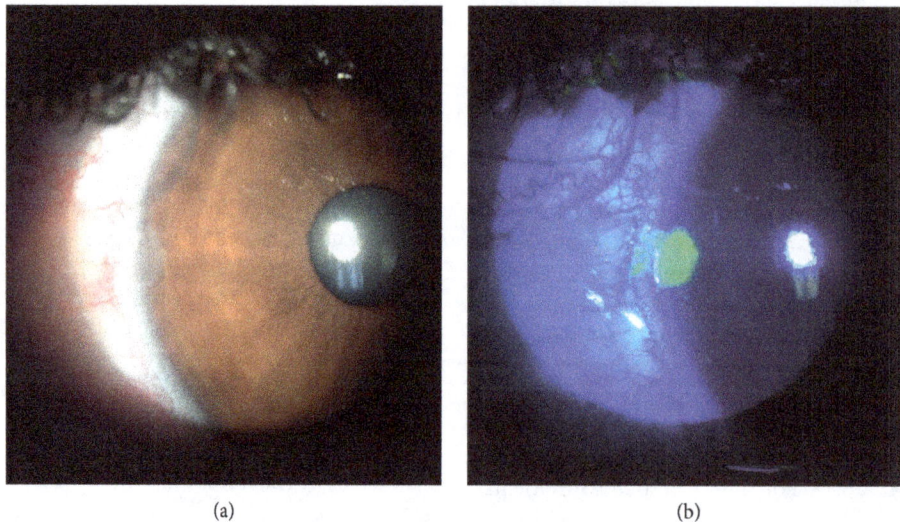

(a)   (b)

FIGURE 2: (a) Epithelial defect and (b) fluorescent staining in a patient with inflamed pinguecula.

TABLE 2: Schirmer 2 and TBUT test results of the groups.

		Patient eyes with inflamed pinguecula ($n = 32$) (Group 1)	Patient eyes without inflamed pinguecula ($n = 32$) (Group 2)	Control eyes ($n = 32$) (Group 3)	p^*	$p^{\#}$ for intergroup comparisons		
						Groups 1 vs 2	Groups 1 vs 3	Groups 2 vs 3
BUT (s)	Mean ± SD	8.1 ± 3.9	9.3 ± 4.3	13.5 ± 4.9	<0.005	0.286	<0.001	0.003
	Median	8.0	8.0	14.0				
	Range	3–19	3–18	4–25				
ST2 (mm)	Mean ± SD	11.6 ± 5.1	11.6 ± 5.3	17.6 ± 7.8	<0.005	0.951	<0.001	0.003
	Median	11.0	10.5	20.0				
	Range	3–22	2–21	4–30				

$^*p$ value for comparison among three groups (Kruskal–Wallis one-way test). $^{\#}p$ values for intergroup comparisons (Mann–Whitney U test). p value <0.05 is statistically significant.

frequently used to assess ocular surface integrity, particularly the cornea [13, 14]. A high rate of nasal corneal PES or epithelial defect was present in the inflamed pinguecula group compared to fellow eyes and control group in our study. This finding was not reported in previous studies. We could not find reports regarding the fluorescein staining of the nasal cornea in pinguecula patients in our literature review. The pathogenesis of this staining may be similar to dellen formation in which corneal thinning occurs usually close to limbus due to reduced tear film spread over a focal corneal area and is usually associated with an adjacent focal conjunctival or corneal elevation. Reduced tear break-up time was also reported to be associated with dellen formation [15]. In dry eye patients, corneal fluorescein staining usually occurs symmetrically on the corneal surface without a predilection for a specific part [16]. Our study suggests that an inflamed and elevated pinguecula may affect the distribution of the tear film and cause a desiccated epithelium in the nasal cornea close to the limbus. Also, impaired tear function evidenced by lower TBUT and ST2 results in these patients may aggravate this situation. These factors together may cause epithelial cell damage and staining in the nasal cornea. There may be other effects of inflammation on the nasal corneal epithelium other than affecting tear film spread since previous reports on pinguecula without inflammation did not report nasal corneal fluorescein staining. The inflammatory cells and mediators may cause epithelial cell damage or may affect the epithelial healing in inflamed pinguecula patients.

Oğuz et al found that eyes with pinguecula have significantly lower TBUT values compared to the healthy controls [11]. Schirmer 1 test (ST1) results were not significantly different between the eyes with pinguecula and control group in their study. Dong et al. found that TBUT values improved after pinguecula excision, but ST1 results did not change [5]. Both TBUT and ST2 results were significantly lower in the eyes with inflamed pinguecula and fellow eyes compared to the control group in our study. TBUT measurements have inherent variability, and taking multiple readings and averaging the results is one way of improving repeatability [17]. Therefore, we used averaging the multiple readings in our study. Similar to these studies, TBUT values were also lower in our study. But unlike them, we also found lower ST2 results. This may be due to difference in study population since we investigated only patients with inflamed pinguecula. The results of our study indicate that both tear film stability and tear production were affected in patients with inflamed pinguecula. Balogun and coworkers compared the TBUT values of pterygium and pinguecula patients and healthy controls. The mean TBUT values were not significantly different between pinguecula group and healthy controls [18]. The inclusion of only inflamed pinguecula patients in our study and the differences in the geographic location and age of the participants may explain the different findings of Bolagun's study and the present one.

To understand whether inflamed pinguecula causes abnormalities of tear film or tear film abnormalities cause inflammation of the pinguecula, we compared the test results of these patients with those of the fellow eyes. We found that the TBUT and ST2 results are not significantly different between the eyes with inflamed pinguecula and fellow eyes. Fellow eyes also had abnormalities of the tear film function, and nearly 50% of these eyes had uninflamed pinguecula (40%) or pterygium (9%). Considering one of our diagnostic criteria of inflamed pinguecula "patients description of a recent increase in ocular redness" together with these results of the fellow eyes, we think that abnormality of the tear film may be present before the inflammation of pinguecula similar to current results of fellow eyes. Our study suggests that impaired tear film together with mechanical irritation of this elevated tissue makes pinguecula prone to inflammation.

Pterygium is a triangular growth of conjunctival fibrovascular tissue onto the cornea. Specific stimulus leading to pterygium formation is still unknown [19]. Although there are similarities in the pathogenesis and histopathological findings of these two ocular surface diseases, it is still unknown if pinguecula is a precursor of pterygium and if so, what causes it to progress to pterygium [1, 6]. Dong et al. reported that abnormal epithelial differentiation is present in pinguecula tissue and that pinguecula epithelium has proliferative capacity exhibiting characteristics of squamous proliferative diseases [5]. There are also several reports indicating the role of inflammatory cytokines and growth factors (GFs) in the pathogenesis of pterygium [19–21]. These GFs and cytokines are also important in the normal corneal wound healing and overexpressed in pterygia. Interleukin-1 and epidermal growth factor were reported to be important, and they have an additive effect on corneal epithelial cell migration in corneal epithelial wounds [22]. Epidermal growth factor was also shown to induce cell migration in pterygium epithelium and fibroblasts [20]. Kim et al. emphasized the importance of myofibroblasts in pterygium formation [23]. They stated that pterygium may be a product of an exaggerated repair process after injury to the ocular surface and prolonged inflammation leading to tissue damage and fibrosis. They also emphasized the importance of stromal cell-derived factor-1 and transforming growth factor-beta with other GFs and inflammatory mediators in the activation of pterygium fibroblasts. These studies mainly emphasize the importance of inflammatory cytokines and GFs in the pterygium formation and that the pterygium may be an exaggerated repair process.

Archila and Arenas stated that exposure to chronic solar radiation causes alteration of conjunctival stroma and leads to pinguecula formation. This causes disruption of tear film and an area of dryness which results in drying of conjunctiva and formation of microulcers on the epithelium. Then, as a part of protective changes, conjunctiva tries to cover erosion and leads to pterygium formation [24]. Based on the literature, our results suggest that abnormal tear film and improper lubrication together with ocular surface irregularity due to pinguecula may cause inflammation of the pinguecula, and these factors cause epithelial defects on the nasal cornea. Inflammation and corneal epithelial damage may cause release of GFs and cytokines which act together to close the wound and relieve the inflammation in these patients. UVR was reported to cause limbal stem cell failure on the nasal cornea [10]. When corneal healing does not occur properly due to limbal stem cell failure, a prolonged inflammatory response and exaggerated wound healing process may occur, and these mediators act on pinguecula epithelium and stroma, leading to proliferation towards the nasal cornea to close the wound. Our study suggests that nasal corneal epithelial damage in inflamed pinguecula patients may be a stimulus for exaggerated wound repair causing the release of GFs leading to growth of conjunctival epithelium onto the cornea. Inflamed pinguecula patients with impaired ocular surface lubrication and nasal corneal epithelial defects may be a subgroup of pinguecula patients who have a propensity to progress to pterygium.

Our study is a cross-sectional study, and it is a limitation of our study. Another limitation is that we did not perform histologic or cytologic examination. The diagnosis of pinguecula is mostly clinical, and due to typical appearance, diagnosis of pinguecula is usually easy but sometimes other pathologies can mimic pinguecula.

In conclusion, to our knowledge, this is the first study evaluating corneal staining properties and tear functions in inflamed pinguecula patients. In a high percentage of inflamed pinguecula groups, we found nasal corneal epithelial staining or epithelial defect. We found lower TBUT and ST2 results in this group. These findings may be important in uncovering the relation of pinguecula and pterygium and also in their pathogenesis. Inflammation, corneal epithelial integrity, and impaired tear film parameters may be important factors in the evolution of the pinguecula to pterygium.

Conflicts of Interest

There are no financial and personal relationships with other people or organizations that could inappropriately influence the present study. The authors have no commercial, proprietary, and financial interest in the material presented in this manuscript.

References

[1] P. A. Jaros and V. P. DeLuise, "Pingueculae and pterygia," *Survey of Ophthalmology*, vol. 33, no. 1, pp. 41–49, 1988.

[2] T. Mimura, T. Usui, H. Obata et al., "Severity and determinants of pinguecula in a hospital-based population," *Eye and Contact Lens: Science and Clinical Practice*, vol. 37, no. 1, pp. 31–35, 2011.

[3] E. S. Perkins, "The association between pinguecula, sunlight and cataract," *Ophthalmic Research*, vol. 17, no. 6, pp. 325–330, 1985.

[4] A. Fotouhi, H. Hashemi, M. Khabazkhoob, and K. Mohammad, "Prevalence and risk factors of pterygium and pinguecula: the Tehran eye study," *Eye*, vol. 23, no. 5, pp. 1125–1129, 2009.

[5] N. Dong, W. Li, H. Lin et al., "Abnormal epithelial differentiation and tear film alteration in pinguecula," *Investigative Ophthalmology and Visual Science*, vol. 50, no. 6, pp. 2710–2715, 2009.

[6] P. Austin, F. A. Jakobiec, and T. Iwamoto, "Elastodysplasia and elastodystrophy as the pathologic bases of ocular pterygia and pinguecula," *Ophthalmology*, vol. 90, no. 1, pp. 96–109, 1983.

[7] Z. Y. Li, R. N. Wallace, B. W. Streeten, B. L. Kuntz, and A. J. Dark, "Elastic fiber components and protease inhibitors in pinguecula," *Investigative Ophthalmology and Visual Science*, vol. 32, no. 5, pp. 1573–1585, 1991.

[8] T. Q. Pham, J. J. Wang, E. Rochtchina, and P. Mitchell, "Pterygium/pinguecula and the five-year incidence of age-related maculopathy," *American Journal of Ophthalmology*, vol. 139, no. 3, pp. 536–537, 2005.

[9] S. C. Tseng, "Concept and application of limbal stem cells," *Eye*, vol. 3, no. 2, pp. 141–157, 1989.

[10] L. S. Kwok and M. T. Coroneo, "A model for pterygium formation," *Cornea*, vol. 13, no. 3, pp. 219–224, 1994.

[11] H. Oguz, S. Karadede, M. Bitiren, B. Gurler, and M. Cakmak, "Tear functions in patients with pinguecula," *Acta Ophthalmologica Scandinavica*, vol. 79, no. 3, pp. 262–265, 2001.

[12] J. Frucht-Pery, C. S. Siganos, A. Solomon, T. Shvartzenberg, C. Richard, and C. Trinquand, "Topical indomethacin solution versus dexamethasone solution for treatment of inflamed pterygium and pinguecula: a prospective randomized clinical study," *American Journal of Ophthalmology*, vol. 127, no. 2, pp. 148–152, 1999.

[13] A. J. Bron, P. Argueso, M. Irkec, and F. V. Bright, "Clinical staining of the ocular surface: mechanisms and interpretations," *Progress in Retinal and Eye Research*, vol. 44, pp. 36–61, 2015.

[14] P. B. Morgan and C. Maldonado-Codina, "Corneal staining: do we really understand what we are seeing?," *Contact Lens and Anterior Eye*, vol. 32, no. 2, pp. 48–54, 2009.

[15] G. Mai and S. Yang, "Relationship between corneal dellen and tearfilm breakup time," *Yan ke Xue Bao = Eye Science*, vol. 7, no. 1, pp. 43–46, 1991.

[16] A. J. Bron, V. E. Evans, and J. A. Smith, "Grading of corneal and conjunctival staining in the context of other dry eye tests," *Cornea*, vol. 22, no. 7, pp. 640–650, 2003.

[17] M. D. P. Willcox, P. Argueso, G. A. Georgiev et al., "TFOS DEWS II tear film report," *Ocular Surface*, vol. 15, no. 3, pp. 366–403, 2017.

[18] M. M. Balogun, A. O. Ashaye, B. G. Ajayi, and O. O. Osuntokun, "Tear break-up time in eyes with pterygia and pingueculae in Ibadan," *West African Journal of Medicine*, vol. 24, no. 2, pp. 162–166, 2005.

[19] J. C. Bradley, W. Yang, R. H. Bradley, T. W. Reid, and I. R. Schwab, "The science of pterygia," *British Journal of Ophthalmology*, vol. 94, no. 7, pp. 815–820, 2010.

[20] N. Di Girolamo, J. Chui, M. T. Coroneo, and D. Wakefield, "Pathogenesis of pterygia: role of cytokines, growth factors, and matrix metalloproteinases," *Progress in Retinal and Eye Research*, vol. 23, no. 2, pp. 195–228, 2004.

[21] T. Liu, Y. Liu, L. Xie, X. He, and J. Bai, "Progress in the pathogenesis of pterygium," *Current Eye Research*, vol. 38, no. 12, pp. 1191–1197, 2013.

[22] H. M. Boisjoly, C. Laplante, S. F. Bernatchez, C. Salesse, M. Giasson, and M. C. Joly, "Effects of EGF, IL-1 and their combination on in vitro corneal epithelial wound closure and cell chemotaxis," *Experimental Eye Research*, vol. 57, no. 3, pp. 293–300, 1993.

[23] K. W. Kim, S. H. Park, and J. C. Kim, "Fibroblast biology in pterygia," *Experimental Eye Research*, vol. 142, pp. 32–39, 2016.

[24] E. A. Archila and M. C. Arenas, "Etiopathology of pinguecula and pterigium," *Cornea*, vol. 14, no. 5, pp. 543–544, 1995.

8

Stereoacuity of Black-White and Red-Green Patterns in Individuals with and without Color Deficiency

Ying Sun [iD],[1] Huang Wu [iD],[2] Yinghong Qiu,[3] and Zhiqiang Yue[3]

[1]*The First Hospital of Jilin University, Changchun, China*
[2]*The Second Hospital of Jilin University, Changchun, China*
[3]*Ophthalmology Hospital of Hebei Province, Hebei, China*

Correspondence should be addressed to Ying Sun; y_sun@jlu.edu.cn

Academic Editor: Lisa Toto

Background. Chromatic contrast may affect stereopsis. Daltonism is a common color deficiency in which the colors red and green are incorrectly detected. The aim of this study was to evaluate the stereoacuity of color-defective individuals presented with color symbols that they see defectively. *Methods.* Ten students diagnosed with daltonism and 10 students with normal color vision were recruited. A stereopsis test system using a phoropter and two 4K smartphones was used. Contour-based graphs and random-dot graphs with black versus white and red versus green patterns were used as test symbols. The Wilcoxon signed rank test was used to test the difference between groups. *Results.* No significant difference in stereoacuity was found between contour-based and random-dot graphs within both daltonism cohort and normal color vision cohort ($P > 0.05$). A significant difference in stereoacuity was found between the black-white ($P = 0.005$) and red-green ($P = 0.007$) graphs for the daltonism cohort, while no significant difference in stereoacuity was found for the normal color vision cohort ($P > 0.05$). *Conclusion.* Chromatic contrast is an influential factor for stereopsis measurement in individuals with color deficiency.

1. Background

Stereopsis facilitates the precise judgment of distance, and stereoacuity is used to evaluate it. Stereoacuity has been measured using the following tests: the Howard-Dolman test [1], the Frisby stereo test [2], the TNO (The Netherlands Optical Society) stereoacuity test [3], and the Titmus stereoacuity test [4]. With the development of information technology, the computer has become a useful tool for evaluating stereopsis, from the cathode ray tube monitor used in the 1980s [5] to the three-dimensional (3D) liquid crystal display or light-emitting diode applied after the twenty-first century [6–8] and finally to the 4K smartphone currently used [9]. The new methods facilitate improved measurement of stereopsis compared with traditional ones. For example, the relationships between chromatic contrast and stereopsis can be evaluated with a computer [5, 6], which is difficult to do using traditional methods.

Color deficiency, commonly called color blindness, is a disorder that causes people to distinguish colors

abnormally. Daltonism is a common color deficiency in which people cannot detect red and green colors correctly. There is a paucity of studies investigating the change in stereoacuity when color blind individuals see symbols in the colors for which their vision is deficient. In the current study, we reevaluated 19 color-deficient freshmen who were preliminarily diagnosed at a school student health center. A newly designed stereopsis test system was used to evaluate the stereoacuity associated with a black-white or a red-green pattern. Students with and without daltonism were tested.

2. Methods

2.1. Participants. Ten students with daltonism diagnosed using a pseudoisochromatic plate test [10] and 10 students with normal color vision were recruited. The correct visual acuity of each eye was no less than 0 logMAR, while the stereoacuity was no less than $40''$ as measured using the Fly Stereo Acuity Test (Vision Assessment Corporation, Elk Grove Village, IL, USA). The other 9 out of the 19 color-deficient students were excluded due to unqualifying stereopsis, or the degree of color deficiency was just red and/or green weakness.

All participants gave their informed written consent before taking part in the study. The research protocol observed the tenets of the Declaration of Helsinki and was approved by the Ethics Committee of the Second Hospital of Jilin University (no. 2017-89).

2.2. Test Equipment. We incorporated a stereopsis measurement system using a phoropter (Topcon VT-10; Topcon Corp., Tokyo, Japan) and two Sony smartphones (Sony Xperia Z5 Premium Dual E6883; resolution, 3840×2160; Sony Mobile Communications Inc., Tokyo, Japan) [9]. The test distance was 65 cm. One pixel disparity represents $10''$ (acrsec) at this distance. With the aid of two 5.5Δ base-out Risley prisms, the subject can fuse the two smartphones into one image (Figure 1). A screen luminance meter (SM208; M&A Instrument Inc., Shenzhen, China) was used to measure the brightness of the display. A program was written using C# to generate all random-dot stereograms. Crossed disparity was used in all test graphs.

2.3. Test Symbols. Two types of symbols, a contour-based graph and a random-dot graph, were used (Figure 2). The shape of the contour-based symbol was similar to that used in the Fly Stereo Acuity Test. One stereo circle stands out from the other three circles if the stereopsis threshold of the subject is better than the disparity of the target circle. The shape of the random-dot symbol was also similar to that used in the Fly Stereo Acuity Test. A circle appears up, down, right, or left in the random-dot graph when the disparity of the stereo target is larger than the stereoacuity of the participant. Eight different groups of disparities were drawn from $80''$ to $10''$. One test page contained $80''$ to $50''$, and the other contained $40''$ to $10''$.

Two types of test pages were used, black versus white and red versus green. The RGB (red, green, and blue) codes of the black, white, red, and green colors used were ($R = 0$, $G = 0$, $B = 0$), ($R = 255$, $G = 255$, $B = 255$), ($R = 255$, $G = 0$, $B = 0$), and ($R = 0$, $G = 255$, $B = 0$), respectively.

2.4. Test Procedure. The sequence of test pages presented was a black-white pattern with $80''$ to $50''$, a black-white pattern with $40''$ to $10''$, a red-green pattern with $80''$ to $50''$, and a red-green pattern with $40''$ to $10''$. The participants pointed out the position of the outstanding circle in the contour-based and random-dot tests, line by line from left to right and from top to bottom, until they could not find the stereo one. The disparities of the last correct identification were recorded as their stereoacuity.

2.5. Statistical Analysis. All data were analyzed using the PASW Statistics 18 software (IBM SPSS Inc., Chicago, IL). The Wilcoxon signed rank test was used to test the difference between groups.

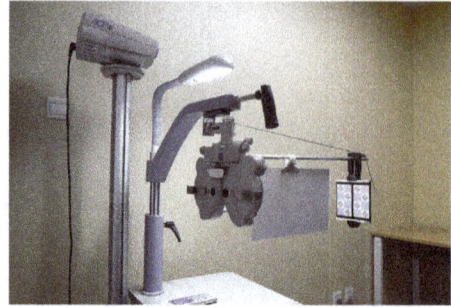

FIGURE 1: The test system used consisted of a phoropter and two Sony smartphones. A pair of smartphone pictures are seen with a black and white pattern.

3. Results

The test results are shown in Table 1 and Figure 3. No significant differences were found between the results for contour-based and random-dot graphs within the cohorts with and without daltonism (Wilcoxon signed rank test: a black-white pattern in the daltonism group: $Z = -1.000, P = 0.317$; a red-green pattern in the daltonism group: $Z = -1.414, P = 0.157$; a black-white pattern in the normal group: $Z = -1.732, P = 0.083$; and a red-green pattern in the normal group: $Z = -1.342, P = 0.180$). A significant difference was found between the results for black-white and red-green test pages in the cohort with daltonism (Wilcoxon signed rank test: contour-based group: $Z = -2.814, P = 0.005$; random-dot group: $Z = -2.714, P = 0.007$). No significant difference was found between the results for the black-white and red-green graphs in the cohort without daltonism (Wilcoxon signed rank test: contour-based group: $Z = -1.414, P = 0.157$; random-dot group: $Z = -1.000, P = 0.317$).

4. Discussion

The relationship between chromatic information and stereopsis has been studied for people with normal color vision [10, 11], although questions still exist. The mechanism of color deficiency, also a conundrum, is still only a hypothesis [12]. People with daltonism can distinguish the difference between red and green, but see red and green differently than people with normal color vision. Chromatic symbols for red and green test pages were used; however, they were not complementary (the complementary color of red ($R = 255$, $G = 0$, $B = 0$) is blue ($R = 0$, $G = 255$, $B = 255$), and the complementary color of green ($R = 0$, $G = 255$, $B = 0$) is magenta ($R = 255$, $G = 0$, $B = 255$)). In both contour-based graphs and random-dot graphs, the contrast of the colors together with the luminant contrast of the symbols against the background (red: luminance = 48 cd/m^2; green: luminance = 146 cd/m^2; Weber contrast = $(I - I_b)/I_b = 67\%$) was obvious enough to keep the stereopsis level from decreasing in people with normal color vision. The situation was different for people with daltonism when observing a red-green pair graph. The luminance contrast of the symbols against the background still existed, but the comparison of the

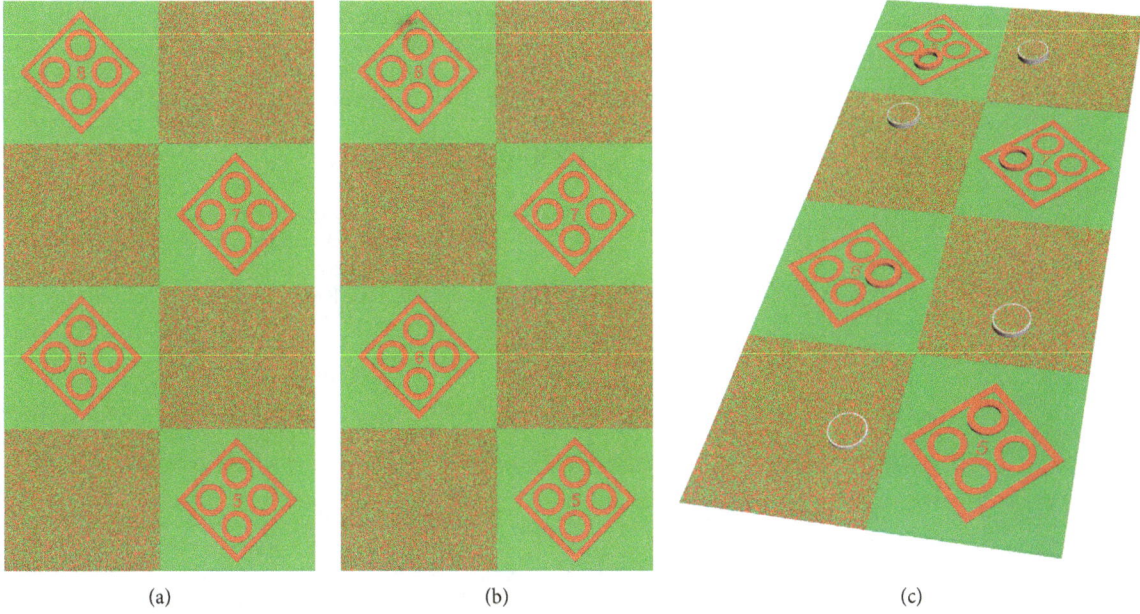

(a)   (b)   (c)

FIGURE 2: Test pages used. A pair with a red and green pattern seen by the (a) left eye and (b) right eye. From top to bottom, the disparity of the stereo targets is 80″, 70″, 60″, and 50″, respectively. From top to end, the stereo symbol in contour-based graphs is left, right, down, and up, respectively, while the stereo symbol in random-dot graphs is down, up, right, and left, respectively. (c) The simulation of the percepts generated by the test images (a, b). This is an attempt to simulate what a subject might perceive when fusing (a) and (b) as one image. The stereo symbols appear to pop out of the background plane.

TABLE 1: Stereoacuity (″) of the participants.

	Daltonism				Normal			
	Black versus white		Red versus green		Black versus white		Red versus green	
ID	Contour-based	Random-dot	Contour-based	Random-dot	Contour-based	Random-dot	Contour-based	Random-dot
1	20	20	60	60	20	10	20	20
2	20	20	30	30	10	10	10	10
3	30	40	60	70	10	10	20	10
4	30	30	50	50	20	10	20	20
5	20	30	70	70	20	20	20	20
6	40	40	80	80	20	20	30	20
7	20	20	80	80	20	30	30	20
8	20	30	30	30	20	10	20	10
9	30	20	60	60	20	20	20	30
10	30	30	60	70	20	20	30	20

colors changed. However, it is hard to interpret why the stereoacuity measured with the red-green pair was significantly lower than that with the black-white pair in the daltonism cohort due to the decrease of color comparison. The luminant contrast in the test was not low enough to affect the stereoacuity result significantly [13]. The positive effect of chromatic contrast for stereopsis evaluation was reported in normal individuals [10, 11].

The literature about binocular vision related to color vision deficiency is rare. Bak et al. evaluated the Worth four-dot test in patients with congenital red-green color vision defects [14]. The red/green anaglyph glasses play an essential role in the Worth four-dot test, and the function of it is to dissociate right and left eyes. So no matter the normal color vision people or red-green color deficiency people, the separate function of the glasses is the same. That is, to evaluate flat fusion, the Worth four-dot test works for both normal color vision and abnormal cohorts. Furthermore, it could be speculated that if using red/green anaglyph glasses as a dissociation tool to evaluate stereopsis, that is, TNO, although no literature be retrieved, it may still work for red-green color vision defects people. If the color elements were not used as a way to separate eyes, but as constituent parts in the test patterns, the situation would change. In our experiment, the color information used in the experiment did not enhance but rather interfered with the stereopsis in individuals with color-defective vision. The difference in stereoacuity between people with normal color vision and people with daltonism when adding chromatic information has not been reported.

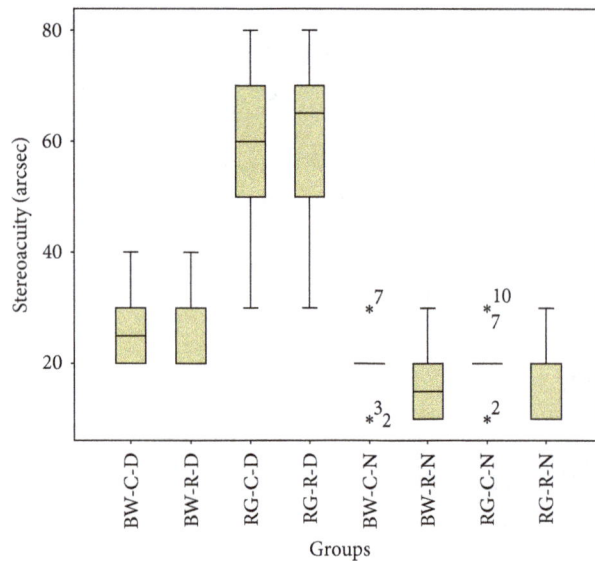

FIGURE 3: Boxplot of the stereoacuity of the following groups: BW-C-D: daltonism cohort tested with black-white contour-based graphs; BW-R-D: daltonism cohort tested with black-white random-dot graphs; RG-C-D: daltonism cohort tested with red-green contour-based graphs; RG-R-D: daltonism cohort tested with red-green random-dot graphs; BW-C-N: normal color vision cohort tested with black-white contour-based graphs; BW-R-N: normal color vision cohort tested with black-white random-dot graphs; RG-C-N: normal color vision cohort tested with red-green contour-based graphs; RG-R-N: normal color vision cohort tested with red-green random-dot graphs. The line perpendicular to the whisker below the box represents the minimum value; the lower edge of the box represents the first quartile; the line in the box is the median; the upper edge of the box represents the third quartile; and the line perpendicular to the whisker above the box represents the maximum value. The stars represent extreme values.

The limitations of our research were the small size of samples and the diagnosing method was not conducted with more quantitative tools, that is, anomaloscope. However, future studies need to be designed to determine the etiology related to why people see color information achromatically in the procedure for measuring stereopsis.

5. Conclusion

The stereoacuity evaluated with red-green and black-white symbols was significantly different for people with daltonism and not significantly different for people with normal color vision. Chromatic contrast influences the stereopsis measurement.

Conflicts of Interest

The authors declare that they have no conflicts of interest.

Acknowledgments

This work was supported by the Jilin Provincial Science and Technology Department, China (Grant no. 20170519004JH).

References

[1] J. J. Saladin, "Phorometry and stereopsis," in *Borish's Clinical Refraction*, W. J. Benjaminpp. 899–960, Butterworth-Heinemann, Oxford, UK, 2nd edition, 2006.

[2] I. Bohr and J. C. Read, "Stereoacuity with Frisby and revised FD2 stereo tests," *PLoS One*, vol. 12, no. 8, Article ID e82999, 2013.

[3] L. L. van Doorn, B. J. Evans, D. F. Edgar, and M. F. Fortuin, "Manufacturer changes lead to clinically important differences between two editions of the TNO stereotest," *Ophthalmic and Physiological Optics*, vol. 34, no. 2, pp. 243–249, 2014.

[4] K. Arnoldi and A. Frenkel, "Modification of the titmus fly test to improve accuracy," *American Orthoptic Journal*, vol. 64, no. 1, pp. 64–70, 2014.

[5] K. Shoji, S. Sumi, and H. Fujita, "Depth perception in moving line patterns," *Perceptual and Motor Skills*, vol. 51, no. 3, pp. 683–687, 1980.

[6] S. B. Han, H. K. Yang, J. Kim, K. Hong, B. Lee, and J. M. Hwang, "New stereoacuity test using a 3-dimensional display system in children," *PLoS One*, vol. 10, no. 2, Article ID e0116626, 2015.

[7] J. Kim, H. K. Yang, Y. Kim, B. Lee, and J. M. Hwang, "Distance stereotest using a 3-dimensional monitor for adult subjects," *American Journal of Ophthalmology*, vol. 151, no. 6, pp. 1081–1086, 2011.

[8] H. Wu, H. Jin, Y. Sun et al., "Evaluating stereoacuity with 3D shutter glasses technology," *BMC Ophthalmology*, vol. 16, p. 45, 2016.

[9] H. Wu, S. Liu, and R. Wang, "Stereoacuity measurement using a phoropter combined with two 4K smartphones," *Clinical and Experimental Optometry*, vol. 101, no. 2, pp. 272–275, 2017.

[10] F. A. Kingdom and D. R. Simmons, "Stereoacuity and colour contrast," *Vision Research*, vol. 36, no. 9, pp. 1311–1319, 1996.

[11] D. R. Simmons and F. A. Kingdom, "Interactions between chromatic- and luminance-contrast-sensitive stereopsis mechanisms," *Vision Research*, vol. 42, no. 12, pp. 1535–1545, 2002.

[12] P. J. Pease, "Color vision," in *Borish's Clinical Refraction*, W. J. Benjamin, Ed., pp. 289–355, Butterworth-Heinemann, Oxford, UK, 2nd edition, 2006.

[13] D. L. Halpern and R. R. Blake, "How contrast affects stereoacuity," *Perception*, vol. 17, no. 4, pp. 483–495, 1988.

[14] E. Bak, H. K. Yang, and J. M. Hwang, "Validity of the Worth 4 dot test in patients with red-green color vision defect," *Optometry and Vision Science*, vol. 94, no. 5, pp. 626–629, 2017.

9

Flt3 Regulation in the Mononuclear Phagocyte System Promotes Ocular Neovascularization

Yushuo Gao ®,[1] Yisheng Zhong ®,[1] Yanji Zhu,[1] Anna M. Demetriades,[2] Yujuan Cai,[1] Jikui Shen,[3] Qing Lu,[1] Xi Shen ®,[1] and Bing Xie ®[1]

[1]Department of Ophthalmology, Ruijin Hospital, Shanghai Jiao Tong University School of Medicine, 197, Ruijin Er Road, Shanghai 200025, China
[2]Department of Ophthalmology, NewYork-Presbyterian Hospital-Cornell, New York, NY, USA
[3]Departments of Ophthalmology and Neuroscience, The Johns Hopkins University School of Medicine, Maumenee 719, 600 N. Wolfe Street, Baltimore, MD, USA

Correspondence should be addressed to Xi Shen; carl_shen2005@126.com and Bing Xie; brinkleybing@126.com

Academic Editor: Terri L. Young

Fms-like tyrosine kinase 3 (Flt3), a tyrosine kinase receptor expressed in CD34+ hematopoietic stem/progenitor cells, is important for both normal myeloid and lymphoid differentiation. It has been implicated in mice and humans for potential multilineage differentiation. We found that mice deficient in Flt3 or mice that received an Flt3 inhibitor (AC220) showed significantly reduced areas of ischemia-induced retinal neovascularization (RNV) and laser-induced choroidal NV (CNV) ($P < 0.05$). Increased Flt3 expression at the protein level was detected in retinas of oxygen-induced retinopathy (OIR) mice at P15 and P18 during retinal NV (RNV) progression. We subsequently found that macrophages (Mphi) polarization was regulated at the site of CNV in Flt3-deficient mice. Flow cytometry analysis demonstrated that Flt3 deficiency shifted Mphi polarization towards an M2 phenotype during RNV with significant reduction in M1 cytokine expression when compared to the wild-type controls ($P < 0.05$). Based on the above findings, we concluded that Flt3 inhibition alleviated ocular NV by promoting a Mphi polarization shift towards the M2 phenotype. Therapies targeting Flt3 may provide a new approach for the treatment of ocular NV.

1. Introduction

Age-related macular degeneration (AMD) represents an ailment whose incidence increases with age and is a leading cause of vision problems in older adults worldwide, affecting approximately 9% of the global population [1–3]. AMD comprises early and advanced types; the latter includes the exudative (characterized by choroidal neovascularization or CNV) and nonneovascular (distinguishable by progressive RPE atrophy) forms [2]. Neovascular AMD progresses rapidly, resulting in 80%–90% of cases with severe vision loss [1]. Currently, <40% of cases show improved vision after clinical therapy [2, 4].

In the past decades, angiogenesis and neovascularization have been studied to a great extent, allowing the development of antiangiogenic products to treat malignancies as well as ocular diseases [5]. Angiogenesis plays a critical role in development, reproduction, and repair; it involves degeneration of the vascular basement membrane, which is normally continuous, and the activation of quiescent endothelial cells (ECs) [6–8]. Vascular tubes are generated and covered with fully formed vascular basement membrane with the involvement of pericytes [7, 9, 10]. Currently, there is an increasing number of patients benefiting from angiogenesis inhibitors such as vascular endothelial growth factor (VEGF), although reduced efficacy and resistance continue to challenge the way we treat the disease [11–14]. At present, several reports have revealed novel molecular mechanisms that provide unique avenues for the improvement of antiangiogenic strategies [14–16].

Fms-like tyrosine kinase 3 (Flt3), expressed in CD34+ hematopoietic stem/progenitor cells, acts as a critical receptor for both normal myeloid and lymphoid differentiation [17]. Phosphorylation of Flt3 receptor activates the intracellular signaling pathways responsible for cell proliferation [18]. Mounting evidence indicates that inflammation, involving dendritic cells (DC) or macrophages (Mphi), accounts for important in neovascularization (NV) [19–21]. Whiteley et al. demonstrated that mesenchymal stromal and circulating angiogenic cells repair the tissues by expanding CD34+ cells [22].

In this study, we used AC220 as an inhibitor of Flt3. Prior first-generation inhibitors of Flt3 were nonselective and developed against additional targets. For instance, semaxanib and sunitinib are tyrosine kinase inhibitors with multiple targets, including VEGFR, c-KIT, and Flt3. AC220, a novel second-generation bis-aryl urea Flt3 inhibitor, has been optimized to inhibit Flt3 with high potency. It is highly selective against other kinases, together with pharmacokinetic properties that afford complete and sustained inhibition of FLT3-ITD and wild-type FLT3 *in vivo*. Moreover, it has shown favorable tolerability and single-agent activity in phase I and II trials [22–24]. Hence, this study assessed the impact of Flt3 on the differentiation of mouse Mphi and ocular NV.

2. Methods and Materials

2.1. Experimental Animals. Animal experiments were performed after approval from the Institutional Animal Care and Use Committee of Shanghai Jiao Tong University School of Medicine and carried out as directed by the Association for Research in Vision and Ophthalmology (ARVO). Pathogen-free C57BL/6 (Charles River, Wilmington, MA), Flt3−/− transgenic, rhodopsin promoter/VEGF (rho/VEGF) transgenic [16, 25], and rho/rtTA-TRE/VEGF double-transgenic [16, 26] mice were used in this study.

2.2. Mouse Model of Laser-Induced CNV. Laser photocoagulation rupture of Bruch's membrane was used to induce CNV in C57BL/6 as described previously [27, 28]. Briefly, laser injury (75 mm spot for 0.1 s at 120 mW) was performed with an OcuLight GL diode laser (Iridex, Mountain View, CA, USA). Only burns with bubbles were assessed and used to confirm breakage of Bruch's membrane [28].

2.3. Flt3 Inhibitor Injections. AC220, a second-generation Flt3 inhibitor, was purchased from Selleck (Selleckchem, Houston, TX) [23, 24]. Mice received intravitreal injections (1 μl) of AC220 and phosphate-buffered saline (PBS) following laser photocoagulation (day 0, D0). This was repeated at 7 days. One microliter AC220 was administered into the vitreous cavity of murine eyes using glass micropipette needles at D0 and D7. Eye analysis was performed at 14 days in order to quantify the area of CNV.

2.4. CNV Flat Mount. After 14 days of modeling, the anesthetized animals underwent perfusion with 1 ml FITC-dextran (Sigma-Aldrich, St. Louis, MO, USA) for the quantification of CNV area. Next, eyes were either stored for cDNA extraction or fixed in 10% buffered formalin, enucleated, and choroid flat mounted for examination. Choroidal lesions were assessed according to previously published

procedures [27, 29–31], as CNV area $(\mu m^2) \pm$ standard error. Groups were compared by Student's *t*-test [31].

2.5. Immunofluorescence Staining and Quantification. Sclerochoroidal flat mounts from CNV mice prepared on D14 after perfusion by FITC-dextran were incubated with phycoerythrin- (PE-) conjugated anti-CD11c antibody (1 : 100) and PE-conjugated anti-CD206 antibody (1 : 100) for staining. After being washed, the specimens were assessed microscopically. The samples were assessed for M1 and M2 using PE-conjugated anti-CD11c and PE-conjugated anti-CD206, respectively.

2.6. Quantitative Real-Time Reverse Transcriptase-Polymerase Chain Reaction (qRT-PCR). After euthanasia of mice with or without laser-induced CNV, the eyes were removed. Total RNA in ocular cup samples was obtained by TRIzol Reagent (Invitrogen, Carlsbad, CA) as directed by the manufacturer [16, 32]. After DNase (Promega, Fitchburg, WI) pretreatment, RNA (2 μg per sample) was submitted to reverse transcription for cDNA synthesis using M-MLV transcriptase and Oligo(dT) Primers (Promega) following the manufacturer's protocol. Quantitative RT-PCR was carried out according to previous reports [16, 33], with iQ SYBR Green mix (Roche, Basel, Switzerland) on an ABI 7500 system; cyclophilin was used for normalization [16, 34]. Samples from two retinas were pooled for analysis by the $\Delta\Delta CT$ method [16]. The following primers were utilized: CD11c, sense 5'-GTGCCCATCAGTTCCT TACA-3' and antisense 5'-GAGAAGAACTGTGGAGCTG AC-3'; CD206, sense 5'-GGAATCAAGGGCACAGAGT TA-3' and antisense 5'-ATTGTGGAGCAGATGGAA-3; F4/80, sense 5'-CGTCAGGTACGGGATGAATATAAG-3' and antisense 5'-CTATGCCATCCACTTCCAAGAT-3'; and cyclophilin A, sense 5'-CAGACGCCACTGTCGCTTT-3' and antisense 5'-TGTCTTTGGAACTTTGTCTGCAA-3'.

2.7. Oxygen-Induced Retinal Neovascularization in Mice and Immunostaining. Wild-type, Flt3+/−, and Flt3−/− transgenic C57BL/6 mice were treated with $75 \pm 3\%$ oxygen from postnatal day 7 (P7) to P12 as discussed in previous reports [16, 35]. C57BL/6 mice were divided into several groups at P12, intravitreal injections of AC220 at 1 μg/μl were performed in one eye, and intravitreal PBS was injected in the contralateral eye, as described in prior studies [36, 37]. After euthanasia at P17, murine eyes were removed and formalin fixation was performed [16]. Retina samples were obtained and stained with fluorescein *Griffonia simplicifolia* lectin-B4 (GSA-Lectin; Vector Laboratories Inc., Burlingame, CA, USA, 1 : 50) as previously described [16]. Analysis was performed by fluorescence microscopy (Nikon Instruments Inc., New York, NY) with Image-Pro Plus (Media Cybernetics, Silver Spring, MD, USA) [16].

2.8. Phospho-Flt3 Enzyme-Linked Immunosorbent Assay. Phosphorylated Flt3 levels were assessed in mouse retina specimens obtained at P13, P15, P18, and P21 by ELISA with a specific kit as previously described [38].

2.9. Isolation of Mouse Retina CD11b+ cells. After intravitreal injection with 1 $\mu g/\mu l$ AC220 (or control vehicle), mouse retinas at P15, P18, and P21 (6–10 retinas per group) were obtained for the isolation of retinal cells as described previously, using antimouse CD11b magnetic beads (Miltenyi Biotec, Bergisch Gladbach, Germany) and a premoistened MS column (BD Biosciences) [16].

2.10. Flow Cytometry Analysis. CD11b+ cells were incubated with PE-conjugated antimouse CD11c, FITC-conjugated F4/80, and Alexa Fluor 647-conjugated CD206 [16]. M1 Mphi were F4/80+/CD11c+, and M2 Mphi were F4/80+/CD206+ [16, 39]. Data analysis was performed with FlowJo (Tree Star, Ashland, OR) [16].

2.11. Mouse Model of VEGF Overexpression. Rho/VEGF transgenic animals were injected intravitreally with 1 $\mu g/\mu l$ AC220 and PBS, in respective eyes, at P12 and submitted to perfusion with fluorescein-labeled dextran under anesthesia [16]. Eye specimens were prepared and assessed by fluorescence microscopy, with Image-Pro Plus used to evaluate the number and total area of NV lesions per retina [16].

Four- to six-week-old double-hemizygous rho/rtTA-TRE/VEGF double-transgenic animals received an intravitreal injection of 1 $\mu g/\mu l$ of AC220 in one eye and intravitreal PBS in the contralateral eye. The mice then received 2 mg/ml doxycycline in drinking water [26] for 5 days. Retinas were examined under a surgical microscope to determine whether there was total retinal detachment (TRD), partial retinal detachment (PRD), or no retinal detachment (no RD) by chi-square test. C57BL/6 mice, rho/rtTA-TRE/VEGF double-transgenic mice, and double-transgenic mice treated with doxycycline were euthanized; the retinas were lysed, and phosphorylated Flt3 amounts were evaluated with PathScan Phospho-Flt3 Sandwich ELISA Kit as described previously [38, 40].

2.12. Immunofluorescence Staining of Flt3, GSA-Lectin, and F4/80. Immunofluorescence staining for Flt3, GSA-Lectin, and F4/80 detection was applied in normal, ischemic, rho/VEGF transgenic, CNV, and rho/rtTA-TRE/VEGF transgenic retinas. OCT- (Miles Laboratories, Elkhart, IN, USA) embedded samples were used to prepare frozen sections (10 μm) [16], which were fixed in acetone at $-20°C$ for 20 minutes and blocked with 5% bovine serum albumin (BSA). After overnight incubation at 4°C with polyclonal rabbit antimouse Flt3 antibody (Cell Signaling Technology Inc., Danvers, MA, USA), the specimens were incubated with Alexa 555 antirabbit IgG (Cell Signaling Technology), GSA-Lectin (Vector Laboratories), and FITC-labeled antimouse F4/80 antibody (eBioscience). The specimens were subsequently assessed by fluorescence microscopy.

2.13. Statistical Analysis. Unless otherwise stated, quantitative data are mean ± SE. The SPSS software was used for statistical analyses. Student's t-test, paired-sample t-test, chi-square test, and one-way ANOVA with the Student-Newman-Keuls (SNK) method (multiple comparisons) were used. Two-tailed $P < 0.05$ indicated statistical significance.

3. Results

3.1. Association of Flt3 with Vascular Endothelial Cells (VEC). Retina samples from normal P18 mice showed faint staining for Flt3 and GSA-Lectin throughout the inner retina (Figure 1(A)). Retinas from P18 mice after oxygen-induced ischemic retinopathy displayed increased Flt3 staining in the inner retina with colocalization of GSA-Lectin on the retinal surface in new vessels (Figure 1(B)). Retina specimens from P21 transgenic animals overexpressing VEGF in photoreceptors (rho/VEGF mice) showed Flt3 expression in inner and intermediate layers with a close association with GSA-Lectin (Figure 1(C)). Sections from a D14 laser-induced CNV mouse showed areas of Flt3 staining closely associated with GSA-Lectin in spite of laser injury (Figure 1(D)). Eyes from 5- to 8-week-old transgenic mice (rho/rtTA-TRE/VEGF) showed areas of Flt3 staining in the inner layers, with a close association with GSA-Lectin (Figure 1(E)).

3.2. Levels of Flt3 in OIR Mouse Retinas. Immunofluorescence staining and ELISA were carried out to assess whether Flt3 was involved in the progression of RNV. Phosphorylated Flt3 levels were significantly increased at P13, P15 and P18 in OIR mouse retina specimens compared with age-matched control samples (Figure 2). Immunofluorescence also revealed higher Flt3 expression in OIR mouse retina specimens at P18 (Figure 1(a)). Merged images showed colocalization of Flt3 and GSA-Lectin (Figure 1). These findings indicated that Flt3 plays an important role in RNV progression.

3.3. Flt3 Effects NV in Both CNV and RNV Mouse Models. Mice lacking Flt3 showed markedly reduced angiogenesis (Figures 3 and 4). Systemic neutralization of Flt3 in C57BL/6 mice starkly decreased CNV (Figure 3), as obtained with Flt3 gene deletion. Representative CNV lesions from an eye of wild-type animals (Figure 3(A)) and Flt3 transgenic mice (Figure 3(B)) showed profound differences in CNV. CNV areas were markedly decreased in Flt3−/− mice, as well as in animals administered 1.0 $\mu g/\mu l$ or 10 $\mu g/\mu l$ AC220; however, the animals treated with 0.1 $\mu g/\mu l$ AC220 and controls showed similar values (Figure 3(E)). RNV areas were significantly decreased in Flt3−/− mice, as well as in animals administered 1.0 $\mu g/\mu l$ AC220, compared with control values (Figure 4).

3.4. The Flt3 Inhibitor AC220 Significantly Reduces Subretinal NV and the Ratio of TRD in VEGF-Overexpressing Mice. Retinal flat mounts assessed by fluorescence microscopy revealed that AC220 inhibited subretinal NV (Figure 5). Rho/rtTA-TRE/VEGF (Tet/opsin/VEGF) animals, compared with those with intraocular injection of 1 μl of PBS and 1 $\mu g/\mu l$ of AC220, respectively, showed significantly less TRDs (Figure 6), suggesting that VEGF-induced ocular NV was closely associated with Flt3.

3.5. Association of Flt3 with Macrophages. Retinal sections were stained with F4/80 and Flt3 antibodies (for labeling of Mphi and Flt3 stained cells, resp.) and evaluated using fluorescence microscopy for visualization and colocalization of immunocompetent retinal cells. Retinas from P18 rodents

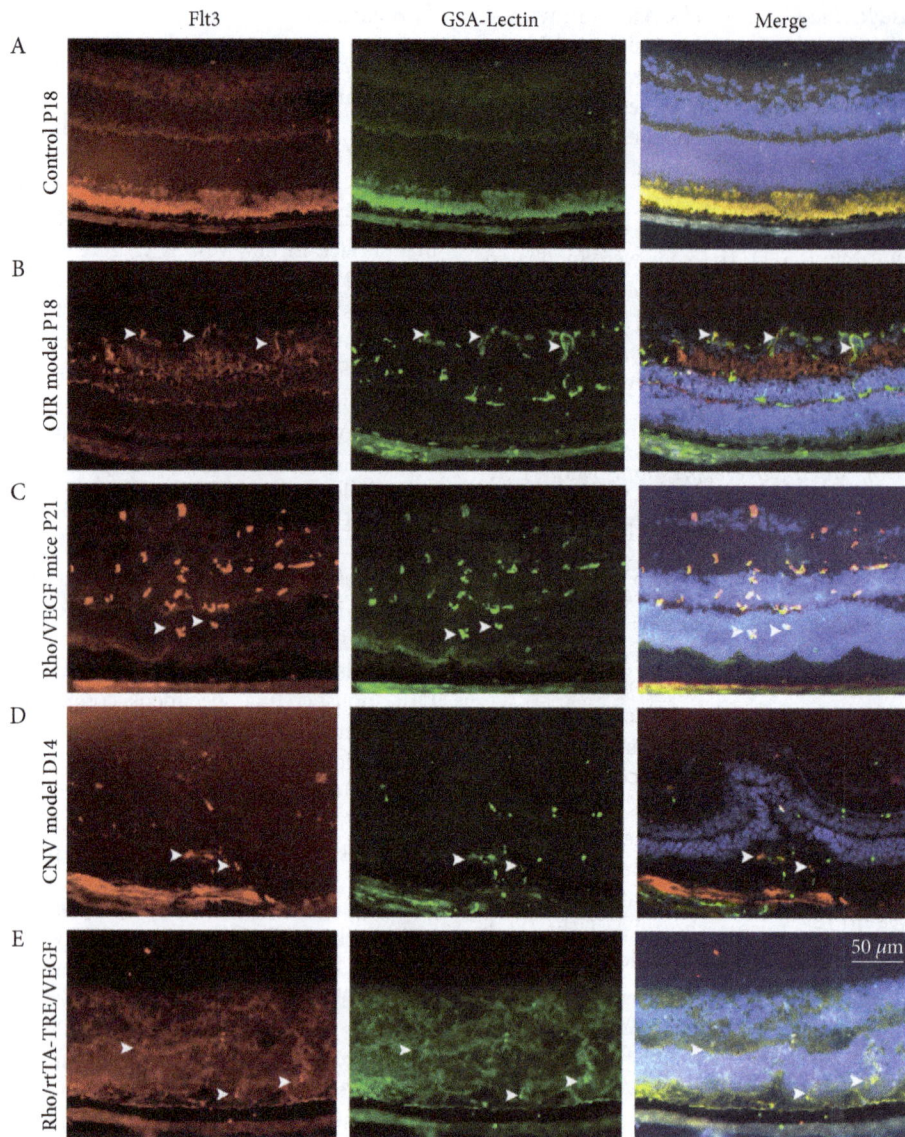

FIGURE 1: Immunofluorescence staining for Flt3 and GSA-Lectin detection in C57BL/6 control, OIR model, rho/VEGF transgenic, CNV model, and rho/rtTA-TRE/VEGF transgenic retinas. Mice were euthanized, and enucleated eyes were submitted to fixation and preparation to generate frozen sections. Immunofluorescence for Flt3 (red) and lectin (green) showed high expression of Flt3 in the OIR model, subretinal NV model, CNV model, and RD model retinas (arrowheads) with NV progression (A–E). Merged images showed colocalization of Flt3 and lectin. Scale bar: 500 μm. (A) Double immunofluorescence staining of Flt3 by Cy3-conjugated secondary antibodies (red) and GSA-Lectin (green) in flat-mounted control retina at P18. (B) Double immunofluorescence staining of Flt3 (red) and GSA-Lectin (green) in flat-mounted OIR retina samples at P18. Areas of staining for Flt3 increased during the pathological progression of OIR. (C) Eye specimens from P21 transgenic mice overexpressing VEGF in photoreceptors (rho/VEGF mice) showed Flt3 staining in the inner plexiform layer and colocalization with GSA-Lectin. (D) Staining of a section from a D14 CNV model showed Flt3 staining, while GSA-Lectin staining of the same section showed vascular staining. (E) Ocular sections from 5- to 8-week-old transgenic mice (rho/rtTA-TRE/VEGF) showed increased Flt3 staining in the inner layer and a close association with vascular staining.

with oxygen-induced ischemic retinopathy displayed areas of enhanced Flt3 expression throughout the inner retina compared with those of samples from normal P18 mice, with colocalization with F4/80 on the surface of the retina in new vessels (Figures 7(A, B)). Eyes from P21 transgenic animals overexpressing VEGF in photoreceptors (rho/VEGF mice) showed Flt3 expression in the inner and intermediate layers, with close association with F4/80 (Figure 7(C)). Ocular sections from D14 choroidal NV models or 5- to

8-week-old transgenic mice (rho/rtTA-TRE/VEGF) also showed areas of Flt3 staining, which were closely associated with F4/80 expression in the same layer (Figures 7(E) and 7(D)), indicating that Flt3 was strongly induced in retinal Mphi.

3.6. Flt3 Regulates M1 and M2 Cytokine Expression in CNV Mouse Model. Retinas of Flt3−/− and wild-type C57BL/6 mice at D14 with CNV were collected for the assessment of

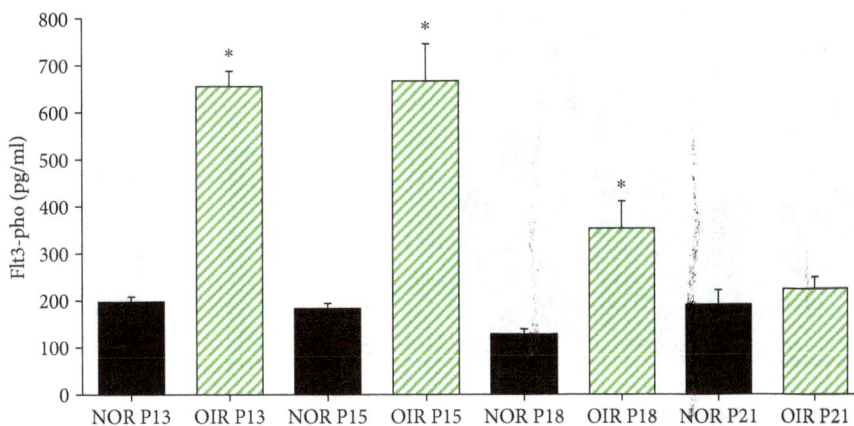

FIGURE 2: Flt3 expression examined by ELISA in retina specimens from OIR animals at P13, P15, P18, and P21. Mice subjected to OIR were sacrificed at P13, P15, P18, and P21; retinas were lysed, and phosphorylated Flt3 levels were measured as described in Methods and Materials. Quantification of phosphorylated Flt3 levels in mice retinas is shown. The asterisk " * " indicates a significant change of phosphorylated Flt3 levels at P13, P15, and P18 in OIR mouse retina specimens compared with age-matched control samples, respectively. Bars represented mean ± SE from 3 independent experiments ($n = 8$, *$P < 0.05$).

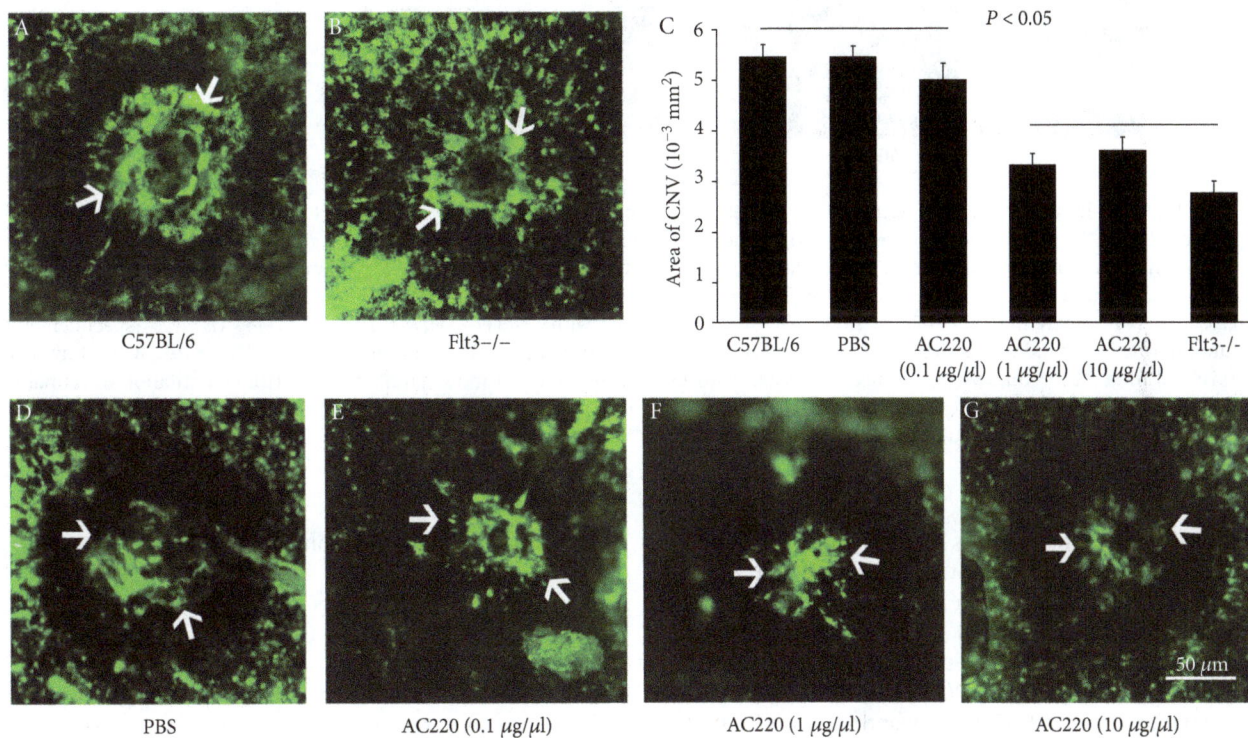

FIGURE 3: CNV at Bruch's membrane rupture sites is decreased in Flt3-deficient animals. Flt3−/− and wild-type C57BL/6 mice were submitted to laser-induced CNV. Wild-type animals were randomly grouped, with intravitreal administration of AC220 in one eye and PBS in the contralateral eye at days one and seven after laser photocoagulation in CNV mice. Choroidal flat mounts for CNV animals were obtained at day 14 (A, B, and D–G, $n = 10$). Areas of CNV were reduced at rupture sites in the Flt3−/− (B) and AC220 treatment (F) groups compared with those of C57BL/6 (A) or PBS treatment group (D). In agreement, image analysis revealed that CNV areas were markedly reduced (ANOVA with SNK) in Flt3−/− animals compared with wild-type mice. AC220-treated eyes exhibited significant inhibitory effects on CNV in comparison to PBS-treated eyes ($P < 0.05$) (C). Dose-effect experiments revealed that 1 μg/μl AC220 reduced CNV significantly at the lowest concentration (C–G).

Mphi polarization-associated molecules. Spiller et al. demonstrated that M1 Mphi appear at early stages of wound healing (1–3 days), later followed by the M2 counterparts (4–7 days) [41]. Therefore, we examined the inflammation related effectors, including CD11c and CD206, most likely involved in M1 and M2 cytokines, respectively. The results suggested that Flt3−/− animals showed relatively reduced amounts of CD11c and elevated levels of CD206, with statistical

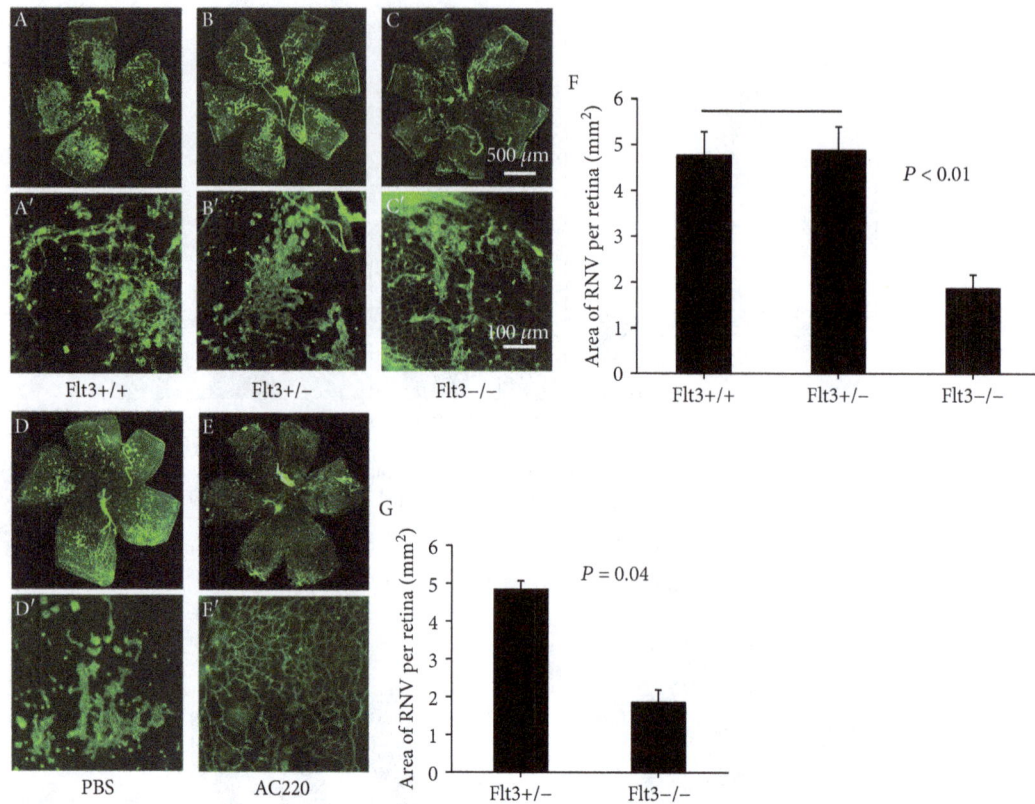

FIGURE 4: Ischemia-induced retinal NV decreases in Flt3-deficient animals. Flt3−/−, Flt3+/−, or Flt3+/+ (C57BL/6) mice were exposed to 75% oxygen from P7 to P12. At P18, retinas were dissected, washed, and incubated in presence of FITC-lectin at room temperature for 45 minutes. Retinal flat mounts were assessed under a fluorescence microscope. Retina samples from Flt3−/− animals (C, C′) showed reduced NV in comparison with those from the Flt3+/− (B, B′) or Flt3+/+ counterparts (A, A′). Quantitation of retinal NV areas confirmed a significant decrease of NV areas in the Flt3$^{-/-}$ group ($n = 12$) compared with Flt3+/− ($n = 12$) or Flt3+/+ ($n = 12$) specimens (F). Immunofluorescence staining of retinal flat mounts of OIR animals after treatment with PBS and AC220. AC220 or PBS was intravitreally administered in at P12; retinas were obtained, incubated with FITC-lectin, and flat mounted at P18 ($n = 12$). Quantitation of retinal NV areas confirmed a significant decrease in the AC220 treatment group ($n = 12$) in comparison with the PBS group (G). Bars represented mean (±SEM); groups were compared by ANOVA with SNK for multiple comparisons.

significance comparable with that of wild-type controls (Figures 8(C, D)). This indicated a potential role for Flt3 inhibitors in Mphi polarization. Immunofluorescence staining of CD11c and CD206 in retina samples from CNV models at D14 also revealed that Flt3 promoted the expression of M1 cytokines (Figures 8(C–F)) and decreased that of M2 cytokines (Figures 8(H–K)). Quantification of CD11c+ staining areas in CNV lesions at 14 days confirmed a substantial decrease in the amounts of these cells in the absence of Flt3 (Figure 8(G)). CD206+ staining areas were significantly increased in the Flt3−/− group (Figure 8(L)).

3.7. Flt3 Deficiency Shifts Macrophage Polarization towards the M2 Phenotype during RNV. Retina samples from AC220- or PBS-treated eyes were assessed by flow cytometry (P15, P18, and P21). There were reduced amounts of M1 Mphi in AC220-treated animals compared with PBS controls (P15 showed more striking differences); however, more M2 Mphi were found in AC220-treated animals compared with PBS controls, with P21 showing more pronounced effects. M1/M2 ratios indicated a shift in Mphi polarization towards

M2 in the AC220 group compared with the PBS group in RNV (Figure 9).

4. Discussion

The area of neovascular complexes penetrating the subretinal space reflects the degree of angiogenesis in CNV. NV pathogenesis has been evaluated by established mouse models, which serve as a tool for preclinical trials assessing therapies for AMD [27, 42]. In this study, inflammation was further characterized by evaluating CNV induction in Flt3-deficient mice. Our working hypothesis was that reduced inflammation and CNV would be found in Flt3-deficient mice. As demonstrated by our findings, mice lacking Flt3 showed a significant decrease in new vessel growth in both transgenic mice and Flt3 inhibitor AC220 injection group. CNV results from damage to Bruch's membrane and RPE defects. In contrast, RNV results from retinal hypoxia, which is found in various ocular diseases, including diabetic retinopathy and retinopathy of prematurity [43]. Interestingly, injection of

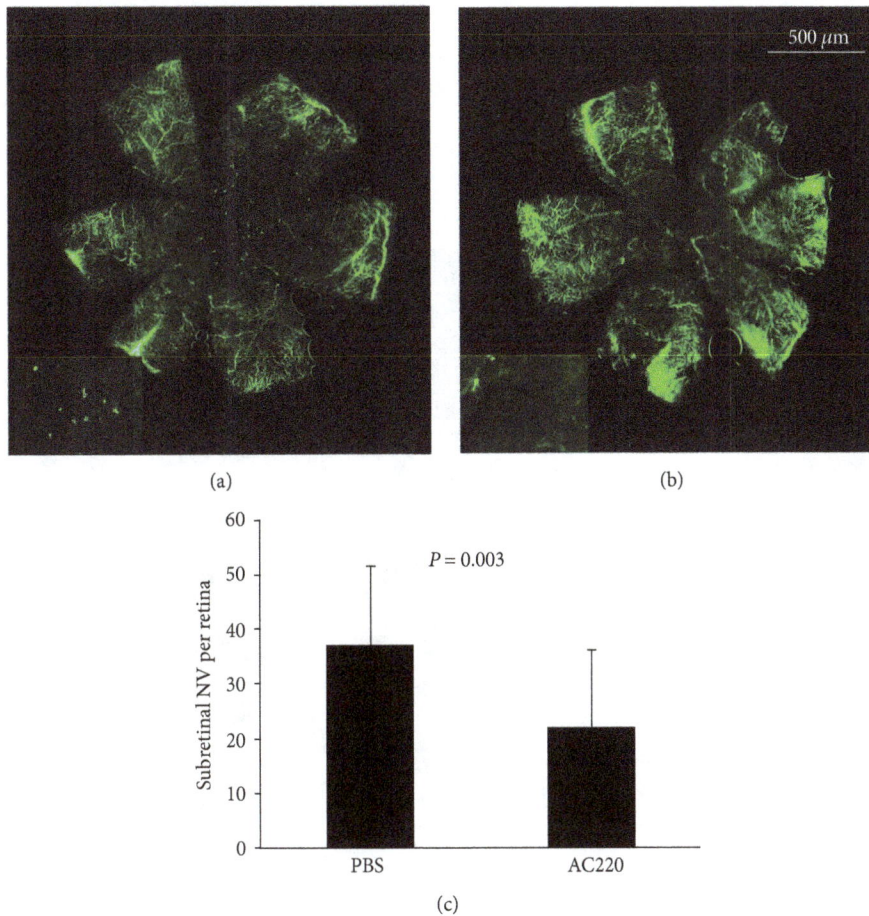

FIGURE 5: Inhibition of Flt3 reduces VEGF-induced subretinal NV. Immunofluorescence staining of retinal flat mounts from rho/VEGF animals after treatment with PBS and AC220. AC220 was intravitreally administered in one eye and PBS in the contralateral eye of rho/VEGF mice at P12, and retinas were obtained, stained, and flat mounted at P21 ($n = 8$). The total number and area of subretinal NV decreased significantly in AC220-treated eyes compared with those in the PBS group (a–c).

the Flt3 inhibitor AC220 resulted in substantially decreased NV areas in our RNV models.

Inflammatory cells, specifically Mphi, produce multiple angiogenic factors and constitute important components in malignancies, heart disease, and ocular disease. However, Mphi functions are rather complex as they induce wound healing [44, 45] while controlling angiogenesis during development [31]. Tsutsumi et al. demonstrated that ocular-infiltrating Mphi were essential for CNV generation, with the influx of Mphi possessing direct angiogenic ability [46]. Caicedo et al. proposed that recruitment of blood-derived Mphi seemed to be more associated with CNV than resident microglia [47].

Flt3 can influence the functions of Mphi. Flt3 ligand exerts potent stimulatory effects on precursors of the monocyte/Mphi lineage [48]. In one study, Flt3 ligand caused whitening of the bone marrow with significant reduction in the number of erythroblastic island Mphi and erythroblasts [49]. Furthermore, Flt3 ligand might be considered a specific marker for IFNγ-differentiated Mphi. Polarizing cytokines such as IFNγ might contribute to the high levels of Flt3 ligand found in rheumatoid arthritis synovium by shifting the Mphi polarization into a M1 phenotype [50]. In our

study, we demonstrate for the first time that Flt3 deficiency results in Mphi switching towards the M2 phenotype in addition to decreased NV. This shows that targeted therapy with the Flt3 inhibitor AC220 is able to reduce local Flt3 function, in turn influencing tissue-specific M2 activity and the controlling NV formation. Mphi are found in two polarization phenotypes, M1 and M2 subsets, which promote and inhibit inflammation, respectively [51, 52]. Brichard et al. demonstrated that M2 cells regulate inflammation and promote tissue repair [53], in turn increasing trophic rescue with heightened clearance of apoptotic cellular debris and promoting tolerance in lieu of autoimmunity [54, 55]. A report by Cao et al. also revealed that an increased number of M2 cells in normal aging eyes compared to M1 Mphi facilitates tissue repair and NV [56].

Transgenic mice with the rhodopsin promoter controlling human VEGF165 levels in photoreceptors (rho/VEGF mice) produce new vessels from the retina's deep capillary bed, starting at P10, which grow into the subretinal space [25, 40]. VEGF production is sustained, and therefore, the new vessels continue to grow and enlarge, forming large nets in the subretinal space similar to the exudative type of AMD [57]. In a retinal detachment model, the Tet/on system was

(a)

(b)

	PBS	AC220
No RD	17.50%	20.00%
PRD	32.50%	55.00%
TRD	50.00%	25.00%

(c)

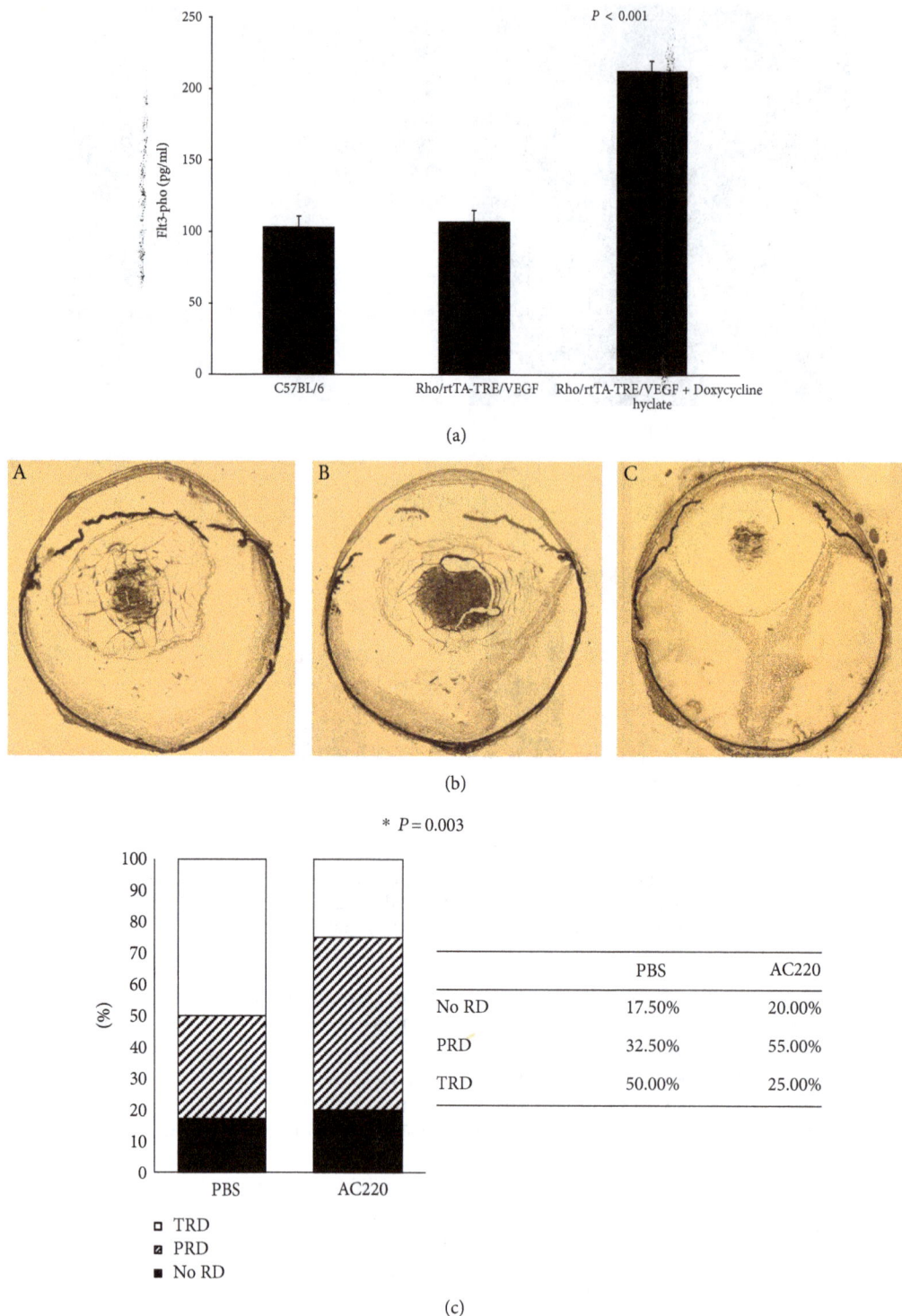

FIGURE 6: Effect of intraocular injection of AC220 in double-transgenic mice overexpressing VEGF in photoreceptors (rho/rtTA-TRE/VEGF mice). Four-week-old adult rho/rtTA-TRE/VEGF mice received an intravitreal injection of 1 μg of AC220 (in 1 μl PBS) in one eye and 1 μl PBS in the contralateral eye. The animals then received doxycycline at 2 mg/ml in drinking water. (a) After five days, non-AC220-treated retinas were lysed, and phosphorylated Flt3 amounts were measured by the ELISA method. Phosphorylated Flt3 amounts in RD model retinas were higher than those in both wild-type and no-doxycycline-treated retinas. (b) Five days after initiation of doxycycline treatment, ocular sections showed no retinal detachment (no RD), partial retinal detachment (PRD), or total retinal detachment (TRD). (c) Intraocular injection of AC220 or PBS in doxycycline-treated rho/rtTA-TRE/VEGF mice. Retina samples were examined under an operating microscope in a blinded manner, to determine if there was TRD, PRD, or no RD. In AC220-treated mice, 25% of eyes had TRD, and 50% of eyes injected with PBS had TRD. The asterisk "$*$" indicates that the incidence of RD in AC220-injected eyes was significantly reduced than that of the PBS-injected counterparts ($P < 0.05$ by chi-square). This suggests that intravitreal injection of 1 μg AC220 significantly reduced TRD.

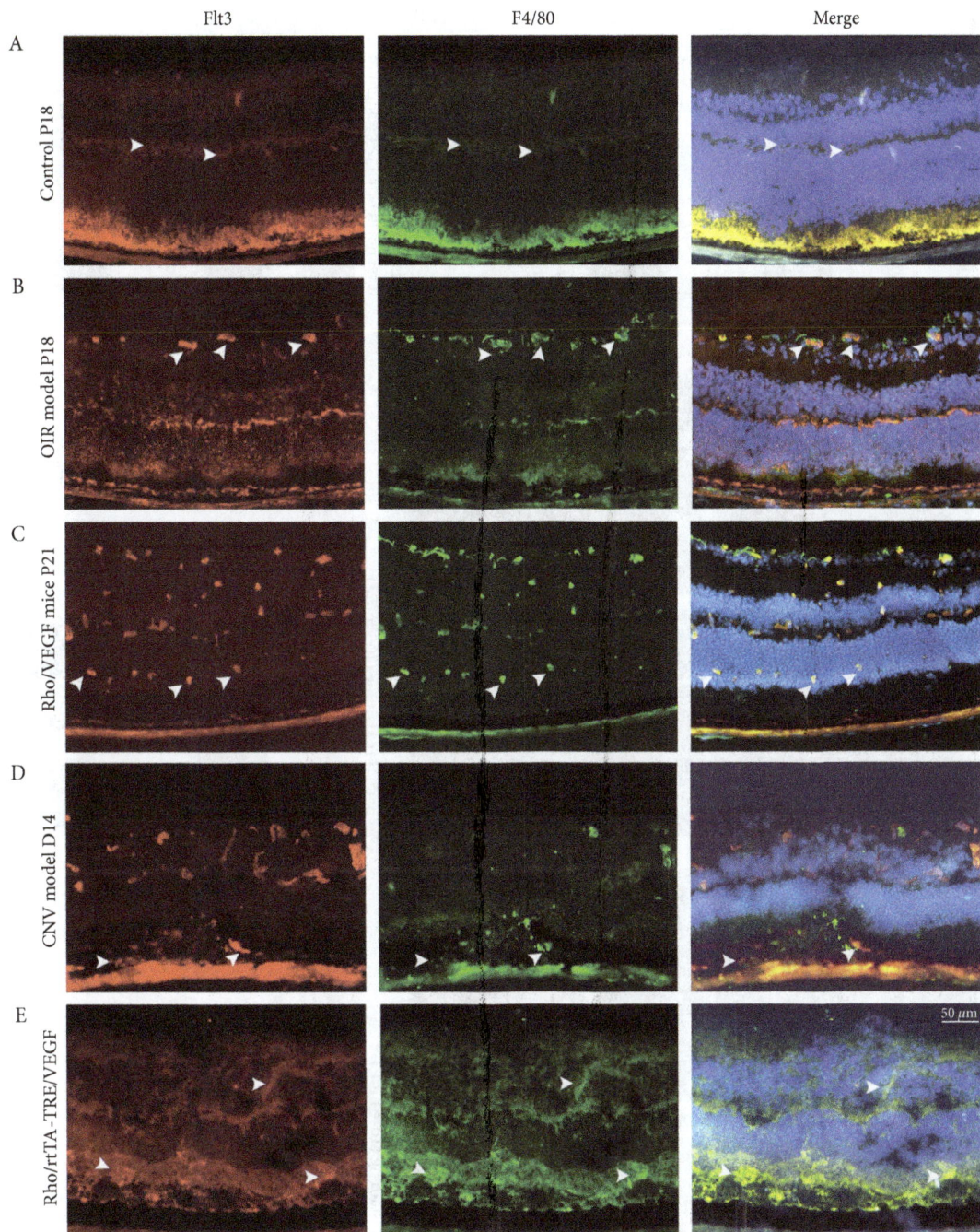

FIGURE 7: Immunofluorescence staining for Flt3 and F4/80 in normal, ischemic retina, rho/VEGF transgenic, CNV, and rho/rtTA-TRE/ VEGF transgenic retinas. Retinal preparation was conducted for staining F4/80 macrophages and Flt3+ cells using the perfusion procedure described earlier. Eyes of OIR mouse model at P18, subretinal NV mouse model at P21, CNV and RD mouse models were enucleated and submitted to fixation and preparation for frozen sections. Immunofluorescence staining of Flt3 (red) showed high expression of Flt3 in OIR, subretinal NV, CNV, and RD model retinas (arrowheads), which colocalized with F4/80 staining. A nonischemic retinal sample from a P18 mouse displayed Flt3 expression areas, as revealed by Cy3-conjugated secondary antibodies (red), throughout the inner retina. F4/80 expression in the same section as in (A) with FITC-conjugated secondary antibodies displayed reduced areas. Ocular section from a P18 mouse after oxygen-induced ischemic retinopathy displayed areas (arrowheads) of increased expression in the whole inner retina colocalizing with F4/80-stained macrophages or closely localized around macrophages in and on the retina (B). Ocular specimens from P21 transgenic mice overexpressing VEGF in photoreceptors (rho/VEGF mice) showing Flt3 expression that colocalizes with F4/80 (C). An ocular section from a D14 CNV mouse model showing Flt3 staining, while F4/80 staining of the same section showed macrophage localization (D). Ocular sections from 5- to 8-week-old transgenic mice (rho/rtTA-TRE/VEGF) showing an area of Flt3 staining in the inner layer (red) and green F4/80 staining (E). Merging of Flt3 and F4/80 staining of all NV model retinas showed colocalization (yellow), indicating that macrophages may express Flt3.

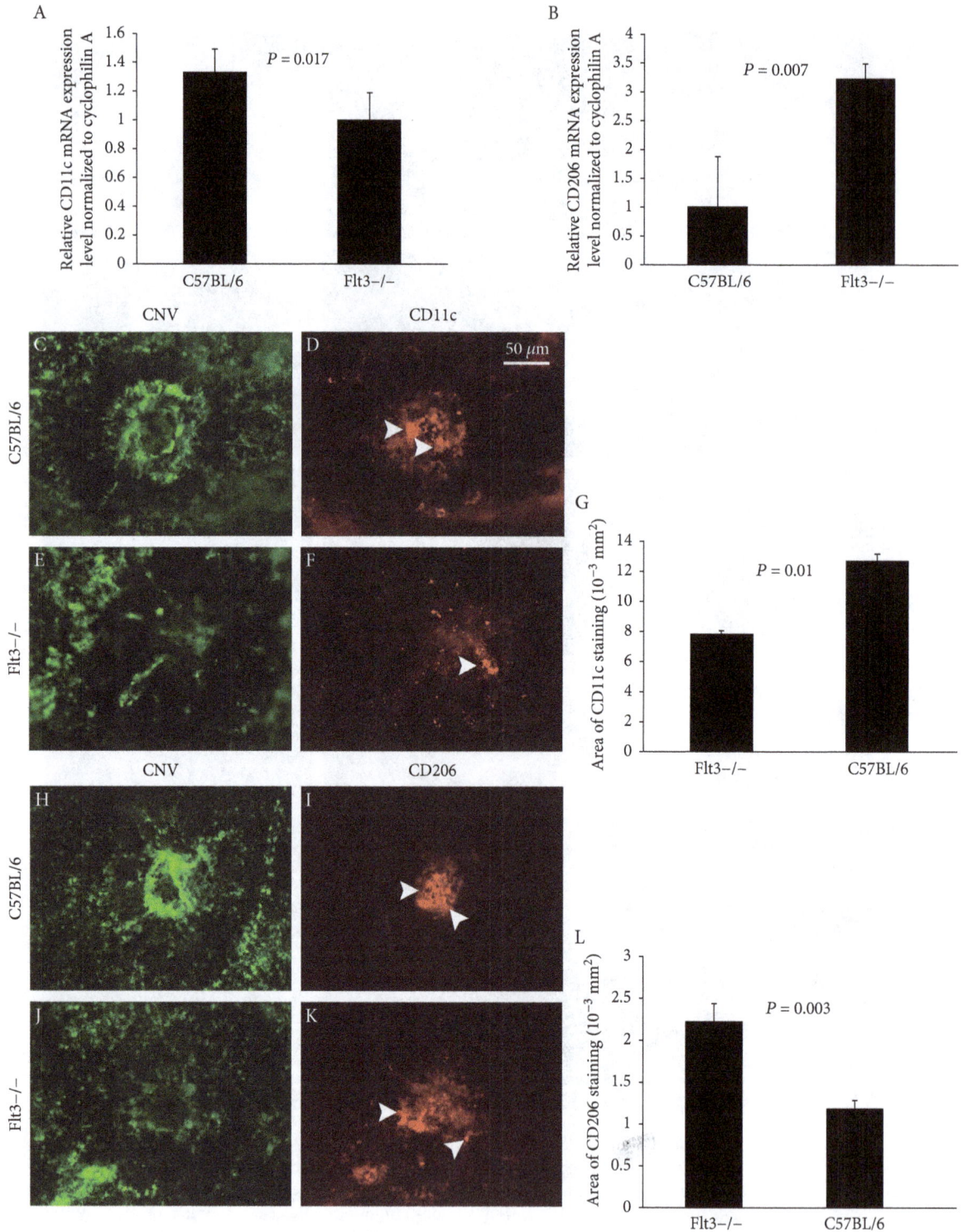

FIGURE 8: CD11c and CD206 levels assessed by quantitative PCR and immunofluorescence in retinas of CNV mouse model at D14. Quantification of CD11c and CD206 levels in mouse retinas are shown, respectively, in (A) and (B). Data are mean ± SE from three independent experiments ($n = 8$, $P < 0.05$). Flt3−/− and wild-type C57BL/6 mice were submitted to laser-induced CNV. Double labeling of NV (green) with CD11c (red) or CD206 (red) was performed on choroidal flat mounts of mice after laser treatment. Immunofluorescence signals of CD11c are shown in (D) and (F); CD206 are shown in (I) and (K). Mean CD11c(+) and CD206(+) cell areas per CNV lesion are presented. Flt3−/− mice exhibited significantly decreased areas of CD11c staining and increased areas of CD206 staining in comparison with controls ($P < 0.05$); similar results were obtained at the mRNA level by real-time RT-PCR.

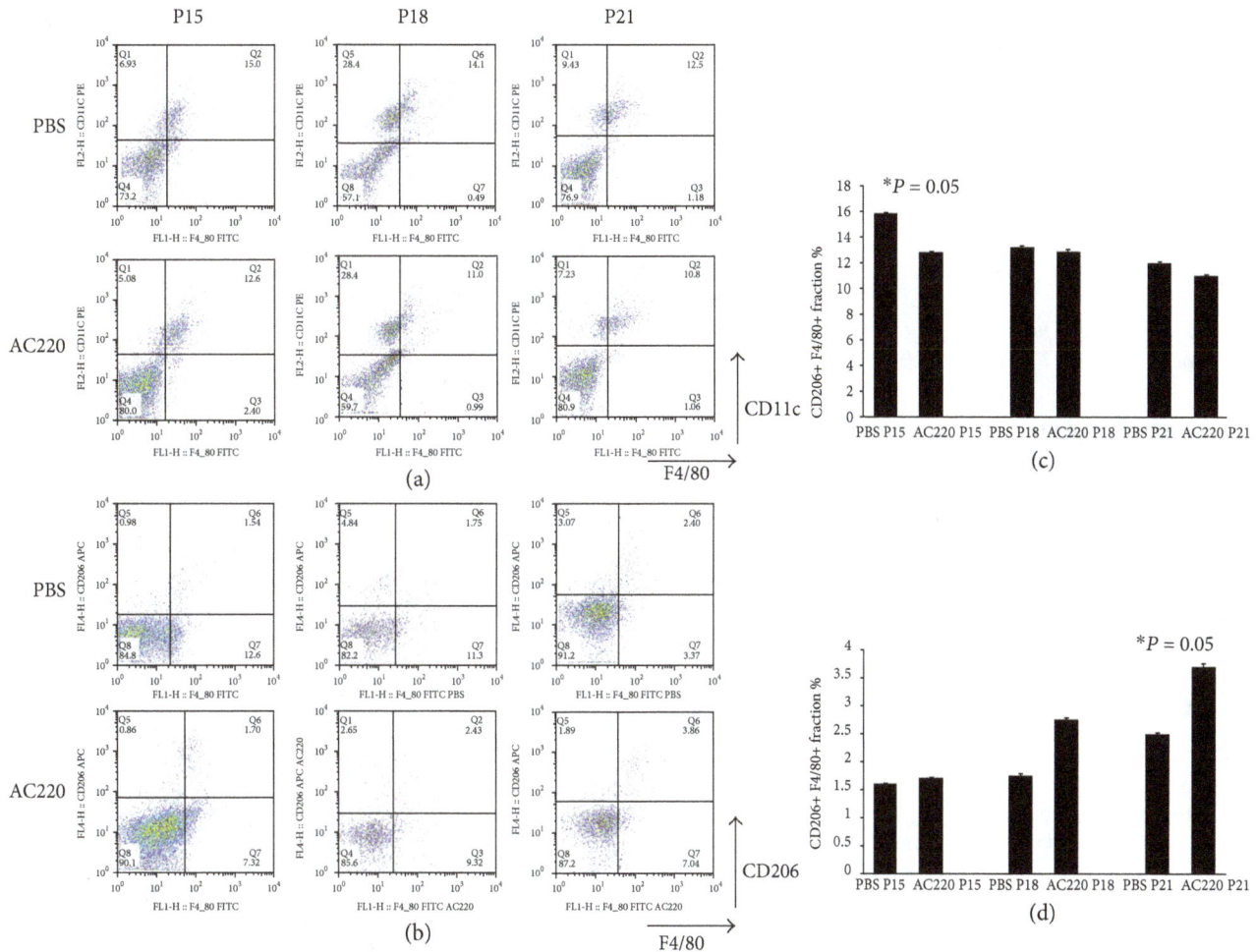

FIGURE 9: Flow cytometry analysis of PBS and AC220-treated OIR mouse model. PBS and AC220 treatments were administered to OIR model mice. At P15, P18, and P21, retina samples were digested with papain, and cells were sorted by CD11b expression before incubation with anti-F4/80, CD11c, and CD206 antibodies. M1 and M2 macrophages were F4/80+/CD11c+ and F4/80+/CD206+, respectively. Representative flow cytograms are shown (A and B). Cycle distribution patterns of F4/80+/CD11c+ and F4/80+/CD206+ cells (C and D). The asterisk " * " indicates a significant change of F4/80+/CD11c+ fraction or F4/80+/CD206+ fraction in AC220 treatment mouse retina specimens compared with PBS control samples. Bars represented mean ± SE from 3 independent experiments ($n = 4 - 6$ mice/group, $p < 0.05$).

employed to produce double-transgenic mice characterized by doxycycline-inducible expression of human VEGF165 in photoreceptors (rho/rtTA-TRE/VEGF or Tet/opsin/VEGF mice) [26]. A dose of 2 mg/ml doxycycline in drinking water highly enhanced VEGF levels in photoreceptors (similar to but higher than those in rho/VEGF mice), causing total exudative retinal detachment in 80–90% of mice within 5 days. Cryosections of retinas were obtained for further assessment from the experimental group and controls [58, 59]. Experiments involving the Flt3 inhibitor AC220, in this study, provided evidence of an association of Flt3 activation with VEGF-induced RNV. Notably, the inhibition of Flt3 induction significantly decreased VEGF-induced RNV in both rho/VEGF and rho/rtTA-TRE/VEGF animals. Furthermore, Flt3 inhibition with AC220 reduced the retinal detachment rate in rho/rtTA-TRE/VEGF mice. These findings support the notion that inhibition of Flt3 by AC220 affects retinal new vessel formation in the retina and detachment induced by VEGF in these models. Markovic et al. showed that

the Flt3-blocking antibody D43 decreased Flt3 tyrosine phosphorylation and reduced Flt3-induced VEGF secretion, indicating that Flt3 signaling is highly involved in VEGF regulation [60].

Further studies are needed to determine the potential mechanisms by which Mphi are polarized in Flt3 deficiency, how Flt3 modulates retinal NV during VEGF overexpression in transgenic mice, and whether Flt3 upregulation can increase NV areas in RNV models. Our study highlights Flt3 as a novel molecular target for the inhibition of neovascularization in murine models of retinopathy. Further evaluation of the antiangiogenic role of Flt3 inhibition in human eyes is needed.

5. Conclusion

In this study, we demonstrated that Flt3 inhibition improved ocular NV by driving Mphi switching towards the M2 phenotype. Our findings revealed Flt3 effects on NV via

Mphi polarization modulation, supporting its potential use for the treatment of NV in ocular disease.

Conflicts of Interest

The authors declare no financial or commercial conflict of interest.

Authors' Contributions

Yushuo Gao and Yisheng Zhong contributed equally to this article.

Acknowledgments

The authors thank the Shanghai Institute of Burns for field and facility assistance. The study was supported by the National Nature Science Foundation of China (81470639, 81570853, and 81670761), the Shanghai Nature Science Foundation (Grant 14411968400), and the Shanghai Charity Cancer Research Center Program 2013.

References

[1] V. R. Cimarolli, R. J. Casten, B. W. Rovner, V. Heyl, S. Sörensen, and A. Horowitz, "Anxiety and depression in patients with advanced macular degeneration: current perspectives," *Clinical Ophthalmology*, vol. 10, pp. 55–63, 2016.

[2] J. N. Cooke Bailey, J. Hoffman, R. Sardell, W. Scott, M. Pericak-Vance, and J. Haines, "The application of genetic risk scores in age-related macular degeneration: a review," *Journal of Clinical Medicine*, vol. 5, no. 12, 2016.

[3] S. Zampatti, F. Ricci, A. Cusumano, L. T. Marsella, G. Novelli, and E. Giardina, "Review of nutrient actions on age-related macular degeneration," *Nutrition Research*, vol. 34, no. 2, pp. 95–105, 2014.

[4] C. Cukras, E. Agrón, M. L. Klein et al., "Natural history of drusenoid pigment epithelial detachment in age-related macular degeneration: Age-Related Eye Disease Study Report No. 28," *Ophthalmology*, vol. 117, no. 3, pp. 489–499, 2010.

[5] S. H. Chang, K. Kanasaki, V. Gocheva et al., "VEGF-A induces angiogenesis by perturbing the cathepsin-cysteine protease inhibitor balance in venules, causing basement membrane degradation and mother vessel formation," *Cancer Research*, vol. 69, no. 10, pp. 4537–4544, 2009.

[6] R. G. Rowe and S. J. Weiss, "Breaching the basement membrane: who, when and how?," *Trends in Cell Biology*, vol. 18, no. 11, pp. 560–574, 2008.

[7] D. R. Senger and G. E. Davis, "Angiogenesis," *Cold Spring Harbor Perspectives in Biology*, vol. 3, no. 8, article a005090, 2011.

[8] C. Sundberg, J. A. Nagy, L. F. Brown et al., "Glomeruloid microvascular proliferation follows adenoviral vascular permeability factor/vascular endothelial growth factor-164 gene delivery," *The American Journal of Pathology*, vol. 158, no. 3, pp. 1145–1160, 2001.

[9] A. N. Stratman, A. E. Schwindt, K. M. Malotte, and G. E. Davis, "Endothelial-derived PDGF-BB and HB-EGF coordinately regulate pericyte recruitment during vasculogenic tube assembly and stabilization," *Blood*, vol. 116, no. 22, pp. 4720–4730, 2010.

[10] A. N. Stratman, K. M. Malotte, R. D. Mahan, M. J. Davis, and G. E. Davis, "Pericyte recruitment during vasculogenic tube assembly stimulates endothelial basement membrane matrix formation," *Blood*, vol. 114, no. 24, pp. 5091–5101, 2009.

[11] E. Allen, P. Miéville, C. M. Warren et al., "Metabolic symbiosis enables adaptive resistance to anti-angiogenic therapy that is dependent on mTOR signaling," *Cell Reports*, vol. 15, no. 6, pp. 1144–1160, 2016.

[12] Z. Deng, J. Zhou, X. Han, and X. Li, "TCEB2 confers resistance to VEGF-targeted therapy in ovarian cancer," *Oncology Reports*, vol. 35, no. 1, pp. 359–365, 2016.

[13] R. N. Gacche and R. J. Meshram, "Angiogenic factors as potential drug target: efficacy and limitations of anti-angiogenic therapy," *Biochimica et Biophysica Acta (BBA) - Reviews on Cancer*, vol. 1846, no. 1, pp. 161–179, 2014.

[14] R. K. Jain, D. Fukumura, and D. G. Duda, "Modes of neovascularization in tumors and clinical translation of antiangiogenic therapy," in *Pathobiology of Human Disease*, pp. 2926–2957, Elsevier Science Publishing Co Inc., San Diego, CA, USA, 2014.

[15] Y. Cai, W. Tan, X. Shen et al., "Neutralization of IL-23 depresses experimental ocular neovascularization," *Experimental Eye Research*, vol. 146, pp. 242–251, 2016.

[16] Y. Zhu, W. Tan, A. M. Demetriades et al., "Interleukin-17A neutralization alleviated ocular neovascularization by promoting M2 and mitigating M1 macrophage polarization," *Immunology*, vol. 147, no. 4, pp. 414–428, 2016.

[17] B. Lowenberg, J. D. Griffin, and M. S. Tallman, "Acute myeloid leukemia and acute promyelocytic leukemia," *Hematology*, vol. 2003, pp. 82–101, 2003.

[18] D. G. Gilliland and J. D. Griffin, "The roles of FLT3 in hematopoiesis and leukemia," *Blood*, vol. 100, no. 5, pp. 1532–1542, 2002.

[19] A. I. Muntyanu, M. Raika, and E. G. Zota, "Immunohistochemical study of the role of mast cells and macrophages in the process of angiogenesis in the atherosclerotic plaques in patients with metabolic syndrome," *Arkhiv Patologii*, vol. 78, no. 2, pp. 19–28, 2016.

[20] H. Iwanishi, N. Fujita, K. Tomoyose et al., "Inhibition of development of laser-induced choroidal neovascularization with suppression of infiltration of macrophages in Smad3-null mice," *Laboratory Investigation*, vol. 96, no. 6, pp. 641–651, 2016.

[21] N. S. Abdelfattah, M. Amgad, and A. A. Zayed, "Host immune cellular reactions in corneal neovascularization," *International Journal of Ophthalmology*, vol. 9, no. 4, pp. 625–633, 2016.

[22] J. Whiteley, R. Bielecki, M. Li et al., "An expanded population of CD34+ cells from frozen banked umbilical cord blood demonstrate tissue repair mechanisms of mesenchymal stromal cells and circulating angiogenic cells in an ischemic hind limb model," *Stem Cell Reviews*, vol. 10, no. 3, pp. 338–350, 2014.

[23] J. Bhullar, K. Natarajan, S. Shukla et al., "The FLT3 inhibitor quizartinib inhibits ABCG2 at pharmacologically relevant concentrations, with implications for both chemosensitization and adverse drug interactions," *PLoS One*, vol. 8, no. 8, article e71266, 2013.

[24] P. P. Zarrinkar, R. N. Gunawardane, M. D. Cramer et al., "AC220 is a uniquely potent and selective inhibitor of FLT3 for the treatment of acute myeloid leukemia (AML)," *Blood*, vol. 114, no. 14, pp. 2984–2992, 2009.

[25] N. Okamoto, T. Tobe, S. F. Hackett et al., "Transgenic mice with increased expression of vascular endothelial growth factor in the retina: a new model of intraretinal and subretinal neovascularization," *The American Journal of Pathology*, vol. 151, no. 1, pp. 281–291, 1997.

[26] K. Ohno-Matsui, A. Hirose, S. Yamamoto et al., "Inducible expression of vascular endothelial growth factor in adult mice causes severe proliferative retinopathy and retinal detachment," *The American Journal of Pathology*, vol. 160, no. 2, pp. 711–719, 2002.

[27] H. Huang, R. Parlier, J. K. Shen, G. A. Lutty, and S. A. Vinores, "VEGF receptor blockade markedly reduces retinal microglia/macrophage infiltration into laser-induced CNV," *PLoS One*, vol. 8, no. 8, article e71808, 2013.

[28] S. Moghaddam-Taaheri, M. Agarwal, and J. Amaral, "Effects of docosahexaenoic acid in preventing experimental choroidal neovascularization in rodents," *Journal of Clinical & Experimental Ophthalmology*, vol. 2, p. 187, 2011.

[29] H. Huang, J. Shen, and S. A. Vinores, "Blockade of VEGFR1 and 2 suppresses pathological angiogenesis and vascular leakage in the eye," *PLoS One*, vol. 6, no. 6, article e21411, 2011.

[30] C. Campa, I. Kasman, W. Ye, W. P. Lee, G. Fuh, and N. Ferrara, "Effects of an anti-VEGF-A monoclonal antibody on laser-induced choroidal neovascularization in mice: optimizing methods to quantify vascular changes," *Investigative Ophthalmology & Visual Science*, vol. 49, no. 3, pp. 1178–1183, 2008.

[31] R. S. Apte, J. Richter, J. Herndon, and T. A. Ferguson, "Macrophages inhibit neovascularization in a murine model of age-related macular degeneration," *PLoS Medicine*, vol. 3, no. 8, article e310, 2006.

[32] J. Shen, X. Yang, B. Xie et al., "MicroRNAs regulate ocular neovascularization," *Molecular Therapy*, vol. 16, no. 7, pp. 1208–1216, 2008.

[33] S. Fujimura, H. Takahashi, K. Yuda et al., "Angiostatic effect of CXCR3 expressed on choroidal neovascularization," *Investigative Ophthalmology & Visual Science*, vol. 53, no. 4, pp. 1999–2006, 2012.

[34] Y. Zhu, Q. Lu, J. Shen et al., "Improvement and optimization of standards for a preclinical animal test model of laser induced choroidal neovascularization," *PLoS One*, vol. 9, no. 4, article e94743, 2014.

[35] J. Shen, B. Xie, A. Dong, M. Swaim, S. F. Hackett, and P. A. Campochiaro, "In vivo immunostaining demonstrates macrophages associate with growing and regressing vessels," *Investigative Ophthalmology & Visual Science*, vol. 48, no. 9, pp. 4335–4341, 2007.

[36] K. Mori, E. Duh, P. Gehlbach et al., "Pigment epithelium-derived factor inhibits retinal and choroidal neovascularization," *Journal of Cellular Physiology*, vol. 188, no. 2, pp. 253–263, 2001.

[37] B. Xie, J. Shen, A. Dong, A. Rashid, G. Stoller, and P. A. Campochiaro, "Blockade of sphingosine-1-phosphate reduces macrophage influx and retinal and choroidal neovascularization," *Journal of Cellular Physiology*, vol. 218, no. 1, pp. 192–198, 2009.

[38] E. Augustin, A. Skwarska, A. Weryszko, I. Pelikant, E. Sankowska, and B. Borowa-Mazgaj, "The antitumor compound triazoloacridinone C-1305 inhibits FLT3 kinase activity and potentiates apoptosis in mutant FLT3-ITD leukemia cells," *Acta Pharmacologica Sinica*, vol. 36, no. 3, pp. 385–399, 2015.

[39] C. N. Lumeng, J. B. DelProposto, D. J. Westcott, and A. R. Saltiel, "Phenotypic switching of adipose tissue macrophages with obesity is generated by spatiotemporal differences in macrophage subtypes," *Diabetes*, vol. 57, no. 12, pp. 3239–3246, 2008.

[40] K. Miki, A. Miki, M. Matsuoka, D. Muramatsu, S. F. Hackett, and P. A. Campochiaro, "Effects of intraocular ranibizumab and bevacizumab in transgenic mice expressing human vascular endothelial growth factor," *Ophthalmology*, vol. 116, no. 9, pp. 1748–1754, 2009.

[41] K. L. Spiller, R. R. Anfang, K. J. Spiller et al., "The role of macrophage phenotype in vascularization of tissue engineering scaffolds," *Biomaterials*, vol. 35, no. 15, pp. 4477–4488, 2014.

[42] S. Jawad, B. Liu, Z. Li et al., "The role of macrophage class a scavenger receptors in a laser-induced murine choroidal neovascularization model," *Investigative Ophthalmology & Visual Science*, vol. 54, no. 9, pp. 5959–5970, 2013.

[43] P. A. Campochiaro, "Retinal and choroidal neovascularization," *Journal of Cellular Physiology*, vol. 184, no. 3, pp. 301–310, 2000.

[44] R. F. Diegelmann and M. C. Evans, "Wound healing: an overview of acute, fibrotic and delayed healing," *Frontiers in Bioscience*, vol. 9, no. 1-3, pp. 283–289, 2004.

[45] J. E. Park and A. Barbul, "Understanding the role of immune regulation in wound healing," *The American Journal of Surgery*, vol. 187, no. 5, Supplement 1, pp. S11–S16, 2004.

[46] C. Tsutsumi, K. H. Sonoda, K. Egashira et al., "The critical role of ocular-infiltrating macrophages in the development of choroidal neovascularization," *Journal of Leukocyte Biology*, vol. 74, no. 1, pp. 25–32, 2003.

[47] A. Caicedo, D. G. Espinosa-Heidmann, Y. Piña, E. P. Hernandez, and S. W. Cousins, "Blood-derived macrophages infiltrate the retina and activate Muller glial cells under experimental choroidal neovascularization," *Experimental Eye Research*, vol. 81, no. 1, pp. 38–47, 2005.

[48] S. E. Nicholls, S. Winter, R. Mottram, J. A. Miyan, and A. D. Whetton, "Flt3 ligand can promote survival and macrophage development without proliferation in myeloid progenitor cells," *Experimental Hematology*, vol. 27, no. 4, pp. 663–672, 1999.

[49] R. N. Jacobsen, B. Nowlan, M. E. Brunck, V. Barbier, I. G. Winkler, and J. P. Levesque, "Fms-like tyrosine kinase 3 (Flt3) ligand depletes erythroid island macrophages and blocks medullar erythropoiesis in the mouse," *Experimental Hematology*, vol. 44, no. 3, pp. 207–212.e4, 2016.

[50] M. I. Ramos, S. G. Perez, S. Aarrass et al., "FMS-related tyrosine kinase 3 ligand (Flt3L)/CD135 axis in rheumatoid arthritis," *Arthritis Research & Therapy*, vol. 15, article R209, no. 6, 2013.

[51] A. Mantovani, S. Sozzani, M. Locati, P. Allavena, and A. Sica, "Macrophage polarization: tumor-associated macrophages as a paradigm for polarized M2 mononuclear phagocytes," *Trends in Immunology*, vol. 23, no. 11, pp. 549–555, 2002.

[52] A. Mantovani, A. Sica, S. Sozzani, P. Allavena, A. Vecchi, and M. Locati, "The chemokine system in diverse forms of macrophage activation and polarization," *Trends in Immunology*, vol. 25, no. 12, pp. 677–686, 2004.

[53] B. Brichard, I. Varis, D. Latinne et al., "Intracellular cytokine profile of cord and adult blood monocytes," *Bone Marrow Transplantation*, vol. 27, no. 10, pp. 1081–1086, 2001.

[54] V. Marchetti, O. Yanes, E. Aguilar et al., "Differential macrophage polarization promotes tissue remodeling and repair in a model of ischemic retinopathy," *Scientific Reports*, vol. 1, no. 1, p. 76, 2011.

[55] S. Gordon and F. O. Martinez, "Alternative activation of macrophages: mechanism and functions," *Immunity*, vol. 32, no. 5, pp. 593–604, 2010.

[56] X. Cao, D. Shen, M. M. Patel et al., "Macrophage polarization in the maculae of age-related macular degeneration: a pilot study," *Pathology International*, vol. 61, no. 9, pp. 528–535, 2011.

[57] T. Tobe, N. Okamoto, M. A. Vinores et al., "Evolution of neovascularization in mice with overexpression of vascular endothelial growth factor in photoreceptors," *Investigative Ophthalmology & Visual Science*, vol. 39, no. 1, pp. 180–188, 1998.

[58] H. Nambu, R. Nambu, Y. Oshima et al., "Angiopoietin 1 inhibits ocular neovascularization and breakdown of the blood-retinal barrier," *Gene Therapy*, vol. 11, no. 10, pp. 865–873, 2004.

[59] K. Takahashi, Y. Saishin, Y. Saishin et al., "Intraocular expression of endostatin reduces VEGF-induced retinal vascular permeability, neovascularization, and retinal detachment," *The FASEB Journal*, vol. 17, no. 8, pp. 896–8, 2003.

[60] A. Markovic, K. L. MacKenzie, and R. B. Lock, "Induction of vascular endothelial growth factor secretion by childhood acute lymphoblastic leukemia cells via the FLT-3 signaling pathway," *Molecular Cancer Therapeutics*, vol. 11, no. 1, pp. 183–193, 2012.

10

Ologen Implantation versus Conjunctival Autograft Transplantation for Treatment of Pterygium

Xiuping Chen ⓘ and Fei Yuan ⓘ

Department of Ophthalmology, Zhongshan Hospital of Fudan University, Shanghai, China

Correspondence should be addressed to Fei Yuan; yuan.fei@zs-hospital.sh.cn

Academic Editor: Cosimo Mazzotta

Purpose. To evaluate the effectiveness and safety of Ologen implantation versus conjunctival autograft transplantation for primary pterygium. *Methods.* A retrospective case-series analysis. Thirty-one eyes of 29 patients were included in the Ologen group and 42 eyes of 35 patients in the autograft group. The patients were followed up for 1 year and evaluated for slit-lamp biomicroscopy, intraocular pressure, and adverse events. Recurrence rate, complications, and final appearance of the cases were evaluated prospectively. *Result.* At 1 year after operation, 2 eyes recurred (6.5%) in the Ologen group and 4 eyes recurred (9.52%) in the autograft group. There was no statistically significant difference between both groups ($P = 0.157$, $\chi^2 = 3.781$). There was no occurrence of serious complications. Two eyes among the 31 eyes of the Ologen group were conjunctivitis; the incidence of complications was 6.45% (2 eyes). There was conjunctivitis in 3 eyes of the autograft group, 1 eye complicated with symblepharon, and 1 eye with conjunctival granuloma; the incidence of complications was 11.90% (5 eyes), and there was no statistically significant difference between both groups ($P = 0.094$). The conjintuva was less vascular and inflamed at 1 month postoperatively in the Ologen group than in the autograft group. *Conclusions.* Ologen transplantation was technically easier, provided short operative time compared with conjunctival autograft transplantation, and preserved healthy conjunctiva with less complication and less recurrence; it may be a new, safe, and effective alternative for improving the short-term success rate of primary surgery.

1. Introduction

Pterygium, a wing-shaped fibrovascular proliferation growth that extends from the conjunctiva onto the cornea, is one of the most common conjunctival surface degenerative disorders [1]. Chronic ultraviolet light exposure, wind, dryness, and other factors may contribute to the formation of pterygium [2, 3]. It can impair vision through altered tear film [4], induced astigmatism, photophobia with a reported prevalence of 0.3% to 29% [3].

Currently, the only effective treatment for pterygia is surgery, but recurrence after surgery remains a great challenge. So, a number of different surgical approaches have been proposed which can be divided into 3 basic types: (1) bare sclera excision, (2) tissue grafting using conjunctival autograft, and (3) amniotic membrane or Ologen transplantation. Among these strategies, variable recurrence rates

have been reported. The simple bare sclera excision is associated with a high recurrence rate up to 88% [5]. Conjunctival autograft transplantation showed low recurrence and complications rates [6]; it prevents recurrence by implanting the conjunctiva harvested from the superior bulbar conjunctiva to the bare sclera, acting as a barrier preventing migration of the nasal conjunctiva [7]. Although tissue grafting is significantly more time consuming and more difficult than leaving bare sclera, it shows a low recurrence rate from 5% to 15% [8]. However, these techniques are associated with their own complications [9].

Ologen (Ologen, Pro Top and Mediking Co./Ologen, Aeon Astron Europe, Netherlands), a 3D collagen-glycosaminoglycan scaffold, is specifically designed to promote wound healing with minimal scarring and low immunogenicity in a wide range of ophthalmic surgeries [10–12]. Our previous [13] study reported that Ologen, compared with mitomycin C for treatment of primary open-angle glaucoma, had a higher success rate and more efficacy bleb. It is considered as a safe, simple and effective alternative to the use of fibrosis disease. Herein, we report the efficacy of recurrence prevention-compared Ologen transplantation with conjunctival autograft surgery in primary pterygium.

2. Materials and Methods

A retrospective medical record review was conducted on patients who underwent pterygium surgery combined with Ologen or conjunctival autograft at Zhongshan Hospital of Fudan University between January 2006 and December 2015. All surgeries were performed by a single surgeon. A total of 136 patients (162 eyes) underwent both pterygium surgeries. Patients fulfilling the following study criteria were enrolled in the study: (a) diagnosis of a single-head primary pterygium on the basis of history and clinical examination; (b) a minimum follow-up period of 12 months; (c) age 18 years or more; and (d) no presence of coexistent ocular surface diseases. This study was conducted in accordance with the declaration of Helsinki and approved by the ethics committee of ZhongShan Hospital of Fudan University.

2.1. Surgical Methods. In the Ologen group, all surgeries were performed by the same surgeon under a surgical microscope in the following manner and sequence: (1) topical anaesthesia was administered with 0.5% proparacaine; (2) the head and body of the pterygium which included the conjunctiva and underlying Tenon's layer was excised by a scissor; (3) removed down to bare sclera from the incision to the cornea limbus and dissected off the head with a surgical blade. The body of the pterygium which included the conjunctiva and underlying Tenon's layer was carefully excised; (4) after removing the remnant tissue on the sclera, put the Ologen under the conjunctival flap; (5) left a 2.0 mm width of bare sclera at the limbus; (6) sutured the flap with 10-0 nylon on the sclera (Figure 1). In conjunctival autograft transplantation group, a conjunctival free graft with similar size was obtained from the superotemporal bulbar conjunctiva. The autograft's limbal side was sutured to the cornea limbal side with 10-0 nylon. Operation did not exceed 30 minutes in all cases, and no complications occurred during surgeries.

Postoperatively, topical tobramycin 0.3% and dexamethasone 0.1% (Tobradex; Alcon Pharmaceuticals, Fort Worth, Texas, USA) was given every four times per day for 2 weeks. 10-0 nylon sutures were removed seven days after surgery. Patients were examined at 1 day, 1 week, 6 months, and 1 year postoperatively. During each visit, routine ocular examination was performed, including external eye photography, slit-lamp biomicroscopy, and intraocular pressure. Recurrence is commonly defined as a recurrent pterygium greater than 1 mm in size anterior to the limbus.

2.2. Statistical Analysis. Categorical variables were analyzed using the chi-square test, and continuous variables were analyzed using the unpaired Student's *t*-test. Continuous variables were presented as mean±standard deviation. Discrete variables were presented as percentages and analyzed using Fisher's exact test. The data were analyzed using SPSS software (version 21.0; SPSS Inc., Chicago, IL, USA). Correlation was considered significant at P value <0.05.

3. Results

The basic profile of patients in the study is shown in Table 1. Thirty-one eyes of 29 patients were included in the Ologen group and 42 eyes of 35 patients in autograft group. The mean age of the Ologen group patients was 56.73 ± 9.04 years (range 45–67 years) and 54.94 ± 10.52 years (range 42–73 years) in the autograft group. There were 10 (32.26%) males and 19 (61.29%) females in the Ologen group and 15 (35.71%) males and 20 (47.62%) females in the autograft group. Pterygium was diagnosed in 18 (58.06%) right eyes and 13 (41.94%) left eyes in the Ologen group. In the autograft group, it was diagnosed in 24 (57.14%) right eyes and 18 (42.86%) left eyes. The pterygium size in the Ologen group varied from 1.5 to 4.2 mm (mean 2.89 ± 0.64 mm). In the autograft group, it varied from 1.7 to 4.5 mm (mean 3.01 ± 0.52 mm). There was no statistically significant difference between both groups.

The postoperative recurrence rates are shown in Table 2. At 1 year after operation, 2 eyes recurred (6.5%) in the 31 eyes of the Ologen group, and 4 eyes recurred (9.52%) in the 41 eyes of the autograft group. There was no statistically significant difference between both groups ($P = 0.157$, $\chi^2 = 3.781$).

The postoperative complications in both groups are shown in Table 3. Two eyes in 31 eyes of the Ologen group were conjunctivitis; the incidence of complications was 6.45% (2 eyes). There were conjunctivitis in 3 eyes of the autograft group, 1 eye concurring with symblepharon, and 1 eye complicated with conjunctival granuloma; the incidence of complications was 11.90% (5 eyes), and there was no statistically significant difference between both groups ($P = 0.094$).

Postoperative slit-lamp photographs are shown in Figure 2. The conjunctiva was less vascular and inflamed at 1 month postoperatively in the Ologen group than in the autograft group.

4. Discussion

Pterygium remains an important health care issue in China. The prevalence of pterygium was 3.7% in northern China and 37.4% in southern China [14], which suggested that ultraviolet exposure and ultraviolet radiation were important risk factors [15]. Up to now, surgery was the main treatment for pterygium [16]. Fibrosis causes adherence of the conjunctiva and Tenon's capsule, which may lead to recurrence, and it is dependent on the patient's inflammatory response [17]. The recurrence rate of simple excision results in high recurrence from 24% to 89%. The use of mitomycin C and other antiproliferative drugs can reduce the recurrence rate, but many complications such as delayed

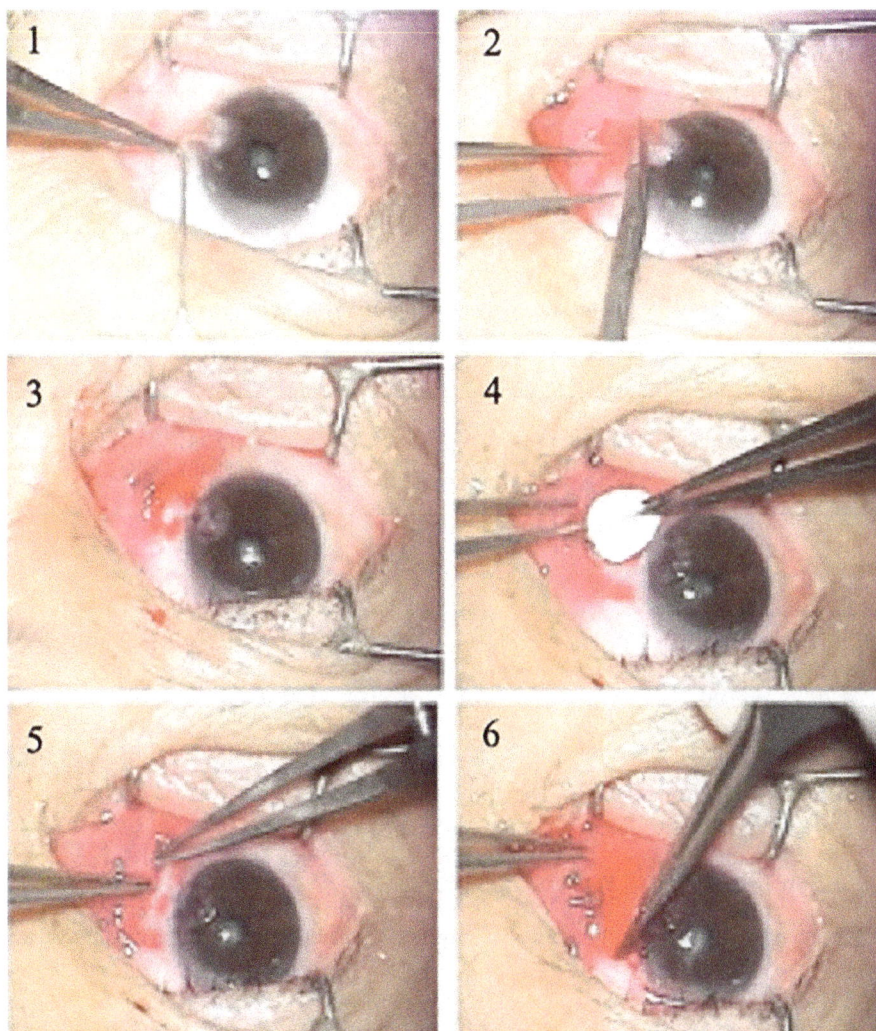

FIGURE 1: The surgery procedure of pterygium excision combined with Ologen implantation. 1: topical anaesthesia. 2: the head and body of the pterygium was excised by a scissor. 3: removed down to bare sclera. 4: put the Ologen under the conjunctival flap. 5: left a 2.0 mm width of bare sclera at the limbus. 6: sutured the flap with 10-0 nylon on the sclera.

TABLE 1: Preoperative characteristics of patients in both groups.

Parameter	Ologen ($n = 31$)	Autograft ($n = 42$)	P value
Age (mean $\pm$ SD)	56.73 ± 9.04	54.94 ± 10.52	0.522^a
Gender (male/female)	10/19	15/20	0.444^b
Eye (right/left)	18/13	24/18	0.212^b
Pterygium size	2.89 ± 0.64 mm	3.01 ± 0.52 mm	0.507^a

[a]Independent Student's t-test. [b]χ^2 test or Fisher's exact test.

healing of the corneal epithelium and scleral ulcers can also be caused. Conjunctival autograft transplantation is a technically difficult and time-consuming procedure and a sacrificed part of the healthy conjunctiva. It may affect the outcome of surgical procedures that require healthy conjunctiva such as trabeculectomy if needed in the future for those patients [18].

Ologen is a three-dimensional porous collagen-glycosaminoglycan copolymer, taken from the matrix of porcine collagen, helps the reorganization of subconjunctival scar formation by separating the subconjunctival and episcleral tissues and inducing fibroblasts and myofibroblasts to grow in the structure after surgical excision of pterygium. It provides a good growth environment for the fibroblasts in the eye and guides the fibroblasts to grow on the pores of the matrix in a discrete manner, so that the wound's healing process will be physiological, and the tissue scar will be inhibited [19]. Remnants between the sclera and conjunctiva may induce recurrence, Ologen was used as a spacer to mechanically separate the subconjunctival and episcleral tissues to prevent fibrosis, it can completely fill this gap and may reduce the recurrence rate. The operation of Ologen implantation is simple.

In this study, Ologen was implanted under the conjunctiva at the same time while pterygium was excised. Two eyes in the 31 eyes were recurred at 1 year postoperatively. The recurrence rate was 6.45%. In the conjunctival autograft group, 4 eyes in the 42 eyes were recurred. The recurrence rate was 9.52%. There was no statistically significant difference between both groups ($P = 0.157$, $\chi^2 = 3.781$). According to the

TABLE 2: The postoperative recurrence rates in both groups.

| Group | Corneal invasion | | | | | | Recurrence (1 y) |
| | <1/2 preoperation | | Between 1/2 and 1 | | Equal to preoperation | | |
	6 m	1 y	6 m	1 y	6 m	1 y	
Ologen	1(3.23)	0(0)	0(0)	1(3.23)	1(3.23)	1(3.23)	2(6.45)
Autograft	1(2.38)	1(2.38)	0(0)	1(2.38)	1(2.38)	2(4.76)	4(9.52)
P value	0.626	0.524	N/A	0.626	N/A	0.431	0.157

TABLE 3: The postoperative complications in both groups.

Complications	Ologen ($n = 31$, n(%))	Autograft ($n = 42$, n(%))	P value
Conjunctivitis	2(6.45)	3(7.14)	0.668
Symblepharon	0(0)	1(2.38)	0.524
Granuloma	0(0)	1(2.38)	0.524
Total	2(6.45)	5(11.90)	0.094

Ologen Autograft

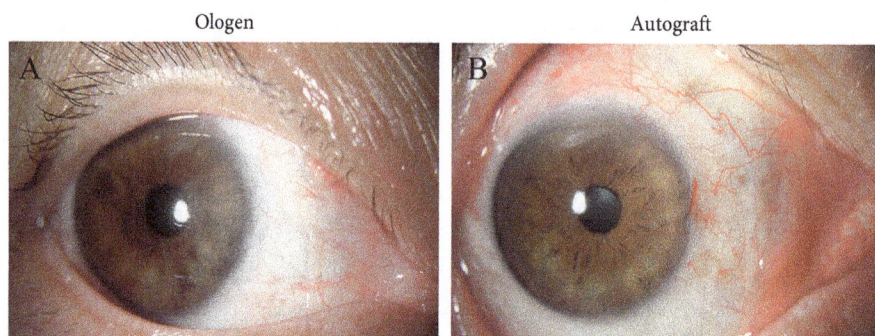

FIGURE 2: (a) Postoperative photo of Ologen group 1 month after surgery. (b) Postoperative photo of conjuntival autograft group 1 month after surgery.

results, the recurrence rate of pterygium after surgery was low in both groups. But in the Ologen group, the recurrence rate is lower than that of the conjunctival autograft group. The surgical complications in the Ologen group are two conjunctivitis; the incidence of complications was 6.45%. In the autograft group, there were three conjunctivitis, one symblepharon, and one granuloma. The incidence of complications was 11.90%. Though there was no statistically significant difference between both groups ($P = 0.094$), in the Ologen group, the complications were less, the safety was higher. It is a safe and effective measure to reduce the postoperative recurrence and complication.

Postoperative inflammation caused by tissue damage induces activation of the fibroblasts of the subconjunctival tissue and induces recurrence [20]. According to the slit-lamp photographs taken 1 month postoperatively, the conjunctiva was less vascular and inflamed in the Ologen group than in the autograft group. This maybe attributed to Ologen's characteristics. Ologen is composed of a porous matrix of cross-linked atelocollagen and glycosaminoglycan. It contains thousands of microscopic pores and can induce fibroblast growth, leading to a minimal scarring and low immunogenicity healing process. Our previous study showed that Ologen created a diffuse bleb in trabeculectomy. It can inhibit scar formation postoperatively. Another

important reason may be that Ologen implantation surgery is a time-saving and less tissue-damaging operation.

We concluded that both techniques used in the current study proved to be effective in reducing the recurrence rate after excision of primary pterygium with minimal complications in the short term postoperatively. Ologen implantation was technically easier, provided short operative time compared with conjunctival autograft transplantation, and preserved healthy conjunctiva. Ologen implantation has the advantage of less complication and less recurrence, it may be a new, safe, and effective alternative for improving the short-term success rate of primary surgery. We will continue to follow up and verify the effectiveness of Ologen. However, larger randomized trials are required to investigate the long-term efficacy and safety of this device.

Conflicts of Interest

The authors have no proprietary or commercial interest in any materials discussed in this article. The authors declare that there are no conflicts of interest regarding the publication of this paper.

Acknowledgments

This study was supported by grants from Beijing Bethune Charitable Foundation (BJ-LM2017001J).

References

[1] L. P. Ang, J. L. Chua, and D. T. Tan, "Current concepts and techniques in pterygium treatment," *Current Opinion in Ophthalmology*, vol. 18, pp. 308–313, 2007.

[2] J. Chui, N. Di Girolamo, D. Wakefield, and M. T. Coroneo, "The pathogenesis of pterygium: current concepts and their therapeutic implications," *Ocular Surface*, vol. 6, no. 1, pp. 24–43, 2008.

[3] L. Liu, J. Wu, J. Geng, Z. Yuan, and D. Huang, "Geographical prevalence and risk factors for pterygium: a systematic review and meta-analysis," *BMJ Open*, vol. 3, no. 11, article e003787, 2013.

[4] M. Ozsutcu, B. Arslan, S. K. Erdur, G. Gulkilik, S. M. Kocabora, and O. Muftuoglu, "Tear osmolarity and tear film parameters in patients with unilateral pterygium," *Cornea*, vol. 33, no. 11, pp. 1174–1178, 2014.

[5] O. Kocamis and M. Bilgec, "Evaluation of the recurrence rate for pterygium treated with conjunctival autograft," *Graefe's Archive for Clinical and Experimental Ophthalmology*, vol. 252, no. 5, pp. 817–820, 2014.

[6] E. Clearfield, V. Muthappan, X. Wang, and I. C. Kuo, "Conjunctival autograft for pterygium," *Cochrane database of Systematic Reviews*, vol. 2, article CD011349, 2016.

[7] H. S. Hwang, K. J. Cho, G. Rand, R. S. Chuck, and J. W. Kwon, "Optimal size of pterygium excision for limbal conjunctival autograft using fibrin glue in primary pterygia," *BMC Ophthalmology*, vol. 18, no. 1, p. 135, 2018.

[8] X. Pan, D. Zhang, Z. Jia, Z. Chen, and Y. Su, "Comparison of hyperdry amniotic membrane transplantation and conjunctival autografting for primary pterygium," *BMC Ophthalmology*, vol. 18, no. 1, p. 119, 2018.

[9] N. S. Aidenloo, Q. Motarjemizadeh, and M. Heidarpanah, "Risk factors for pterygium recurrence after limbal-conjunctival autografting: a retrospective, single-centre investigation," *Japanese Journal of Ophthalmology*, vol. 62, no. 3, pp. 349–356, 2018.

[10] H. M. Marey, S. S. Mandour, and A. F. Ellakwa, "Subscleral trabeculectomy with mitomycin-C versus ologen for treatment of glaucoma," *Journal of Ocular Pharmacology and Therapeutics*, vol. 29, no. 3, pp. 330–334, 2013.

[11] S. Cillino, F. Di Pace, G. Cillino, and A. Casuccio, "Biodegradable collagen matrix implant vs mitomycin-C as an adjuvant in trabeculectomy: a 24-month, randomized clinical trial," *Eye*, vol. 25, no. 12, pp. 1598–1606, 2011.

[12] C. H. Cho and S. B. Lee, "Biodegradable collagen matrix (Ologen™) implant and conjunctival autograft for scleral necrosis after pterygium excision: two case reports," *BMC Ophthalmology*, vol. 15, no. 1, p. 140, 2015.

[13] F. Yuan, L. Li, X. Chen, X. Yan, and L. Wang, "Biodegradable 3D-porous collagen matrix (ologen) compared with mitomycin C for treatment of primary open-angle glaucoma: results at 5 years," *Journal of Ophthalmology*, vol. 2015, Article ID 637537, 2015.

[14] Z. Li and H. Cui, "Prevalence and associated factors for pterygium in a rural adult population (the Southern Harbin Eye Study)," *Cornea*, vol. 32, no. 6, pp. 806–809, 2013.

[15] W. P. Zhou, Y. F. Zhu, B. Zhang, W. Y. Qiu, and Y. F. Yao, "The role of ultraviolet radiation in the pathogenesis of pterygia (Review)," *Molecular Medicine Reports*, vol. 14, no. 1, pp. 3–15, 2016.

[16] A. V. Petrayevsky and K. S. Trishkin, "Surgical treatment of pterygium," *Vestnik oftal'mologii*, vol. 134, no. 1, pp. 85–88, 2018.

[17] Y. Y. Chen, C. F. Tsai, M. C. Tsai, W. K. Chen, and Y. W. Hsu, "Anti-fibrotic effect of rosmarinic acid on inhibition of pterygium epithelial cells," *International Journal of Ophthalmology*, vol. 11, no. 2, pp. 189–195, 2018.

[18] J. S. Lee, S. W. Ha, S. Yu, G. J. Lee, and Y. J. Park, "Efficacy and safety of a large conjunctival autograft for recurrent pterygium," *Korean Journal of Ophthalmology*, vol. 31, no. 6, pp. 469–478, 2017.

[19] K. E. Han, S. Yoon, R. M. Jun, T. I. Kim, and E. K. Kim, "Conjunctival flap with biodegradable collagen matrix implantation for the treatment of scleromalacia after periocular surgery," *Ocular Immunology and Inflammation*, pp. 1–8, 2018.

[20] C. Da Costa Paula, G. Julio, P. Campos, P. Pujol, and M. Asaad, "Effects of mitomycin C in early conjunctival inflammation after pterygium surgery," *Current Eye Research*, vol. 42, no. 5, pp. 696–700, 2017.

11

Descriptive Study of Conjunctival Cysts: A Rare Complication after Strabismus Surgery

Xiaoshan Min ⑩,[1] Hui Jiang,[2] and Lingyan Shi[1]

[1]Department of Ophthalmology, Xiangya Hospital, Central South University, Changsha, Hunan Province, China
[2]Department of Ophthalmology, The Second Affiliated Hospital of Hunan University of Chinese Medicine, Changsha, Hunan Province, China

Correspondence should be addressed to Xiaoshan Min; minxiaoshan@csu.edu.cn

Academic Editor: Enrique Mencía-Gutiérrez

Aim. Conjunctival cyst is one of the uncommon complications of strabismus surgery. It is important for surgeons and patients to be aware of and take precautions to minimize the risk. This study aimed to explore the clinical manifestations, etiology, and prognosis of conjunctival cyst at the operative site after strabismus surgery. *Methods.* The data of 1675 patients were included in our retrospective analysis, who underwent strabismus surgery at the Xiangya Hospital of Central South University between 2010 and 2016. During the postoperative follow-up, conjunctival cyst was found in 7 cases (7 eyes; 0.4% detective rate of all cases). The clinical characteristics, prognosis, and follow-up data were recorded together with the results of pathological and bacteriological tests. *Results.* Seven patients between the age of 3 years 8 months and 39 years, with the mean age of 12.71 years (12.71 ± 12.59, years of age), were included in the study. Strabismus surgery affected 13 recti, 8 medial and 5 lateral recti, and 3 obliques (all inferior oblique). Conjunctival cyst was detected in seven patients between 10 days and 6 months postoperatively (42.57 ± 61.11, detected days). In six cases, the cyst was detected at the nasal (3 cases) or temporal side (other 3 cases), and at the fornix in one case. Four out of 7 patients underwent cyst excision, and methicillin-resistant Staphylococcus aureus (MRSA) was detected in one patient. *Conclusions.* Conjunctival cyst is a rare postoperative complication of strabismus surgery, conjunctival epithelium implantation should be the primary cause, and infection might exaggerate the situation. A longer duration of the surgical procedure could increase the possibility of infection, which could be accompanied with a greater tendency to the occurrence of conjunctival cyst.

1. Introduction

Strabismus is a common ocular disorder occurring at all ages, with an estimated prevalence of 2–5% in the general population [1–4]. The purpose of strabismus treatment is to improve ocular alignment and make bilateral eye movement concordant, as well as to recover or rebuild comfortable binocular vision [5]. Surgery is a common and effective cure for treatment of strabismus [6]. Combined with glasses, prisms-wearing, and visual training before and after surgery, strabismus surgery creates the opportunity of building and restoring binocular vision function and eventually improves the possibility of increasing of visual acuity, or even patients' quality of life [7, 8]. Strabismus surgery is also called extraocular muscle surgery; it is a minimally invasive surgery

under direct vision, with limited complications and quick recovery [9].

Conjunctival cyst is a rare complication after strabismus surgery; according to the time of onset, it is primarily caused by infection, conjunctival epithelial implantation, and chronic allergic response (probably a response to the suture). It typically manifests as a conjunctival abscess, granuloma or an epithelial inclusion cyst, and chronic or nonspecific inflammation [10, 11]. Most conjunctival cysts subside spontaneously, whereas surgery should be considered for cases not going into remission after a long period of time or those with symptoms, such as foreign body sensation, redness, swelling, hot, and painful eye [10, 11]. In this report, clinical data for 7 cases of conjunctival cyst, recorded by a strabismus surgeon at the Department of Pediatric

Ophthalmology, Xiangya Hospital of Central South University, were analyzed. The purpose of the study was to utilize the data and summarize the existing literature to provide an overview of the pathogenesis, progression, management, and prevention of this rare complication.

2. Subjects and Methods

2.1. Participants. This is a retrospective clinical study of 1675 patients who underwent strabismus surgery between 2010 and 2016 at the Department of Ophthalmology, Xiangya Hospital of Central South University, were included in the present study. The study was approved by the Medical Ethics Committee of the Xiangya Hospital of the Central South University.

2.2. Inclusion and Exclusion Criteria. Patients who met the following criteria were included in the study: (i) diagnosed with strabismus and underwent strabismus surgery; (ii) had a clinical examination performed once suspicious manifestations of conjunctival cyst were discovered during follow-up; and (iii) had conjunctival cyst located at the surgical site.

Patients who had other ocular conjunctiva-associated tumors or conjunctival hyperplasia were excluded from the study.

2.3. Methods

2.3.1. Surgical Modality. Surgery in all patients was performed by a surgeon with more than 20 years of specialization in strabismus and amblyopia treatment. All adults, as well as adolescents who understood the procedure and were cooperative, were given topical anesthesia (qxybuprocaine hydrochloride eye drops, Benoxil®, Santen Pharmaceutical Co. Ltd., Japen) only. No sedation was used. General anesthesia was given to the remaining patients. Park's conjunctival incision was made in parallel on and below the limbus, and the broken end of the muscle was fixated with the double-loop suture technique by an absorbable suture 6-0 (6-0 Coated Coated Vicryl® absorbable, Ethicon, INC, Ethicon, INC), one suture for one muscle, seamed to the designed site on scleral, followed by suturing of the conjunctival incision with absorbable 8-0 (8-0 Coated Vicryl® absorbable, Ethicon, INC). Postoperative local antibiotics (tobramycin/ofloxacin) and steroid (dexamethasone) eye drops were administered to all patients three times daily for 2 weeks.

2.3.2. Follow-Up. All patients were subjected to a follow-up schedule of 6 weeks, 3 months, 6 months' postsurgery, and every 6 months afterwards. In order to remind the patients of timely follow-up, trained nurses would ask the patients about the condition of the incision, vision status, adherence to the medication regimen, and other types of discomfort at one and three months after surgery. A QR code for access to the surgeon's personal web page at Good Doctor website was provided to every patient to facilitate direct communication with the primary surgeon. The patients or the parents were

all informed of possible occurrence of conjunctival cyst and its main symptoms. Once the chief complaint from patients was identified as a conjunctival cyst, an appointment was made at the hospital immediately.

3. Results

Seven patients (7 eyes; 7out of 1675), between the ages of 3 years and 8 months and 39 years (mean age of 12.71 years (12.71 ± 12.59 years old)), presented with conjunctival cyst at different time points postoperatively. Strabismus surgery affected 13 recti, including 8 medial and 5 lateral recti, and 3 obliques (all inferior obliques). Conjunctival cysts were located at the nasal in 3 cases and temporal side in other 3 cases and at the fornix with inferior oblique surgery in 1 case. The time of discovery of the conjunctival cyst ranged from 10 days to 6 months postoperatively (the detected days, mean time of 42.57 ± 61.11 days). According to the sequence of operation on muscles, there are 2 cases affected at the first or the only operated muscle, 3 cases affected at the second muscle of the first eye, while 2 other cases affected at the second operated eye, as summarized in Table 1.

3.1. Case 1. A 39-year-old female patient underwent surgery under local anesthesia following the diagnosis of concomitant exotropia. In the month following the surgery, the patient complained of a foreign body sensation. A conjunctival cyst was visualized at the middle nasal side of the right eye, with severe conjunctival congestion (Figure 1(a)). Tobramycin and dexamethasone eye drops (Tobradex®, SA Alcon-Couvreur NV, Belgium) were applied 4 times daily for 1 week, together with deproteinized calf blood extract eye gel (Shenyang Xing Qi Ophthalmic Limited by Share Ltd, China) for 2 weeks. The conjunctival cyst resolved in the next 1 month.

3.2. Case 2. A 10-year-old male patient underwent strabismus surgery twice (in 2009 and 2015) under general anesthesia following the diagnosis of concomitant exotropia. At 2 weeks postoperatively in 2015, the patient complained of redness affecting the left eye (the second operated eye) and a conjunctival cyst was found at the nasal side. Postoperative medication was further administered for one week, and the cyst resolved in the 1st month follow-up examination.

3.3. Case 3. A 4-year-old male patient underwent surgery under general anesthesia following the diagnosis of concomitant exotropia. There weeks postoperatively, his mother found a hyaline cyst of the conjunctiva at the inferior temporal right eye next to the fornix, without evidence of congestion. The patient showed no obvious discomfort, and no specific treatment was applied. At the 5-year follow-up, no change has been reported (Figure 1(b)).

3.4. Case 4. A 14-year-old male patient underwent surgery under local anesthesia following the diagnosis of concomitant exotropia. Two weeks later, a conjunctival cyst

TABLE 1: Patient characteristics.

Case number	Sex	Age (yrs)	Surgical modality	Cyst site	Discovery time	Primary symptoms	The operated sequence of affected muscle	Treatment and prognosis	Pathology	Bacteria culture
1	Female	39	Right lateral rectus recession and medial rectus resection	Middle right nasal	1 month	Foreign object sense	Sole surgical eye, the 2nd muscle	Spontaneous remission	NA	NA
2	Male	10	Right lateral rectus recession and medial rectus resection in 2009, bilateral inferior oblique myectomy + medial rectus recession in 2015	Left subnosal	2 weeks	Redness	The 2nd surgical eye	Spontaneous remission	NA	NA
3	Male	4	Right lateral rectus recession and medial rectus resection	Inferior temporal fornix	>20 days	Conjunctival cyst found	Sole operated eye, the 1st muscle	Asymptomatic persistent	NA	Negative
4	Male	14	Right medial rectus recession and lateral rectus resection	Right temporal	2 weeks	Foreign body sense and cyst found	The 2nd muscle of operated eye	Excision at 6 weeks postoperative	NA	Negative
5	Female	15	Bilateral rectus recession and right medial rectus resection	5 × 5 mm, middle right temporal	6 months	Foreign body sense and cyst found	The 2nd operated eye	Excision at 2 years postoperative	Squamous epithelium	Negative
6	Female	3	Inferior oblique myectomy	Right inferior fornix	1 month	Restriction of eye movement, swelling of the eyelid.	Sole operated eye, the only muscle	Excision at 4 months postoperative	Dermoid cyst	Negative
7	Female	4	Bilateral medial rectus recession	Left nasal	10 days	Cyst found	The 2nd operated eye, the 2nd muscle	Excision at 6 months postoperative	Inflammation, single-layer epithelium	MRSA+

was found at the left temporal side, with evidence of conjunctival congestion. Tobramycin and dexamethasone eye drops and ointment (Tobradex, SA Alcon-Couvreur NV, Belgium) were applied for 1 week, and the cyst remained unresolved. The patient stopped treatment by himself. Although he showed no symptoms, exploratory surgery of the cyst was performed at the 6th week follow-up (Figure 1(c)). No purulent fluid was detected in the cyst, and mild necrosis was found in the adjacent soft tissues; the suture was not fully absorbed. The suture segment was completely removed and tested negative in bacterial culture.

3.5. Case 5. A 15-year-old female patient underwent surgery under local anesthesia following the diagnosis of concomitant exotropia. Six months postoperatively, the patient complained of foreign body sensation, and a conjunctival cyst, 5 × 5 mm, was found at the right middle temporal side (Figure 2(a)). The cyst was surgically excised 2 years

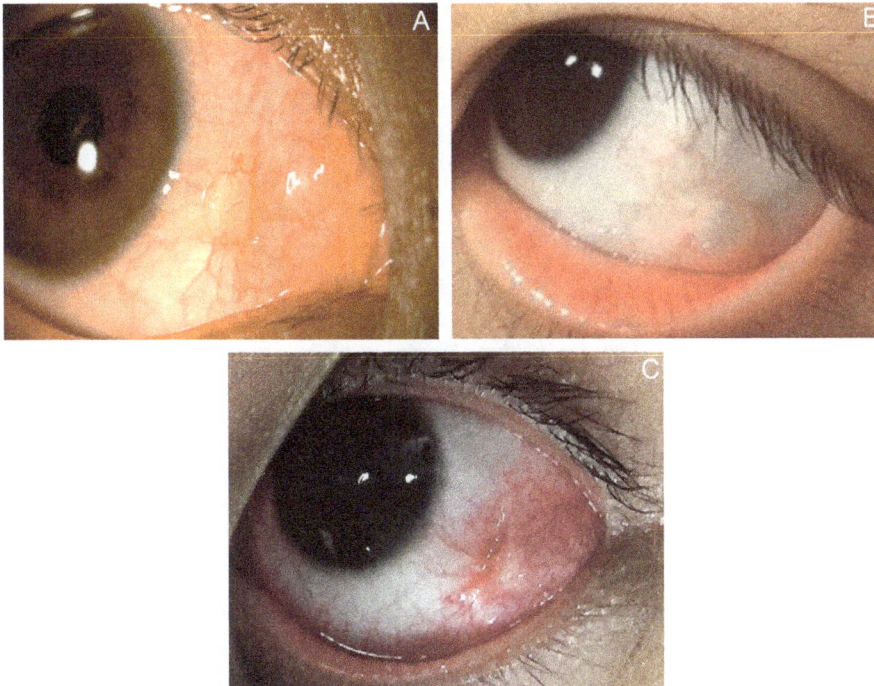

FIGURE 1: Conjunctival cysts at the left temporal side for Case 1 (a), Case 3 (b), and Case 4 (c).

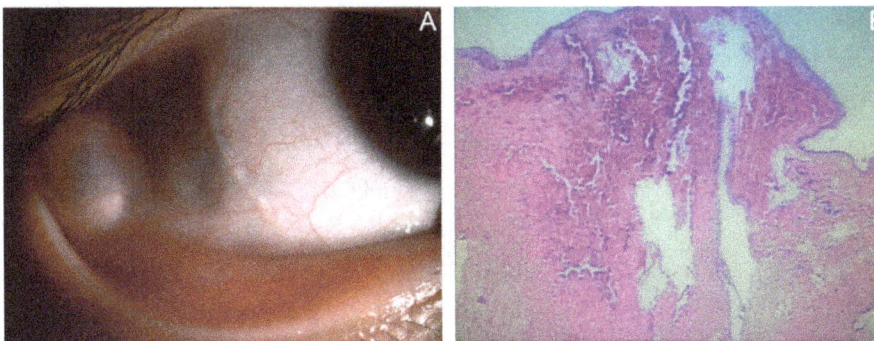

FIGURE 2: (a) Conjunctival cyst at the right temporal side in Case 5; (b) histopathological picture of right conjunctival cyst.

postoperatively. Pathological results showed that the cyst wall was coated with stratified squamous epithelium, with fibrous connective tissue in the cyst cavity (Figure 2(b)).

3.6. Case 6. A 3-year, 8-month-old female patient underwent disinsertion of right inferior oblique and general anesthesia and following the diagnosis of "right superior oblique muscle paralysis." During the first postoperative month, the patient's mother found her eye showed a restricted up-gaze and limited inferior turn (Figure 3(a)), and swelling of the lower right eyelid was also evident due to the massive size of the cyst. But the patient did not report any discomfort. Conjunctival cyst was found at the inferior fornix conjunctiva. A B-ultrasound scan found cystic degeneration area, irregular in shape, at the subcutaneous region of the lower right eyelid, with clear boundaries, intracystic compartments, and multiple uneven medium to strong echoic masses. Computed tomography (CT) images revealed irregular high-density foci inferior and

external to the right eyeball, with uneven internal density and no enhanced signal. Furthermore, signs of evident compression and superior dislocation of the right eyeball and optic nerve were present, as well as an intact eye ring without bone damage. The image diagnosis was recommended as "hematoma considered." Local application of Levofloxacin eye drops (0.5%, Santen Pharmaceutical Co. Ltd., Japen) combined with tobramycin and dexamethasone eye drops (Tobradex, SA Alcon-Couvreur NV, Belgium) 3 times per day for 2 weeks, resulted in no relief. The cyst was then surgically excised at 4 months postoperatively (Figure 3(b)). Intraoperative findings showed a cystic mass on the surface of the right inferior rectus, with intact cystic wall enclosing caviar-like particles and transparent cystic fluid. The dimensions of the cyst were approximately $6 \times 5 \times 4$ mm, and it was not tightly attached to adjacent tissues. Pathological results revealed a cyst wall coated with stratified squamous epithelium, with fibrous connective tissue in the cyst cavity. The diagnosis of a benign conjunctival cyst was made (Figure 3(c)). Gram

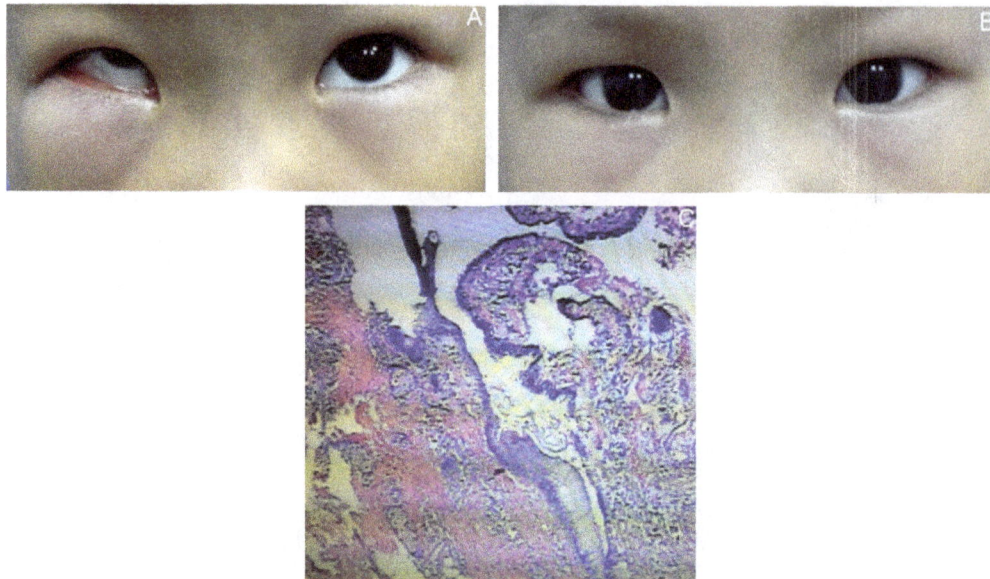

FIGURE 3: (a) Conjunctival cyst at right inferior fornix in Case 6; (b) four months after surgical excision of conjunctival cyst; (c) histopathological picture of conjunctival cyst.

staining revealed occasional G⁻ bacilli, but bacterial culture was negative.

3.7. Case 7. A 4-year-old female patient underwent surgery under general anesthesia following the diagnosis of concomitant exotropia. Ten days following the strabismus surgery, the patient showed subconjunctival cyst in the left eye, without evident symptoms (Figure 4(a)). Surgical exploration discovered thin purulent fluid in the subconjunctival cyst, with no evident capsule and an unclear boundary mostly made up of necrotic soft tissue. The broken end of medial rectus was firmly attached to the sclera surface (surgical design: 5 mm posterior insertion) and the initial muscle suture (6-0 Coated Vicryl absorbable, Ethicon, INC) was intact but loose; therefore, it was removed. A portion of necrotic tissue was extracted for bacterial and fungal culture tests, as well as a pathological test which revealed (left subconjunctival) chronic suppurative inflammation (Figure 4(b)). Postoperative bacterial culture was positive for methicillin-resistant Staphylococcus aureus (MRSA) infection. According to a drug sensitivity test, vancomycin (0.25 g, q8h) was administered via intravenous drip, combined with local antibiotic and corticosteroid eye drops (Tobradex, SA Alcon-Couvreur NV, Belgium). Five days postoperatively, scant mucous discharge was present at the conjunctival incision suture (Figure 4(c)). Therefore, the conjunctival suture was removed. At the first postoperative follow-up 1 month after the surgery, a complete recovery of conjunctival incision (Figure 4(d)) with right binocular alignment was shown.

4. Discussion

We can find sporadic reports of surgical implantation cysts involve patients who had strabismus surgery [12], retinal detachment surgery with scleral buckling [13], or previous enucleation [14]. Conjunctival cyst is a rare complication of strabismus surgery, with a reported incidence of 0.25% [15]; in our study, we detected 7 cases in 1675 patients, and the rate of detection is 0.4%, which might not be the actual incidence rate of conjunctival cysts. There are several types of conjunctival cyst following surgery: conjunctival epithelium implantation, subconjunctival abscess, chronic granuloma, and conjunctival stress edema [6].

It is generally believed that conjunctival epithelium implantation was the main cause for conjunctival cyst after strabismus surgery. Our observation reported similar results. Three cases (Case 5, Case 6, and Case 7) were confirmed by pathological analysis to be epithelial cysts, which may be associated with conjunctival epithelium implantation. One case (Case 3) had a persistent existence of conjunctival cysts for several years, and the cysts did not resolve after antibiotic eye drops and anti-inflammatory treatments. It is highly possible that conjunctival epithelium implantation played a major role in these cases.

Khan et al. [16] reported a misdiagnosis of infected epithelial inclusion cyst and proposed that presumed subconjunctival abscess after strabismus surgery could all be infected epithelial inclusion cyst. In our study, the pathological section of Case 7 showed the cyst wall was composed of epithelium, and a history of living in kindergarten shortly after operation, which might indicate the possibility of an exogenous infection with epithelial encapsulated cyst formation. Song et al. [12] suggested that a massive conjunctival inclusion cyst may form rapidly when serious infection, such as orbital cellulitis, endophthalmitis takes place due to severe pollution or immune hypofunction. Several groups reported orbital cellulitis occurred days after strabismus surgery [17–19].

Surgery is usually a frequent cause of acquired infection. In the seven cases analyzed in this study, all strabismus surgeries were performed in a laminar flow operation room,

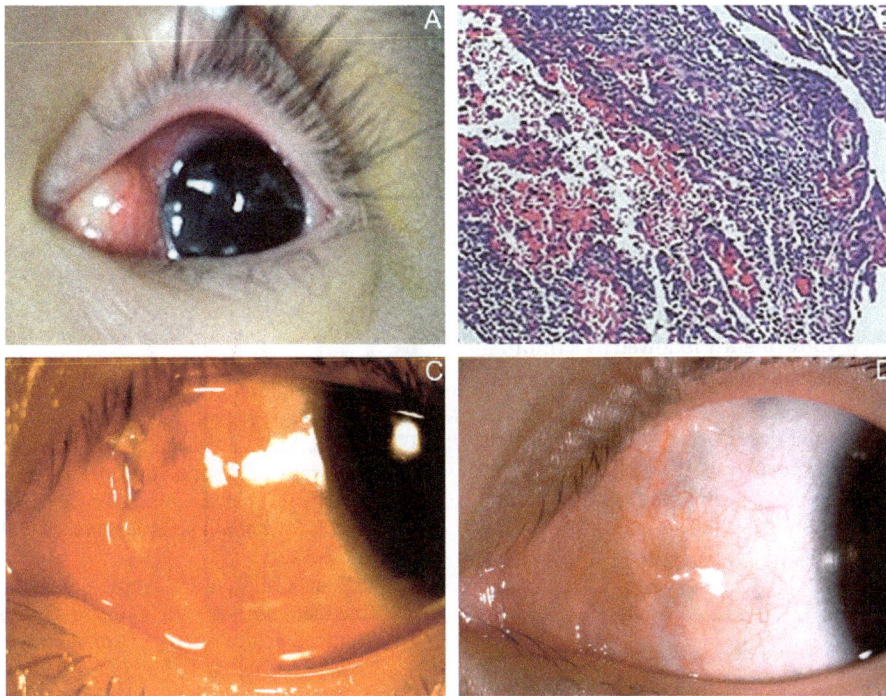

FIGURE 4: (a) A 7 × 8 mm conjunctival cyst at the left nasal side prior to exploratory surgery in Case 7; (b) postoperative histopathological picture; (c) suture extending out of incision at the left side; (d) wound resolved after left conjunctival suture removal.

and antibiotic eye drops were administered for 3 days before surgery and two weeks after surgery as a precaution. Also, a routine preoperative rinse of the conjunctival cyst was performed with povidone-iodine antibacterial eyewash. Therefore, we suggest a possible cause of early-stage (first month after operation) inflammation is suture response, which is a pathological reaction to suture material in susceptible individuals. A foreign body may induce an immunological rejection, or inflammation, or other factors resulting in a suture response. It has been reported that Vicryl absorptive suture can cause a serious response in the early period after suturing [20]. Absorptive suture is made by multistrand cross knitting and multistrand braiding around one main line, which makes it susceptible to bacterial attachment.

In their randomized, controlled study, Eustis and coworkers [21] found a higher than estimated incidence of needle and suture contamination after strabismus surgery, a 28% bacterial contamination rate for sterile sutures, which is close to the 15–25.2% contamination rate reported by Olitsky et al. [22] and Carothers and coworkers [23]. Even though absorptive sutures used in strabismus surgery are stored in sterile packages, they can touch the eyelashes and skin during operation and get contaminated by germs (mostly conditional pathogenic bacteria) from the hair follicles adjacent to the incision.

A different study found that the same bacterial colony causes infection post cataract surgery as the one residing in the patient's extraocular tissue [24]. Also, the possibility of bacterial contamination of the operative environment cannot be excluded either. During surgery, the 6-0 Vicryl absorbable suture is preset at the broken end of muscle; its distal end can touch the margins of the eyelid and the

eyelashes, even the regions outside of the operative field. In agreement with this hypothesis, coagulase-negative Staphylococci were found on the eyelid and eyelashes in a previous study [23]. In Cases 4 and 7, nonabsorbent suture segment was visualized floating in the cystic fluid during resection of the conjunctival cyst. The culture of the suture segment was negative for Case 4 and positive for MRSA for Case 7. The negative bacteria culture result of Case 4 could be affected by the effective antibiotic eye drops used before surgery.

Common pathogenic bacteria causing infection after strabismus surgery include Staphylococcus aureus, Staphylococcus epidermidis, Streptococcus pneumoniae, and Haemophilus influenzae. Statistical data from a comprehensive hospital trial (all departments) revealed that the primary pathogens causing acquired hospital infection include Escherichia coli [24], Staphylococcus aureus, and Proteus mirabilis [23]. Among them, anaerobic bacteria, such as Pseudomonas aeruginosa and MRSA, are particularly common in a surgery setting. In a large-scale survey, Kivlin and Wilson [17] reported 308 forms of postoperative infection after strabismus surgery, which was carried out at multiple hospitals affiliated with the American Academy of Strabismus and Pediatric Ophthalmology. Staphylococcus aureus was isolated in 56% of 25 cases. Among the 25 cases, sub-Tenon's abscess was found in 3 cases. All three cases experienced symptoms in the first week after the surgery, with positive cultures for Proteus mirabilis and Staphylococcus aureus obtained. Since 1988, MRSA incidence has been on the rise. One study uncovered type II coagulase as the only coagulase type in MRSA, which is also one of the most common colonies causing acquired hospital infection [25]. Since the late 1990s, the incidence rate of community-associated MRSA (CA-MRSA) has increased on an annual basis, particularly in children and adolescents [18, 19], mainly because of frequent physical contact in schools and kindergartens. In order to prevent postoperative infection, Ing and coworkers [26] highlighted the importance of personal hygiene in patients undergoing eye surgery. Case 7 is a child who developed conjunctival cyst two days after returning to kindergarten, with a positive MRSA culture of the excised specimen. In this case, the suture was found separated free from the muscle with some necrotic adjacent tissue around. Therefore, we inferred that reaction between the suture and the muscle might be the primary cause of inflammatory. During the process, inflammatory secretion accumulated and the cyst got enlarged, subsequently followed by a thinning or cracks of the wall, which made it susceptible for exogenous MRSA infection.

Another risk factor is the duration of surgery. A longer procedure entails longer exposure of the instruments and suture to the air and thus is accompanied with a greater chance of bacterial infection at the incision site [23]. In our study, 7 diseased eyes from 7 cases were categorized according to the sequence of muscle which was operated on; the first muscle was affected in 2 cases (the first and sole operated muscle in 1 case), while the second or above muscle was affected in 5 cases. We inferred that infection might be more common in the muscle of the eye which is operated later. However, the small sample size and use of routine antibiotic eye drops before surgery highlighted the necessity of future study to confirm our hypothesis.

Al-Shehah [27] noted that conjunctival cyst tends to enlarge gradually and more treatment is required to eliminate the enlargement. Therefore, he recommended early excision. Hawkins recommended thermal cautery under the ophthalmic slit lamp [28], while some specialists tried ethanol injection into the cyst [10]. Other studies documented the role of povidone-iodine in the reduction of suture colonization [29] while antibiotic-embedding of the suture was reported to reduce postoperative infection after strabismus surgery [21].

The limitations of our study include a retrospective data set obtained only from one hospital unit and one surgeon. Furthermore, not all patients were adhering to the follow-up schedule. It is possible that some conjunctival cysts were not discovered due to their tiny size, hidden position, or spontaneous regression in the early short period of time after surgery. Therefore, the actual incidence rate of conjunctival cysts after strabismus surgery is likely to be higher than what is reported here. Even though most of them are not considered serious complications, conjunctival cysts can interfere with postoperative recovery and need multiple intervention in severe cases, such as Case 6 and Case 7.

In summary, conjunctival cyst is a rare complication of strabismus surgery. Conjunctival epithelium implantation is the primary cause, and infection might exaggerate the situation. Suture contamination, poor personal hygiene, or longer duration of surgical procedure increases the possibility of infection.

Conflicts of Interest

All authors declared that they have no conflicts of interest.

Acknowledgments

This study was supported by the 2015 Medical Big Data Project of Central South University.

References

[1] American Optometric Association, *Optometric Clinical Practice Guideline: Care of the Patient with Strabismus: Esotropia and Exotropia*, American Optometric Association, St. Louis, MO, USA, 2011.

[2] X. Chen, Z. Fu, J. Yu et al., "Prevalence of amblyopia and strabismus in Eastern China: results from screening of preschool children aged 36-72 months," *British Journal of Ophthalmology*, vol. 100, no. 4, pp. 515–519, 2016.

[3] J. Fu, S. M. Li, L. R. Liu et al., "Prevalence of amblyopia and strabismus in a population of 7th-grade junior high school students in Central China: the Anyang Childhood Eye Study (ACES)," *Ophthalmic Epidemiology*, vol. 21, no. 3, pp. 197–203, 2014.

[4] National Children Amblyopia and Strabismus Prevention and Treatment Group and Chinese Ophthalmological Society, "Epidemiological survey of amblyopia in children (Chinese)," *Chinese Journal of Ophthalmology*, vol. 21, p. 31, 1985.

[5] W. Zhang and K. Zhao, "Some problems needing attention in the treatment of strabismus and amblyopia (Chinese)," *Ophthalmology*, vol. 18, no. 5, pp. 293–296, 2009.

[6] M. Aroichane, "Planning strabismus surgery: how to avoid pitfalls and complications," *American Orthoptic Journal*, vol. 66, no. 1, pp. 63–78, 2016.

[7] Q. Xiao, M. Xu, H. Yu, Y. Wang, and X. Yu, "Postoperative shifts in adult strabismus patients with visual deficits," *Current Eye Research*, vol. 41, no. 8, pp. 1016–1020, 2016.

[8] X. Wang, X. Gao, M. Xiao et al., "Effectiveness of strabismus surgery on the health-related quality of life assessment of children with intermittent exotropia and their parents: a randomized clinical trial," *Journal of American Association for Pediatric Ophthalmology and Strabismus*, vol. 19, no. 4, pp. 298–303, 2015.

[9] I. Asproudis, N. Kozeis, A. Katsanos, S. Jain, P. G. Tranos, and A. G. Konstas, "A Review of Minimally Invasive Strabismus Surgery (MISS): is this the way forward?," *Advances in Therapy*, vol. 34, no. 4, pp. 826–833, 2017.

[10] J. W. Simon, "Complications of strabismus surgery," *Current Opinion in Ophthalmology*, vol. 21, no. 5, pp. 361–366, 2010.

[11] K. Nath, R. Gogi, and N. Zaidi, "Cystic lesions of conjunctiva," *Indian Journal of Ophthalmology*, vol. 31, pp. 1–4, 1983.

[12] J. J. Song, P. T. Finger, M. Kurli, H. J. Wisnicki, and C. E. Iacob, "Giant secondary conjunctival inclusion cysts: a late complication of strabismus surgery," *Ophthalmology*, vol. 113, no. 6, pp. 1045–1049.e2, 2006.

[13] D. W. Johnson, G. B. Bartley, J. A. Garrity, and D. M. Robertson, "Massive epithelium-lined inclusion cysts after scleral buckling," *American Journal of Ophthalmology*, vol. 113, no. 4, pp. 439–442, 1992.

[14] A. Junemann and L. M. Holbach, "[Epithelial giant inclusion cyst 50 years after enucleation without orbital implant]," *Klinische Monatsblätter für Augenheilkunde*, vol. 212, no. 2, pp. 127-128, 1998.

[15] A. M. Guadilla, P. G. de Liano, P. Merino, and G. Franco, "Conjunctival cysts as a complication after strabismus surgery," *Journal of Pediatric Ophthalmology and Strabismus*, vol. 48, no. 5, pp. 298–300, 2011.

[16] A. O. Khan, H. Al-Katan, I. Al-Baharna, and F. Al-Wadani, "Infected epithelial inclusion cyst mimicking subconjunctival

abscess after strabismus surgery," *Journal of American Association for Pediatric Ophthalmology and Strabismus*, vol. 11, no. 3, pp. 303-304, 2007.

[17] J. D. Kivlin and M. E. Wilson Jr., "Periocular infection after strabismus surgery. The Periocular Infection Study Group," *Journal of Pediatric Ophthalmology and Strabismus*, vol. 32, no. 1, pp. 42–49, 1995.

[18] M. Mikhail, R. K. Koenekoop, and A. Khan, "Orbital cellulitis and multiple abscess formation after strabismus surgery," *Canadian Journal of Ophthalmology*, vol. 51, no. 2, pp. e60–e62, 2016.

[19] A. Basheikh and R. Superstein, "A child with bilateral orbital cellulitis one day after strabismus surgery," *Journal of American Association for Pediatric Ophthalmology and Strabismus*, vol. 13, no. 5, pp. 488–490, 2009.

[20] H. Flick, "Synthetic, absorbable suture in eye-muscle surgery (author's transl)," *Albrecht von Graefes Archiv für Klinische und Experimentelle Ophthalmologie*, vol. 205, no. 1, pp. 1–8, 1977.

[21] H. S. Eustis and A. Rhodes, "Suture contamination in strabismus surgery," *Journal of Pediatric Ophthalmology and Strabismus*, vol. 49, no. 4, pp. 206–209, 2012.

[22] S. E. Olitsky, M. Vilardo, S. Awner, and J. D. Reynolds, "Needle sterility during strabismus surgery," *Journal of American Association for Pediatric Ophthalmology and Strabismus*, vol. 2, no. 3, pp. 151-152, 1998.

[23] T. S. Carothers, D. K. Coats, K. M. McCreery et al., "Quantification of incidental needle and suture contamination during strabismus surgery," *Binocular Vision and Strabismus Quarterly*, vol. 18, no. 2, pp. 75–79, 2003.

[24] D. Liang and Z. Yang, "Analysis of causes of increased incision infection in patients with open surgery in a hospital (Chinese)," *Modern Preventive Medicine*, vol. 36, no. 18, pp. 3586-3587, 2009.

[25] S. Strul, M. S. McCracken, and K. Cunin, "Orbital cellulitis and intraconal abscess formation after strabismus surgery in an adult patient," *Journal of American Association for Pediatric Ophthalmology and Strabismus*, vol. 18, no. 1, pp. 82–84, 2014.

[26] M. R. Ing, "Infection following strabismus surgery," *Ophthalmic Surgery*, vol. 22, no. 1, pp. 41–43, 1991.

[27] A. Al-Shehah and A. O. Khan, "Subconjunctival epithelial inclusion cyst complicating strabismus surgery: Early excision is better," *Saudi Journal of Ophthalmology*, vol. 24, no. 1, pp. 27–30, 2010.

[28] A. S. Hawkins and N. A. Hamming, "Thermal cautery as a treatment for conjunctival inclusion cyst after strabismus surgery," *Journal of American Association for Pediatric Ophthalmology and Strabismus*, vol. 5, no. 1, pp. 48-49, 2001.

[29] J. D. Rossetto, S. Suwannaraj, K. M. Cavuoto et al., "Evaluation of postoperative povidone-iodine in adjustable suture strabismus surgery to reduce suture colonization: a randomized clinical trial," *JAMA Ophthalmology*, vol. 134, no. 10, pp. 1151–1155, 2016.

12

Modern Corneal Eye-Banking using a Software-Based IT Management Solution

C. Kern [ID],[1] K. Kortuem [ID],[1,2] C. Wertheimer,[1] O. Nilmayer,[1] M. Dirisamer,[1] S. Priglinger,[1] and W. J. Mayer[1]

[1]*Department of Ophthalmology, University Hospital LMU, Munich, Germany*
[2]*Moorfields Eye Hospital, London, UK*

Correspondence should be addressed to C. Kern; christoph.kern@med.uni-muenchen.de

Academic Editor: Yu-Chi Liu

Background. Increasing government legislation and regulations in manufacturing have led to additional documentation regarding the pharmaceutical product requirements of corneal grafts in the European Union. The aim of this project was to develop a software within a hospital information system (HIS) to support the documentation process, to improve the management of the patient waiting list and to increase informational flow between the clinic and eye bank. *Materials and Methods.* After an analysis of the current documentation process, a new workflow and software were implemented in our electronic health record (EHR) system. *Results.* The software takes over most of the documentation and reduces the time required for record keeping. It guarantees real-time tracing of all steps during human corneal tissue processing from the start of production until allocation during surgery and includes follow-up within the HIS. Moreover, listing of the patient for surgery as well as waiting list management takes place in the same system. *Conclusion.* The new software for corneal eye banking supports the whole process chain by taking over both most of the required documentation and the management of the transplant waiting list. It may provide a standardized IT-based solution for German eye banks working within the same HIS.

1. Introduction

A global survey showed that keratoplasty is the most common tissue transplantation in the world, with 184.576 performed procedures involving 283.530 grafts in 2016 [1]. The regulations for the processing of human corneal grafts, which are regulated as pharmaceutical products, have increased in Germany within the last years because of new European and national regulations. In 2007, new legislation on the Quality and Safety of Human Tissues and Cells (Tissue law) incorporating amended European directives was passed by the German government. This resulted in major changes in medical law, transplant law and drug law. To define and control the quality requirements of donor tissue, corneal grafts were classified as a drug and not a human transplant. Therefore, this tissue is now regulated not only by tissue and transplant law, but also by drug law. The changes in the law generated increased documentation,

processing costs and more thorough tests [2]. All regulations were reviewed and summarized by the "Deutsche Ärztekammer" (German medical council) and the "Paul-Ehrlich Institute" and led to new national guidelines [3, 4]. Because of the change in the laws, we adapted quality management and other regulations at our Cornea Bank accordingly to meet the new criteria [5]. As most of the documentation during processing at our tissue bank was paper-based or relied on the manual input of data into software such as Microsoft Excel, we observed an increase in the documentation time required during the processing of corneal grafts.

In 2013, to improve patient-related documentation at the university eye clinic, we started to develop a custom-made electronic health record (EHR) adjusted to the needs of ophthalmology based on the hospital information system (HIS) i.s.h.med (Cerner AG, Erlangen, Germany). This system is now used for the entire clinical documentation at our hospital [6, 7]. Using a Picture Archiving and Communication System (PACS), we linked diagnostic data from diagnostic devices to the clinical data of patients and built a data-warehouse including clinical and diagnostic data from more than 350,000 patients [8].

The processing of corneal grafts is documented on quality-audited paper forms. Manual repetitive documentation and manual data transfer between the eye hospital and the eye bank risk processing errors and do not guarantee a high safety level or auditability. Efficient, complete and comprehensible record-keeping is listed as one of the key features of eye banks in the literature [9].

Special requirements for electronic documentation were defined by the Bavarian Medical Council: safety of the network against access from outside, daily data and documentation back-up, long-term data storage, assignment of all entries to a responsible employee and, of course, proof of later additional changes in the patient's documentation [10]. These requirements can be achieved and guaranteed by using an established, professionally secured and backed-up HIS [11].

The aim of this project was to develop custom-made documentation algorithm based on our HIS, not only to improve documentation, but also to link waiting list management with transplant allocation. These data could enrich clinical information of importance concerning the number and quality of performed corneal transplantations at our clinic and should additionally simplify data analysis.

2. Material and Methods

2.1. Process Analysis. As a first step, the documentation process during corneal graft processing, together with waiting list management and allocation, was analysed and transferred into a process flow chart to guarantee the proper implementation and functionality of the new custom-made documentation software. Time measurements before and after introduction of the new system were recorded for three different steps: initial documentation on arrival of the donor tissue at the eye bank, documentation of nutritional liquid change of the graft and documentation for final clearance.

2.2. Software Requirements. Many requirements had to be considered before the development process was initiated. First, the software had to meet the criteria for documentation as defined in the "Good manufacturing practice" guideline provided by the Paul-Ehrlich Institute [3]. This involves the legibility and the auditability of the documentation. All changes in the documentation must be clearly visible and linked to the working user. Moreover, according to national guidelines, all documentation must be stored for at least 30 years after the expiry date of the product. These requirements are met by the well-established hospital IT platform run by the university hospital's IT department [12]. Access to the software must be limited for normal users as they should not be aware of links between donor and receiver identities.

Another requirement was the support of the employees of the eye banks during the documentation process, as most of their time was now used for documentation and not processing. In addition to the automatically performed timestamps, user logging, audit trails and lot numbers of the used material, the software must simplify the documentation process itself through pre-allocation.

2.3. Software Implementation. The development of the necessary user interface was performed within our HIS (i.s.h.med, Cerner AG, Erlangen, Germany), which is based on a SAP (SAP SE, Walldorf, Germany) platform by using Advanced Business Application Programming (ABAP) programming language [13]. The development process started in the late summer of 2016, with a first version being available in a HIS testing environment in spring 2017 during which functionality and stability were assessed. After several revisions to the software, the system was launched in December 2017.

3. Results

3.1. Process Analysis. Every single documentation step of the old process was identified and a data input structure was developed to define the requirements of the custom-made information input algorithm.

Several quality-managed Word files (Microsoft Corporation, Redmond, USA) were necessary for the monitoring and documenting of processing in the old workflow (Figure 1). After printing one set of documents per graft, a medical technical assistant (MTA) manually filled in the ongoing process documentation on paper. Once the processing was completed, the paper documents were archived in a folder and stored in an office.

The previous processing documentation and the listing and transplant allocation process were analysed (Figure 1). In the past, the waiting list was managed by using Microsoft Excel Spreadsheets (Microsoft Corporation, Redmond, USA) for which no audit trail was available. The whole process therefore needed to be optimized at every step and was subsequently defined in a detailed development plan of the new software.

3.2. Software Implementation. The software was implemented in the hospital's HIS by creating a new working environment for the eye bank and contained three different views: an overview of the processed transplants, the waiting list and a history of transplanted grafts for both our own and externally provided grafts (Figure 2). Based on assigned access rights, only eye bank employees can access the new working environment. All data are stored in the hospital's professionally managed redundant data centre, which guarantees data protection, high availability and regular data back-ups. Real-time data is stored on six different servers and weekly back-ups of the whole database are stored on servers using redundant array of independent disks technology (RAID-servers). Moreover, the data containing graft

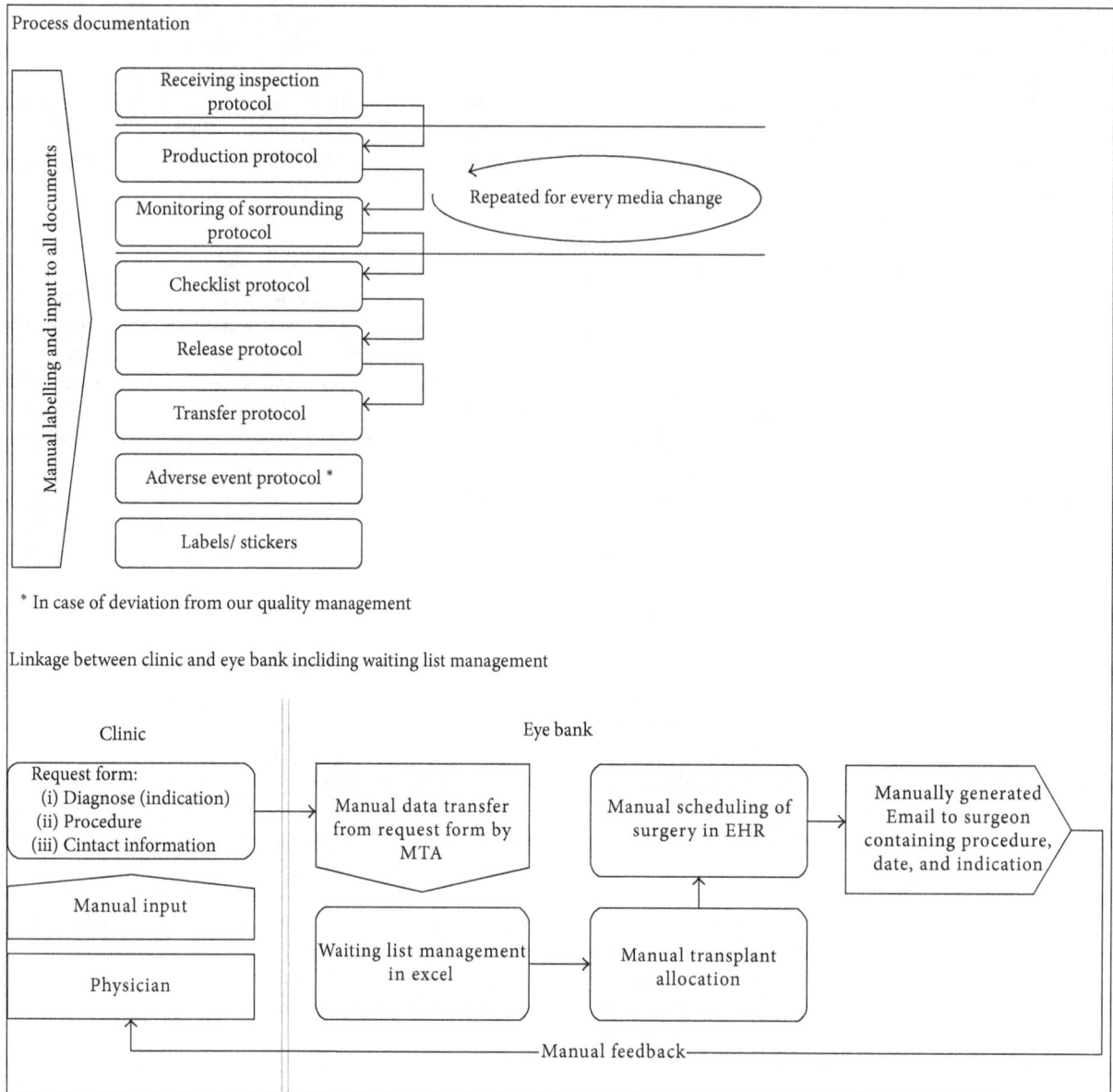

FIGURE 1: Process analysis before implementation of new software solution.

information are stored in the data-warehouse of the clinic to simplify data access for research and statistics.

3.3. Documentation of the Tissue-Processing Process.

Five new user interfaces (HIS-term: parametric medical documents (PMD)) have been developed to allow process documentation. All PMDs are linked to a patient within the HIS patient master index. Therefore, all donors are registered, if they have not been a patient during their lifetime, in the category "cornea donor." This categorization allows data access to be limited to those employees with special access rights. The processing protocol including the graft ID is linked to the recipient's EHR. This allows the linking of graft ID and the donor's identity for eye bank staff (special access rights) in cases of any adverse events. Graft and surgery complications are recorded in the recipient's EHR and can be

queried by the eye bank staff at any time from the data warehouse. Figure 3 shows the data structure of the new processing documentation process. In a university setting, final clearance for all grafts is provided by a responsible consultant with the necessary access rights. Follow-up documentation within the recipient's EHR is guaranteed by this data structure, even though, due to information governance issues, backtracking of the graft's origin is not possible for the treating physician. To provide a better overview of multiple processed transplants, all data appear in a view in the working environment (Figure 4). This contains the graft's ID, the donor's information and clearance following various microbiological tests.

3.4. Linkage between Clinic and Eye Bank.

Improvements in the listing of patients for corneal transplantation and in the feedback loop were further objectives of this software

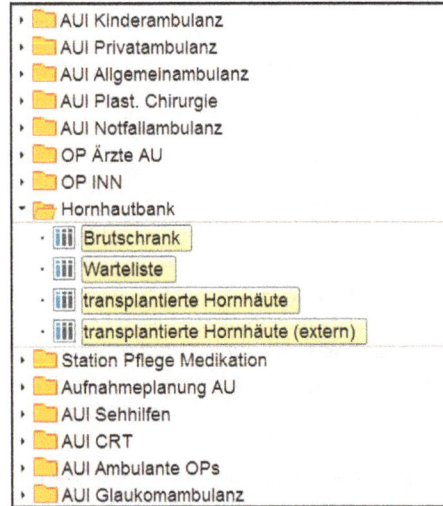

FIGURE 2: New eye bank working environment within the clinical HIS user interface. Translations related to corneal grafts only: Hornhautbank = Eyebank; Brutschrank = transplants in production; Warteliste = Waiting list; transplantierte Hornhäute = history of transplanted grafts; transplantiert Hornhäute (extern) = history of externally obtained transplanted grafts.

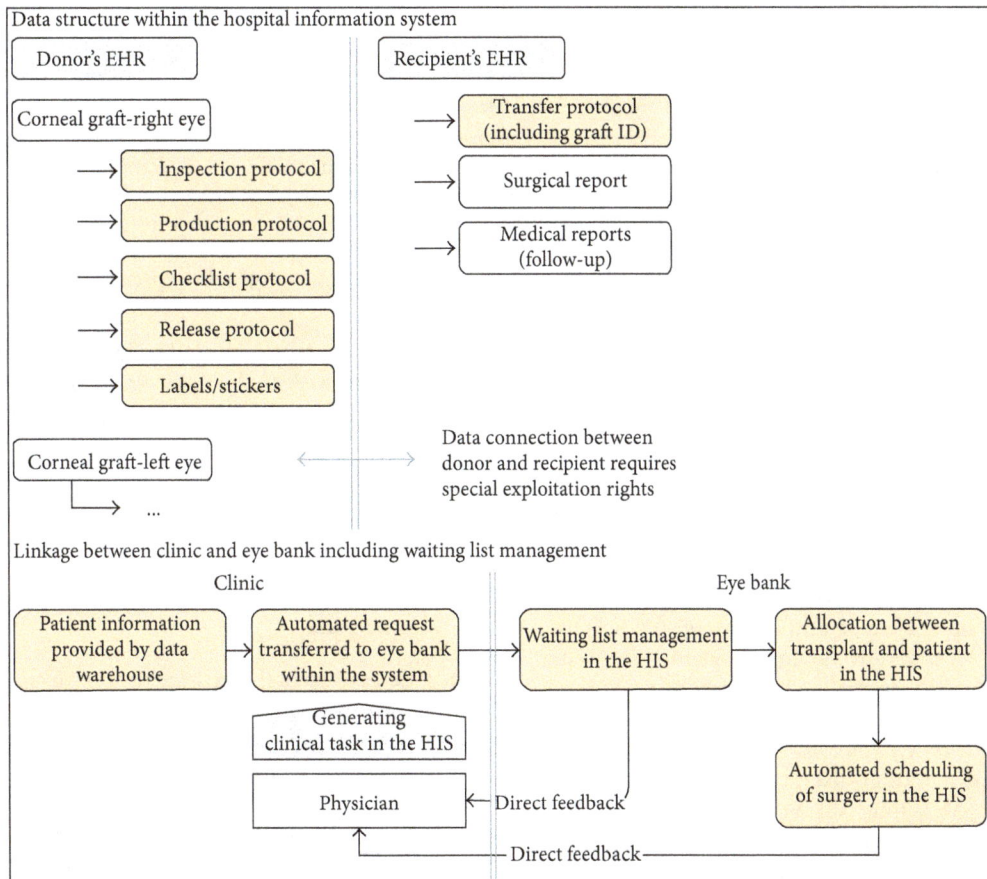

FIGURE 3: Process analysis after implementation of new software. All documents and steps shaded in peach are supported by the new software.

solution. A new item in the entry management part of the HIS was developed to enable the safe and rapid listing of patients for the physician. The clinical and contact information of the patient is automatically added to data fields before the inclusion of the patient to the waiting list. This step replaces the manually filled-in request form (Figure 3). After the allocation of a transplant to a recipient, a new surgical procedure in the theatre diary will be generated providing the surgeon with direct feedback about the date, time and relevant procedure. Relevant parameters about the

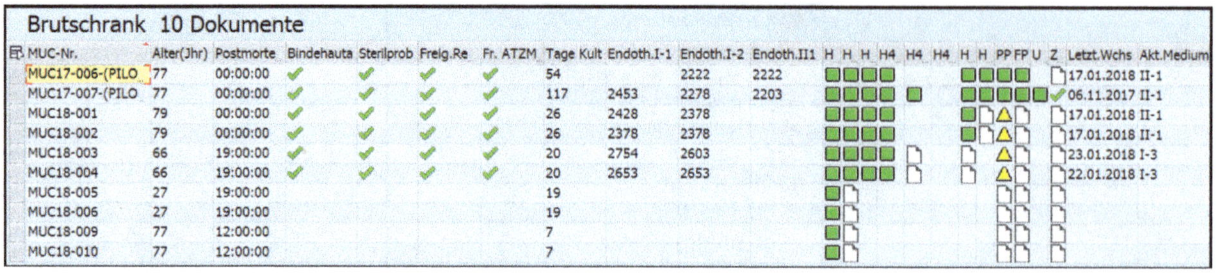

FIGURE 4: Working environment "Transplants in production." Headings of columns starting on the left side: Graft ID, age donor, time between donor's death and explantation of the corneal graft, microbiological testing of conjunctiva, microbiological testing of first medium, clearance by forensic medicine, clearance by serological testing, number of days cultivated, endothelial count I-1, I-2 and II-1, status of documents (blank sheets means the document can be set up, a yellow triangle symbolizes a document without final clearance (changes still possible) and the green square indicates a finished document), last medium change, actual medium.

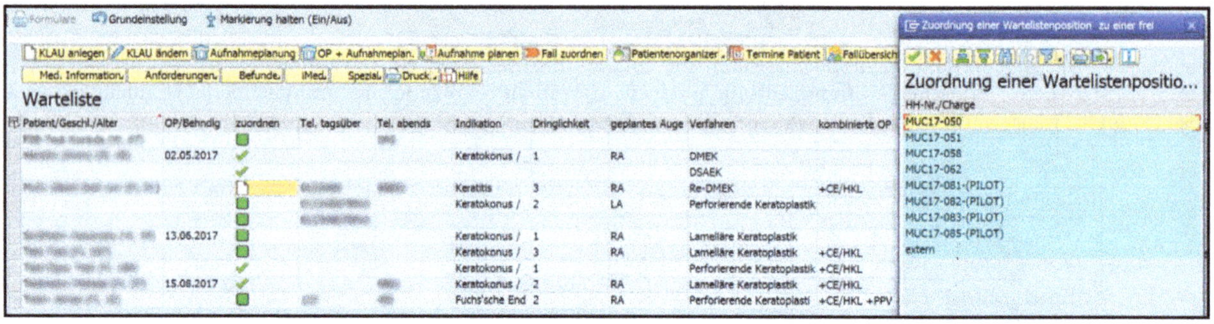

FIGURE 5: Working environment "waiting list." The process of linking a patient from the waiting list to a graft is shown. Headings of the columns starting on the left: patient/sex/age if available, scheduled surgery, connection, daytime phone number, evening phone number, indication, side, procedure, combined procedure. The column headed connection shows a green tick if the surgery has been performed, a green square if it is scheduled and a blank sheet of paper if no connection between this patient and a graft exists. Clicking on the blank paper, you can see a selection of the available grafts from the working environment of "transplants in production."

graft are provided to the surgeon in the operation theatre on an automatically filled in checklist, which is printed and attached to the graft package. The whole waiting list management takes now place within the user interface of the HIS (Figure 5). To provide a transparent system of allocating tissues in the waiting list, we defined three different urgency groups based on clinical criteria: "elective," "urgent," "emergency." For the first group, grafts are provided depending on the patients' overall waiting time, for the second group within 4 weeks and an emergency listed patient will receive the next available transplant. After a processed transplant has been matched to a patient on the waiting list, all stickers and forms are generated automatically by using previously entered data. After the removal of the patient from a waiting list position, the transplanted cornea is moved to a third subfolder of the eye bank environment, where information about the donor, the processing process and the recipient is visualized. This enables employees with the necessary rights to obtain a rapid overview of donors, corneal graft IDs, recipients, indications and the date and type of surgery. Data can be also filtered by date to simplify annual statistics for internal or official use.

3.5. Time Measurements. Before the introduction of the new system, the time consumed during initial documentation was 30 minutes per graft. Changing the nutritional liquid

took 20 minutes and final clearance 60 minutes of documentation time. With the new system, initial documentation time decreased to 10 minutes per graft. Changing the graft liquid only took 5 minutes and the final clearance 20 minutes of documentation per graft. This equals a reduction of 66% for initial documentation, 75% for liquid change and 66% for final clearance.

4. Discussion

After the analysis of the existing process and the definition of certain documentation requirements as legally specified, new software has been implemented to streamline our corneal graft processing. The new software features a high degree of automation and supports the linkage of clinics and our eye bank. Compared with former paper-based and handwritten documentation, many tasks have been automated (e.g., time, date and lot numbers). The implementation within the leading HIS has made a transparent and clear tissue allocation process with the highest amount of information being available to all involved staff to guarantee patient safety. All processing and transplant allocation data are now safely stored on hospital servers according to German/European data safety and storage guidelines [14].

The generation of a waiting list order position via a patient EHR is one of the key features of the new software.

It guarantees easy access from every clinic desk and immediate listing during clinical examination. The automatic addition of each patient's personal and clinical data into the list should eliminate errors during the listing of patients. Moreover, this system simplifies the workflow as the generation of a list position within the EHR replaces the previously used paper-based versions. Subjectively, the data quality within EHR-based listing form has increased through the new system by providing all the necessary clinical information and the correct contact information. After a request for a graft by a physician, the eye bank employee receives immediate feedback through the sending of the clinical task to the worklist as explained by Kortuem et al. [7]. Within the HIS, comments can be added and waiting list positions can be edited and, thus, all information is clearly visible to managing employees.

In 2016, a survey was performed by the "Deutsche Ophthalmologische Gesellschaft" (German ophthalmologic society). It covered questions related to IT infrastructure at eye hospitals. The results have shown that the most commonly used system is i.s.h. med in 13 German eye hospitals [11]. Worldwide, more than 500 hospitals participate in Cerners' HIS solution [15]. Developed as a module of i.s.h. med, our eye bank software can easily be transferred to other clinics by using the same HIS. This will expand the usability spectrum of the systems at other clinics.

Recently, a corneal transplant registry was set up at India's National Eye Bank including the follow-up data of graft recipients. According to the authors, the database simplified data collection for follow-up compared with former paper-based outcome analysis [16]. The connection of the corneal graft documentation process to the EHR simplifies access to data regarding the processing of the tissue and the graft itself [8, 11]. This provides further helpful information about the graft to the surgeon prior surgery. Within the existing data-warehouse, graft-specific data can be easily matched to the clinical data of the follow-up examinations of the recipients. This provides easy access to data for further statistical analysis, quality control, research, recipient follow-up and the correlation of graft data to clinical outcome and possible complications.

Many legal and professional regulations exist concerning the safety assessment of donor and recipient electronic records [10]. In addition to tracking changes in the records made by users and the identification of changes in the existing documentation, network safety must be guaranteed [14]. The used HIS should however provide regular back-up and long-term data storage and, moreover, the servers running the system should receive clearance from a data protection officer [11]. By implementing the software within an established HIS, all mandatory points concerning data protection and auditability have been met. Furthermore, in cases of any required inspections by the responsible authorities, access to the whole documentation can be granted through a digital system.

By the development of a custom-made documentation software into out HIS, we improved the dataflow between the clinic and eye bank, with a saving of 66% of documentation time. Electronic documentation systems can thus reduce the workload for employees and even increase patient safety because of the automatic, less error-prone transfer of data between the clinic and tissue bank.

Conflicts of Interest

The authors declare that there are no conflicts of interest regarding the publication of this paper.

References

[1] P. Gain, R. Jullienne, Z. He et al., "Global survey of corneal transplantation and eye banking," *JAMA Ophthalmology*, vol. 134, no. 2, pp. 167–173, 2016.

[2] C. Hauswald and T. Bredehorn-Mayr, "Practical implications of the law on tissues for cornea banks in Germany," *Developments in Ophthalmology*, vol. 43, pp. 125–130, 2009.

[3] Beschluss der Bundesärztekammer über die Richtlinie zur Gewinnung von Spenderhornhäuten und zum Führen einer Augenhornhautbank," *Deutsches Arzteblatt International*, vol. 115, no. 6, p. 262, 2018.

[4] Richtlinie zur Gewinnung von Spenderhornhäuten und zum Führen einer Augenhornhautbank, Erste Fortbeschreibung," *Deutsches Ärzteblatt*, vol. 115, no. 6, p. 262, 2018.

[5] M. Toniolo, D. Camposampiero, C. Griffoni, and G. L. Jones, "Quality management in European eye banks," *Developments in Ophthalmology*, vol. 43, pp. 70–86, 2009.

[6] K. Kortuem, M. Muller, C. Hirneiss et al., "Smart eye data: development of a foundation for medical research using smart data applications," *Der Ophthalmologe*, vol. 113, no. 6, pp. 469–477, 2016.

[7] K. U. Kortuem, M. Müller, A. Babenko, A. Kampik, and T. C. Kreutzer, "Entwicklung eines augenärztlichen klinischen Informationssystems für bettenführende Augenkliniken," *Der Ophthalmologe*, vol. 112, no. 12, pp. 995–1001, 2015.

[8] K. U. Kortuem, M. Muller, C. Kern et al., "Using electronic health records to build an ophthalmologic data warehouse and visualize patients' data," *American Journal of Ophthalmology*, vol. 178, pp. 84–93, 2017.

[9] R. Tandon, A. Singh, N. Gupta, M. Vanathi, and V. Gupta, "Upgradation and modernization of eye banking services: Integrating tradition with innovative policies and current best practices," *Indian Journal of Ophthalmology*, vol. 65, no. 2, pp. 109–115, 2017.

[10] Berufsordnung für die Ärzte Bayerns–Bekanntmachung vom 09. Januar 2012 i.d.F. der Änderungsbeschlüsse vom 21 Oktober 2017," *Bayerisches Ärzteblatt*, 2017, http://www.blaek.de/docs/epaper/berufsordnung_2015_2016/html5/index.html?&locale=DEU.

[11] K. Kortum, C. Kern, G. Meyer, S. Priglinger, and C. Hirneiss, "Required framework for the collection of real-life data: an example from University Eye Hospital Munich," *Klinische Monatsblätter für Augenheilkunde*, vol. 234, no. 12, pp. 1477–1482, 2017.

[12] *Services Provided by the Departement of "Medizintechnik und IT" (MIT)*, http://www.klinikum.uni-muenchen.de/Medizintechnik-und-IT/de/ueber-uns/index.html.

[13] J. Wendt, *Grundlagen der COBOL-Programmierung. COBOL: Einführung mit PC-Spracherweiterungen und Übungen*, Gabler Verlag, Wiesbaden, Germany, 1994.

[14] Empfehlungen zur ärztlichen Schweigepflicht, Datenschutz und Datenverarbeitung in der Arztpraxis," *Dtsch Arztebl International*, vol. 115, no. 10, p. 453, 2018.

[15] Cerner Health Services, *i.s.h. med–die klinische Welt in SAP for Healthcare*, Cerner Health Services, North Kansas City, MO, USA, 2016.

[16] V. Gogia, S. Gupta, J. S. Titiyal, A. Panda, R. M. Pandey, and R. Tandon, "A preliminary descriptive analysis of Corneal Transplant Registry of National Eye Bank in India," *Contact Lens and Anterior Eye*, vol. 37, no. 2, pp. 111–115, 2014.

13

Comparison of the Effect of Intravitreal Dexamethasone Implant in Vitrectomized and Nonvitrectomized Eyes for the Treatment of Diabetic Macular Edema

Sadık Görkem Çevik(ID),[1] Sami Yılmaz,[2] Mediha Tok Çevik,[3] Fatma Düriye Akalp,[4] and Remzi Avcı[2]

[1]Department of Ophthalmology, Yüksek Ihtisas Research and Training Hospital, Bursa, Turkey
[2]Retina Eye Hospital, Bursa, Turkey
[3]Sisli Hamidiye Etfal Research and Training Hospital, İstanbul, Turkey
[4]Department of Ophthalmology, Acıbadem Hospital, Bursa, Turkey

Correspondence should be addressed to Sadık Görkem Çevik; gorkemcevik@hotmail.com

Academic Editor: Dirk Sandner

Purpose. To compare the effectiveness of sustained-release dexamethasone (DEX) intravitreal implant in nonvitrectomized eyes and vitrectomized eyes with diabetic macular edema (DME). *Methods.* A retrospective review of the medical records of 40 eyes of 30 consecutive patients with diabetic macular edema who underwent intravitreal DEX implant injection. Patients were divided into 2 subgroups: 31 eyes that were nonvitrectomized (group 1) and 9 eyes that had previously undergone standard pars plana vitrectomy (group 2). The main outcome measures were BCVA and foveal thickness (FT). *Results.* A significant improvement was seen in BCVA in both group 1 and group 2 at the 1st, 2nd, and 6th months after treatment with DEX implant ($p < 0.05$). In group 1, a significant reduction in FT was observed at the 1st, 2nd, and 6th months ($p < 0.05$). In group 2, a significant reduction in FT was seen at the 1st and 2nd months ($p < 0.05$), but the reduction rate at the 6th month after the injection was not statistically significant ($p = 0.06$). *Conclusion.* DEX implant is effective for the treatment of diabetic macular edema, and the effectiveness of the drug is similar in vitrectomized and nonvitrectomized eyes.

1. Introduction

Diabetic macular edema is one of the most important causes of blindness worldwide particularly affecting those individuals of working age [1–3]. Since the recognition of the role of inflammation and importance of the vascular endothelial growth factor (VEGF) in the pathogenesis of diabetic retinopathy, treatment options have been altered with anti-VEGF drugs, and corticosteroids have taken an active role in the treatment of diabetic retinopathy [4–7]. Dexamethasone and triamcinolone are the most frequently used corticosteroids. Although dexamethasone is powerful, it remains in the vitreous for a limited amount of time; therefore, attempts have been made to support it with carriers which can remain longer in the vitreous [8, 9].

Despite the many new treatments that are available, a pars plana vitrectomy (PPV) is still required in some diabetic patients. The vitreoretinal tractions can be released, and the inflammatory stimulators that cause macular edema can be removed via PPV [10]. By its very nature, repeated intravitreal injections may be required in post-PPV patients. Anti-VEGF drugs, 5-FU, triamcinolone, and amphotericin B have been observed to clear out more rapidly in patients who have undergone PPV; thus, the effective duration has been reported to be shorter than expected [11–15].

The positive effects of corticosteroids in cases of diabetic macular edema have been known for many years. The effect of corticosteroids is achieved through the lowering of ICAM-1 gene expression and the VEGF level [17–19]. To prolong the corticosteroid half-life, carrier platforms which dissolve within the vitreous over a longer period of time have been developed, with Ozurdex being a significant long-term release dexamethasone implant. Ozurdex contains 0.7 mg of dexamethasone within its carrying system (Novadur® Styrolution; Aurora, Illinois, USA). It dissolves into lactic and glycolic acid in the vitreous, and this dissolution generates a slow dexamethasone release [20–22]. Following the implantation, an intense effect occurs during the first 2 months, which continues for 6 months [23].

This research aimed to compare the effective duration of a slow-release dexamethasone implant (Ozurdex) in vitrectomized and nonvitrectomized eyes for the treatment of diabetic macular edema.

2. Materials and Methods

This study was conducted in accordance with the Declaration of Helsinki, and informed consent forms were obtained from all of the patients. Our study involved a retrospective review of 40 eyes of 30 patients who were treated with Ozurdex implant injections for diabetic macular edema under operating room conditions at the Bursa Retina Eye Hospital between January 2012 and May 2015. Each intravitreal implant was applied under topical anesthesia with a 22 G applicator, 3.5 mm posterior to the limbus. The patients were divided into two: group 1 ($n = 31$), patients who were not operated on, and group 2 ($n = 9$), patients who had undergone vitrectomy surgery. The patients in group 1 had diabetic retinopathy, and those patients were previously treated with panretinal laser photocoagulation, intravitreal anti-VEGF (bevacizumab), or triamcinolone injections. Combined vitrectomy surgeries (phacoemulsification + PPV + endolaser treatment + gas tamponade + ILM peeling) were performed due to complications of diabetic retinopathy in all of the group 2 patients.

The age, gender, lens status of the patients, and previous treatments like focal-grid laser or other intravitreal therapies like anti-VEGF and triamcinolone were recorded. We used bevacizumab as anti-VEGF drug, and we did not switch throughout the study period. The inclusion criteria were the presence of intraretinal fluid demonstrated by optical coherence tomography (OCT) and at least 60 days since the last treatment. The exclusion criteria were a history of glaucoma, any kind of vitreomacular traction, uncontrolled diabetes (HbA1c > 8), incomplete laser treatment, and cases which required vitreous surgery during the follow-up. Recurrence of DME was defined as new intraretinal fluid showed by OCT after the final injection.

For each patient, the best-corrected visual acuity (BCVA) (Snellen converted logMAR) and macular thickness on OCT at baseline visit and within the 1st, 2nd, 6th months, and during follow-up visits were obtained. The OCT measurements were taken with a spectral domain OCT device (Heidelberg, Germany). Those patients who presented with complaints of visual impairment were measured for visual acuity and macular thickness. The changes in the BCVA, the presence of intraretinal fluid and intraocular pressure (IOP), the complications, and the time to recurrence were evaluated. When

recurrence of DME was observed, a second injection was performed after the 6th month.

The statistical analyses were performed using IBM SPSS 22.0 statistics software. The Wilcoxon signed-rank test was used for the determination of the visual acuity and the changes in foveal thickness in the groups. The Chi-squared test was used in the evaluation of the distribution of the patients with recurrence, while the Mann–Whitney U test was used in the evaluation of the time to recurrence. A value of $p < 0.05$ was accepted as statistically significant.

3. Results

The mean age of patients was 63.1 ± 8.1 (47–85) years in group 1 and 60.4 ± 9.2 (47–77) years in group 2. The mean follow-up time was 19.7 ± 11.2 (6–36) months in group 1 and 15.8 ± 9.3 (6–36) months in group 2. Focal laser photocoagulation treatment was performed before the intravitreal Ozurdex therapy in 25 eyes (71%) in group 1 and in 9 eyes (100%) in group 2. The intravitreal steroid (except Ozurdex) and/or anti-VEGF (bevacizumab) injections were given before the intravitreal Ozurdex therapy in 27 eyes (87%) in group 1 and in 8 eyes (88%) in group 2. Fourteen eyes (45%) in group 1 and 9 eyes (100%) in group 2 had pseudophakia (Table 1).

In group 1, the best-corrected visual acuity (BCVA) was 0.88 ± 0.46 at the baseline visit, 0.60 ± 0.38 at the 1st month, 0.56 ± 0.32 at the 2nd month, and 0.58 ± 0.41 at the 6th month (logMAR). In group 2, the BCVA was 0.98 ± 0.66 at the baseline visit, 0.67 ± 0.48 at the 1st month, 0.54 ± 0.26 at the 2nd month, and 0.77 ± 0.58 at the 6th month (logMAR). When compared to the baseline values, the increases in the BCVA in group 1 within the 1st, 2nd, and 6th months were statistically significant ($p < 0.001$, $p < 0.001$, and $p < 0.001$, resp.). In group 2, the increases in the BCVA were also statistically significant at the 1st, 2nd, and 6th months when compared to the baseline levels ($p = 0.011$, $p < 0.001$, and $p = 0.048$, resp.).

In group 1, the macular thickness was 596 ± 170 (265–1004) microns prior to injection, 403 ± 108 (160–575) microns at the 1st, 304 ± 74 (190–440) microns at the 2nd, and 339 ± 176 (88–835) microns at the 6th month. In group 1, the changes in the macular thickness were statistically significant at the 1st, 2nd, and 6th months when compared to the baseline visit values ($p < 0.05$). The macular thickness in group 2 at baseline visit was 547 ± 166 (354–810) microns, and it was 358 ± 99 (200–505) microns at the 1st, 221 ± 105 (150–350) microns at the 2nd, and 349 ± 178 (164–700) microns at the 6th month. The changes in the macular thickness within the 1st and 2nd months in group 2 were statistically significant ($p = 0.012$ and $p < 0.011$, resp.) when compared to the baseline values, but the change at the 6th month was not statistically significant ($p = 0.06$) (Table 2).

During the first 6-month period, the time to recurrence of macular edema was 20.2 ± 2.2 weeks in group 1 and 17.5 ± 4.4 weeks in group 2, but there was no statistically significant difference between the 2 groups ($p = 0.082$). Recurrences were observed in 16 eyes in group 1 and in 4 eyes in group

TABLE 1: Results of the current study.

Eye	Patient age	Focal laser treatment	Intravitreal injection	Preoperative lens status	Complication	Vitrectomy surgery	Usage of treatment after recurrence (patients who accepted the treatment)
1	53	N	7	N	Ø	N	Dex
2	55	N	2	P	Ø	N	Dex
3	60	Y	4	N	Ø	N	
4	68	Y	2	N	Ø	N	
5	55	Y	4	P	Ø	N	Dex
6	55	Y	Ø	P	Ø	N	
7	68	Y	1	P	Ø	N	
8	68	Y	1	P	Ø	N	
9	77	Y	1	P	Ø	N	
10	67	Y	1	P	Ø	N	
11	67	Y	3	N	Ø	N	Dex
12	67	Y	3	N	Ø	N	Dex
13	67	Y	3	N	Ø	N	
14	85	Y	3	P	Ocular HT	N	Anti-VEGF
15	52	Y	1	N	Ø	N	
16	69	Y	7	N	Cataract	N	
17	71	N	2	P	Ø	N	
18	54	N	1	P	Ø	N	
19	54	Y	1	N	Ø	N	
20	60	Y	1	N	Ø	N	
21	77	Y	1	P	Ø	N	
22	58	N	2	N	Ocular HT	N	Anti-VEGF
23	47	Y	1	N	Ø	N	
24	65	Y	1	N	Ø	N	Dex
25	65	Y	2	N	Cataract	N	Dex
26	60	Y	2	N	Ø	N	Dex
27	67	Y	1	N	Ø	N	
28	57	Y	1	N	Ø	N	
29	65	N	Ø	P	Ø	N	
30	63	Y	Ø	P	Ø	N	
31	63	Y	Ø	P	Ø	N	
32	55	Y	1	P	Ø	Y	
33	51	Y	1	P	Ø	Y	
34	47	Y	1	P	Ø	Y	Dex
35	77	Y	2	P	Ø	Y	Dex
36	65	Y	1	P	Ø	Y	
37	60	Y	Ø	P	Ø	Y	
38	60	Y	1	P	Ø	Y	
39	59	Y	2	P	Ø	Y	
40	70	Y	3	P	Glaucoma	Y	

Y: yes; N: no; P: pseudophakic; N: natural; Dex: dexamethasone implant.

2, but there was no statistically significant difference between the 2 groups ($p = 0.076$).

High IOP (HIP) values, which can be brought under control with medical treatment, were measured as >25 mmHg in 2 eyes in group 1 and in 1 eye in group 2, although none of these measurements exceeded 30 mmHg. Within the first 6-month period, cataract development was observed in 2 eyes in group 1. Moreover, all of the group 2 patients had pseudophakia. Cataract progression was clinically observed. Visual acuities of the cases with cataract were removed from statistical analysis.

Of the patients with recurrence, a second dexamethasone implant was applied to 8 of the patients who accepted treatment in group 1 and to 2 of the patients in group 2. The

TABLE 2: Results of the current study.

Eye	Prein. VA (Snellen)	Postin. 1st month VA (Snellen)	Postin. 2nd month VA (Snellen)	Postin. 6th month VA (Snellen)	Prein. foveal thickness (μ)	Postin. 1st month foveal thickness (μ)	Postin. 2nd month foveal thickness (μ)	Postin. 6th month foveal thickness (μ)	Time to recurrence (week)	Group
1	20/2000	20/800	20/400	20/2000	752	575	300	380	16	1
2	20/1600	20/400	20/400	20/1600	550	368	280	471	20	1
3	20/100	20/80	20/80	20/40	577	270	244	200	Ø	1
4	20/100	20/100	20/100	20/100	454	438	350	476	22	1
5	20/200	20/100	20/100	20/125	662	291	190	835	19	1
6	20/40	20/32	Ø	20/25	350	242	200	240	Ø	1
7	20/40	20/40	Ø	20/25	383	364	Ø	300	Ø	1
8	20/400	20/400	Ø	20/200	853	563	Ø	104	Ø	1
9	20/200	20/100	Ø	20/125	413	400	Ø	163	Ø	1
10	20/100	20/50	Ø	20/40	642	400	Ø	485	20	1
11	20/40	20/40	20/40	20/125	662	540	265	481	24	1
12	20/40	20/32	20/32	20/63	550	432	380	463	20	1
13	20/200	20/125	20/125	20/125	1004	560	390	204	Ø	1
14	20/2000	20/400	20/400	20/200	330	200	200	250	22	1
15	20/125	20/40	20/40	20/80	607	400	305	334	Ø	1
16	20/125	20/40	20/40	20/80	529	356	290	200	Ø	1
17	20/50	20/32	20/32	20/25	525	390	280	173	Ø	1
18	20/125	20/100	Ø	20/40	496	337	Ø	490	20	1
19	20/400	20/125	Ø	20/63	884	540	Ø	150	Ø	1
20	20/200	20/50	20/50	20/40	826	550	350	88	Ø	1
21	20/200	20/125	20/200	20/200	525	332	300	118	Ø	1
22	20/50	20/40	20/40	20/63	716	505	440	553	16	1
23	20/200	20/125	20/100	20/200	808	510	430	162	Ø	1
24	20/63	20/40	20/125	20/40	741	450	400	450	21	1
25	20/200	20/125	20/125	20/63	592	480	190	363	20	1
26	20/200	20/63	20/63	20/50	516	440	320	419	24	1
27	20/200	20/100	Ø	20/125	479	400	Ø	186	Ø	1
28	20/200	20/63	Ø	20/63	265	160	Ø	302	20	1
29	20/40	20/40	20/63	20/25	620	325	300	600	20	1
30	20/40	Ø	Ø	20/25	590	364	Ø	317	Ø	1
31	20/125	Ø	Ø	20/100	598	335	300	560	20	1
32	20/200	20/100	20/100	20/125	810	387	350	283	Ø	2
33	20/40	Ø	20/32	20/32	463	Ø	Ø	358	Ø	2
34	20/50	20/40	20/40	20/40	449	250	210	700	16	2
35	20/200	20/100	20/50	20/100	708	505	310	468	22	2
36	20/200	20/50	20/50	20/125	768	450	150	164	Ø	2
37	20/200	20/50	20/40	20/50	456	375	180	165	Ø	2
38	20/2000	20/500	20/400	20/500	457	374	200	166	Ø	2
39	20/2000	20/500	20/500	20/2000	458	323	180	389	20	2
40	20/32	20/25	20/32	20/50	354	200	190	450	12	2

remaining patients with recurrence did not accept another intravitreal injection. Intravitreal anti-VEGF (bevacizumab) treatments were applied to 2 patients following recurrence in group 1 because of the HIP. The recurrences of diabetic macular edema were observed in 6 eyes that had undergone second dexamethasone implant injections in group 1. In those eyes, the mean recurrence time was 21 ± 2.6 (19–25) weeks. We observed a recurrence of diabetic macular edema during the 21st week in 1 patient who had undergone a second intravitreal injection of a dexamethasone implant in group 2. A third dexamethasone implant was injected into 2 patients in group 1. Following repeated Ozurdex injections,

TABLE 3: Recurrence and retreatment number and times.

	Total	Retreatment	Avg. recurrence time	Second retreatment	Secondary recurrence	Avg. recurrence time 2	Retreatment
Recurrence in 6 months							
Group 1	16 eyes	8 (out of 16)	21 ± 2.6 weeks	8 eyes	6 eyes	25 ± 1.3 weeks	2 eyes
Group 2	4 eyes	2 eyes	21 weeks	1 eye			
Recurrence > 6 month							
		6–12 months					
Group 1	20 eyes						
Group 2	6 eyes						
Recurrence > 6 month							
Group 1	20	9	24.2 ± 1.3 weeks	9 eyes	6 eyes	26.4 ± 1.8 weeks	3 eyes
Group 2	6	4	24.16 ± 1.83 weeks	2 eyes	2 eyes	25.1 ± 1.3 weeks	1 eye

the time to recurrence of DME extended from 21 ± 2.6 weeks to 25 ± 1.3 weeks (Table 3).

When we looked at the final results of those patients without recurrence during the first 6 months of follow-up, we saw recurrence in both group1 and group 2 during the following 6 months. In group 1, recurrence was observed in 8 of 15 eyes within 6 to 9 months of follow-up and in 5 eyes within 9 to 12 months. No recurrence was observed in 2 eyes in 36 months of total follow-up. Of those 9 eyes (out of 13) in which recurrence was observed after 6 months, 6 of them were treated with Ozurdex and 3 of them were treated with anti-VEGF (bevacizumab). Four eyes left untreated due to the patients' disapproval. In group 2, recurrence was observed in 4 eyes after 6 months, which were retreated with Ozurdex. No recurrence was observed within 36 months in only 1 eye.

4. Discussion

Following PPV surgery, frequently repeated application of intravitreal medication may be required; therefore, it is important to know how these medications will act on the eyes which have undergone vitrectomy surgery [16]. The results of this study showed that a dexamethasone implant was effective in both vitrectomized and nonvitrectomized eyes. After the removal of the vitreous, the eye becomes less viscous; therefore, a clearance of intravitreal drugs from the vitreus cavity is accelerated [11, 24, 25]. It is well known that the clearance of triamcinolone particles is much faster in vitrectomized eyes [26, 27]. Previous studies have shown a shorter half-life of anti-VEGF drugs in the eyes which have undergone PPV, and a 60% decrease has been observed in the half-life of bevacizumab in monkey eyes following PPV [28]. In a study by Niwa et al., comparing the half-lives of ranibizumab and aflibercept in vitrectomized and nonvitrectomized eyes, the half-lives of both molecules were decreased in vitrectomized eyes [29]. Moisseiev et al. calculated the half-life of bevacizumab on vitrectomized and nonvitrectomized eyes and reported that the half-life was 4.9 days in the nonvitrectomized eyes and 0.66 days in the vitrectomized eyes [30]. However, the Diabetic Retinopathy Clinical Research Network trial had shown favorable responses to

intravitreal ranibizumab treatment in the management of DME among patients with prior vitrectomy [43].

In the current study, the increases in the BCVA during the 1st, 2nd, and 6th months, when compared to the baseline levels, were statistically significant in the nonvitrectomized and vitrectomized eyes, and all of the medications were seen to have similar effects in both groups. In a study comprised of 24 vitrectomized and 34 nonvitrectomized eyes by Dutra Medeiros et al., statistically significantly increases were observed in BCVA during the 1st, 3rd, and 6th months after the intravitreal Ozurdex injection. In the same study, statistically significant improvements in the foveal thicknesses of both the vitrectomized and nonvitrectomized eyes were observed during the 1st, 3rd, and 6th months when compared with the baseline levels [31]. Although we have found similar results in our study, the change in macular thickness in vitrectomized eyes at 6 months was not statistically significant. This nonstatistically significant result was attributed to the lower number of patients in group 2 ($p = 0.06$), which was a significant drawback of our study. Given the small number of cases in group 2, this condition may be interpreted as clinically significant.

The detection time of recurrent macular edema was an average of 17.5 weeks in the vitrectomized eyes and 20 weeks in the nonvitrectomized eyes, and this period was determined to be similar between the 2 groups. In a study by Escobar-Barranco et al., Ozurdex implants were applied to refractory and treatment naïve patients with diffuse diabetic macular edema, and the median time for reinjection was 4 months [32]. Hattenbach et al. studied 24 patients (25 eyes) who had undergone PPV and had persistent postoperative macular edema. The macular thickness decreased within 4 to 8 weeks after the Ozurdex implantation, and the visual improvement was observed in 79% of the patients. In the same study, the macular thickness was observed to increase between 10 and 16 weeks, and the dexamethasone implant was reapplied to 12 of 25 eyes [33]. In another study by Hattenbach et al., the medical records of 37 patients (39 eyes) who had been treated with intravitreal DEX implant for postoperative persistent cystoid macular edema following vitrectomy and peeling of idiopathic epiretinal membranes were retrospectively reviewed [39]. And they reported that

17 of 39 eyes (43.6%) necessitated minimum 1 repeat injection of DEX implant. Klamann et al. reported that intravitreal DEX implant is an effective treatment among patients with postoperative macular edema after cataract surgery or pars plana vitrectomy. They observed recurrence of macular edema in 8 patients 8.1 ± 5.3 months after the first injection of DEX which responded to reinjection [40]. In an experimental study, the behavior of Ozurdex implants injected into vitrectomized eyes was modeled, and Ozurdex was injected into a BSS-filled box at different release angles (15°, 30°, and 45°) [41]. They found that the implant injected at 15° reached the highest mean initial velocity and mean initial normalized energy. The combination of intravitreal DEX injection with pars plana vitrectomy had been shown to be safe and effective for some underlying conditions that result in macular edema, like diabetic retinopathy, retinal vein occlusion, and uveitis [42].

The results obtained in this study showed no statistically significant difference regarding recurrence of macular edema time between vitrectomized and nonvitrectomized eyes. The time to recurrence of macular edema was 20.2 ± 2.2 weeks in nonvitrectomized group and 17.5 ± 4.4 weeks in vitrectomized group.

Shah et al. evaluated the efficacy of intravitreal dexamethasone implants among 8 vitrectomized eyes with persistent diabetic macular edema, which were previously treated with intravitreal anti-VEGF therapy [37]. They observed an increase in the visual acuity and a decrease in the macular thickness 1 month after treatment. Additionally, that effect lasted for at least 3 months. Thanos et al. injected intravitreal Ozurdex implant to patients who had recalcitrant macular edema after a successful rhegmatogenous retinal detachment repair surgery. They observed recurrence of the edema in all patients at the end of 3 months [38]. In that study, the average number of implants to treat macular edema in their set of patients was 4 (range 1–14). In our study, we observed longer duration of the effect. Also, the second injection had greater efficacy than the first.

In a study by the Ozurdex CHAMPLAIN study group, a 26-week evaluation of the safety and efficacy of Ozurdex was conducted on 55 vitrectomized eyes via OCT scanning and foveal thickness examination. The findings showed a decrease in the maximum foveal thickness and an increase in vision in the 8th week, and these effects continued for 26 weeks. In the current study, the maximum increases in vision and decreases in the foveal thickness were observed in both patient groups in the postoperative 1st and 2nd months. The most frequently seen side effects in the Ozurdex CHAMPLAIN study group were conjunctival bleeding, an increase in the IOP, and pain; however, the medication was deemed to be safe [34]. In the current study, an increase in the IOP possibly requiring medical treatment was observed in 1 vitrectomized eye and 2 nonvitrectomized eyes. When the side effect profile of Ozurdex was evaluated, the increase in the IOP and development of cataract became prominent.

In the BEVORDEX study in which Ozurdex and bevacizumab were compared for 12 months, the IOP levels of 26% of the patients in the Ozurdex group were ≥25 mmHg, but they were lowered with medical treatment [35]. In the current study, all of the HIP cases were brought under control with medical treatment. In addition, cataract development is an important side effect of steroids that are applied intraocularly. In the MEAD study, in which dosages of 0.7 mg and 0.35 mg were compared, cataract development was determined at the rates of 67.9%, 64.1%, and 20.4%, respectively, for the 3 groups (including a 3rd control group) over a 3-year period. The rates of cataract surgery were 59.2%, 52.3%, and 7.2%, respectively, while in the dexamethasone implant group, cataract surgery was performed between 18 and 30 months in 75% of the patients [36]. In the current study, cataract development was observed in 2 eyes within the first 6-month period, with an expected increase at the longer term follow-up visits.

Our study had certain limitations, such as its retrospective nature, the small sample of eyes in group 2, and that the refusal of reinjection by some patients with recurrent macular edema. However, our follow-up time is long enough to evaluate the long-term effectiveness and safety of Ozurdex. In addition, we observed the period of recurrence extended as the number of injections increased in vitrectomized and nonvitrectomized eyes.

5. Conclusion

Overall, the sustained-release dexamethasone implant was shown to be similarly effective in both vitrectomized and nonvitrectomized eyes. When the duration of the effect on vitrectomized eyes in particular is taken into consideration, sooner, reinjection may be required in vitrectomized eyes to achieve the same results.

Disclosure

This study was presented as a poster in EuRetina 2016 meeting.

Conflicts of Interest

The authors do not have any conflict of interest.

References

[1] T. A. Ciulla, A. G. Amador, and B. Zinman, "Diabetic retinopathy and diabetic macular edema: pathophysiology, screening, and novel therapies," *Diabetes Care*, vol. 26, no. 9, pp. 2653–2664, 2003.

[2] S. Resnikoff, D. Pascolini, D. Etya'ale et al., "Global data on visual impairment in the year 2002," *Bulletin of the World Health Organization*, vol. 82, no. 11, pp. 844–851, 2004.

[3] I. Kocur and S. Resnikoff, "Visual impairment and blindness in Europe and their prevention," *British Journal of Ophthalmology*, vol. 86, no. 7, pp. 716–722, 2002.

[4] H. A. Al Dhibi and J. F. Arevalo, "Clinical trials on corticosteroids for diabetic macular edema," *World Journal of Diabetes*, vol. 4, no. 6, pp. 295–302, 2013.

[5] Early Treatment Diabetic Retinopathy Study Research Group, "Photocoagulation for diabetic macular edema. Early Treatment Diabetic Retinopathy Study report number 1," *Archives of Ophthalmology*, vol. 103, no. 12, pp. 1796–1806, 1985.

[6] P. Romero-Aroca, J. Reyes-Torres, M. Baget-Bernaldiz, and C. Blasco-Sune, "Laser treatment for diabetic macular edema in the 21st century," *Current Diabetes Reviews*, vol. 10, no. 2, pp. 100–112, 2014.

[7] N. Cheung, I. Y. Wong, and T. Y. Wong, "Ocular anti-VEGF therapy for diabetic retinopathy: overview of clinical efficacy and evolving applications," *Diabetes Care*, vol. 37, no. 4, pp. 900–905, 2014.

[8] I. M. Gan, L. C. Ugahary, J. T. van Dissel, and J. C. van Meurs, "Effect of intravitreal dexamethasone on vitreous vancomycin concentrations in patients with suspected postoperative bacterial endophthalmitis," *Graefe's Archive for Clinical and Experimental Ophthalmology*, vol. 243, no. 11, pp. 1186–1189, 2005.

[9] L. Zhang, W. Shen, J. Luan et al., "Sustained intravitreal delivery of dexamethasone using an injectable and biodegradable thermogel," *Acta Biomaterialia*, vol. 23, pp. 271–281, 2015.

[10] E. Stefánsson, "Physiology of vitreous surgery," *Graefe's Archive for Clinical and Experimental Ophthalmology*, vol. 247, no. 2, pp. 147–163, 2009.

[11] S. S. Lee, C. Ghosn, Z. Yu et al., "Vitreous VEGF clearance is increased after vitrectomy," *Investigative Ophthalmology & Visual Science*, vol. 51, no. 4, pp. 2135–2138, 2010.

[12] H.-S. Chin, T.-S. Park, Y.-S. Moon, and J.-H. Oh, "Difference in clearance of intravitreal triamcinolone acetonide between vitrectomized and nonvitrectomized eyes," *Retina*, vol. 25, no. 5, pp. 556–560, 2005.

[13] R. H. Schindler, D. Chandler, R. Thresher, and R. Machemer, "The clearance of intravitreal triamcinolone acetonide," *American Journal of Ophthalmology*, vol. 93, no. 4, pp. 415–417, 1982.

[14] B. H. Doft, J. Weiskopf, I. Nilsson-Ehle, and L. B. Wingard Jr., "Amphotericin clearance in vitrectomized versus nonvitrectomized eyes," *Ophthalmology*, vol. 92, no. 11, pp. 1601–1605, 1985.

[15] G. Jarus, M. Blumenkranz, E. Hernandez, and N. Sossi, "Clearance of intravitreal fluorouracil: normal and aphakic vitrectomized eyes," *Ophthalmology*, vol. 92, no. 1, pp. 91–96, 1985.

[16] D. A. H. Laidlaw, "Vitrectomy for diabetic macular oedema," *Eye*, vol. 22, no. 10, pp. 1337–1341, 2008.

[17] S. G. Schwartz, H. W. Flynn, and I. U. Scott, "Intravitreal corticosteroids in the management of diabetic macular edema," *Current Ophthalmology Reports*, vol. 1, no. 3, pp. 144–149, 2013.

[18] M. Nauck, G. Karakiulakis, A. P. Perruchoud, E. Papakonstantinou, and M. Roth, "Corticosteroids inhibit the expression of the vascular endothelial growth factor gene in human vascular smooth muscle cells," *European Journal of Pharmacology*, vol. 341, no. 2-3, pp. 309–315, 1998.

[19] J. L. Edelman, D. Lutz, and M. R. Castro, "Corticosteroids inhibit VEGF-induced vascular leakage in a rabbit model of blood–retinal and blood–aqueous barrier breakdown," *Experimental Eye Research*, vol. 80, no. 2, pp. 249–258, 2005.

[20] D. P. Hainsworth, P. A. Pearson, J. D. Conklin, and P. Ashton, "Sustained release intravitreal dexamethasone," *Journal of Ocular Pharmacology and Therapeutics*, vol. 12, no. 1, pp. 57–63, 1996.

[21] L. Zhang, Y. Li, C. Zhang, Y. Wang, and C. Song, "Pharmacokinetics and tolerance study of intravitreal injection of dexamethasone-loaded nanoparticles in rabbits," *International Journal of Nanomedicine*, vol. 4, pp. 175–183, 2009.

[22] B. D. Kuppermann, M. S. Blumenkranz, J. A. Haller et al., "Randomized controlled study of an intravitreous dexamethasone drug delivery system in patients with persistent macular edema," *Archives of Ophthalmology*, vol. 125, no. 3, pp. 309–317, 2007.

[23] J.-E. Chang-Lin, M. Attar, A. A. Acheampong et al., "Pharmacokinetics and pharmacodynamics of a sustained-release dexamethasone intravitreal implant," *Investigative Opthalmology & Visual Science*, vol. 52, no. 1, p. 80, 2011.

[24] J. I. Patel, P. G. Hykin, M. Schadt, V. Luong, F. Fitzke, and Z. J. Gregor, "Pars plana vitrectomy for diabetic macular oedema: OCT and functional correlations," *Eye*, vol. 20, no. 6, pp. 674–680, 2006.

[25] Diabetic Retinopathy Clinical Research Network Writing Committee, "Vitrectomy outcomes in eyes with diabetic macular edema and vitreomacular traction," *Ophthalmology*, vol. 117, no. 6, pp. 1087–1093.e3, 2010.

[26] P. M. Beer, S. J. Bakri, R. J. Singh, W. Liu, G. B. Peters III, and M. Miller, "Intraocular concentration and pharmacokinetics of triamcinolone acetonide after a single intravitreal injection," *Ophthalmology*, vol. 110, no. 4, pp. 681–686, 2003.

[27] S. Gisladottir, T. Loftsson, and E. Stefansson, "Diffusion characteristics of vitreous humour and saline solution follow the Stokes Einstein equation," *Graefe's Archive for Clinical and Experimental Ophthalmology*, vol. 247, no. 12, pp. 1677–1684, 2009.

[28] M. Kakinoki, T. Miyake, O. Sawada, T. Sawada, H. Kawamura, and M. Ohji, "The clearance of intravitreal bevacizumab in vitrectomized macaque eyes," *Investigative Ophthalmology & Visual Science*, vol. 52, no. 14, p. 5630, 2011.

[29] Y. Niwa, M. Kakinoki, T. Sawada, X. Wang, and M. Ohji, "Ranibizumab and aflibercept: intraocular pharmacokinetics and their effects on aqueous VEGF level in vitrectomized and nonvitrectomized macaque eyes," *Investigative Ophthalmology & Visual Science*, vol. 56, no. 11, p. 6501, 2015.

[30] E. Moisseiev, M. Waisbourd, E. Ben-Artsi et al., "Pharmacokinetics of bevacizumab after topical and intravitreal administration in human eyes," *Graefe's Archive for Clinical and Experimental Ophthalmology*, vol. 252, no. 2, pp. 331–337, 2014.

[31] M. Dutra Medeiros, M. Alkabes, R. Navarro, J. Garcia-Arumí, C. Mateo, and B. Corcóstegui, "Dexamethasone intravitreal implant in vitrectomized versus nonvitrectomized eyes for treatment of patients with persistent diabetic macular edema," *Journal of Ocular Pharmacology and Therapeutics*, vol. 30, no. 9, pp. 709–716, 2014.

[32] J. J. Escobar-Barranco, B. Pina-Marín, and M. Fernández-Bonet, "Dexamethasone implants in patients with naïve or refractory diffuse diabetic macular edema," *Ophthalmologica*, vol. 233, no. 3-4, pp. 176–185, 2015.

[33] L. O. Hattenbach, C. Kuhli-Hattenbach, C. Springer, J. Callizo, and H. Hoerauf, "Intravitreales dexamethason-implantat zur behandlung des persistierenden postoperativen makulaödems nach vitrektomie," *Der Ophthalmologe*, vol. 113, no. 7, pp. 581–588, 2016.

[34] D. S. Boyer, D. Faber, S. Gupta et al., "Dexamethasone intravitreal implant for treatment of diabetic macular edema in vitrectomized patients," *Retina*, vol. 31, no. 5, pp. 915–923, 2011.

[35] M. C. Gillies, L. L. Lim, A. Campain et al., "A randomized clinical trial of intravitreal bevacizumab versus intravitreal dexamethasone for diabetic macular edema: the BEVORDEX study," *Ophthalmology*, vol. 121, no. 12, pp. 2473–2481, 2014.

[36] D. S. Boyer, Y. H. Yoon, Belfort R Jr et al., "Three-year, randomized, sham-controlled trial of dexamethasone intravitreal
implant in patients with diabetic macular edema," *Ophthalmology*, vol. 121, no. 10, pp. 1904–1914, 2014.

[37] A. R. Shah, M. Xi, A. M. Abbey et al., "Short-term efficacy of
intravitreal dexamethasone implant in vitrectomized eyes with
recalcitrant diabetic macular edema and prior anti-VEGF
therapy," *Journal of Ophthalmic & Vision Research*, vol. 11,
no. 2, pp. 183–187, 2016.

[38] A. Thanos, B. Todorich, Y. Yonekawa et al., "Dexamethasone
intravitreal implant for the treatment of recalcitrant macular
edema after rhegmatogenous retinal detachment repair,"
Retina, p. 1, 2017.

[39] L. O. Hattenbach, C. Springer-Wanner, H. Hoerauf et al.,
"Intravitreal sustained-release steroid implants for the
treatment of macular edema following surgical removal of
epiretinal membranes," *Ophthalmologica*, vol. 237, no. 4,
pp. 232–237, 2017.

[40] A. Klamann, K. Böttcher, P. Ackermann, G. Geerling,
M. Schargus, and R. Guthoff, "Intravitreal dexamethasone
implant for the treatment of postoperative macular edema,"
Ophthalmologica, vol. 236, no. 4, pp. 181–185, 2016.

[41] R. Panjaphongse, W. Liu, P. Pongsachareonnont, and J. M.
Stewart, "Kinematic study of Ozurdex injection in balanced
salt solution: modeling the behavior of an injectable drug
delivery device in vitrectomized eyes," *Journal of Ocular Pharmacology and Therapeutics*, vol. 31, no. 3, pp. 174–178, 2015.

[42] A. Zheng, E. K. Chin, D. R. P. Almeida, S. H. Tsang, and
V. B. Mahajan, "Combined vitrectomy and intravitreal dexamethasone (Ozurdex) sustained-release implant," *Retina*,
vol. 36, no. 11, pp. 2087–2092, 2016.

[43] S. B. Bressler, M. Melia, A. R. Glassman et al., "Ranibizumab
plus prompt or deferred laser for diabetic macular edema in
eyes with vitrectomy before anti-vascular endothelial growth
factor therapy," *Retina*, vol. 35, no. 12, pp. 2516–2528, 2015.

14

Assessment of Ocular Surface Damage during the Course of Type 2 Diabetes Mellitus

Fanglin He,[1,2] **Zhanlin Zhao,**[1,2] **Yan Liu,**[1,2] **Linna Lu** ⓘ,[1,2] **and Yao Fu** ⓘ[1,2]

[1]*Department of Ophthalmology, Shanghai Ninth People's Hospital, Shanghai Jiaotong University School of Medicine, Shanghai, China*
[2]*Shanghai Key Laboratory of Orbital Disease and Ocular Oncology, Shanghai, China*

Correspondence should be addressed to Linna Lu; drlulinna@126.com and Yao Fu; drfuyaofy@sina.com

Fanglin He and Zhanlin Zhao equally contributed to this work.

Academic Editor: Steven F. Abcouwer

Purpose. To investigate the impact of disease duration on the ocular surface during the course of type 2 diabetes mellitus compared with nondiabetic controls. *Methods.* One hundred twenty diabetic patients were divided into three groups according to disease duration: less than 5 years, 5–10 years, and over 10 years. All eyes were imaged using a corneal topographer (Oculus Keratograph 5M). Tear film measurements and meibography were also recorded. Meibomian gland changes were scored from 0 to 6 (meiboscore). *Results.* The noninvasive breakup time first (NIKBUT-1st) and noninvasive breakup time average (NIKBUT-avg) were significantly shorter in the over 10 years diabetic group compared with the control group ($P = 0.0056$ and $P = 0.010$, resp.). Tear meniscus height (TMH) was significantly lower in the over 10 years diabetic group compared with the control group ($P = 0.0016$) and the 5 years group ($P = 0.0061$). We also found that more patients in the over 10 years diabetic group showed bulbar and limbal hyperemia compared with the control group (bulbar hyperemia: $P = 0.049$; limbal hyperemia: $P = 0.026$). The meiboscore in the over 10 years diabetic group was significantly higher compared with the other three groups ($P < 0.05$). Bulbar hyperemia showed a significant negative correlation with NIKBUT-1st in the over 10 years diabetic group ($r = -0.35$ and $P < 0.05$). *Conclusion.* Ocular surface damage in long-term type 2 diabetes is more severe than that in patients with shorter disease duration.

1. Introduction

Type 2 diabetes mellitus is one of the largest public health problems worldwide, especially in developing nations such as China [1], due to changes in lifestyle and diet preferences in recent years. Diabetes is often associated with macrovascular abnormalities. Although retinal complications of diabetes are well recognized and can act as a predictive index for the disease course [2], the effects of diabetes on the ocular surface are poorly understood.

However, according to a clinical study, up to 73.6% of type 2 diabetic patients suffer from corneal complications, such as punctate keratopathy, endothelial dystrophy, and recurrent erosions [3]. In particular, diabetic patients often complain of dry eye symptoms, including dryness, burning,

redness, pain, ocular irritation, and easily fatigued eyes. The International Dry Eye Workshop 2017 classified diabetes as a risk factor for aqueous-deficient dry eye [4]. During the course of diabetes, microvascular damage to the lacrimal gland due to hyperglycemia, reduced lacrimal innervation as a result of autonomic neuropathy, reduced trophic support to lacrimal tissue, and reduced reflex tearing due to impairment of corneal sensitivity all contribute to the altered tear film status in diabetic patients [4].

In contrast to aqueous-deficient dry eye, which is usually caused by a lack of tear production, evaporative dry eye is due to lid-related and ocular surface-related causes such as meibomian gland dysfunction (MGD) and is more frequent [5]. It is acknowledged that the clinical characteristics of both aqueous-deficient and evaporative dry eye are present in patients as dry eye disease progresses. In addition, a large epidemiologic study in Spain [6] suggested that diabetes was associated with MGD, the major contributor to dry eye according to clinical studies [7, 8].

Corneal changes usually depend on the type, duration, and compensation of diabetes mellitus. In this study, we aimed to analyze the tear film stability and morphological changes in meibomian glands using keratography in diabetic patients compared with nondiabetic controls and to better understand the impact of disease duration on the ocular surface during the course of type 2 diabetes mellitus.

2. Materials and Methods

2.1. Subjects. The study was approved by the Investigational Review Board of Shanghai Ninth People's Hospital, Shanghai Jiaotong University School of Medicine, Shanghai, China. All subjects enrolled were informed of the aims of this study.

One hundred twenty patients diagnosed with type 2 diabetes mellitus met the inclusion criteria and were enrolled in the study at the Shanghai Ninth People's Hospital between April 2016 and January 2017. Data were obtained from the right eye of each subject unless this eye was excluded, in which case data were collected from the left eye. The inclusion criteria were as follows: at least 40 years of age and willingness to participate in the study. Patients were excluded if they used topical medications; wore contact lenses; had undergone ocular surgery in the past year or had evidence of other ocular surface diseases; had active ocular infection, inflammation, or systemic disease; or were taking medications that would alter the ocular surface. All diabetic patients had a blood glucose level within the normal range. Diabetic patients were divided into the following three groups according to duration of diabetes since the first diagnosis: less than 5 years, 5–10 years, or more than 10 years. Forty subjects were recruited as nondiabetic controls. The exclusion criteria were similar to those of the control group. Fasting blood glucose was measured to rule out diabetes even in those without a history of diabetes. All patients underwent noninvasive ocular surface examinations in the following order: tear meniscus height (TMH), noninvasive tear film breakup time, bulbar and limbal hyperemia, and grading of meibomian gland loss with the Oculus Keratograph 5M (Wetzlar, Germany). All patients were examined by the same physician (He FL).

All diabetic patients were from the Department of Endocrinology in our hospital. These patients had been followed up over a long period, and disease duration was confirmed by their professional endocrinologists. The data in this article are reliable and were obtained from medical files. The groups were matched by age.

2.2. Oculus Keratograph 5M. Oculus Keratograph 5M can provide automated measurements of tear film dynamics and meibographic images using infrared light without topical anesthetic, fluorescein staining, cobalt blue light, or manual timing. Measurements of noninvasive breakup time

(NIKBUT) obtained with the advanced corneal topographer provide a simple, noninvasive screening test for dry eyes with acceptable sensitivity, specificity, and repeatability [9]. Meibography highlights a glandular architecture, which can be used to analyze glandular density and glandular atrophy [10].

2.3. Tear Film Measurements

2.3.1. TMH. TMH was measured twice in each eye using infrared images obtained from the keratograph. The lower tear film meniscus images were captured 5 s after blinking, and the values were graded perpendicular to the lower eyelid margin at the central point.

2.3.2. NIKBUT. NIKBUT was measured twice in each eye using the Oculus noninvasive Keratograph tear breakup time (NIKBUT) tool. The participants were instructed to blink twice before screening and to keep their eyes open to the best of their ability when recording. The NIKBUT was then determined by Keratograph 5M, which automatically generated two measures for NIKBUT: NIKBUT first (NIKBUT-1st) and NIKBUT average (NIKBUT-avg). NIKBUT-1st represents the time point at which the tear film starts to break up. NIKBUT-avg represents the average time for the overall tear film to break up.

2.4. Bulbar and Limbal Hyperemia. Increased conjunctival redness is often one of the first signs indicating abnormal strain or pathological changes in the eye. Patients were required to open their eyes as wide as possible and focus on a point inside the camera while a keratograph image was captured. The images were then analyzed by the R-SCAN tool following the evaluation protocol. The software analyzed the image automatically and assigned a red eye index (accurate to 0.1 unit).

2.5. Meibography. The upper and lower eyelids were ectropionized, and their respective infrared images were captured. Meibomian gland loss was graded as described by Arita et al. [11]. The meiboscore was as follows: grade 0, no dropout; grade 1, dropout of <1/3 of the lid area; grade 2, dropout of 1/3-2/3 of the lid area; and grade 3, dropout of >2/3 of the lid area. The sum of the upper and lower lid scores was calculated, and the total meiboscore ranged from 0 to 6 [11].

2.6. Statistical Analysis. Pearson's chi-squared test was applied to analyze sex and age differences between the groups. The Shapiro–Wilk test or Kruskal–Wallis test was performed accordingly. Normally distributed continuous parameters were analyzed between the groups by one-way ANOVA and Welch ANOVA tests. The Spearman correlation test was used to calculate correlations. All analyses were performed using the statistical software package GraphPad Prism (version 6.00 for Mac). All P values less than 0.05 were

TABLE 1: Clinical parameters of the four study groups.

Parameter	Control	<5 years	5–10 years	>10 years
Age (yr)	64.88 ± 7.04	64.75 ± 8.20	65.03 ± 7.14	66.11 ± 7.44
Sex ratio (male/female)	18/22	20/24	17/23	16/20
TMH (mm)	0.23 ± 0.06	0.23 ± 0.05	0.21 ± 0.07	0.18 ± 0.06
NIKBUT-1st (s)	6.86 ± 2.20	6.76 ± 2.24	6.25 ± 2.53	5.13 ± 1.77
NIKBUT-avg (s)	9.33 ± 3.68	8.32 ± 2.63	8.21 ± 2.60	7.30 ± 1.63
Bulbar hyperemia	1.53 ± 0.69	1.57 ± 0.69	1.56 ± 0.57	1.92 ± 0.66
Limbal hyperemia	1.52 ± 0.67	1.57 ± 0.64	1.56 ± 0.55	1.93 ± 0.64
Meibography score	3.15 ± 1.09	3.13 ± 1.08	3.53 ± 1.05	4.25 ± 1.14

considered statistically significant. Data are presented as mean $\pm$ SD.

3. Results

3.1. Description of Enrolled Subjects. From April 2016 to January 2017, 120 eyes of 120 type 2 diabetic patients and 40 eyes of 40 nondiabetic patients (22 women and 18 men; aged 64.88 ± 7.04 years) were included in this study. In the diabetic group, the duration of diabetes ranged from 1 to 25 years: in 44 eyes of 44 patients (24 women and 20 men; aged 64.75 ± 8.20 years), the duration was less than 5 years; in 40 eyes of 40 patients (23 women and 17 men; aged 65.03 ± 7.141 years), the duration was 5–10 years; and the duration was more than10 years in 36 eyes of 36 patients (20 women and 16 men; aged $66.11 + 7.44$ years). Table 1 summarizes the demographic and clinical characteristics of the participants. Age and gender did not differ significantly between the subject groups.

3.2. Clinical Parameters of the Ocular Surface. Medians and ranges of clinical parameters in the control group and diabetic groups are shown in Figures 1(a)–(f), respectively. Meibomian glands were almost intact in the control group (Figure 2(a)), and only minimal meibomian gland changes were observed in the 5 years and 5–10 years diabetic groups (Figures 2(b) and 2(c)). In contrast, various meibomian gland changes, including dropouts, shortening, distortion, and dilation were apparent in the over 10 years diabetic patients (Figure 2(d)).

3.3. Comparison of Tear Film Parameters and Meiboscore between the Diabetic and Nondiabetic Groups. The results of clinical parameters in each group and P values for pairwise comparisons between the groups are presented in Tables 1 and 2. Significant differences were observed in TMH, NIKBUT, bulbar and limbal hyperemia, and meiboscore between the control group and the over 10 years diabetic group.

The NIKBUT-1st was significantly shorter in the over 10 years diabetic group compared with the control group (5.13 ± 1.77 versus 6.86 ± 2.20, $P < 0.01$) and the 5 years group (5.13 ± 1.77 versus 6.76 ± 2.24, $P < 0.01$). Similarly, NIKBUT-avg was significantly shorter in the over 10 years diabetic group compared with the control group (7.30 ± 1.63 versus 9.33 ± 3.68, $P < 0.05$). The association between

NIKBUT-1st and time from diagnosis was calculated and indicated a slightly negative Spearman correlation ($r_s = -0.41$ and $P < 0.0001$; Figure 3). The TMH value was significantly lower in the over 10 years diabetic group compared with the control group (0.18 ± 0.06 versus 0.23 ± 0.06, $P < 0.01$) and the 5 years group (0.18 ± 0.06 versus 0.23 ± 0.05, $P < 0.01$). The association between TMH and time from diagnosis was also calculated and indicated a slightly negative Spearman correlation ($r_s = -0.26$ and $P < 0.01$; Figure 4).

The bulbar and limbal redness scan found that more patients in the over 10 years diabetic group showed bulbar and limbal hyperemia compared with the control group (bulbar hyperemia: 1.92 ± 0.66 versus 1.53 ± 0.69, $P < 0.05$; limbal hyperemia: 1.93 ± 0.64 versus 1.53 ± 0.69, $P < 0.05$).

The over 10 years diabetic group showed more meibomian gland changes including dropouts, shortening, distortion, and dilation. The meiboscore in this group was significantly higher compared with the other three groups (the control group versus the over 10 years group, $P = 0.0001$; the 5 years group versus the over 10 years group, $P < 0.0001$; and the 5–10 years group versus the over 10 years group, $P < 0.05$), which indicated that the over 10 years diabetic patients suffered a loss of meibomian glands.

In addition to the significant difference in tear film parameters observed between the over 10 years diabetic group and the control group, we also observed a tendency for ocular surface damage in the three diabetic groups as disease duration increased.

3.4. Correlations between Clinical Parameters. In addition to higher bulbar hyperemia and shorter NIKBUT-1st in the over 10 years diabetic group compared with the nondiabetic group, we also found that bulbar hyperemia had a significant negative correlation with NIKBUT-1st in the over 10 years diabetic group ($r = -0.35$ and $P < 0.05$), which is shown in Figure 5. Thus, the over 10 years diabetic patients who had a less stable tear film were also likely to have higher bulbar hyperemia.

4. Discussion

Diabetic eye disease is well known due to its retinal microvascular disorder, diabetic retinopathy. However, diabetes also has an impact on tear film dynamics and can lead to dry eye. The loss of tear film homeostasis in diabetes may be involved and induce dry eye disease [12]. Given that

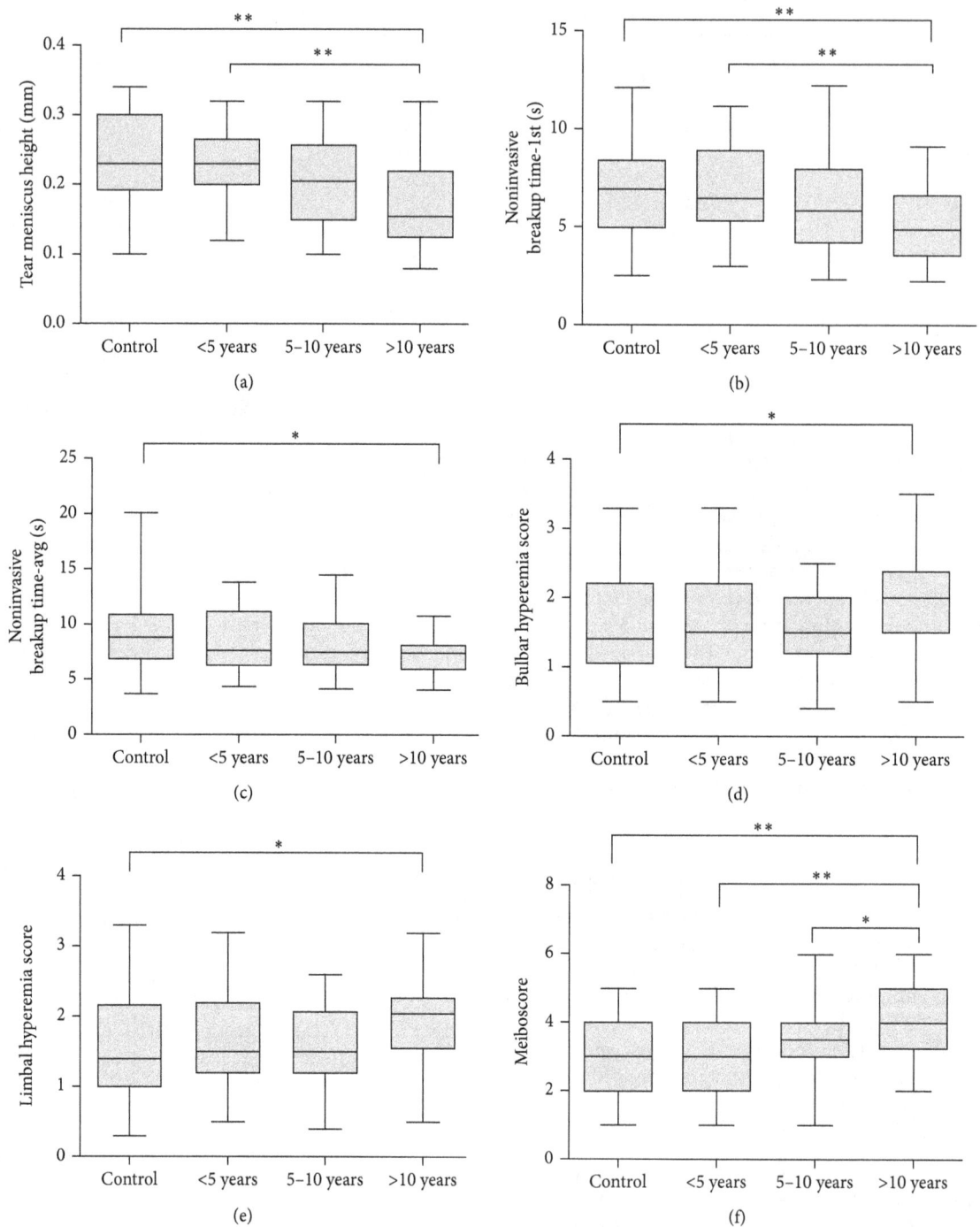

FIGURE 1: (a) Tear meniscus height (mm) in each group ($^*P < 0.05$; $^{**}P < 0.01$). (b) Noninvasive breakup time first (s) in each group ($^*P < 0.05$; $^{**}P < 0.01$). (c) Noninvasive breakup time average (s) in each group ($^*P < 0.05$). (d) Bulbar hyperemia score in each group ($^*P < 0.05$). (e) Limbal hyperemia score in each group ($^*P < 0.05$). (f) Meiboscore in each group ($^*P < 0.05$; $^{**}P < 0.01$). For all, results are presented as medians and ranges (min to max).

major attention is paid to retinopathy, tear stability changes are merely diagnosed. Therefore, this study was conducted to assess changes of tear film parameters during the course of diabetes and found a shorter tear breakup time, greater conjunctival redness, and severe meibomian gland changes in long-term diabetic patients compared to healthy controls, and a tendency for deterioration was observed with increased disease duration.

Our study found that NIKBUT-1st and NIKBUT-avg in the over 10 years diabetic group decreased significantly compared with the normal control group, reflecting instability of the tear film in these patients. These results correlated with previous studies [13–15]. In addition, the TMH value was significantly lower in the over 10 years diabetic group compared with the control group. A decreasing tendency was also noted in the 5 years diabetic

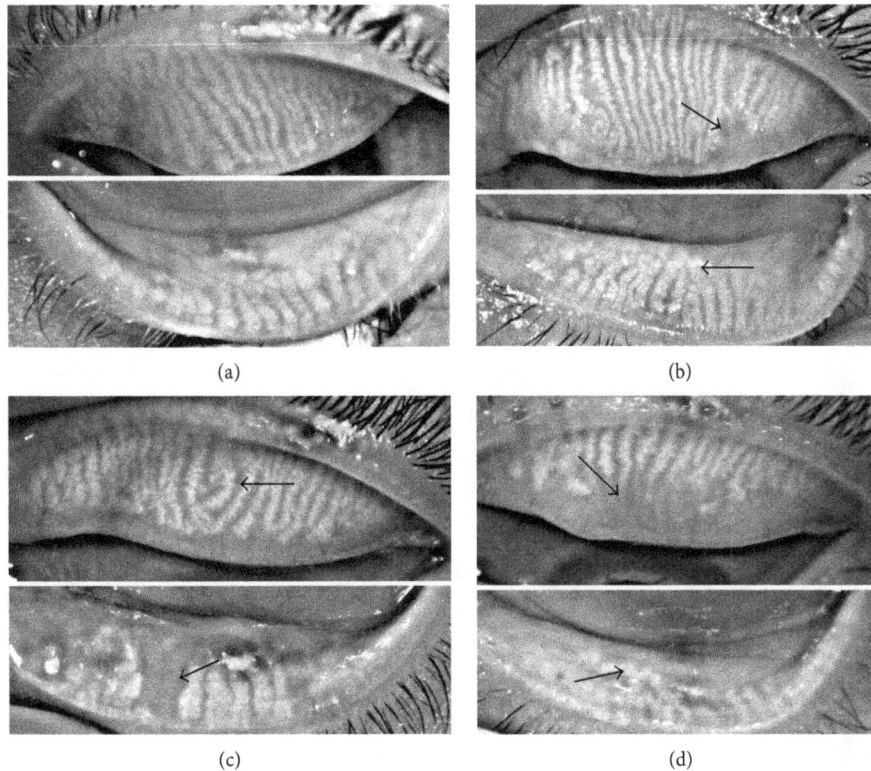

FIGURE 2: Noninvasive meibographic images of the upper and lower eyelids, respectively. (a) No morphologic changes of meibomian glands in either eyelid were apparent (meiboscore of 0). (b) Minor morphologic changes of meibomian glands in both upper and lower eyelids were apparent (meiboscore of 1). The arrow in the upper eyelid shows the partial absence of meibomian glands, and the arrow in the lower eyelid shows a minor distortion of meibomian glands. (c) Less than 1/3 of the meibomian gland loss and minor morphologic changes in both upper and lower eyelids were apparent (meiboscore of 2). The arrow in the upper eyelid shows partial distortion of meibomian glands, and the arrow in the lower eyelid shows an obvious meibomian gland loss. (d) More than 2/3 of shortening, distortion, and dilation of meibomian glands were observed in both eyelids (meiboscore of 5). The arrow in the upper eyelid shows a large area of meibomian gland loss, and the arrow in the lower eyelid shows a significant distortion and dilatation of meibomian glands.

TABLE 2: Statistical comparison (P values) of clinical parameters among the study groups using the ANOVA test.

Parameter	Control versus <5 years	Control versus 5–10 years	Control versus >10 years	<5 years versus 5–10 years	<5 years versus >10 years	>10 years versus 5–10 years
TMH (mm)	0.9617	0.3517	0.0016	0.6246	0.0061	0.1561
NIKBUT-1st (s)	0.9977	0.6299	0.0056	0.7274	0.0079	0.1327
NIKBUT-avg (s)	0.5321	0.4151	0.0100	0.9958	0.2234	0.3468
Bulbar hyperemia	0.9839	0.9937	0.0490	0.9997	0.0996	0.0912
Limbal hyperemia	0.9726	0.9888	0.0262	0.9995	0.0672	0.0595
Meibography score	>0.9999	0.4259	0.0001	0.3725	<0.0001	0.0241

group and 5–10 years diabetic group compared with the control group. Patients with longer duration of diabetes showed reduced TMH and tear film breakup was quicker. Considering that patients often have the disease for a variable amount of time before it is diagnosed, it is really hard to determine the exact disease duration of those patients. We selected data of the two tear film parameters (NIKBUT-1st and TMII) whose P value was less than 0.01, and the data of the two parameters were analyzed with time from diagnosis as a linear variable. It showed that the stability of tear film was negatively correlated with the duration of disease in diabetic patients. The result was consistent with the categorical results. Multiple factors in diabetes could contribute

to reduced tear film stability. It is possible that damage to the lacrimal gland microvasculature together with autonomic neuropathy may contribute to impaired gland function. In particular, peripheral neuropathy in diabetes leads to abnormalities in corneal nerve density and function [16]. Reduced corneal innervation has been found to correlate with a reduced number of goblet cells and reduced mucin protein [15, 17], resulting in altered tear film.

The bulbar conjunctiva and anterior episclera are nourished by vessels from the anterior and long posterior ciliary arteries [18], and the limbal conjunctiva is supplied by superficial arcades of the anterior ciliary vessels [19]. Our study found that the over 10 years diabetic group showed

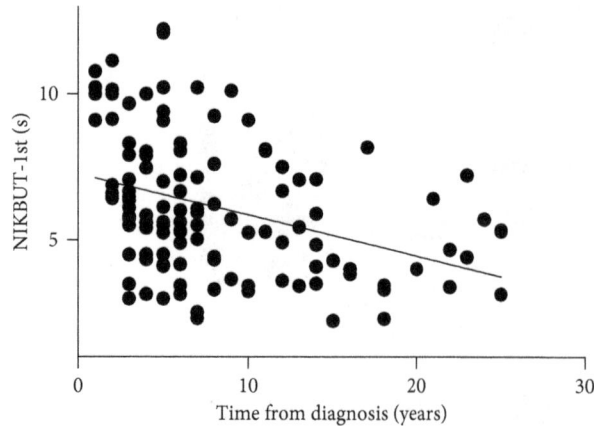

FIGURE 3: Scatterplot graph showing a slight negative Spearman correlation ($r_s = -0.41$ and $P < 0.0001$) between NIKBUT-1st and time from diagnosis.

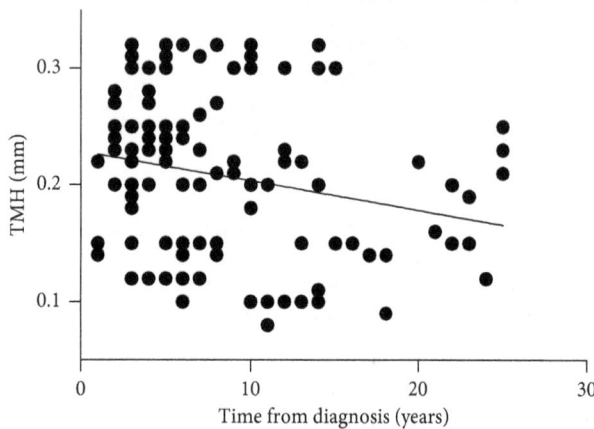

FIGURE 4: Scatterplot graph showing a slight negative Spearman correlation ($r_s = -0.26$ and $P < 0.01$) between TMH and time from diagnosis.

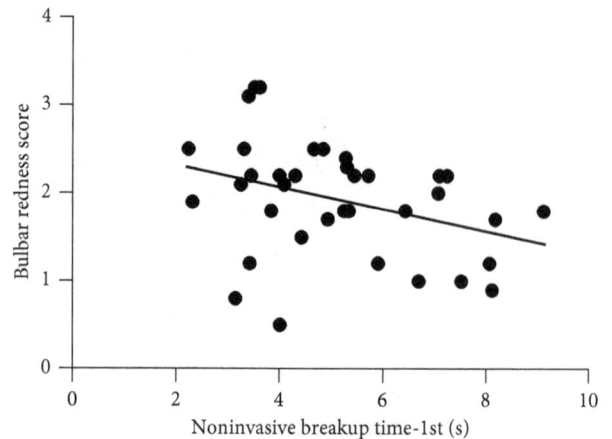

FIGURE 5: Scatterplot graph showing a negative correlation between bulbar hyperemia and NIKBUT-1st ($r = -0.36$, $r^2 = 0.12$, and $P = 0.039$) in the over 10 years group.

significant conjunctival redness compared with the healthy controls ($P < 0.05$), and bulbar hyperemia had a significant negative correlation with NIKBUT-1st in the over 10 years diabetic group ($r = -0.35$ and $P < 0.05$). Conjunctival inflammation is a hallmark of dry eyes [20, 21]. We deduced that increased conjunctival redness may be compensatory to conjunctival inflammation as vasodilation of these vessels results in enhanced blood flow and edema with leakage of fluid and protein from capillaries [22]. In addition, tear evaporation may accelerate when the preconjunctival tear layer temperature rises due to hyperemia. These disorders are associated with signs and symptoms of ocular discomfort such as irritation and foreign body sensation, which can also lead to conjunctival redness.

We compared meibographic findings in the 4 groups, and a significant difference in the meiboscore was found between the control patients and the over 10 years diabetic patients. This was consistent with previous findings [23, 24] where diabetes was associated with MGD. Our data showed that duration of diabetes was closely related to the severity of meibomian gland abnormality (as reflected by the meiboscore, which indicates meibomian gland loss). Several studies have reported that dry eye in diabetes was related to the duration of diabetes [25, 26], but there have been few clinical studies examining meibomian gland function. To the best of our knowledge, the present investigation is the first study to focus on duration of disease in diabetic patients and provides additional evidence for the correlation between the meibomian gland and type 2 diabetes mellitus.

The meibomian gland synthesizes and produces lipids and proteins which form the outermost layer of the tear film. These lipids decrease evaporation and promote stability of the tear film. The International Workshop on Meibomian Gland Dysfunction suggested that MGD is the most prevalent cause of evaporative dry eye and may play a role in aqueous-deficient dry eye [27]. The meiboscore also indicates the thickness of the lipidic layer of the tear film [28], with a higher meiboscore corresponding to a thinner lipidic layer and consequent tear film instability. Although our study provides evidence that meibomian gland function was impaired in long-term diabetic patients, the mechanism of this impairment is unknown and requires further investigation. Recently, a study by Ding et al. demonstrated that insulin stimulated the proliferation of immortalized human meibomian gland epithelial cells (HMGECs), whereas high glucose was found to be toxic to HMGECs [29]. This suggests that insulin resistance/deficiency and hyperglycemia are deleterious to HMGECs, which supports our hypothesis that long-term duration of the disease and insufficient control of blood glucose may be associated with MGD. Moreover, the various medications prescribed to diabetic patients may exacerbate the dry eye state, which may have contributed to the association between duration of diabetes and meibomian gland function in our study. Furthermore, the concomitant inflammatory response in diabetes may also induce MGD. Suzuki et al. suggested that obstructive MGD is a precursor of meibomitis [30].

In addition, Oculus Keratograph 5M is a corneal topographer with additional noninvasive imaging tools for the assessment of tear film kinetics and meibography. It includes the ability to capture clear images of the meibomian gland architecture using infrared light, eliminating the need for instillation of sodium fluorescein into the tear film or the use of white light that exacerbates photophobia in patients with ocular surface disturbance. However, there is no consistent method for meibographic analysis in clinical practice. Our results provide an objective grading method to illustrate complementary data of glandular density.

In summary, our data suggest that long-term type 2 diabetes predisposes to various changes on the ocular surface, which should be noted at an early stage and treated appropriately in order to prevent more severe eye complications. Therefore, close attention should be paid to the ocular surface, especially in long-term diabetics. Further studies are needed to expand the sample size and include fluctuations in blood sugar as a key factor in studying the ocular surface.

Conflicts of Interest

The authors report no conflicts of interest.

Acknowledgments

This study was supported by the National Natural Science Foundation of China (nos. 81370992, 81570812, and 81500765), the Shanghai Municipal Education Commission-Gaofeng Clinical Medicine Grant Support (Grant no. 20161421), the Science and Technology Commission of Shanghai (17DZ2260100), and the Fundamental Research Program Funding of Ninth People's Hospital affiliated to the Shanghai Jiao Tong University School of Medicine (JYZZ001).

References

[1] Y. Xu, L. Wang, J. He et al., "Prevalence and control of diabetes in Chinese adults," *JAMA*, vol. 310, no. 9, pp. 948–959, 2013.

[2] D. S. W. Ting, G. C. M. Cheung, and T. Y. Wong, "Diabetic retinopathy: global prevalence, major risk factors, screening practices and public health challenges: a review," *Clinical & Experimental Ophthalmology*, vol. 44, no. 4, pp. 260–277, 2016.

[3] D. L. DeMill, M. Hussain, R. Pop-Busui, and R. M. Shtein, "Ocular surface disease in patients with diabetic peripheral neuropathy," *British Journal of Ophthalmology*, vol. 100, no. 7, pp. 924–928, 2016.

[4] A. J. Bron, P. C. S. De, S. K. Chauhan et al., "The ocular surface TFOS DEWS II pathophysiology report," *Ocular Surface*, vol. 15, no. 3, pp. 438–510, 2017.

[5] F. Stapleton, M. Alves, V. Y. Bunya et al., "The ocular surface TFOS DEWS II epidemiology report," *Ocular Surface*, vol. 15, no. 3, pp. 334–365, 2017.

[6] E. Viso, M. T. Rodriguez-Ares, D. Abelenda et al., "Prevalence of asymptomatic and symptomatic meibomian gland dysfunction in the general population of Spain," *Investigative Ophthalmology and Visual Science*, vol. 53, no. 6, pp. 2601–2606, 2012.

[7] M. A. Lemp, L. A. Crews, A. J. Bron et al., "Distribution of aqueous-deficient and evaporative dry eye in a clinic-based patient cohort: a retrospective study," *Cornea*, vol. 31, no. 5, pp. 472–478, 2012.

[8] E. Viso, F. Gude, M. T. Rodríguez-Ares et al., "The association of meibomian gland dysfunction and other common ocular diseases with dry eye: a population-based study in Spain," *Cornea*, vol. 30, no. 1, pp. 1-6, 2011.

[9] J. Hong, X. Sun, A. Wei et al., "Assessment of tear film stability in dry eye with a newly developed keratograph," *Cornea*, vol. 32, no. 5, pp. 716–721, 2013.

[10] N. S. Abdelfattah, A. Dastiridou, S. R. Sadda, and O. L. Lee, "Non-invasive imaging of tear film dynamics in eyes with ocular surface disease," *Cornea*, vol. 32, no. 10, pp. 716–721, 2013.

[11] R. Arita, K. Itoh, K. Inoue, S. Amano et al., "Noncontact infrared meibography to document age-related changes of the meibomian glands in a normal population," *Ophthalmology*, vol. 115, no. 5, pp. 911–915, 2008.

[12] J. P. Craig, K. K. Nichols, E. K. Akpek et al., "The ocular surface TFOS DEWS II definition and classification report," *Ocular Surface*, vol. 15, no. 3, pp. 276–283, 2017.

[13] M. Goebbels, "Tear secretion and tear film function in insulin dependent diabetics," *British Journal of Ophthalmology*, vol. 84, no. 1, pp. 19–21, 2000.

[14] P. Cousen, P. Cackett, H. Bennett et al., "Tear production and corneal sensitivity in diabetes," *Journal of Diabetes and Its Complications*, vol. 21, no. 6, pp. 371–373, 2007.

[15] K. A. Beckman, "Characterization of dry eye disease in diabetic patients versus nondiabetic patients," *Cornea*, vol. 33, no. 8, pp. 851–854, 2014.

[16] E. M. Messmer, C. Schmid-Tannwald, D. Zapp et al., "In vivo confocal microscopy of corneal small fiber damage in diabetes mellitus," *Graefe's Archive for Clinical and Experimental Ophthalmology*, vol. 248, no. 9, pp. 1307–1312, 2010.

[17] M. Dogru, C. Katakami, and M. Inoue, "Tear function and ocular surface changes in noninsulin-dependent diabetes mellitus," *Ophthalmology*, vol. 108, no. 3, pp. 586–592, 2001.

[18] M. B. Abelson, "Code red: the key feature of hyperemia," *Review of Ophthalmology*, vol. 22, pp. 1–12, 2010.

[19] E. M. Van Buskirk, "The anatomy of the limbus," *Eye*, vol. 3, no. 2, pp. 101–108, 1989.

[20] M. E. Stern and S. C. Pflugfelder, "Inflammation in dry eye," *Ocular Surface*, vol. 2, no. 2, pp. 124–130, 2004.

[21] M. Hessen and E. K. Akpek, "Dry eye: an inflammatory ocular disease," *Journal of Ophthalmic and Vision Research*, vol. 9, no. 2, pp. 240–250, 2014.

[22] C. W. McMonnies, "Conjunctival tear layer temperature, evaporation, hyperosmolarity, inflammation, hyperemia, tissue damage, and symptoms: a review of an amplifying cascade," *Current Eye Research*, vol. 42, no. 12, pp. 1574–1584, 2017.

[23] X. L. Lin, B. Xu, Y. Zheng et al., "Meibomian gland dysfunction in type 2 diabetic patients," *Journal of Ophthalmology*, vol. 2017, Article ID 3047867, 7 pages, 2017.

[24] R. P. Shamsheer and C. Arunachalam, "A clinical study of meibomian gland dysfunction in patients with diabetes," *Middle East African Journal of Ophthalmology*, vol. 22, no. 4, pp. 462–466, 2015.

[25] M. R. Manaviat, M. Rashidi, M. Afkhami-Ardekani, and M. R. Shoja, "Prevalence of dry eye syndrome and diabetic retinopathy in type 2 diabetic patients," *BMC Ophthalmology*, vol. 8, no. 1, p. 10, 2008.

[26] L. Yu, X. Chen, G. Qin et al., "Tear film function in type 2 diabetic patients with retinopathy," *Ophthalmologica*, vol. 222, no. 4, pp. 284–291, 2008.

[27] K. K. Nichols, "The International Workshop on Meibomian Gland Dysfunction: introduction," *Investigative Ophthalmology and Visual Science*, vol. 52, no. 4, pp. 1917–1921, 2011.

[28] Y. Eom, J. S. Lee, S. Y. Kang et al., "Correlation between quantitative measurements of tear film lipid layer thickness and meibomian gland loss in patients with obstructive meibomian gland dysfunction and normal controls," *American Journal of Ophthalmology*, vol. 155, no. 6, pp. 1104–1110.e2, 2013.

[29] J. Ding, Y. Liu, and D. A. Sullivan, "Effects of insulin and high glucose on human meibomian gland epithelial cells," *Investigative Ophthalmology and Visual Science*, vol. 56, no. 13, pp. 7814–7820, 2015.

[30] T. Suzuki, S. Teramukai, and S. Kinoshita, "Meibomian glands and ocular surface inflammation," *Ocular Surface*, vol. 13, no. 2, pp. 133–149, 2015.

15

Effect of Age on Pentacam Keratoconus Indices

Maged Maher Salib Roshdy [iD],[1,2] **Sherine Shafik Wahba** [iD],[1,2] **Rania Serag Elkitkat** [iD],[1,2] **Amira Maurice Hakim,**[2] and **Ramy Riad Fikry** [iD][2,3]

[1]*Ophthalmology Department, Ain Shams University, Cairo, Egypt*
[2]*Al Watany Eye Hospital, Cairo, Egypt*
[3]*Ophthalmology Department, Cairo University, Cairo, Egypt*

Correspondence should be addressed to Rania Serag Elkitkat; raniaselkitkat@med.asu.edu.eg

Academic Editor: Flavio Mantelli

Purpose. To assess the effect of age on elevation and pachymetric Pentacam keratoconus (KC) detection indices, and the need to adjust normative values accordingly. *Methods.* In a retrospective study, 95 eyes of myopic normal subjects without KC were evaluated using the OCULUS Pentacam, with an age range of 17.4 to 46.8 years. Subjects were categorised into three groups according to their age: the first included those younger than 21 years (19 eyes), the second was for the age range of 21–40 years (65 eyes), and the third comprised subjects older than 40 years (11 eyes). *Results.* There were statistically significant differences among the three groups regarding many elevation indices: AE from BFS, PE from BFS, and PE minus AE from BFS ($P = 0.003$, 0.010, and <0.001, resp.), and pachymetric indices: PPI avg, PPI max, ART avg, ART max, and diagonal decentration of the thinnest point ($P = $ <0.001, 0.024, 0.003, 0.026, and 0.026, resp.). On comparing subjects below 21 years to those above 40 years, there was a statistically significant decrease of both PE from BFS and PE minus AE ($P = 0.005$ and <0.001, resp.) and statistically significant increase in AE from BFS ($P = 0.001$). *Conclusions.* Age is an important determinant of elevation indices, significantly altering their normative values. The use of the more robust pachymetry, rather than elevation, indices is recommended in subjects below 21 or above 40 years of age.

1. Introduction

As corneal refractive surgery evolves, professional expectations increase and require continuous refinements of preoperative screening and interpretation [1]. Currently, Scheimpflug tomography devices, such as the Pentacam (OCULUS Optikgerate GmbH, Wetzlar, Germany), are the most popular techniques providing anterior and posterior corneal surface elevations, together with a detailed thickness profile [2]. Early and accurate keratoconus (KC) detection using variable indices has been widely discussed, comparing the sensitivities and specificities of various parameters [3–5]. Furthermore, new algorithms and combined indices have been introduced, aiming at earlier and more precise KC detection [6, 7].

Ageing can alter the human corneal topography, with a detected increase in aberrations [8] and an altered pattern of corneal astigmatism [9]. The possible effect of age on

corneal elevation and pachymetric profiles has been sparsely discussed [10].

Moreover, the spherical refractive error effect on tomographic corneal values is an issue that deserves proper analysis. Most of the topographic screening values were initially based on a predominantly myopic population [11], rendering it obviously inaccurate to apply the normative values on the hyperopic population, as emphasized in Kim et al.'s study [1].

This study aims at assessing the effect of age on elevation and pachymetry-based KC diagnostic indices and at studying this age effect after controlling for the spherical refractive error, using the OCULUS Pentacam, and the possible need to adjust the normative values accordingly.

2. Materials and Methods

This is a retrospective study including 95 consecutive myopic normal corneas imaged in the time interval between June

2008 and December 2009, using the Pentacam branded as Allegro Oculyzer (WaveLight, GmbH, Erlangen, Germany) [12] with software version 1.16r12, at Al Watany Eye Hospital, Cairo, Egypt. The study adhered to the tenets of the Declaration of Helsinki and was approved by the local institutional review board.

We excluded candidates with any detected corneal pathology, previous ocular surgery, contact lens wear within the last two weeks, or narrow palpebral fissure precluding proper imaging. Moreover, the participants were followed up annually until December 2016 to confirm that no ectasia developed along the years, either in eyes that underwent laser refractive surgeries (88 eyes) or in those who were unsuitable due to inconvenient myopic refractive error values (7 eyes). Hence, we made sure that any determined changes in index values were not due to forme fruste KC. Corneal evaluation on follow-up included the evaluation of refraction stability and, in query cases, by assessing the posterior elevation values, using the same Pentacam device.

Subjective refraction and spherical equivalent (SE) calculation were performed. All eyes were scanned at least thrice by Pentacam according to the recommendations of the device manual. Each scan included 25 Scheimpflug images. Despite good repeatability, data were collected from the most reliable scan as stated by the "QS" pop-up box (i.e., the largest analysed area, valid data percent, and good alignment). The data were collected from the automatically calculated indices for a reference surface shape 8 mm in diameter, then getting the elevation values on mouse click at the thinnest point. The investigated indices included:

  (i) Elevation-based indices:

    (a) Anterior elevations (AE) from BFS

    (b) Posterior elevations (PE) from BFS

    (c) PE from the best-fit toric ellipsoid (BFTE)

    (d) PE minus AE from BFS

  (ii) Pachymetry-based indices:

    (a) Apex thickness, thickness at pupil centroid (CCT), and the thinnest-point thickness (TCT)

    (b) Minimum, average, and maximum corneal pachymetry progression indices (PPI min, PPI avg, and PPI max, resp.)

    (c) Minimum, average, and maximum Ambrosio's relational thickness indices (ART min, ART avg, and ART max, resp.)

    (d) Thinnest-point displacement at x- and y-axes (thinnest dX and thinnest dY, resp.) and diagonal decentration index

Subjects were then categorised into three groups according to their age on the day of Pentacam evaluation: the first included those younger than 21 years (19 eyes), the second

was for the age range of 21–40 years (65 eyes), and the third comprised subjects older than 40 years (11 eyes).

2.1. Statistical Analysis. Data were collected and verified, and the compound indices were calculated using Microsoft Excel 2010 (Redmond, Washington, USA). Statistical analyses were performed using IBM SPSS Statistics (v19; Armonk, NY, USA). The following tests were performed: calculation of the mean, standard deviation (SD), one-sample Kolmogorov-Smirnov test to test normality, independent-sample Kruskal-Wallis test for comparison of the three groups, independent-sample Mann–Whitney U test for comparing each pair of groups, Spearman correlation coefficient, and partial correlation coefficients controlling for SE and age one at a time. Values were considered statistically significant if the P value was less than 0.05.

3. Results

3.1. Demographics. The study included 95 participants, with an average age of 28.7 ± 7.8 years (ranging from 17.4 to 46.8). Forty-nine right eyes and 46 left eyes were examined. Participants' spherical equivalent had a mean of -4.6 ± 3.0 D (ranging from −0.375 to −16.625).

3.2. Age Grouping Effect. The SE was evenly represented in the three age groups ($P = 0.912$). There were statistically significant differences among the three groups regarding many elevation (AE from BFS, PE from BFS, and PE minus AE from BFS) and pachymetric indices (PPI avg, PPI max, ART avg, ART max, and diagonal decentration of the thinnest point). On the other hand, some indices did not show statistically significant differences as regard age grouping, including a single elevation-based index (PE from BFTE) and some pachymetric indices (apex thickness, CCT, TCT, PPI min, ART min, thinnest dX, and thinnest dY) (Table 1).

The indices showing statistical significance among the three groups were then compared between every 2 groups (Table 2).

The 2 and 3 SD limits (of the indices showing statistical significance) for each of the three age groups are shown in Table 3. For ART avg and ART max, the alarming values are those less than the mean − 2 or −3 SD, while for other indices, the alarming values are those greater than the mean + 2 or +3 SD.

3.3. Refraction versus Age Effect. Most of indices were found correlated with SE alone (when calculating the partial correlation controlling for age). However, only the elevation indices from BFS were found correlated with age. Furthermore, on excluding the SE effect (controlling for SE), all the elevation indices from either BFS or BFTE were correlated with age (Table 4). Age was not found correlated to any of the pachymetric indices.

4. Discussion

Higher expectations for corneal refractive surgeries mandate better screening strategies and data analysis to avoid inappropriately permitting or excluding candidates [2]. This

TABLE 1: Mean, standard deviation, and statistical significance of different indices among the three age groups.

| | <21 years | | 21 to 40 years | | >40 years | | Kruskal-Wallis |
	Mean	SD	Mean	SD	Mean	SD	test (P value)
Age	19.5	1.2	28.7	4.5	44.6	1.8	
SE	−5.24	5.01	−4.51	2.26	−4.31	2.71	
AE from BFS	2.9	1.2	2.7	1.4	1.3	1.1	0.003*
PE from BFS	1.4	3.0	3.9	4.2	5.3	3.3	0.010*
PE from BFTE	3.3	2.7	4.0	3.9	5.7	5.0	0.427
PE minus AE from BFS	−1.5	2.9	1.2	3.9	4.0	3.0	<0.001*
Apex thickness	541.6	35.9	547.3	30.4	559.3	36.9	0.602
CCT	541.5	35.6	547.7	30.5	560.1	37.3	0.632
TCT	540.3	35.4	545.6	31.1	558.0	36.9	0.623
PPI min	0.505	0.151	0.548	0.150	0.482	0.108	0.218
PPI avg	0.779	0.132	0.845	0.129	0.700	0.089	<0.001*
PPI max	1.021	0.132	1.086	0.168	0.964	0.129	0.024*
ART min	1184.9	423.9	1103.7	443.5	1236.8	400.0	0.26
ART avg	713.7	134.4	661.1	110.2	812.6	143.6	0.003*
ART max	538.3	81.4	513.6	82.4	588.8	90.5	0.026*
Thinnest dX	0.059	0.488	0.021	0.595	−0.028	0.413	0.877
Thinnest dY	−0.222	0.159	−0.286	0.210	−0.237	0.207	0.41
Diagonal decentration	0.522	0.175	0.645	0.244	0.465	0.190	0.026*

AE from BFS: anterior elevation from the best-fit sphere, PE from BFS: posterior elevation from the best-fit sphere, PE from BFTE: posterior elevation from the best-fit toric ellipsoid, CCT: thickness at pupil centroid, TCT: the thinnest-point thickness, PPI min: minimum corneal pachymetry progression index, PPI avg: average corneal pachymetry progression index, PPI max: maximum corneal pachymetry progression index, ART min: minimum Ambrosio's relational thickness index, ART avg: average Ambrosio's relational thickness index, ART max: maximum Ambrosio's relational thickness index, thinnest dX: the thinnest-point displacement at x-axis, thinnest dY: the thinnest-point displacement at y-axis. *Values flagged as statistically significant differences.

TABLE 2: The significance (P value) of comparing indices between every 2 groups.

Compared groups Test	(<21 years) versus (21–40 years) Mann–Whitney	(<21 years) versus (>40 years) Mann–Whitney with exact significance	(21–40 years) versus (>40 years) Mann–Whitney
AE from BFS	0.624	0.001*	0.002*
PE from BFS	0.022*	0.005*	0.092
PE minus AE from BFS	0.008*	0.001*	0.004*
PPI avg	0.038*	0.094	0.001*
PPI max	0.106	0.268	0.015*
ART avg	0.080	0.112	0.002*
ART max	0.194	0.145	0.012*
Diagonal decentration	0.061	0.471	0.025*

AE from BFS: anterior elevation from the best-fit sphere, PE from BFS: posterior elevation from the best-fit sphere, PPI avg: average corneal pachymetry progression index, PPI max: maximum corneal pachymetry progression index, ART avg: average Ambrosio's relational thickness index, ART max: maximum Ambrosio's relational thickness index. *Statistical significance ($P < 0.05$).

necessitates continuous refinements for any parameter that can cause falsely positive or negative diagnosis. Although there is a consensus on the absence of a single index robustly detecting KC and that KC diagnosis requires multiple index interpretation, adjusting and comparing the accuracies of individual indices remain an issue that deserves proper investigation. It would be highly valuable to highlight the indices to rely upon, in which cases, and their normal range.

The human cornea, together with other parts of the eye, suffers age-related changes. Some corneal topographic age changes have been previously highlighted [8, 9]. Likewise, the corneal tomographic parameters, pachymetric and elevation indices, need proper evaluation regarding their possible changes with age [10].

Most of the Pentacam normative database was obtained from refractive surgery candidates, with an age range of 21

TABLE 3: Mean ± two and three standard deviation values of the indices having statistically significant differences among different age groups.

	<21 years		21–40 years		>40 years	
	M ± 2 SD	M ± 3 SD	M ± 2 SD	M ± 3 SD	M ± 2 SD	M ± 3 SD
AE from BFS	5.4	6.6	5.6	7.0	3.5	4.6
PE from BFS	7.5	10.5	12.4	16.6	11.9	15.1
PE minus AE from BFS	4.2	7.1	9.0	12.9	10.1	13.1
PPI avg	1.042	1.174	1.102	1.231	0.879	0.968
PPI max	1.284	1.416	1.421	1.589	1.221	1.350
ART avg	444.9	310.4	440.7	330.5	525.4	381.7
ART max	375.5	294.1	348.8	266.3	407.8	317.2
Diagonal decentration	0.871	1.046	1.133	1.377	0.846	1.037

TABLE 4: Correlation of age with other indices, partial correlation with SE after controlling for age effect, and partial correlation with age after controlling for SE effect.

	Correlation of age		Correlation of SE controlled for age		Correlation of age controlled for SE	
	Spearman's rho	P value	Partial correlation	P value	Partial correlation	P value
AE from BFS	−0.217	0.035	0.241	0.019	−0.294	0.004
PE from BFS	0.419	0.001	0.299	0.003	0.378	0.001
PE from BFTE	0.135	0.192	0.203	0.050	0.227	0.028
PE minus AE from BFS	0.498	0.001	0.231	0.025	0.493	0.001
Apex thickness	−0.004	0.971	−0.241	0.019	0.127	0.224
CCT	0.013	0.898	−0.245	0.017	0.138	0.185
TCT	−0.013	0.899	−0.249	0.015	0.114	0.272
PPI min	0.184	0.074	0.190	0.067	0.121	0.247
PPI avg	0.062	0.553	0.285	0.005	−0.030	0.774
PPI max	0.133	0.197	0.240	0.020	0.056	0.595
ART min	−0.190	0.065	−0.200	0.053	−0.101	0.334
ART mid	−0.070	0.499	−0.364	0.001	0.125	0.232
ART max	−0.111	0.284	−0.339	0.001	0.036	0.729
Thinnest dX	−0.039	0.707	0.002	0.982	−0.039	0.711
Thinnest dY	−0.036	0.729	0.135	0.195	0.016	0.878
Resultant decentration	−0.017	0.870	0.188	0.070	−0.118	0.258

to 40 years. The present study evaluated many pachymetry and elevation indices not only for this age range, but also for the late teenagers below 21 and for older subjects above 40 years of age, hence including a wide age range, aiming at investigating the correlation between age and various KC detection indices.

To be sure that the observed difference is not a fallacy caused by the refraction as a covariant, we performed partial correlation analyses controlled for the SE effect. This confirmed that the observed changes in indices were caused by the age effect and not only a fallacy due to refractive variation among the recruited subjects.

Regarding elevation indices, they showed statistically significant differences among groups, except for PE from BFTE. However, after controlling for the SE effect, the latter index did not stand robust in correlation to age. Thus, our results highlight a significant correlation between age and all the studied elevation indices and hence the

inaccuracy of relying upon them using usual cutoff values in evaluating refractive candidates.

On evaluating elevation indices in late teenagers below 21 years, we detected a statistically significant decrease of most of the elevation indices: PE from BFS and PE minus and a statistically significant increase in AE from BFS. In the elevation indices that showed statistically significant differences among groups, the effect of age was most highlighted on comparing subjects below 21 years to those above 40 years, where all the elevation indices were statistically significant between them. Therefore, extremes of age are the most sensitive cohorts to elevation index fallacies. Regarding the older age group, more than 40 years of age, there was a tendency for higher PE and lower AE compared with younger subjects. However, this did not reach statistical significance in all cases.

Hashemi et al. [10] found a significant correlation of age with the maximum AE within the central 6 mm zone

($P < 0.001$), but not with the maximum PE ($P = 0.476$). However, their study included a heterogeneous group of patients with KC and forme fruste KC together with healthy subjects. As the values of indices in KC and forme fruste KC are highly variable, and these conditions are a confounding factor on their own, we preferred to include normal corneas only.

As regard pachymetric indices, our results revealed significant differences among groups in many of them, while some others did not show any statistical significance (apex thickness, CCT, TCT, PPI min, ART min, thinnest dX, and thinnest dY). This declares the robustness of the mentioned indices. Furthermore, on comparing every two groups, all the pachymetric indices were statistically insignificant between late teenagers below 21 and older age > 40 years. Moreover, after controlling for the SE effect, all the pachymetric indices showed no statistical significance in correlation to age. This important finding poses a recommendation of relying on pachymetric rather than elevation parameters in prerefractive surgery assessment for candidates below the age of 21 and those above 40 years of age.

Elevation-based indices were the parameters that showed a statistically significant difference across studied age groups. Hence, our study presented the two and three SD values in patients for these indices, where values outside the 2 SD limit represent less than 5% of corneas and values outside the 3 SD represent less than 0.3% of corneas. Values above 3 SD are suggestive of a probable pathology (Table 3).

Although the primary aim of our study was not to evaluate the refractive error effect, our results revealed that after controlling for the SE effect, all the elevation indices, from either BFS or BFTE, were correlated with age. This finding reaffirmed our suggestion of relying on pachymetric indices rather than elevation indices for extremes of age.

The evaluation of KC indices in relation to the SE effect has been previously discussed. Kim et al. [1] assessed corneal elevation and pachymetry in hyperopes compared to myopes, where they concluded that when adjusted for age, the PE changes remained statistically significant between hyperopic and myopic patients, but AE changes lost significance. On the contrary, Hashemi et al. [13] found that values of both maximum AE and PE within the central 4 mm circle in myopes were significantly higher than in hyperopic eyes, in a collaborative study evaluating the various effects of refractive errors on anterior segment Pentacam parameters. However, these studies analysed the SE effect between myopic and hyperopic cohorts. To the best of our knowledge, no studies analysed the effect of both age and refraction within the myopic range.

In our study, we followed up the subjects for several years, either with or without performing laser refractive surgeries, aiming to absolutely exclude forme fruste KC, an issue that may lead to fallacies in results. However, in other studies, including Kim et al. [1], they tried to avoid undiagnosed or forme fruste KC merely by excluding subjects with a family history of KC. We believe that following up patients is more reliable.

5. Conclusion

We recommend the use of pachymetry-based indices, or the elevation indices with altered normative data, when assessing corneas of patients outside the usual 21–40 years range.

Conflicts of Interest

Maged Maher Salib Roshdy received travel support from Novartis, Orchidia Pharma, and Bayer. Sherine Shafik Wahba, Rania Serag Elkitkat, and Amira Maurice Hakim have nothing to declare. Ramy Riad Fikry received travel support from Novartis.

References

[1] J. T. Kim, M. Cortese, M. W. Belin, R. Ambrosio Jr, and S. S. Khachikian, "Tomographic normal values for corneal elevation and pachymetry in a hyperopic population," *Journal of Clinical & Experimental Ophthalmology*, vol. 02, no. 2, pp. 130–133, 2011.

[2] M. Dubbelman, V. A. Sicam, and G. L. Van der Heijde, "The shape of the anterior and posterior surface of the aging human cornea," *Vision Research*, vol. 46, no. 6-7, pp. 993–1001, 2006.

[3] P. R. Vazquez, J. D. Galetti, N. Minguez et al., "Pentacam Scheimpflug tomography findings in topographically normal patients and subclinical keratoconus cases," *American Journal of Ophthalmology*, vol. 158, no. 1, pp. 32–40.e2, 2014.

[4] P. R. Vazquez, M. Delrivo, F. F. Bonthoux, T. Pfortner, P. Chiaradia, and J. Galletti, "Subclinical keratoconus detection based on Pentacam Scheimpflug tomography indices," *Investigative Ophthalmology & Visual Science*, vol. 54, no. 15, p. 534, 2013.

[5] S. S. Wahba, M. M. Roshdy, R. S. Elkitkat, and K. M. Naguib, "Rotating Scheimpflug imaging indices in different grades of keratoconus," *Journal of Ophthalmology*, vol. 2016, Article ID 6392472, 9 pages, 2016.

[6] R. Vinciguerra, R. Ambrosio, A. Elsheikh et al., "Detection of keratoconus with a new biomechanical index," *Journal of Refractive Surgery*, vol. 32, no. 12, pp. 803–810, 2016.

[7] M. K. Arbelaez, F. Versaci, G. Vestri, P. Barboni, and G. Savini, "Use of a support vector machine for keratoconus and subclinical keratoconus detection by topographic and tomographic data," *Ophthalmology*, vol. 119, no. 11, pp. 2231–2238, 2012.

[8] A. Guirao, M. Redondo, and P. Artal, "Optical aberrations of the human cornea as a function of age," *Journal of the Optical Society of America*, vol. 17, no. 10, pp. 1697–1702, 2000.

[9] J. D. Ho, S. W. Liou, R. J. Tsai, and C.-Y. Tsai, "Effects of aging on anterior and posterior corneal astigmatism," *Cornea*, vol. 29, no. 6, pp. 632–637, 2010.

[10] H. Hashemi, A. Beiranvand, M. Khabazkhoob et al., "Corneal elevation and keratoconus indices in a 40- to 64-year-old population, Shahroud Eye Study," *Journal of Current Ophthalmology*, vol. 27, no. 3-4, pp. 92–98, 2015.

[11] R. H. Wei, L. Lim, W. K. Chan, and D. Tan, "Evaluation of Orbscan II corneal topography in individuals with myopia," *Ophthalmology*, vol. 113, no. 2, pp. 177–183, 2006.

[12] J. J. Holladay, *Allegro Oculyzer User Manual. The Holladay Report. In the Pentacam: Precision, Confidence, Results, and Accurate K's. Insert to Cataract and Refractive Surgery Today*, p. 20, 2007.

[13] M. Hashemi, K. G. Falavarjani, G. H. Aghai, K. A. Aghdam, and A. Gordiz, "Anterior segment study with the Pentacam Scheimpflug camera in refractive surgery candidates," *Middle East African Journal of Ophthalmology*, vol. 20, no. 3, pp. 212–216, 2013.

16

Medial Rectus Tendon Elongation with Bovine Pericard (Tutopatch®) in Thyroid-Associated Orbitopathy: A Long-Term Follow-Up including Oculodynamic MRI

Monika Wipf ⑩,[1] Britt-Isabelle Berg ⑩,[2,3] and Anja Palmowski-Wolfe ⑩[1]

[1]*University Eye Hospital, University of Basel, Mittlere Strasse 91, 4031 Basel, Switzerland*
[2]*Department of Cranio-Maxillofacial Surgery, University of Basel, Spitalstrasse 21, 4031 Basel, Switzerland*
[3]*Division of Oral and Maxillofacial Radiology, Columbia University Medical Center, 622 W. 168th St., New York, NY 10032, USA*

Correspondence should be addressed to Britt-Isabelle Berg; isabelle.berg@usb.ch

Academic Editor: Achim Langenbucher

Introduction. To assess long-term efficacy of bimedial rectus tendon elongation with Tutopatch in thyroid-associated orbitopathy (TAO). *Materials and Methods.* Retrospective chart review of 5 patients with TAO undergoing bimedial rectus recession with Tutopatch tendon elongation between 2009 and 2015. We analyzed horizontal squint angles, motility, field of binocular single vision, dose effect of surgery, and when possible oculodynamic MRI (OD-MRI). Dose effect and motility were compared to 4 TAO patients with conventional bimedial recession. *Results and Discussion.* In the Tutopatch group, preoperative angles ranged from 14 to 120Δ (prism diopters) at distance and 12–120Δ at near. Mean dose effect was 3.63Δ/mm for the distance and 3.43Δ/mm for the near angle. All patients were orthotropic at final FU (ranging from 1 to 10 years). OD-MRI showed the elasticity of Tutopatch. In the conventional recession group, preoperative angles ranged between 18 and 35Δ at distance and 12–33Δ at near. At final FU, 2 patients had reverted to their underlying microesotropia <2Δ, 1 patient was orthophor, and one was reoperated for a remaining esotropia of 14Δ. Dose effect was 2.95Δ/mm for the distance and 2.18Δ/mm for the near angle. Motility improved in both groups even after 3 months. *Conclusions.* Dose effect for medial rectus recessions with Tutopatch in TAO was higher than previously reported, presenting a good alternative to treat large squint angles while preserving good motility.

1. Introduction

In patients with thyroid-associated orbitopathy (TAO), inflammation and fibrotic changes of the extraocular muscles may cause restriction of eye movements with strabismus and diplopia. The inferior rectus muscle is most commonly affected, followed by the medial rectus muscle [1, 2]. Restrictive strabismus is corrected by recession of the fibrotic muscle. Generally, the medial rectus muscle may be recessed up to 5 mm and the inferior rectus muscle up to 6 mm without causing additional weakening in the direction of muscle action [3]. In TAO, the mean dose effect (DE) reported for bilateral medial rectus recession is 1.56–1.59°/mm (≈2.7Δ/mm) [1]. Thus, in angles exceeding 20° (≈40Δ), conventional bilateral recession alone does not yield enough reduction of angle.

Large angles occur more commonly in patients following orbital decompression surgery, as the orbital content may shift to the side following removal of an orbital wall. This is especially common after medial wall recessions [1]. Following orbital decompression, the reported mean DE of a bilateral medial rectus recession is reduced to 1.2°/mm (≈2.1Δ/mm), which means that the maximal effect of a bilateral 6.5 mm recession is only 15.6° (≈27.3Δ) [1]. For patients with larger angles, a tendon elongation procedure using bovine pericard, Tutopatch, has been suggested for the inferior rectus muscle [4].

This study focuses on the less frequently performed medial rectus recession with tendon elongation using Tutopatch. The technique is discussed elsewhere [4] and schematically represented in Figure 1. Further, we compare the DE of these individuals with those of other patients with

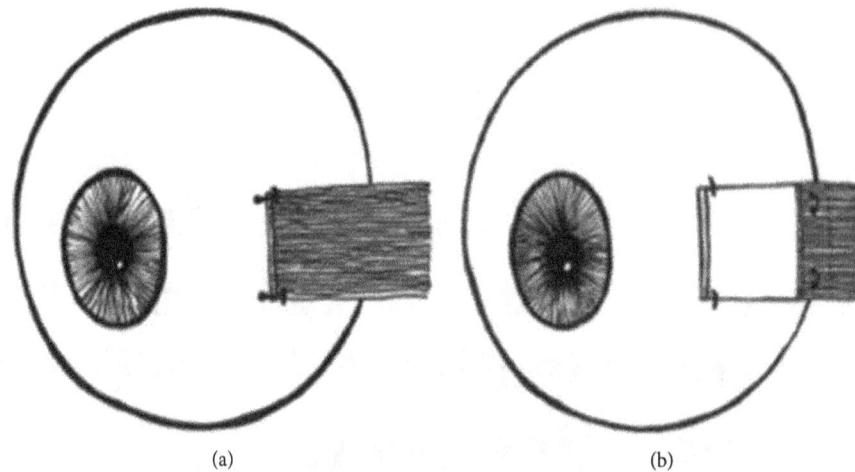

(a)   (b)

FIGURE 1: Schematic representation of conventional rectus muscle recession (a) and medial rectus muscle recession with Tutopatch tendon elongation (b). Note that the extraocular muscle comes to lie over Tutopatch, so that there is no direct contact between the tendon stump and the sclera.

TAO that underwent conventional bimedial recession at our hospital. These DEs are compared to those found in the literature. Additionally, we made use of oculodynamic MRI (OD-MRI) performed on four patients of the Tutopatch group to analyze the postoperative motility.

2. Materials and Methods

Approval of the Institutional Review Board to undertake this study was obtained in August 2015. The study was conducted in adherence to the Declaration of Helsinki.

The charts of all patients with TAO who underwent bilateral recession of the medial rectus muscle and tendon elongation with Tutopatch between 2006 and 2015 in our institution were retrospectively reviewed.

In addition, the charts of all patients with TAO who underwent a conventional bilateral medial rectus muscle recession between 2006 and 2015 were retrospectively reviewed for comparison. This resulted in a total number of 9 patients, 5 of whom received a tendon elongation with Tutopatch and 4 of whom underwent conventional muscle recession.

2.1. Patients. Patient details are summarized in Table 1

(1) Patient 1, female, aged 60 at strabismus surgery with tendon elongation. She was diagnosed with TAO 3 years prior to surgery and had had no previous orbital decompression. FU was 84 months.

(2) Patient 2A, female, aged 53 at strabismus surgery with tendon elongation. She was diagnosed with TAO 2 years prior to surgery, underwent bilateral orbital decompression consisting of an endonasal osteotomy of the medial orbital wall followed by a resection of the lateral orbital wall via coronary access, and developed a consecutive esotropia. She had also undergone radioiodine treatment. She had had a conventional bilateral recession of the medial rectus muscle 7.5 months prior to tendon elongation with Tutopatch with insufficient effect and a remaining

manifest angle of 14Δ (data shown as patient 2B below). In addition to the tendon elongation, the scleral attachment of the right medial rectus muscle was readvanced by 1.5 mm, resulting in a total recession of 6 mm. FU was 130 months.

(3) Patient 3, male, aged 43 at strabismus surgery with tendon elongation, was diagnosed with TAO 1 year before surgery. He underwent orbital decompression (same procedure as patient 2, with endonasal medial decompression and lateral orbitotomy via coronary access) with an increase of his squint angle from $+20\Delta$ to $+120\Delta$. He had an early strabismus surgery one month after systemic treatment with i.v. steroids according to Kahaly et al. [5]. FU was 41 months.

(4) Patient 4, male, aged 42 at surgery, was diagnosed with TAO 2 years before strabismus surgery with tendon elongation. He had orbital decompression (same procedure as patients 2 and 3) 1.5 years prior to surgery and also underwent radioiodine therapy. FU was 36 months.

(5) Patient 5, female, aged 66 at strabismus surgery with tendon elongation, diagnosed with TAO 1 year prior to surgery underwent orbital decompression of the medial orbital wall only (via endonasal access). This was the only patient in the Tutopatch group with no history of smoking. This case has been described with a 7-month FU in a previous case report [6]. Here, we are able to follow up to 13 months and present her OD-MRI.

(6) Patient 6, female, aged 56 at surgery, diagnosed with TAO 1 year prior to conventional strabismus surgery. She had undergone bilateral orbital decompression 15 months previously via endonasal access with ethmoidectomy and underwent bilateral radiation of the orbit. FU was 47 months.

(7) Patient 7, female, aged 35 at conventional strabismus surgery. She had no previous radiation of the orbit and was the only patient of the conventional recession group with no history of smoking. She was diagnosed

TABLE 1: Patients' characteristics.

Case	Age @ surgery	Radioiodine therapy	Current medication	Orbital decompression	Medial rectus recession with Tutopatch	Sutures
P1	60	No	No	No	OU[b] Σ 17 mm: OU[b] MRR[f] 4 mm + Tutopatch 4.5 mm	Mersilene 5-0
P2A	53	Yes	Eltroxin	1 year prior to first surgery	OU[b] Σ 6 mm: OU[b] Tutopatch tendon elongation 3.75 mm OD[c] anteroposition 1.5 mm	Safil 6-0
P3	43	No	Carbimazol	9 mo prior to surgery	OU[b] Σ 35 mm: OU[b] MRR[f] 4 mm + Tutopatch 13.5 mm	Mersilene 5-0
P4	42	Yes	Levothyroxin-natrium	1.5 years prior to surgery	OU[b] Σ 18 mm: OD[c] MRR[f] 4 mm + Tutopatch 5.5 mm SRR[h] 3 mm OS[d] MRR[f] 3 mm + Tutopatch 5.5 mm	Polysorb 6-0
P5	66	No	Carbimazol	5 mo prior to surgery	OU[b] Σ 21 mm: OD[c] Tutopatch tendon elongation 10 mm, IRR[i] 11 mm OS[d] Tutopatch tendon elongation 11 mm IRR[i] 8 mm	Polysorb 6-0

Case	Age @ surgery	Radioiodine therapy	Current medication	Orbital decompression	Conventional bimedial rectus recession	Sutures
P2B[a]	52	Yes	Eltroxin	1 year prior to surgery	OU[b] Σ 10.5 mm OD[c] 6 mm OS[d] 4.5 mm	Not specified
P6	56	Yes	None	15 mo prior to surgery	OU[b] Σ 7.5 mm	Safil 6-0
P7	35	No	Eltroxin	12 mo prior to surgery	OU[b] Σ 7 mm OS[d] SOR[e]	Safil 6-0
P8	50	Yes	Eltroxin	12 mo prior to surgery	OU[b] Σ 7 mm OD[c] MRR[f] 3 mm IOR[g] OS[d] MRR[f] 4 mm IOR[g]	Safil 6-0

[a]Patient 2B is the same patient as 2A who had subsequent bimedial recession with Tutopatch due to a residual angle of 14 PD; [b]OU = both eyes; [c]OD = right eye; [d]OS = left eye; [e]SOR = superior oblique recession to the nasal side of the superior rectus 4 mm distal to its insertion; [f]MRR = medial rectus recession; [g]IOR = inferior oblique recession; [h]SRR = superior rectus recession; [i]IRR = inferior rectus recession.

with TAO 1 year before surgery at the age of 34 years, whereas she had been diagnosed with Morbus Basedow at the age of 27 years. She had undergone orbital decompression 1 year before eye muscle surgery. FU was 81 months.

(8) Patient 8, female, aged 50 at conventional strabism surgery. She was diagnosed with TAO 3 years prior to surgery and an orbital decompression had been performed 12 months prior to eye muscle surgery, as well as radioiodine therapy two years prior to surgery. FU was 87 months.

Findings obtained preoperatively and at postoperative weeks one and twelve and at final follow-up (FU) were evaluated. Orthoptic measures included were Snellen visual acuity, squint angle at near and distance, adduction and abduction measured with the Kestenbaum limbus test [7], binocular single vision (Harms tangent screen), and stereo vision (Bagolini, Lang, TNO, and Titmus test) [3].

We made use of OD-MRI performed on four patients of the Tutopatch group to further analyze postoperative motility. Details of the OD-MRI technique have been described by Berg et al. [8].

TAO-specific data analyzed were as follows: presence of diplopia and clinical activity score (CAS) [9], information on previous surgeries (extraocular muscles and orbital decompression), previous and current treatment of the TAO (steroids)/Graves' disease (GD) (thyroid surgery and radioiodine treatment), patient's age at onset of TAO, and history of tobacco use.

Collected surgical data included the amount of muscle recessed, length of tendon elongation, complications reported, and patient satisfaction.

The dose effect was calculated separately for the angles at distance and near fixation. DE = (presurgical manifest angle in prism diopters – angle at last follow-up in prism diopters)/total recession in millimeters.

3. Results

3.1. Patients with Bimedial Recession with Tutopatch. All patients had undergone intravenous steroid treatment according to Kahaly et al. [5] at some point of their TAO.

TABLE 2: Recession with Tutopatch: development of horizontal squint angles.

Patient			1	2A (Figure 2)	3 (Figure 3)	4	5
Duration of follow up (months)			84	130	41	36	13
Total recession $\sum$ OD[b] + OS[c] (mm)			17	6	35	18	21
Angle @ distance	FU[d]	Baseline	78[e]	14[e]	120[e]	59[e]	95[e]
		1 week	20[e]	−9[f]	—	25[e]	2.5[f]
		3 months	13[e]	−5[f]	2[f]	12[e]	−12[f]
		Last visit	0	−2[f]	0	4[f]	−11[f]
		DE[g] (PD/mm)	4.59	2.33	3.428	3.3	4.52
Angle @ near	FU[d]	Baseline	70[e]	12[e]	120[e]	54[e]	95[e]
		1 week	16[e]	−14[f]	−12[e]	20[e]	—
		3 months	3[e]	−16[f]	−14[f]	6[f]	−12
		Last visit	−3[f,h]	−9[f]	−8[f]	−8[f]	−28[f]
		DE[g] (PD/mm)	4.12	2	3.428	3.11	4.52

[b]OD = right eye; [c]OS = left eye; [d]FU = follow-up; [e]manifest angle; [f]latent angle; [g]DE = dose effect; [h]following correcting the vertical angle.

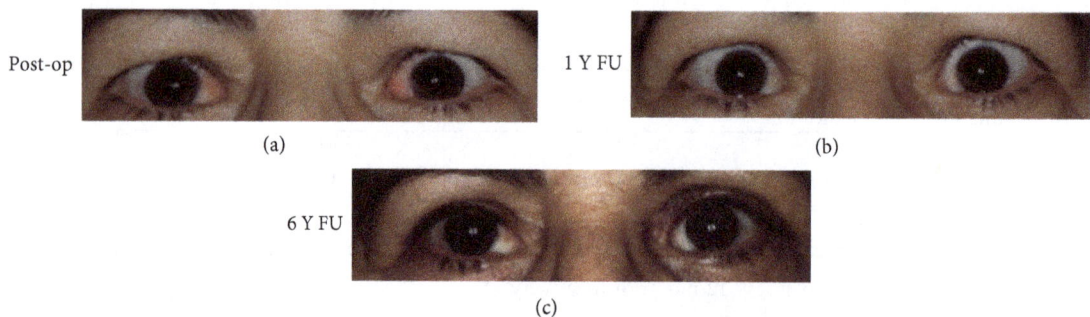

(a)

(b)

(c)

FIGURE 2: Patient 2 after surgery with Tutopatch (a) and 1 year later (b). (c) The same patient following lid surgery to correct her retraction of the upper eye lid.

Prior to strabismus surgery with Tutopatch, patients did not show signs of clinical activity for at least six months, with the exception of P3 and P5 with large incapacitating squint angles.

The mean age at the time of surgery was 52.8 years. Follow-up ranged from 13 to 130 months. For each patient, Table 2 describes the development of the horizontal deviation at distance, the dosage, and DE of surgery. Figures 2 and 3 show examples of individual patients. Before surgery, all patients showed a manifest esodeviation with angles between 14Δ (prism diopters), in the patient with previous conventional medial recession, and 120Δ at distance. At near fixation, angles ranged between 12 and 120Δ. This compared to a mean postoperative manifest deviation of 0Δ at distance as well as at near fixation. The mean length of tendon elongation per muscle was 7.55 mm, ranging from 3.75 mm to 13.5 mm with a mean total recession of 9.7 mm per muscle, ranging from 2.25 mm to 17.5 mm. The mean DE at the last FU was 3.63, ranging from 2.33 to 4.59Δ/mm for the distance angle and 3.43 ranging from 2 to 4.52Δ/mm for the near angle.

Table 3 shows the development of the horizontal motility: at baseline, mean abduction per eye was 3.05 mm (range: 0–6 mm). At the 3-month FU, mean abduction had increased by about 2 mm. At final FU, abduction had increased further to 5.7 (2.5–8.5) mm.

Mean adduction at baseline was 7.95 mm (range: 5–11 mm). As expected this was decreased at the 3-month FU by about 2.6 mm. At final FU, adduction improved slightly to 5.9 (2–9) mm.

3.2. Conventional Bimedial Recession Group. Mean age at surgery was 48.25 years. The patients were followed for a mean of 55.6 (7.5–87) months (Table 4). Mean preoperative esodeviation was 27 (18–35)Δ at distance and 21 (12–33)Δ at near fixation. At the last follow-up, two patients with underlying microesotropia still had a manifest deviation, ranging from 0 to 2Δ (Table 4). In patient 2B, a manifest angle of 14Δ at distance remained, which resulted in further recession of the medial recti with Tutopatch (=patient 2A). Total recession was on average 8 (7–10.5) mm. The mean DE was 2.95Δ/mm at distance and 2.18Δ/mm at near fixation.

Preoperative mean abduction and mean adduction in patients 6–8 were 6.0 and 9.38 mm, respectively. At three months, abduction had increased to 6.82 mm, and adduction had decreased to 8 mm. At the final follow-up, abduction increased further to 7.56 mm, and adduction increased as well to 8.81 mm (Table 3).

4. Discussion

Our results confirm that tendon elongation of the medial rectus muscle with Tutopatch is a valid option in patients with severe restriction of ocular motility due to TAO.

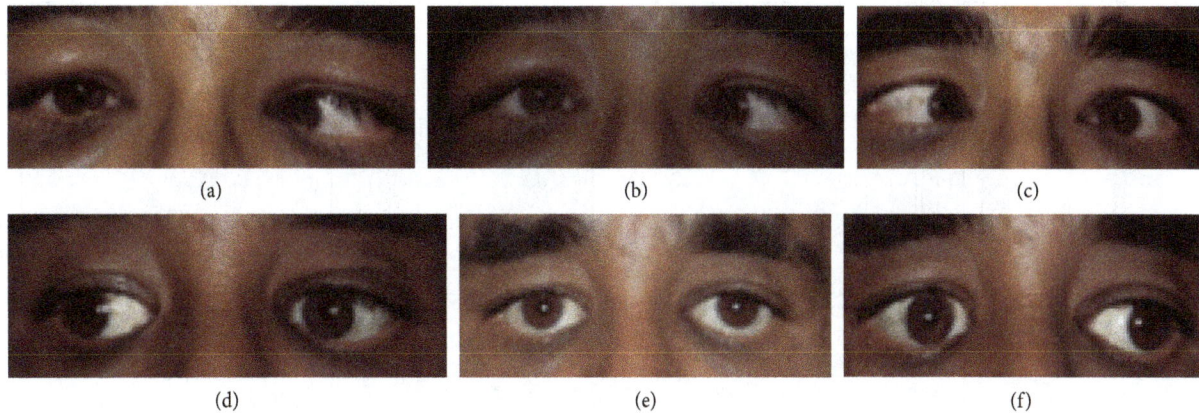

FIGURE 3: Images showing patient 3 before surgery in rightgaze (a), primary position (b), and leftgaze (c). The patient 4 years after bimedial rectus recession with Tutopatch in rightgaze (d), in primary position (e), and in leftgaze (f). Considering the large recession of 17.5 mm per medial rectus muscle, the patient shows excellent motility with some restriction of adduction on the right eye > left eye.

TABLE 3: Development of motility (mm).

| | Tutopatch: P1–P5 | | | | Conventional recession: P2B, P6–P8 | | | |
| | Abduction | | Adduction | | Abduction | | Adduction | |
	Mean	Range	Mean	Range	Mean	Range	Mean	Range
Baseline	3.05	0–6[a]	7.95	5–11[b]	6.0	3–8.5	9.375	3.5–11
FU[c] 3 months	5.25	2–8	5.3	2.5–7.5	6.83	5–9	8	7–9.5
FU[c] last visit	5.7	2.5–8.5	5.9	2–9	7.56	4.5–10	8.81	7.5–10

[a]Abduction assumed to be zero in P3 and P5 because midline could not be reached; [b]adduction measured as the possible motility from the starting point, not primary position; [c]FU = follow up.

TABLE 4: Conventional bimedial recession: development of horizontal squint angles.

Patient			2B[a]	6	7	8
Duration of follow-up (months)			7.5	47	81	87
Total recession $\sum$ OD[b] + OS[c] (mm)			10.5	7.5	7	7
Angle @ distance	FU[d]	Baseline	35[e]	30[e]	18[e]	25[e]
		1 week	18[e]	4[f]	7[e]	5[e]
		3 months	17[e]	0	14[f]	3[e]
		Last visit	14[e]	2[f]	2e,h	0.5e,h
	DE[g] (PD/mm)		2	4	2.29	3.5
Angle @ near	FU[d]	Baseline	33[e]	23[e]	12[e]	16[e]
		1 week	12	0	—	0
		3 months	14[e]	-2[f]	6[f]	3[f]
		Last visit	12[e]	2[f]	2e,h	0.5e,h
	DE[g] (PD/mm)		2	3.06	1.43	2.21

[a]Patient 2B is the same patient as 2A who had subsequent bimedial recession with Tutopatch due to a residual angle of 14 PD; [b]OD = right eye; [c]OS = left eye; [d]FU = follow-up; [e]manifest angle; [f]latent angle; [g]DE = dose effect; [h]underlying microesotropia with latent esophoria.

Esser et al. [4] have reported on the recession of the inferior rectus muscle using tendon elongation with Tutopatch in TAO with good results (FU up to 6 months). Eckstein et al. [10] reported on bilateral medial rectus recession with Tutopatch tendon elongation in 30 patients with TAO following different types of orbital decompression. In that study, patients were followed up to 3 months. While we report on fewer patients, we report a longer follow-up of up to

10 years and the inclusion of OD-MRI videos that allow appreciation of extraocular muscle motility in vivo.

A successful outcome of strabismus surgery is frequently defined as an angle under 5Δ–10Δ and absence of diplopia in primary position. Following these criteria, all our patients who underwent bimedial tendon elongation with Tutopatch had a successful outcome, as all of them were orthotropic at near and at distance, without diplopia in primary position of gaze and with a reasonable field of binocular single vision. Figure 4 displays the fields of binocular single vision (FBSV) obtained from the patients with Tutopatch before and after surgery: all patients had double vision in all directions of gaze before surgery, and all had at least a central field of binocular single vision after surgery. This was seen at the 3-month FU in 3 patients and in the other two patients after 11 months (P1) or 18 months (P4). Thus, in tendon elongation with Tutopatch, improvement may be seen over a longer period of time than generally expected.

Table 5 compares our DE to those of the literature. Generally, the DE for recession of the medial rectus is lower than for the inferior rectus muscle. It is even lower following orbital decompression [1]. Comparing our DE to the literature is difficult, as it is often not specified if the DE relates to angles at distance or at near fixation.

In conventional bimedial recession, our DE compared well to the literature: we found a mean DE of 2.95Δ/mm at distance and 2.18Δ/mm at near fixation. This corresponds to ≈1.69°/mm and 1.25°/mm, respectively. In bimedial recession, the DE has previously been reported as

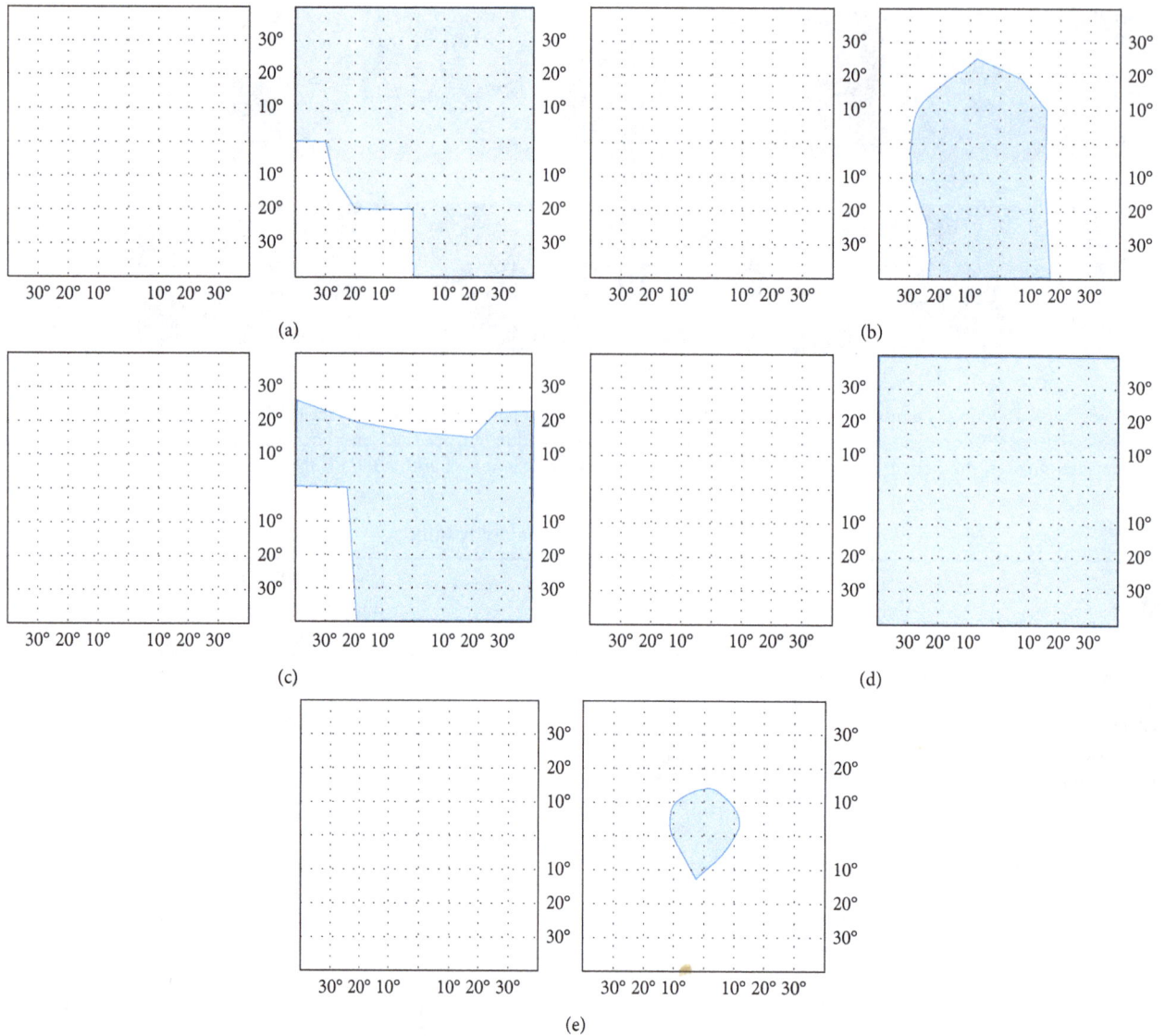

FIGURE 4: The field of binocular single vision (FBSV, blue area) of the patients with bimedial rectus recession with Tutopatch. The left column shows the FBSV before and the right column at the last FU after bimedial rectus recession with Tutopatch. Rows depict individual patients.

TABLE 5: Dose effect (PD/mm): comparison with the literature.

Method		Our results	Results in literature[a]
Recession with Tutopatch	Bilateral M. rectus medialis	@ distance: 3.63 @ near fixation: 3.43	1.57–1.75[b,c] 1.39–1.57[b,d]
	Unilateral M. rectus inferior	—	3.46–3.58[b,c]
Conventional recession	Bilateral M. rectus medialis	@ distance: 2.95 @ near fixation: 2.18	2.72–2.77[c,e] 1.92–2.27[b,c]
	Unilateral M. rectus inferior	—	3.49[b,c]

[a]Not specified if angle at near fixation or distance, degrees converted to prism diopters (rate: °/0.5729); [b]with prior decompression; [c]Eckstein, Schittkowski et al.[1]; [d]Eckstein et al. [10]; [e]without prior decompression.

1.56–1.59°/mm without prior decompression and 1.1–1.3°/mm with prior decompression [1].

The DE in our Tutopatch group was higher than previously reported [10] and also higher than in our patients with conventional bimedial recession (Table 5). This is in contrast to reports of a lower DE in bimedial recessions with Tutopatch compared to conventional bimedial recession [10].

Figure 5 depicts the dependency of the DE on the angle at baseline in our Tutopatch group. The different DE found in our Tutopatch group may be explained by the larger angles at

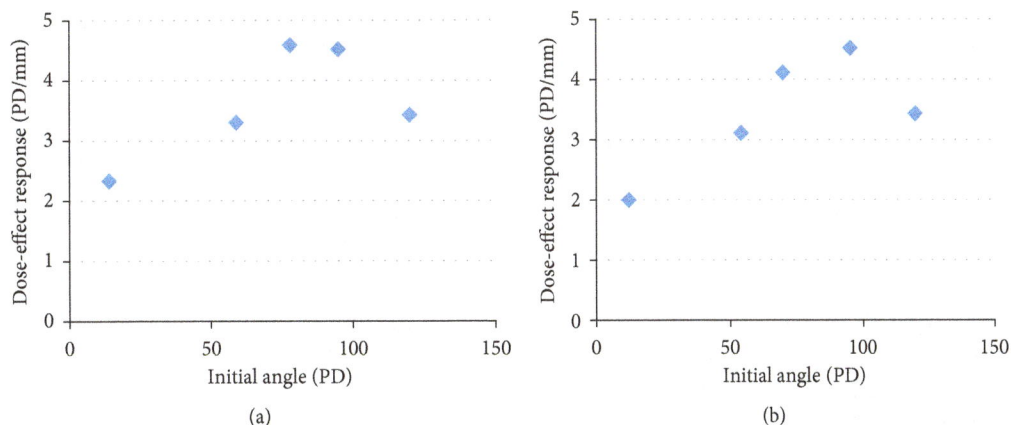

FIGURE 5: Dose effect at the last follow-up in relation to angle at baseline in the patients with bimedial recession with Tutopatch.

baseline in our Tutopatch group compared to our patients who received conventional bimedial recession. In our Tutopatch group, angles at baseline were also larger than in the patients reported by Eckstein et al. [10], where the maximum angle was 69Δ. This is supported by findings in unilateral medial rectus recessions where the DE appears independent of the presurgical angle as long as the latter is <15° [11, 12].

Bimedial rectus recession in TAO resulted in an increase of abduction while decreasing adduction. This held true for bimedial recession with or without tendon elongation. The motility at baseline and consequently at follow-up was better in the group with conventional bimedial recession, reflecting a lesser degree of restrictive disease and also a lesser angle at baseline. Interestingly, both groups showed an initial decrease in adduction at 3 months followed by a slight and similar improvement of adduction and abduction by 0.5–0.8 mm at final follow-up. Overall, good motility was preserved, even in the patients with an extremely large initial angle.

An alternative technique to treat larger squint angles is the use of hang-back sutures. These require the use of nonabsorbable sutures which may be rejected [13]. Time has shown that tendon elongation with Tutopatch has the advantage of allowing the use of absorbable sutures (Table 1) [14]. Also, the Tutopatch graft has been shown to resemble normal tendon on revision surgery [10, 14]. This suggests that in patients requiring further elongation, a revision would appear easier than with hang-back sutures.

A study evaluating the reattachment site of the superior rectus muscle after hang-back recession in rabbits showed that, the higher the amount of recession, the bigger the risk and amount of muscle advancement [15]. In the procedure using Tutopatch, it is not to be expected that the muscle will reattach to the globe posteriorly, as the end of the muscle comes to lie over the interponate (Figure 1). OD-MRI could confirm that the recessed medial rectus was still attached to Tutopatch and not to the globe. In the one patient where scarring was seen, this did not affect the globe. In addition, OD-MRI allowed the appreciation of the elasticity of Tutopatch, allowing for a good passive movement with minimal leash effects.

Strabismus surgery with tendon elongation using Tutopatch is a good alternative to treat large squint angles while preserving good motility. It is worthwhile to expand on this study to include more patients in order to establish more meaningful DE relations. In individual patients, improvement may occur up to 11 months following surgery.

Disclosure

Parts of these findings have been presented at the Annual ARVO Meeting 2015 and at the Meeting of the Swiss Ophthalmological Society 2016. Patient 5 has been published in parts as a case report in Klinische Monatsblätter für Augenheilkunde with a shorter FU and without oculodynamic MRI findings.

Conflicts of Interest

The authors declare that they have no conflicts of interest.

Authors' Contributions

Britt-Isablle Berg and Anja Palmowski-Wolfe contributed equally as last authors.

Acknowledgments

This study has been supported in part by the Smith-Kettlewell Eye Research Institute, San Francisco, CA, USA (to Anja Palmowski-Wolfe). The authors wish to thank Nisha Dissanayake, University Eye Hospital, University of Basel, for her assistance in data collection.

Supplementary 2. Video 2: patient 2: OD-MRI of patient 2 shows smooth horizontal motility without apparent restrictions (supplementary video 2).

Supplementary 3. Video 3: patient 4: OD-MRI (supplementary video 3) shows the swollen orbital tissue (OS > OD) displaced medially following medial and lateral wall decompression. In agreement with the Kestenbaum measures, adduction is impaired in OD compared to OS, and abduction is impaired in OS compared to OD.

Supplementary 4. Video 4: patient 5: OD-MRI supplementary videos 4–6 show the dramatically improved horizontal and vertical motility. The swollen orbital tissue (OS > OD) is displaced nasally following medial wall decompression. On the horizontal OD-MRI (supplementary video 4), the asymmetry of the Tutopatch elongation (OS > OD) can be appreciated. In contrast to P1, P2, and P4, a second proximal thickening in the area of Tutopatch is indicative of adhesions (scar tissue) to the surrounding connective tissue in the area of the suture between Tutopatch and the muscle. As a consequence, abduction is noticeably impaired and comes to a more abrupt stop, which may also reflect the greater amount of orbital fat.

References

[1] A. Eckstein, M. Schittkowski, and J. Esser, "Surgical treatment of Graves' ophthalmopathy," *Best Practice and Research Clinical Endocrinology and Metabolism*, vol. 26, no. 3, pp. 339–358, 2012.

[2] A. Eckstein and J. Esser, "Endocrine orbit disorders. Pathogenesis, clinical presentation and examination, stage-dependent therapy," *Der Ophthalmologe*, vol. 100, no. 10, pp. 857–880, 2003.

[3] H. Kaufmann, *Strabismus*, Georg Thieme Verlag, Stuttgart, Germany, 2004.

[4] J. Esser, M. Schittkowski, and A. Eckstein, "Graves' orbitopaty: inferior rectus tendon elongation for large vertical squint angles that cannot be corrected by simple muscle recession," *Klinische Monatsblatter fur Augenheilkunde*, vol. 228, no. 10, pp. 880–886, 2011.

[5] G. J. Kahaly, K. A. Ponto, S. Pitz, W. J. Mann, M. M. Weber, and N. Pfeiffer, "Management of Graves' orbitopathy: evidence-based recommendations," *Deutsche medizinische Wochenschrift*.vol. 134, no. 49, pp. 2521–2524, 2009.

[6] M. Wipf and A. Palmowski-Wolfe, "Treatment of extreme strabismus in TAO (thyroid associated orbitopathy): medial rectus and inferior rectus tendon elongation with Tutopatch®, an alternative to conventional strabismus surgery: a case report," *Klinische Monatsblätter für Augenheilkunde*, vol. 234, no. 4, pp. 588–590, 2017.

[7] A. Kestenbaum, *Clinical Methods of Neuro-Ophthalmologic Examination*, William Heinemann Medical Books Ltd., London, UK, 1947.

[8] I. Berg, A. Palmowski-Wolfe, K. Schwenzer-Zimmerer et al., "Near-real time oculodynamic MRI: a feasibility study for evaluation of diplopia in comparison with clinical testing," *European Radiology*, vol. 22, no. 2, pp. 358–363, 2012.

[9] M. P. Mourits, M. F. Prummel, W. M. Wiersinga, and L. Koornneef, "Clinical activity score as a guide in the management of patients with Graves' ophthalmopathy," *Clinical Endocrinology*, vol. 47, no. 1, pp. 9–14, 1997.

[10] A Eckstein, C. Weiermüller, M. Holdt et al., "Schielformen und augenmuskeloperationen nach orbitadekompression," *Zeitschrift für Praktische Augenheilkunde*, vol. 32, pp. 335–344, 2011.

[11] J. Esser and A. Eckstein, "Ocular muscle and eyelid surgery in thyroid-associated orbitopathy," *Experimental and Clinical Endocrinology and Diabetes*, vol. 107, no. S5, pp. S214–S221, 1999.

[12] J. Esser, "Endocrine orbitopathy. Interventions on the external eye muscles," *Der Ophthalmologe*, vol. 91, no. 1, pp. 3–19, 1994.

[13] H. S. Eustis, T. R. Elmer Jr., and G. Ellis Jr., "Postoperative results of absorbable, subconjunctival adjustable sutures," *Journal of American Association for Pediatric Ophthalmology and Strabismus*, vol. 8, no. 3, pp. 240–242, 2004.

[14] L. J. van Rijn, S. J. van De Ven, J. S. Krijnen, S. M. Jansen, A. J. Bakels, and A. M. Langenhorst, "Tendon elongation with bovine pericardium (Tutopatch®) when conventional strabismus surgery is not possible," *European Journal of Ophthalmology*, vol. 26, no. 3, pp. 193–202, 2016.

[15] Y. Wysenbeek, T. Wygnanski-Jaffe, M. Rosner, and A. Spierer, "Evaluation of superior rectus muscle attachment following hang-back recession in rabbit eyes," *European Journal of Ophthalmology*, vol. 14, no. 6, pp. 464–466, 2004.

17

Peripheral Cone Dystrophy: Expanded Clinical Spectrum, Multimodal and Ultrawide-Field Imaging, and Genomic Analysis

Robert A. Sisk ⓘ,[1,2,3] Robert B. Hufnagel,[4] Ailee Laham,[1] Elizabeth S. Wohler,[5] Nara Sobreira,[5] and Zubair M. Ahmed[6]

[1]Department of Ophthalmology, University of Cincinnati College of Medicine, Cincinnati, OH, USA
[2]Cincinnati Eye Institute, Cincinnati, OH, USA
[3]Division of Pediatric Ophthalmology, Cincinnati Children's Hospital Medical Center, Cincinnati, OH, USA
[4]Division of Human Genetics, Cincinnati Children's Hospital Medical Center, Cincinnati, OH, USA
[5]McKusick-Nathans Institute of Genetic Medicine, Johns Hopkins University School of Medicine, Baltimore, MD, USA
[6]Department of Otorhinolaryngology, School of Medicine, University of Maryland, Baltimore, MD, USA

Correspondence should be addressed to Robert A. Sisk; rsisk@cincinnatieye.com

Robert A. Sisk and Robert B. Hufnagel contributed equally to this work.

Academic Editor: Hyeong Gon Yu

Purpose. To present new clinical features, multimodal and ultrawide-field imaging characteristics of peripheral cone dystrophy (PCD), and results of laboratory and genetic investigation to decipher the etiology. *Methods.* Retrospective observational case-series. *Results.* Three patients with PCD presented with bilateral paracentral scotomas and a mean visual acuity of 20/25. All exhibited confluent macular hyperautofluorescence with a central bull's eye lesion. Spectral-domain optical coherence tomography revealed loss of outer retinal elements, particularly the inner segment ellipsoid band and external limiting membrane, within the area of macular hyperautofluorescence. This area corresponded with a lightened fundus appearance and variable retinal pigment epithelium (RPE) abnormalities. Full field and multifocal electroretinography distinguished PCD from other photoreceptor dystrophies. Ultrawide-field imaging revealed irregular peripheral retinal lesions in a distribution greater nasally than temporally and not contiguous with the macular lesion. Functional and anatomic testing remained stable over a mean follow-up of 3 years. Laboratory investigation for causes of uveitis was negative. Whole exome sequencing identified rare variants in genes associated with macular or cone dystrophy or degeneration. *Conclusions.* In contrast to the original description, the funduscopic and fluorescein angiographic appearance of PCD is abnormal, although the defects are subtle. Peripheral lesions may be observed in some patients. Bilateral, symmetric, macular hyperautofluorescence associated with outer retinal atrophy that spares the fovea is a characteristic of PCD. Pathogenic variants in the same gene were not shared across the cohort, suggesting genetic heterogeneity. Further evaluation is warranted.

1. Introduction

Cone dystrophy is a slowly progressive, diffuse photoreceptor dystrophy that presents as hemeralopia, reduced visual acuity, and nystagmus associated with macular cone photoreceptor and retinal pigment epithelium (RPE) atrophy [1–6]. Two forms of localized cone dysfunction syndromes have been described: occult macular dystrophy (OCMD; MIM 613587) and peripheral cone dystrophy (PCD; MIM 609021) [7–16]. OCMD and PCD can be segregated by electrophysiologic responses to full field electroretinography (ffERG) and multifocal electroretinography (mfERG). OCMD displays normal photopic waveforms on ffERG and reduced mfERG responses only at the fovea, which correlates clinically with reduced visual acuities and foveal cone photoreceptor atrophy seen on spectral-domain optical coherence tomography (SDOCT). OCMD is inherited in a dominant fashion and is usually associated with mutations in *RP1L1* [17].

PCD is a very rare retinal disease originally characterized by normal fundoscopic appearance, normal fluorescein angiographic imaging, mildly reduced photopic potentials with preserved scotopic potentials on ffERG, and relative preservation of foveal cone function by mfERG. The name "peripheral cone dystrophy" is unfortunately a misnomer, as central rather than peripheral cone involvement is a prominent feature, but the name was selected to contrast "central" cone dystrophy, or OCMD, because the foveola is preserved. Kondo and Miyake, who also first described OCMD, first reported three cases of PCD, who presented with bilateral ring scotomas and near-normal visual acuity [7, 12]. These seminal cases included a pair of affected siblings, suggesting autosomal recessive inheritance or autosomal dominant inheritance with parental germline mosaicism. However, no genetic cause has been associated with this disorder.

PCD is a diagnosis of exclusion. The differential diagnosis includes Stargardt disease, cone dystrophy, enhanced S-cone syndrome, pericentral retinitis pigmentosa, syphilitic placoid chorioretinitis, acute zonal occult outer retinopathy (AZOOR), posterior scleritis, traumatic retinopathy (commotio retinae), posterior uveitis, hydroxychloroquine toxicity, and autoimmune retinopathy [18–22]. Here, we report previously undescribed funduscopic, fundus autofluorescence (FAF), infrared imaging, fluorescein angiography (FA), and SDOCT abnormalities in three probands with PCD. We also describe results of our investigation using whole exome sequencing (WES) to identify a causative gene among our three unrelated probands.

2. Methods

2.1. Human Subjects Research. Institutional Review Board (IRB) approval was obtained for retrospective and prospective evaluation of all cases of PCD diagnosed at the Cincinnati Eye Institute between September 1, 2009, and May 1, 2013. Records were reviewed for patient age, sex, demographics, family history, medical history, toxic and infectious exposures, and ocular examination findings. Patients underwent extensive ophthalmic testing including fundus imaging with standard (TRC-50DX®, Topcon Medical Systems, Oakland, NJ) and ultrawide-field cameras (Optos 200Tx®, Optos, Marlborough, MA). Multimodal imaging (Spectralis® HRA-OCT, Heidelberg Engineering, Dossenheim, Germany) was utilized including red-free imaging, infrared imaging (IR), FAF, FA, and SDOCT. Full field and multifocal electroretinography (Diagnosys D218, Software V6.0.47 with 61 hexagon array, Lowell, MA) was performed to meet ISCEV standards. B-scan ultrasonography (Eye Cubed I³® unit, Ellex, Minneapolis, MN) was performed to exclude posterior scleritis or infiltrative choroidal disease. Laboratory testing was performed for infectious and noninfectious causes of uveitis, including syphilis, tuberculosis, cat-scratch disease, Lyme disease, toxoplasmosis, ANCA-associated uveitides, systemic lupus erythematosus, and sarcoidosis. HLA testing was performed to evaluate for HLA-B27-associated uveitis and birdshot chorioretinopathy.

2.2. Molecular Genetic Investigation. After informed consent was obtained to participate in genetic research, whole blood samples were obtained from all patients. Genetic analysis was performed through the BHCMG and the National Eye Institute (eyeGENE®, National Ophthalmic Genotyping and Phenotyping Network, Stage 1—Creation of DNA Repository for Inherited Ophthalmic Diseases). Sanger sequencing for *ABCA4*, *PRPH2*, and *ELOVL4* was performed on one proband (case 1), and *PRPH2*/RDS-peripherin was sequenced in all cases. The Baylor-Hopkins Center for Mendelian Genomics (BHCMG) performed WES and analysis on all three probands. The aforementioned testing, clinical histories, and family histories were provided to these organizations with the patients' permission using PhenoDB [23].

We used WES to investigate both for variations in retinal dystrophy genes in each proband and for genes commonly mutated in the 3 affected individuals. The Agilent SureSelect HumanAllExonV4_51MbKit_S03723314 was used for exome capture. Libraries were sequenced on the HiSeq2500 platform with onboard clustering using 100 bp paired end runs and sequencing chemistry kits TruSeq Rapid PE Cluster Kit-HS and TruSeq Rapid SBS-HS. FASTQ files were aligned with BWA [24] version 0.5.10-tpx to the 1000 genomes phase 2 (GRCh37) human genome reference. Duplicate reads were flagged with Picard version 1.74. Local realignment around indels and base call quality score recalibration were performed using the Genome Analysis Toolkit (GATK) 2.3–9 multisample calling with a Unified Genotyper [25]. Variant filtering was done using the variant quality score recalibration (VQSR) method [26]. The variant prioritization strategy was designed using the Variant Analysis Tool of PhenoDB [27] and Ingenuity Variant Analysis (Qiagen, Redwood City, CA). Rare functional variants (missense, nonsense, splice site variants, and indels) with a MAF ≤0.01 in the Exome Variant Server (release ESP6500SI-V2) or 1000 Genomes Project were prioritized [28]. We also excluded all variants found in in-house controls for PhenoDB (CIDRVar 51 Mb) and Cincinnati Children's Hospital Medical Center (CCHMC). Postanalysis, PCR primers were designed to amplify exons and flanking intronic splice sites followed by direct Sanger sequencing to validate the candidate causative variants.

3. Results

3.1. Case Descriptions. Three patients (two female and one male) were identified at a median age of 51 years (range 42 to 57 years) with visual symptoms that began at a mean of 9 years prior. Mean best-corrected visual acuity was 20/25, and it remained stable throughout the mean follow-up of 3 years. All complained of paracentral visual field loss and mildly reduced best-corrected visual acuities, and no patient described progression beyond their initial presentation. No patient could attribute a precipitating event, injury, or illness to the onset of symptoms, yet none described their vision loss as acute. Only case 2 had any family history of retinal dystrophy or blindness or exposure to any medication known to be toxic to the retina or RPE. Laboratory investigation for causes of infectious and noninfectious uveitis was negative in all patients.

(a)

(b)

(c)

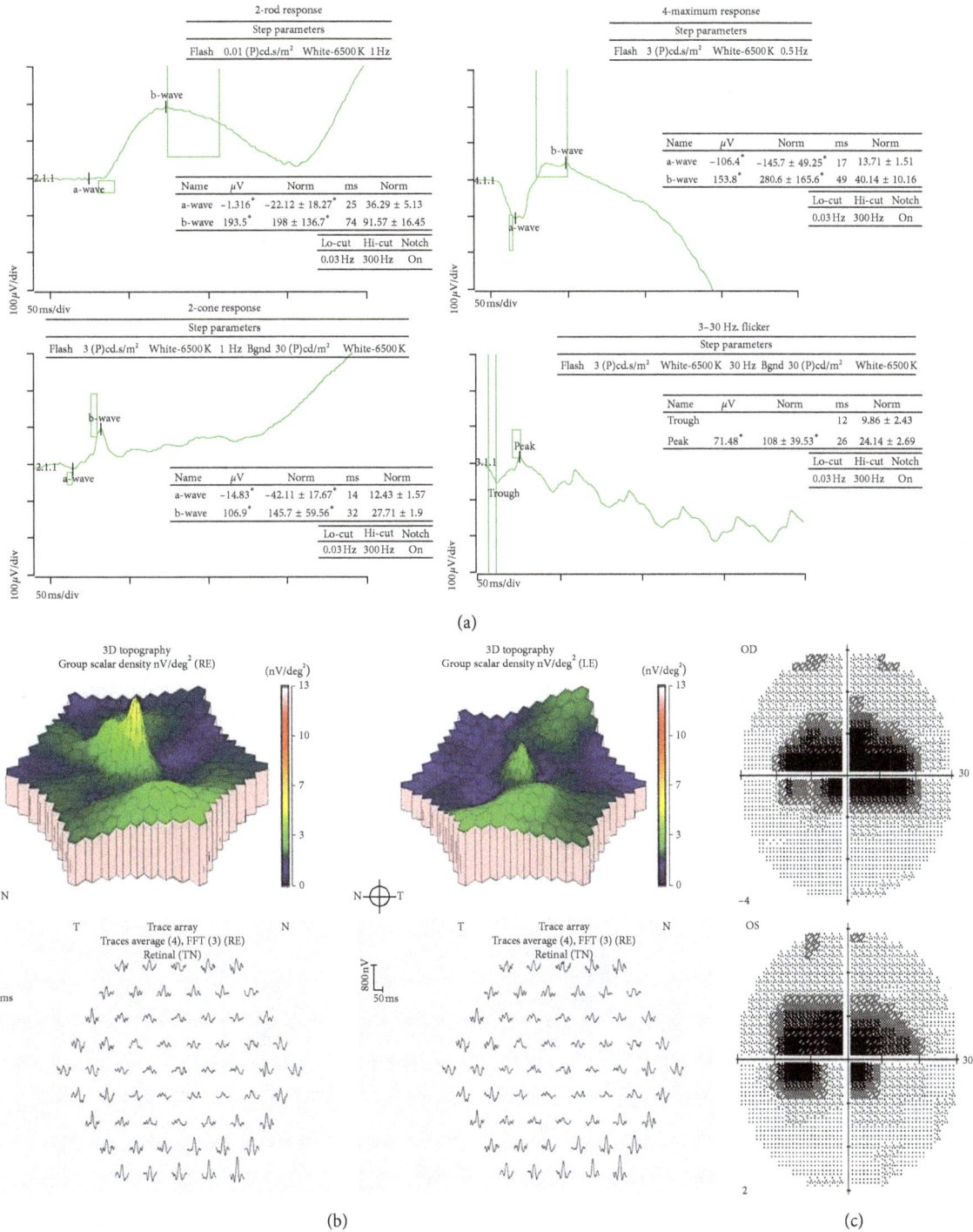

FIGURE 1: Full field electroretinography (ffERG), multifocal electroretinography (mfERG), and visual field testing of case 1. (a) Full field electroretinography demonstrated low normal a- and b-wave amplitudes and implicit times on scotopic testing. Photopic testing showed moderately reduced a- and b-wave amplitudes with mildly delayed implicit times. See Supplementary Figure 1 for normal reference and ffERG for cases 2 and 3. (b) Central amplitudes were reduced in the central and paracentral 15° with relative sparing of the fovea on multifocal electroretinography. See Supplementary Figure 2 for normal reference and mfERG testing for cases 2 and 3. (c) Humphrey Sita-Standard protocol with size III stimulus revealed bilateral dense paracentral scotomas that spared foveal sensitivities. See Supplementary Figure 3 for visual field testing of cases 2 and 3.

3.1.1. Case 1. A 57-year-old Caucasian male presented with a ten-year history of nonprogressive ring scotomas OU (Figure 1). He denied other ocular- or nonocular-associated symptoms or any prior ocular trauma. Family history was negative for any retinal disease, uncorrectable vision loss, hemeralopia, or nystagmus. Best-corrected visual acuities on presentation were 20/25-2 OU. Ishihara color vision testing was diminished to four out of eleven plates in each eye.

Anterior segment examination was unremarkable except for mild nuclear sclerotic cataracts in both eyes. He exhibited typical funduscopic findings for pathologic myopia including staphylomatous changes, parapapillary atrophy, and inferotemporal lacquer cracks in the left eye and areas of chorioretinal atrophy in both the posterior pole and periphery OU.

3.1.2. Case 2.
A 52-year-old African American female was referred for evaluation after three years of hydroxychloroquine treatment for rheumatoid arthritis. The medication dosage was never supratherapeutic, and she denied visual changes on the medication. Interestingly, her visual complaints predated the use of the medication by two years, but no baseline visual field testing had been performed. She described her mother as having "macular degeneration and retinitis pigmentosa" that began as central vision loss in her forties and progressed to nyctalopia and peripheral vision loss. Visual acuities were 20/20 OU, and anterior segment examination was unremarkable. Ishihara color vision testing was diminished to ten out of fifteen plates in the right eye and eleven out of fifteen plates in the left eye. The right eye had received laser retinopexy after posterior vitreous detachment for symptomatic retinal holes associated with lattice degeneration.

3.1.3. Case 3.
A 42-year-old Caucasian female who originally presented 22 years prior with perimacular pigmentary changes had been diagnosed with bilateral choroidal osteomas, although neither eye had an orange choroidal lesion nor hyperreflective plaque by B-scan ultrasonography on any prior testing. She denied progression of vision loss, although visual acuities at original presentation were 20/20 OD and 20/30 OS and declined to 20/30 OU when diagnosed with PCD. Ishihara color vision testing was diminished to three out of fifteen plates in each eye. Her family history was negative for eye-related phenotypes. Anterior segment examination was normal, but fundus examination showed perimacular arcuate and circumferential nasal retinal lightening with central pigmentary clumping OU.

3.2. Electroretinography.
Full field electroretinography (ffERG) showed a pattern consistent with cone dystrophy for cases 1 and 3 (Supplementary Figure 1). There were relatively preserved (at the lower limit of our normal reference range) a- and b-wave amplitudes with normal implicit times on scotopic testing and moderately reduced amplitudes with mildly increased implicit times on photopic testing. ffERG resembled cone-rod dystrophy for case 2 with moderate reductions in a- and b-wave amplitudes and delayed implicit times on scotopic and photopic testing (Supplementary Figure 2). Responses were symmetrical between OD and OS in most recorded waveforms in all patients. Waveforms had otherwise typical architecture and specifically did not have a sinusoidal appearance. Multifocal electroretinography demonstrated diffusely reduced amplitudes and increased

implicit times with relative sparing of the foveal spike OU (Supplementary Figure 2).

3.3. Visual Fields.
Humphrey 30-2 Sita Standard and Goldmann threshold visual field testing confirmed bilateral paracentral scotomas in all patients that remained stable throughout follow-up (Supplementary Figure 3). The macular appearance was unremarkable funduscopically in all cases except for the myopic fundus changes in case 1. Peripheral RPE alterations were observed in the nasal peripheral retina in all patients. These were unilateral in case 2 and attributable to a history of laser retinopexy for retinal breaks associated with posterior vitreous detachment. Scotomas were not observed corresponding to these peripheral lesions.

3.4. Blue-Light Fundus Autofluorescence.
All probands had bilateral, relatively symmetric, central, geographic areas of confluent macular hyperautofluorescence with rounded or scalloped borders that extended nasally past the optic disc (Figure 2). In cases 1 and 3, this area was sharply delineated from the surrounding isoautofluorescence by a narrow border of hyperautofluorescence of greater intensity than the central confluence. This transition could be observed funduscopically by a subtle color change best appreciated on the laser-generated ultrawide-field images (Figure 3). Case 2 had a gradual transition in FAF and no funduscopically visible transition. The caliber of retinal vessels was reduced with the areas of central FAF alterations in all patients. Focal curvilinear hypoautofluorescent interruptions were present in two probands with funduscopically visible RPE alterations (lacquer cracks of high myopia in case 1 and a superior, symmetrical, serpiginous band of RPE thinning and clumping extending away from the disc in case 3). Centrally, a bull's eye lesion of alternating rings centripetally of hypoautofluorescence and hyperautofluorescence surrounding normal foveal hypoautofluorescence was observed in all patients, although the bull's eye lesion was least distinct in case 2.

Peripheral autofluorescence abnormalities were appreciated on ultrawide-field imaging in cases 1 and 3 (Figure 4). These ranged from clustered patches of arcuate, amoeboid hyperautofluorescence with variable central hypoautofluorescence to discrete, isolated ovoid areas of hyperautofluorescence of variable size. The location of peripheral lesions was variable but tended to involve the nasal hemiretina, producing a bifocal appearance when viewed against the macula on the ultrawide-field images. Funduscopically, this corresponded to lightened areas of the nasal fundus (cases 1 and 3) with central RPE pigment clumping and intraretinal migration (case 3).

3.5. Fluorescein Angiography.
FA demonstrated a subtle hyperfluorescence at the area of confluent macular hyperautofluorescence. Areas of funduscopically visible RPE thinning and atrophy demonstrated anticipated window defects. Areas of RPE clumping exhibited blockage. No patient had

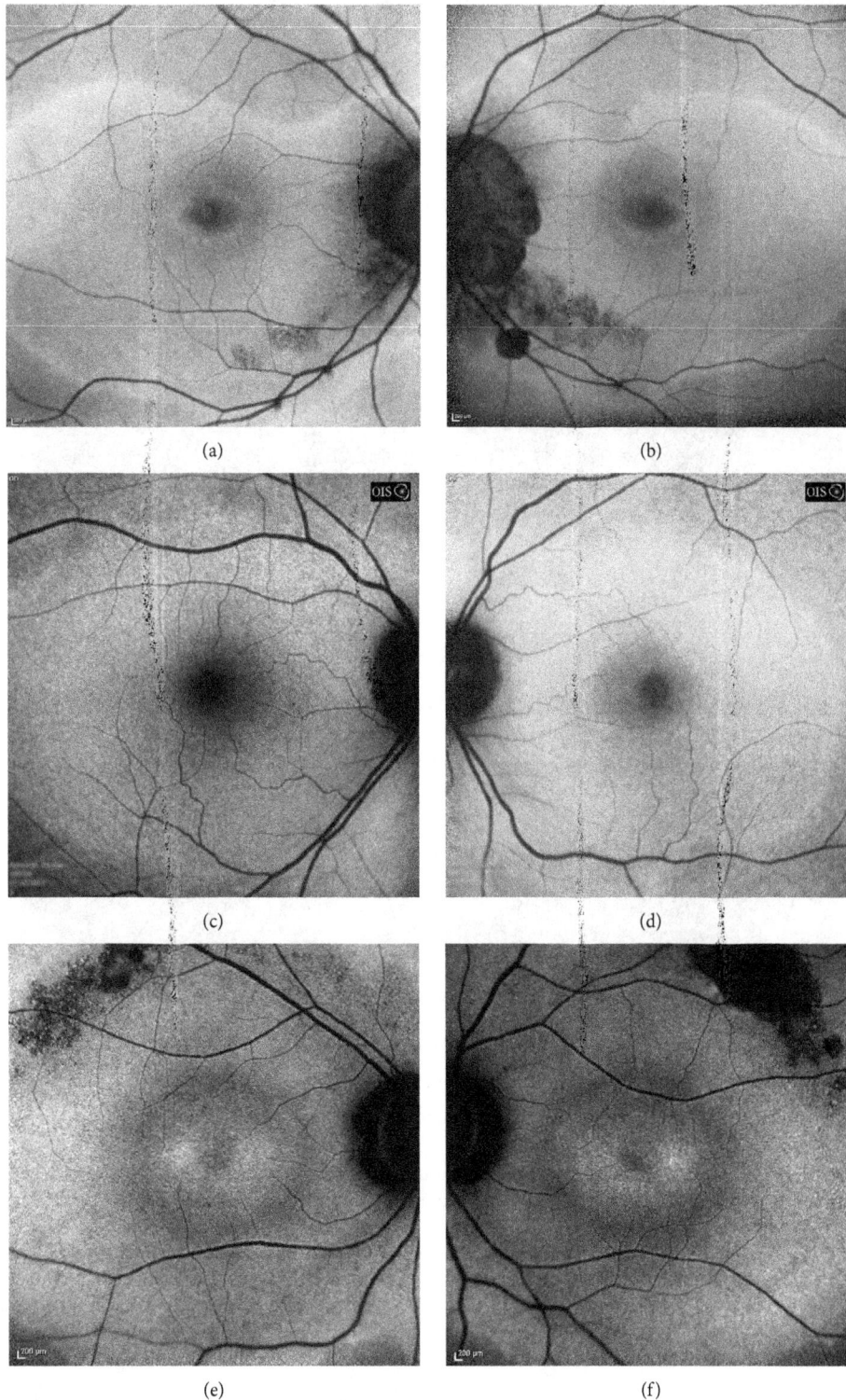

Figure 2: Thirty degree confocal scanning laser ophthalmoscope-based fundus autofluorescence by 488 nm argon blue laser excitation and emission filtered less than 500 nm. (a, b) Right and left maculas of case 1 had a geographic area of hyperautofluorescence with uniform hyperautofluorescent scalloped border that encompassed the majority of the macula and parapapillary retina outside alpha zone atrophy (seen as intensely hypoautofluorescent). A central ovoid bull's eye lesion of alternating hyper- and hypoautofluorescence was centered on the fovea. Linear granular hypoautofluorescence from lacquer cracks was observed in this patient with high myopia. (c, d) Right and left maculas of case 2 showed similar features, except the outer hyperautofluorescent border and bull's eye lesions were not as prominent. (e, f) Right and left maculas of case 3 also exhibited coarse, densely hypoautofluorescent arcs along the superotemporal arcades and a larger central bull's eye lesion in each eye.

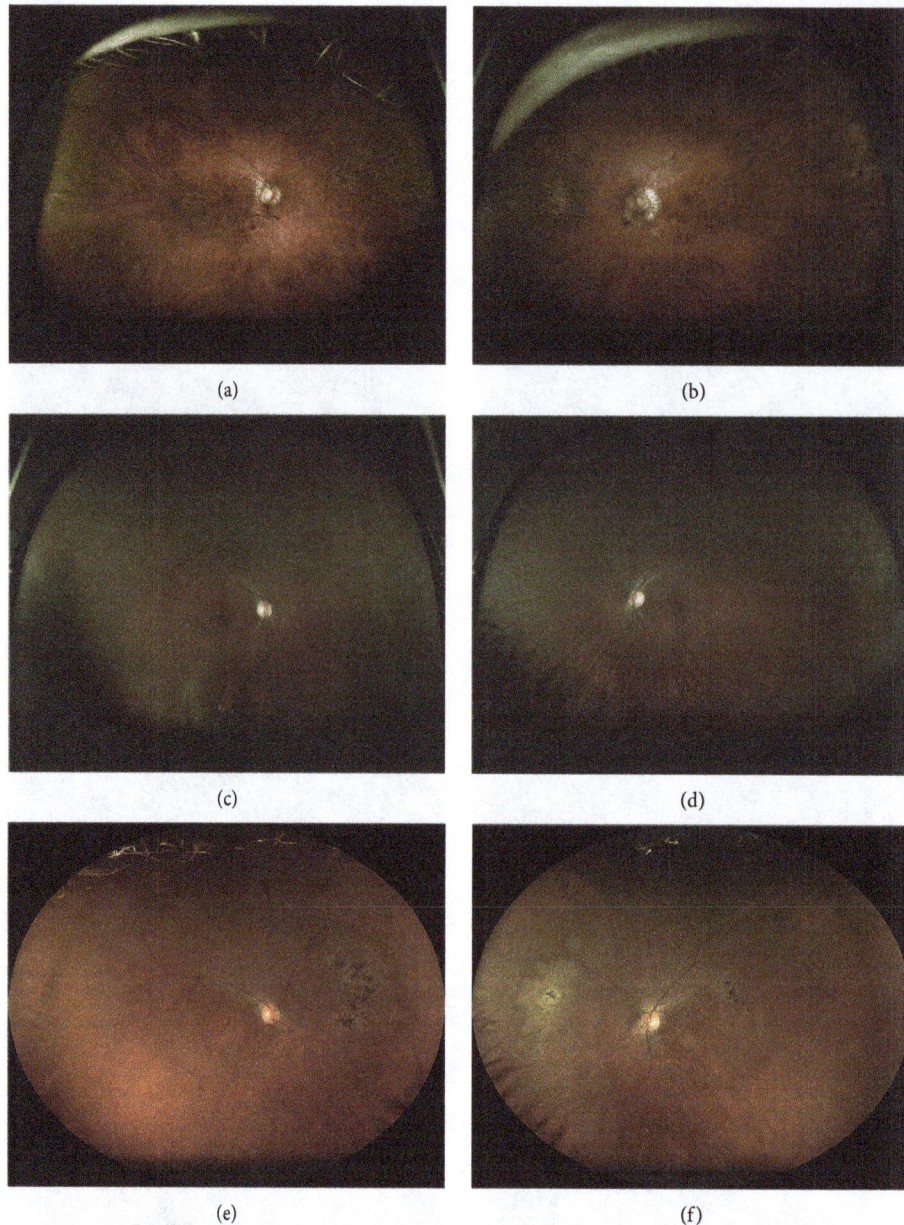

FIGURE 3: Two hundred degree ultrawide-field color retinal imaging using 633 nm, 532 nm, and 488 nm lasers demonstrate subtle retinal whitening in all patients corresponding to the geographic areas of hyperautofluorescence observed in Figure 2. Peripheral retinal pigment epithelial abnormalities were seen in the nasal periphery in all patients, although these were attributable to prior laser retinopexy in case 2. (a, b) Right and left fundi of case 1 exhibited alpha zone parapapillary atrophy and surrounding fundus lightening associated with high myopia. A nasal tongue of pigmentary changes extended from the peripheral retina posteriorly along the horizontal midline in each eye. (c, d) Right and left fundi of case 2 showed areas of lattice degeneration in both eyes surrounded by chorioretinal scarring from laser treatment. (e, f) Right and left fundi of case 3 had prominent posterior rings of retinal whitening and pigmentary alterations centered around the maculas. Irregular circumferential lesions with central reticular intraretinal pigment migration were observed nasally in both eyes.

vascular filling defects or leakage. Case 2 had blocked choroidal fluorescence. Interestingly, case 1, who had a single pathologic *ABCA4* mutation, did not have blocked choroidal fluorescence.

3.6. Infrared Imaging.
Infrared imaging was less useful for discerning the transition from abnormal to intact outer retinal architecture, although there was a subtle intensity change that mirrored the transition zone on FAF imaging.

3.7. Ultrasonography.
B-scan ultrasonography excluded posterior scleritis, choroidal thickening or infiltration, or retrobulbar disease (data not shown).

3.8. Spectral-Domain Optical Coherence Tomography.
SDOCT demonstrated reduced macular thickness and volume measurements in all probands due to loss of outer retinal elements (Figure 5). Inner retinal thickness and architecture were undisturbed. The inner segment ellipsoid

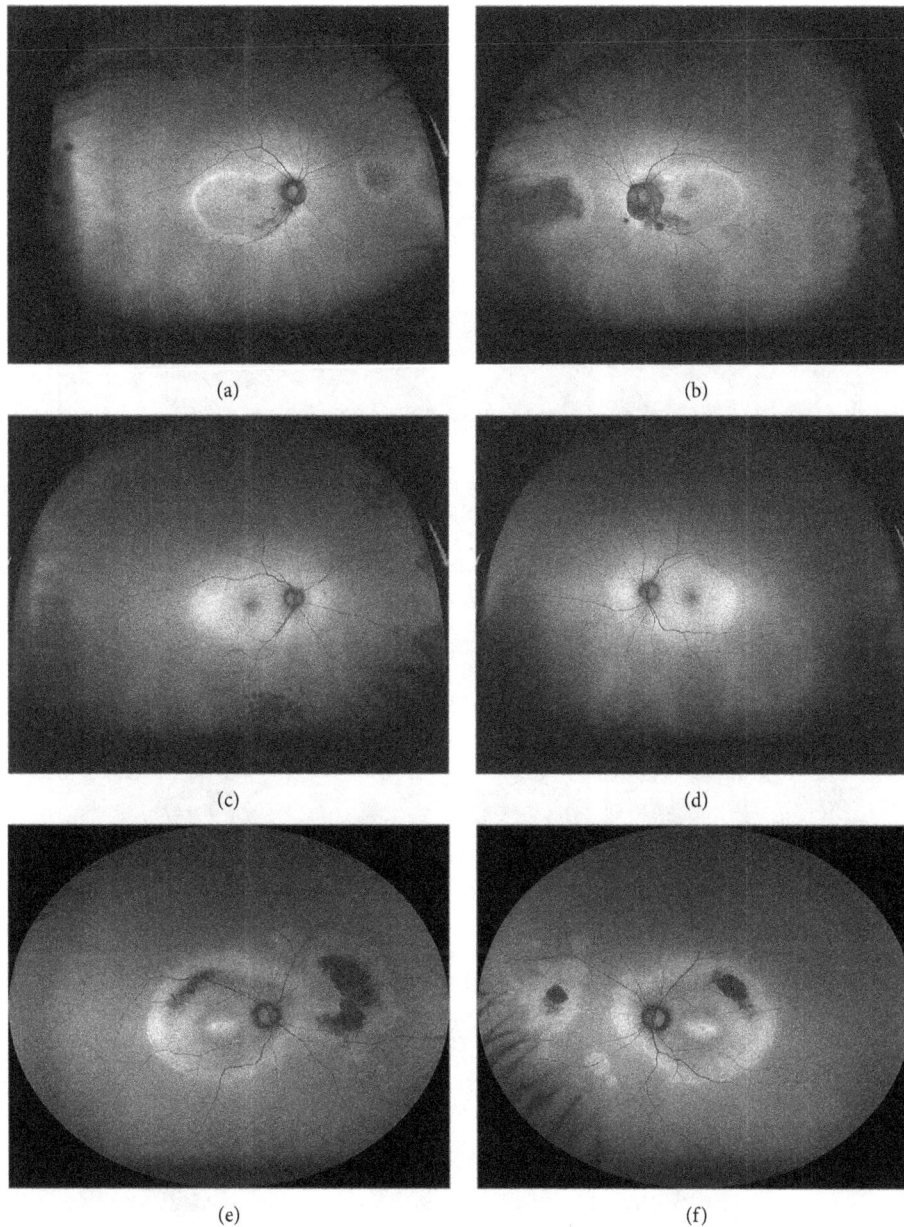

FIGURE 4: Two hundred degree ultrawide-field fundus autofluorescence with 488 nm laser excitation demonstrates macular changes as described in Figure 2 but reveals additional peripheral autofluorescence abnormalities in all patients. (a, b) Right and left fundi of case 1 had grouped nummular hypoautofluorescent areas anterior to the equator from cobblestone degeneration. A hypoautofluorescent tongue with hyperautofluorescent borders extended posteriorly towards the optic nerve in both eyes. Areas of funduscopically visible black pigment clumping appeared densely hypoautofluorescent. (c, d) Hypoautofluorescence from prior laser treatment of lattice degeneration in the right eye was the only evident peripheral autofluorescence abnormality seen in case 2. (e, f) A bifocal area of hyperautofluorescence with central hypoautofluorescence to the nasal portion was observed in the right and left fundi of case 3. In the right eye, the lesions were contiguous and the area of hypoautofluorescence was larger.

(iSE) band, external limiting membrane (ELM), and even photoreceptor cell bodies were diminished or absent within the well-defined area of confluent macular hyperautofluorescence. The external border between hyperautofluorescence and iso-autofluorescence marked the transition from abnormal to intact outer retinal architecture and lamination. The central bull's eye lesion on FAF imaging represented a transition from diminished to intact iSE and ELM bands, a pattern previously observed with other photoreceptor dystrophies. Within the

macula, retinal architecture was most intact at the fovea, consistent with the sparing of central visual acuities relative to the surrounding paracentral scotomas. The choroid was normal in thickness, except for an anticipated amount of thinning in case 1 related to high myopia.

3.9. Genetic Analysis. Genetic testing for genes associated with cone dysfunction, retinitis pigmentosa, or lipofuscin

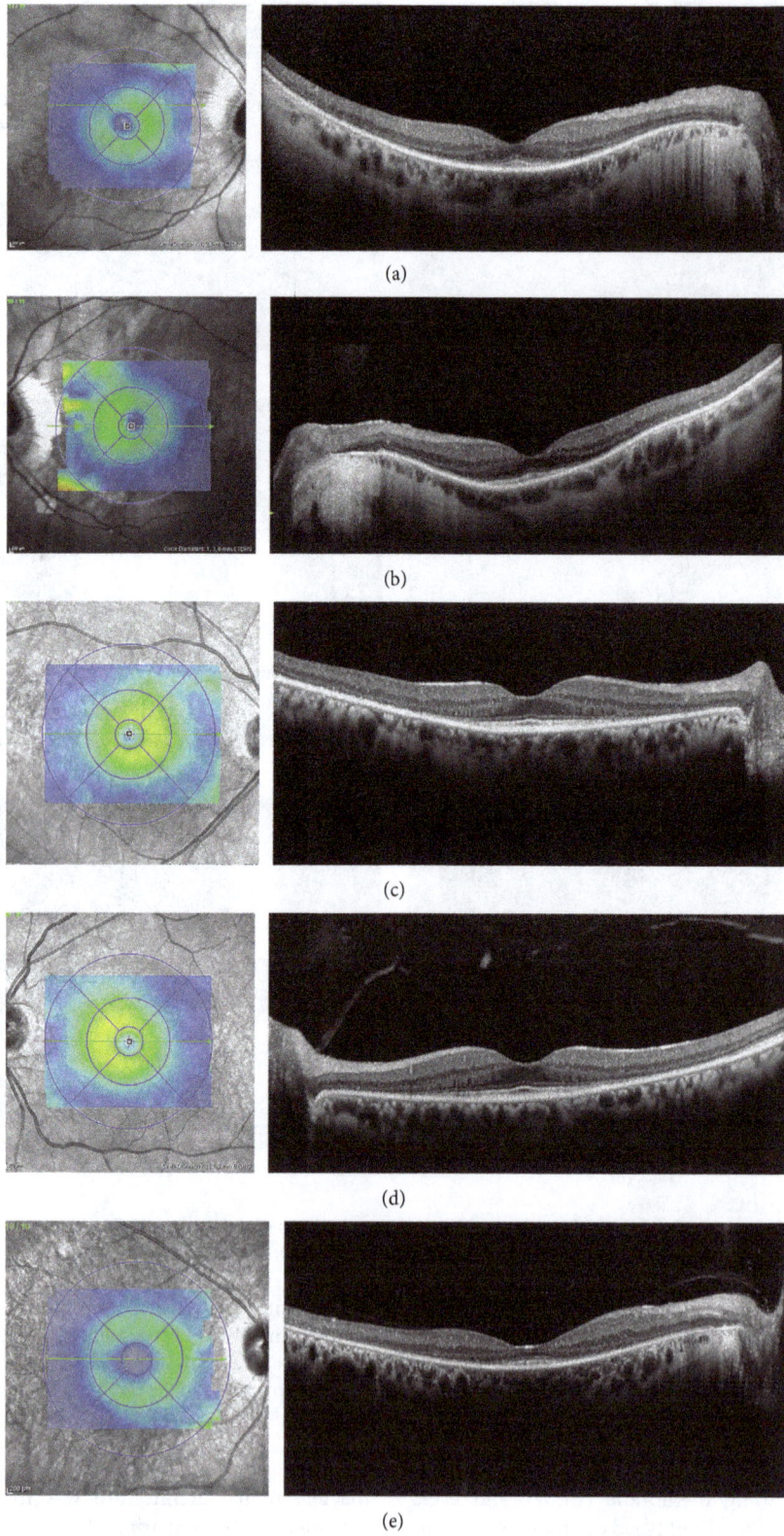

(a)

(b)

(c)

(d)

(e)

Figure 5: Continued.

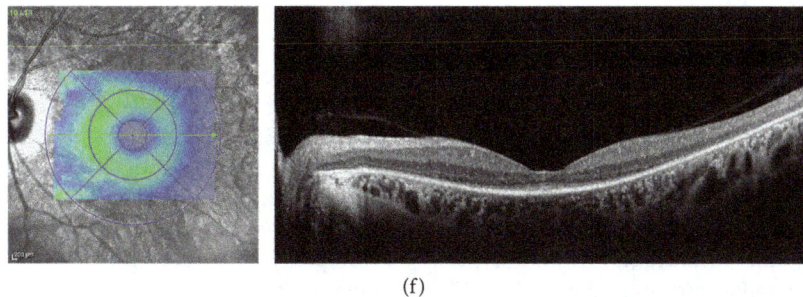

(f)

FIGURE 5: Spectral-domain optical coherence tomography registration thickness maps (left column) exhibited severe retinal thinning in all eyes. Accompanying foveal horizontal raster scans (right column) demonstrated outer retinal loss sparing the foveola in both eyes of all patients. The external limiting membrane, inner segment ellipsoid band, and photoreceptor outer segments were lost centrifugally until the hyperautofluorescent border of the macular lesions in Figure 2, where there was transition to normal retinal architecture. All cases had normal choroidal thickness, except case 1, who had pathologic myopia. (a, b) Right and left maculas of case 1 had staphylomatous posterior pole curvature, alpha zone parapapillary RPE atrophy, and choroidal thinning associated with pathologic myopia. (c, d) Right and left maculas of case 2 had the greatest preservation of outer retinal layers at the fovea and the nerve fiber layer throughout the macula compared to the other two cases. (e, f) Right and left maculas of case 3 had reduced inner retinal thickness with preservation of inner retinal lamination, similar to case 1.

accumulation revealed no pathogenic variants in a pattern consistent with a monogenic cause for disease. Specifically, Sanger sequencing of *ABCA4*, *PRPH2*/RDS-peripherin, and *ELOVL4* was negative except for Proband 1, who had a heterozygous *ABCA4* missense variant (c.2588G>C; p.Gly863Ala) and no family history of Stargardt disease or cone-rod dystrophy. This substitution has been previously reported as disease-causing (rs76157638; HGMD ID CS024003), but not associated with pericentral retinal degeneration (PRD) [29–32].

WES was then performed on the three probands. Details of bioinformatics analysis are available in Methods. Briefly, we prioritized rare functional variants (missense, nonsense, splice site variants, and indels) that were heterozygous, homozygous, or compound heterozygous in each of the 3 probands and excluded variants with a MAF >0.01 in the Exome Variant Server (release ESP6500SI-V2), 1000 Genomes Project, or Exome Aggregation Consortium (ExAC) [28, 33]. We also excluded all variants with a frequency of >0.01 found in in-house controls for BHCMG (CIDRVar 51 Mb) and CCHMC. This allele frequency cutoff was used to account for variants causing autosomal recessive disease. Parent and sibling samples were not available for segregation analysis.

Variant lists generated for each proband were first screened for rare variants (<1% minor allele frequency) in 52 genes related to pattern dystrophy, macular dystrophy, cone dystrophy, cone-rod dystrophy, rod-cone dystrophy, and cone photoreceptor development and function, including cone opsin genes (Supplementary Table 1). Supplementary Table 2 lists the 7 variants that were validated by Sanger sequencing. The *ABCA4* variant in case 1 was also detected by the WES. In cases 1 and 2, missense variants were identified in *IMPG2*, p.Leu842Met, and p.Ser11Tyr, respectively. *IMPG2* is associated with autosomal dominant vitelliform macular dystrophy 5 [MIM #616152] [34]. Both variants were predicted pathogenic by SIFT and Polyphen-2 [35, 36]. In case 2, a rare, predicted-pathogenic variant was noted in the protein kinase domain of *GUCY2D*

(p.Glu779Lys), associated with autosomal dominant cone-rod dystrophy 6 [MIM #601777] [37, 38]. Additionally in case 2, we identified two variants in *RP1L1*, p.Ala624Thr, and p.Trp2306Arg. However, neither were predicted pathogenic by Polyphen-2, and only p.Trp2306Arg was predicted pathogenic by SIFT. In case 3, we identified one predicted-pathogenic variant in *ADAM9* (p.Gln800His), associated with cone-rod dystrophy 9 [MIM #612775] [39]. We then searched for genes with rare variants in other retinal dystrophy genes (Supplementary Table 3) and rare variants in all 3 probands (not shown), though no common candidate gene was identified with rare variants. These variants are all considered variants of uncertain significance (VOUSs).

4. Discussion

At the time of its initial description a decade ago, PCD was an electrophysiologic diagnosis in individuals with normal fundus appearance and fluorescein angiography [12]. OCT and FAF had limited clinical applications and lacked the resolution available with conventional scanning laser ophthalmoscope-based platforms. Yet review of the fundus photography and fluorescein angiography images from the report by Kondo and coauthors demonstrates the same features we describe in our cohort: (a) a lightened macular color funduscopically that transitions at the temporal arcades, (b) narrowing of retinal vessels within the affected macular region, (c) macular hyperfluorescence on FA that transitions at the same location as the funduscopic color change, and (d) variable blocked choroidal fluorescence outside the macular lesion. In our cohort, two of the three probands also had nasal RPE and retinal changes that were not described in the original report. From the findings presented, we assert that PCD has features on ophthalmoscopy and multimodal imaging that distinguishes this diagnosis from other rare diseases.

SDOCT and FAF clarify the functional deficits observed by visual field and electroretinographic testing. The total macular volume is reduced, and the photoreceptor layer within the macular lesion, except of the fovea, is thinned and disorganized. The iSE and ELM bands particularly are diminished or absent with greater involvement of cone photoreceptor cell bodies centrifugally until the border of the hyperautofluorescent lesion. This unveiling of outer retinal elements was associated with the observed window defect of confluent macular hyperautofluorescence [40]. The transition between affected and unaffected outer retina correlated well with the transition from hyperautofluorescence to isoautofluorescence. Unlike SDOCT changes observed in retinitis pigmentosa and typical cone-rod dystrophies, choroidal thickness was not reduced, and the RPE remained largely intact except focal disruptions which were also evident funduscopically [41–49]. These findings corroborate that the photoreceptor layer is primarily affected, and the RPE may be secondarily affected. Ultrawide-field FAF imaging revealed large affected regions nasally that produced a bifocal appearance and helped explain the greater reduction in cone amplitudes than would be expected for a purely macular disease. Despite no reduction in inner retinal thickness by SDOCT, retinal arterioles within the central hyperautofluorescent region with photoreceptor disease were thinned. There was no evidence from SDOCT or FA imaging of a primary vascular disease. Without photoreceptor-generated impulses from affected areas, presumably, there is a reduced activity of inner retinal layers, reduced oxygen demand, and a resultant reduction in vessel caliber by autoregulation. This has been observed commonly in other photoreceptor dystrophies [50]. We observed greater variation in full field electroretinographic findings than the original series presented by Kondo et al., with cases 1 and 3 displaying the typical pattern reported for PCD and case 2 having a cone-rod dystrophy pattern.

PCD can be distinguished from pericentral retinal degeneration (PRD), which shares many clinical features, and has heterogeneous genetic causes, particularly genes causing retinitis pigmentosa and Stargardt disease. Foremost, the electrophysiologic profile for PRD resembles rod-cone dystrophy rather than cone or cone-rod dystrophy. Annular visual field loss is complete in PRD and may be incomplete in PCD. Peripheral retinal pigmentary changes are not observed in PRD, so annular or curvilinear visual field deficits are not observed beyond forty degrees, as are seen in our cases of PCD. Cases of ABCA4-related PRD involve mutations that prevent production of a protein product and produce photoreceptor dysfunction. Heterozygous mutations in ABCA4 can produce bull's eye lesions or occult macular dystrophy, but photoreceptor loss does not extend past the arcades and is accompanied by progressive RPE atrophy.

PCD may be a nonspecific rare presentation of cone dystrophy, and this is supported by pathogenic variants associated with macular dystrophy in all patients without a consensus candidate gene among them. Although WES did not reveal the leading candidate gene(s) among the probands, all probands harbored VOUSs in known photoreceptor dystrophy genes. We observed rare and predicted pathogenic variants in IMPG2 in cases 1 and 2, which is associated with autosomal dominant vitelliform macular

dystrophy, and variants in RP1L1 in case 2, which is associated with autosomal dominant occult macular dystrophy [17, 34]. Both genes cause a variable macular phenotype overlapping with peripheral cone dystrophy. The manifestations of RP1L1 pathogenic variants are complex and include both limited and diffuse forms of cone dystrophy [17, 51, 52]. We speculate that RP1L1 may modulate the effects of another cone dystrophy gene or autoimmune retinopathy contributing to allow sparing of the foveolar cones in the PCD phenotype. In case 2, the previously unreported variant in GUCY2D, associated with autosomal dominant cone-rod dystrophy, was considered as potentially contributing to this phenotype given the cone-rod pattern on ffERG and her mother's end stage cone-rod dystrophy phenotype. Given foveal sparing in both case 2 and her mother, the phenotype may be modulated by the RP1L1 variant. No prior report of GUCY2D or ADAM9-related cone dystrophy involves broad macular involvement sparing the foveola [39, 53–55]. Rather, those diseases typically involve the fovea early and have prominent macular RPE changes, and those with bull's eye lesions sparing the umbo do not extend beyond the parafovea.

Several features of PCD could also be consistent with postinflammatory changes of a retinal white dot syndrome [19, 56–65]. The geographic and racial backgrounds were variable, and two cases were sporadic. The regional clustering of both cohorts in the peer-reviewed literature against time and geography favors an autoimmune disease incited by a local pathogen or toxin. The lack of progression observed by anatomical and electrophysiological testing is atypical for retinal dystrophy, although follow-up with high-resolution anatomic testing was performed after three years and may represent the end stage of disease progression. Case 3 was noted to have nonprogressive symptoms and stable fundus appearance when compared with her original retinal drawings from twenty years prior. The Japanese cohort has exhibited similar stability after the publication (Kondo, personal communication 2013). The variable involvement of the peripheral retina resembles the random pattern observed in inflammation more than the predictable patterns observed in retinal dystrophies. The peripheral hyperautofluorescent lesions with central hypofluorescent RPE disruption are similar to those observed in other retinal white dot syndromes (MEWDS, AZOOR, and PIC). On the contrary, specific sparing of the fovea while the surrounding outer retina is decimated would be unexpected for an inflammatory disease. With the exception of MEWDS, severe RPE alterations and persistent scotomas usually accompany preceding chorioretinal inflammation, and these were not observed with the peripheral lesions. The presence of tapetal sheen, seen intermittently in case 2 and not previously described with PCD, is a characteristic for a retinal dystrophy rather than inflammation or drug toxicity.

A third explanation is that both genetic and environmental factors play a role in the development and manifestations of PCD. An environmental agent or pathogen may create an autoimmune response against short wavelength (S-cone) photoreceptors modulated by a pathogenic variant in cone dystrophy genes like RP1L1. In case 2, we cannot rule out the contribution of hydroxychloroquine toxicity to her phenotype, although photoreceptor damage to the arcades would be unusual without prominent RPE changes.

In summary, PCD is a distinct clinical entity with ring scotomas, outer retinal attenuation relatively sparing the foveola, macular hyperautofluorescence with bull's eye lesions, and variable peripheral lesions. However, the etiology remains unknown. Studies of human and primate retinas demonstrate absence of S-cone photoreceptors within the foveola, greater S-cone concentrations within the macula than peripheral retina, and greater concentrations in the retinal periphery nasally than temporally [66–68]. This pattern highly correlates with the location of disease observed in our cohort. Given the limitation of patient numbers for this rare disease, further investigation is warranted, including whole exome sequencing of other probands, investigation of trios, animal models, and serum analysis from more recently affected individuals, and a search for an infectious homologue or compound with selective toxicity to S-cone proteins.

Disclosure

One case was presented as an unknown at the 45th Annual Retina Society Conference in Washington, DC, October 4, 2012. The full cohort was presented at the 32nd annual meeting of the American Society of Retina Specialists in San Diego, CA, August 9–13, 2014.

Conflicts of Interest

The authors declare that they have no conflicts of interest.

Acknowledgments

The Baylor-Hopkins Center for Mendelian Genomics (BHCMG) and the National Ophthalmic Disease Genotyping and Phenotyping Network (eyeGENE) performed genetic analysis at no cost to the patients or the authors. Grants from the National Human Genome Research Institute, (1U54HG006542) and National Institute for Deafness and Communication Disorders (R01DC016295) provided support for this work.

Supplementary Materials

This article contains additional online-only material. The following should appear online only: Supplementary Tables 1–3. Supplementary Figure 1: results of full field electroretinography of the right eye for the 3 probands and a normal age-matched control. Waveforms were symmetrical between the two eyes of each patient and the control. Supplementary Figure 2: multifocal electroretinography of the right eye for the 3 probands and a normal age-matched control. Waveforms and 3D topography plots were symmetrical between the two eyes of each patient and the control. Supplementary Figure 3: visual field testing for the 3 probands. Humphrey visual field testing using a 30-2 Sita-Standard protocol with a size III stimulus was used for case 1. Cases 2 and 3 were tested using Goldmann threshold perimetry. Paracentral scotomas were identified by the smallest isopter. Case 2 could not discern I2E targets and had constricted I3E within 30°. Case 3 could not discern I3E targets. Supplementary Table 1: candidate photoreceptor and macular dystrophy genes. Supplementary Table 2: variants detected in candidate photoreceptor or macular dystrophy genes. Supplementary Table 3: variants detected in 2 of 3 probands in genes with known retinal expression. (*Supplementary Materials*)

References

[1] S. Roosing, A. A. Thiadens, C. B. Hoyng et al., "Causes and consequences of inherited cone disorders," *Progress in Retinal and Eye Research*, vol. 42, pp. 1–26, 2014.

[2] G. A. Fishman, "Electrophysiology and inherited retinal disorders," *Documenta Ophthalmologica*, vol. 60, no. 2, pp. 107–119, 1985.

[3] M. P. Simunovic and A. T. Moore, "The cone dystrophies," *Eye*, vol. 12, no. 3, pp. 553–565, 1998.

[4] M. Michaelides, D. M. Hunt, and A. T. Moore, "The cone dysfunction syndromes," *British Journal of Ophthalmology*, vol. 88, no. 2, pp. 291–297, 2004.

[5] M. Michaelides, A. J. Hardcastle, D. M. Hunt, and A. T. Moore, "Progressive cone and cone-rod dystrophies: phenotypes and underlying molecular genetic basis," *Survey of Ophthalmology*, vol. 51, no. 3, pp. 232–258, 2006.

[6] C. P. Hamel, "Cone rod dystrophies," *Orphanet Journal of Rare Diseases*, vol. 2, p. 7, 2007.

[7] Y. Miyake, M. Horiguchi, N. Tomita et al., "Occult macular dystrophy," *American Journal of Ophthalmology*, vol. 122, no. 5, pp. 644–653, 1996.

[8] Y. Miyake, K. Ichikawa, Y. Shiose, and Y. Kawase, "Hereditary macular dystrophy without visible fundus abnormality," *American Journal of Ophthalmology*, vol. 108, no. 3, pp. 292–299, 1989.

[9] R. A. Sisk, A. M. Berrocal, and B. L. Lam, "Loss of foveal cone photoreceptor outer segments in occult macular dystrophy," *Ophthalmic Surgery, Lasers and Imaging*, vol. 9, pp. 1–3, 2010.

[10] S. J. Park, S. J. Woo, K. H. Park et al., "Morphologic photoreceptor abnormality in occult macular dystrophy on spectral-domain optical coherence tomography," *Investigative Ophthalmology & Visual Science*, vol. 51, no. 7, pp. 3673–3679, 2010.

[11] K. Fujinami, K. Tsunoda, G. Hanazono et al., "Fundus autofluorescence in autosomal dominant occult macular dystrophy," *Archives of Ophthalmology*, vol. 129, no. 5, pp. 597–602, 2011.

[12] M. Kondo, Y. Miyake, N. Kondo et al., "Peripheral cone dystrophy: a variant of cone dystrophy with predominant dysfunction in the peripheral cone system," *Ophthalmology*, vol. 111, no. 4, pp. 732–739, 2004.

[13] T. Okuno, H. Oku, T. Kurimoto, S. Oono, and T. Ikeda, "Peripheral cone dystrophy in an elderly man," *Clinical and Experimental Ophthalmology*, vol. 36, no. 9, pp. 897–899, 2008.

[14] M. S. Vaphiades and J. I. Doyle, "Peripheral cone dystrophy: a diagnostic improbability?," *Journal of Neuro-Ophthalmology*, vol. 34, no. 4, pp. 366–368, 2014.

[15] Y. Mochizuki, K. Shinoda, C. S. Matsumoto et al., "Case of unilateral peripheral cone dysfunction," *Case Reports in Ophthalmology*, vol. 3, no. 2, pp. 162–168, 2012.

[16] J. Baek, H. K. Lee, and U. S. Kim, "Spectral domain optical coherence tomography findings in bilateral peripheral cone dystrophy," *Documenta Ophthalmologica*, vol. 126, no. 3, pp. 247–251, 2013.

[17] M. Akahori, K. Tsunoda, Y. Miyake et al., "Dominant mutations in *RP1L1* are responsible for occult macular dystrophy," *American Journal of Human Genetics*, vol. 87, no. 3, pp. 424–429, 2010.

[18] I. Cima, J. Brecelj, M. Sustar et al., "Enhanced S-cone syndrome with preserved macular structure and severely depressed retinal function," *Documenta Ophthalmologica*, vol. 125, no. 2, pp. 161–168, 2012.

[19] T. Fujiwara, Y. Imamura, V. J. Giovinazzo, and R. F. Spaide, "Fundus autofluorescence and optical coherence tomographic findings in acute zonal occult outer retinopathy," *Retina*, vol. 30, no. 8, pp. 1206–1216, 2010.

[20] R. F. Spaide, "Collateral damage in acute zonal occult outer retinopathy," *American Journal of Ophthalmology*, vol. 138, no. 5, pp. 887–889, 2004.

[21] J. T. Pearlman, J. Saxton, and G. Hoffman, "Unilateral retinitis pigmentosa sine pigmento," *British Journal of Ophthalmology*, vol. 60, no. 5, pp. 354–360, 1976.

[22] M. Mititelu, B. J. Wong, M. Brenner et al., "Progression of hydroxychloroquine toxic effects after drug therapy cessation: new evidence from multimodal imaging," *JAMA Ophthalmology*, vol. 131, no. 9, pp. 1187–1197, 2013.

[23] A. Hamosh, N. Sobreira, J. Hoover-Fong et al., "PhenoDB: a new web-based tool for the collection, storage, and analysis of phenotypic features," *Human Mutation*, vol. 34, no. 4, pp. 566–571, 2013.

[24] H. Li and R. Durbin, "Fast and accurate long-read alignment with Burrows-Wheeler transform," *Bioinformatics*, vol. 26, no. 5, pp. 589–595, 2010.

[25] A. McKenna, M. Hanna, E. Banks et al., "The Genome Analysis Toolkit: a MapReduce framework for analyzing next-generation DNA sequencing data," *Genome Research*, vol. 20, no. 9, pp. 1297–1303, 2010.

[26] M. A. DePristo, E. Banks, R. Poplin et al., "A framework for variation discovery and genotyping using next-generation DNA sequencing data," *Nature Genetics*, vol. 43, no. 5, pp. 491–498, 2011.

[27] N. Sobreira, F. Schiettecatte, C. Boehm et al., "New tools for Mendelian disease gene identification: PhenoDB variant analysis module; and GeneMatcher, a web-based tool for linking investigators with an interest in the same gene," *Human Mutation*, vol. 36, no. 4, pp. 425–431, 2015.

[28] G. R. Abecasis, A. Auton, L. D. Brooks et al., "An integrated map of genetic variation from 1,092 human genomes," *Nature*, vol. 491, no. 7422, pp. 56–65, 2012.

[29] C. E. Briggs, D. Rucinski, P. J. Rosenfeld, T. Hirose, E. L. Berson, and T. P. Dryja, "Mutations in ABCR (ABCA4) in patients with Stargardt macular degeneration or cone-rod degeneration," *Investigative Ophthalmology & Visual Science*, vol. 42, no. 10, pp. 2229–2236, 2001.

[30] A. Maugeri, M. A. van Driel, D. J. van de Pol et al., "The 2588G-->C mutation in the ABCR gene is a mild frequent founder mutation in the Western European population and allows the classification of ABCR mutations in patients with

Stargardt disease," *American Journal of Human Genetics*, vol. 64, no. 4, pp. 1024–1035, 1999.

[31] J. Comander, C. Weigel-DiFranco, M. Maher et al., "The genetic basis of pericentral retinitis pigmentosa-a form of mild retinitis pigmentosa," *Genes*, vol. 8, no. 10, 2017.

[32] R. Matsui, A. V. Cideciyan, S. B. Schwartz et al., "Molecular heterogeneity within the clinical diagnosis of pericentral retinal degeneration," *Investigative Ophthalmology & Visual Science*, vol. 56, no. 10, pp. 6007–6018, 2015.

[33] M. Lek, K. J. Karczewski, E. V. Minikel et al., "Analysis of protein-coding genetic variation in 60,706 humans," *Nature*, vol. 536, no. 7616, pp. 285–291, 2016.

[34] I. Meunier, G. Manes, B. Bocquet et al., "Frequency and clinical pattern of vitelliform macular dystrophy caused by mutations of interphotoreceptor matrix IMPG1 and IMPG2 genes," *Ophthalmology*, vol. 121, no. 12, pp. 2406–2414, 2014.

[35] P. C. Ng and S. Henikoff, "Predicting deleterious amino acid substitutions," *Genome Research*, vol. 11, no. 5, pp. 863–874, 2001.

[36] I. A. Adzhubei, S. Schmidt, L. Peshkin et al., "A method and server for predicting damaging missense mutations," *Nature Methods*, vol. 7, no. 4, pp. 248–249, 2010.

[37] R. E. Kelsell, K. Gregory-Evans, A. M. Payne et al., "Mutations in the retinal guanylate cyclase (RETGC-1) gene in dominant cone-rod dystrophy," *Human Molecular Genetics*, vol. 7, no. 7, pp. 1179–1184, 1998.

[38] I. Perrault, J. M. Rozet, S. Gerber et al., "A retGC-1 mutation in autosomal dominant cone-rod dystrophy," *American Journal of Human Genetics*, vol. 63, no. 2, pp. 651–654, 1998.

[39] D. A. Parry, C. Toomes, L. Bida et al., "Loss of the metalloprotease ADAM9 leads to cone-rod dystrophy in humans and retinal degeneration in mice," *American Journal of Human Genetics*, vol. 84, no. 5, pp. 683–691, 2009.

[40] K. B. Freund, S. Mrejen, J. Jung et al., "Increased fundus autofluorescence related to outer retinal disruption," *JAMA Ophthalmology*, vol. 131, no. 12, pp. 1645–1649, 2013.

[41] Y. Makiyama, S. Ooto, M. Hangai et al., "Macular cone abnormalities in retinitis pigmentosa with preserved central vision using adaptive optics scanning laser ophthalmoscopy," *PLoS One*, vol. 8, no. 11, Article ID e79447, 2013.

[42] A. Oishi, K. Ogino, Y. Makiyama et al., "Wide-field fundus autofluorescence imaging of retinitis pigmentosa," *Ophthalmology*, vol. 120, no. 9, pp. 1827–1834, 2013.

[43] M. Oishi, A. Oishi, K. Ogino et al., "Wide-field fundus autofluorescence abnormalities and visual function in patients with cone and cone-rod dystrophies," *Investigative Ophthalmology and Visual Science*, vol. 55, no. 6, pp. 3572–3577, 2014.

[44] A. G. Robson, Z. Saihan, S. A. Jenkins et al., "Functional characterisation and serial imaging of abnormal fundus autofluorescence in patients with retinitis pigmentosa and normal visual acuity," *British Journal of Ophthalmology*, vol. 90, no. 4, pp. 472–479, 2006.

[45] A. G. Robson, M. Michaelides, V. A. Luong et al., "Functional correlates of fundus autofluorescence abnormalities in patients with *RPGR* or *RIMS1* mutations causing cone or cone rod dystrophy," *British Journal of Ophthalmology*, vol. 92, no. 1, pp. 95–102, 2008.

[46] N. Tojo, T. Nakamura, C. Fuchizawa et al., "Adaptive optics fundus images of cone photoreceptors in the macula of patients with retinitis pigmentosa," *Clinical Ophthalmology*, vol. 7, pp. 203–210, 2013.

[47] A. G. Robson, E. Lenassi, Z. Saihan et al., "Comparison of fundus autofluorescence with photopic and scotopic fine

matrix mapping in patients with retinitis pigmentosa: 4- to 8-year follow-up," *Investigative Ophthalmology & Visual Science*, vol. 53, no. 10, pp. 6187–6195, 2012.

[48] L. H. Lima, J. M. Sallum, and R. F. Spaide, "Outer retina analysis by optical coherence tomography in cone-rod dystrophy patients," *Retina*, vol. 33, no. 9, pp. 1877–1880, 2013.

[49] S. C. Cho, S. J. Woo, K. H. Park, and J. M. Hwang, "Morphologic characteristics of the outer retina in cone dystrophy on spectral-domain optical coherence tomography," *Korean Journal of Ophthalmology*, vol. 27, no. 1, pp. 19–27, 2013.

[50] D. Y. Yu and S. J. Cringle, "Retinal degeneration and local oxygen metabolism," *Experimental Eye Research*, vol. 80, no. 6, pp. 745–751, 2005.

[51] S. Kikuchi, S. Kameya, K. Gocho et al., "Cone dystrophy in patient with homozygous RP1L1 mutation," *Biomed Research International*, vol. 2015, Article ID 545243, 13 pages, 2015.

[52] Y. Miyake and K. Tsunoda, "Occult macular dystrophy," *Japanese Journal of Ophthalmology*, vol. 59, no. 2, pp. 71–80, 2015.

[53] S. Hull, G. Arno, V. Plagnol, A. Robson, A. R. Webster, and A. T. Moore, "Exome sequencing reveals ADAM9 mutations in a child with cone-rod dystrophy," *Acta Ophthalmologica*, vol. 93, no. 5, pp. e392–e393, 2014.

[54] O. Goldstein, J. G. Mezey, A. R. Boyko et al., "An ADAM9 mutation in canine cone-rod dystrophy 3 establishes homology with human cone-rod dystrophy 9," *Molecular Vision*, vol. 16, pp. 1549–1569, 2010.

[55] D. Zobor, E. Zrenner, B. Wissinger et al., "GUCY2D- or GUCA1A-related autosomal dominant cone-rod dystrophy: is there a phenotypic difference?," *Retina*, vol. 34, no. 8, pp. 1576–1587, 2014.

[56] A. Joseph, E. Rahimy, K. B. Freund et al., "Fundus autofluorescence and photoreceptor bleaching in multiple evanescent white dot syndrome," *Ophthalmic Surgery, Lasers and Imaging Retina*, vol. 44, no. 6, pp. 588–592, 2013.

[57] B. J. Thomas, T. A. Albini, and H. W. Flynn, "Multiple evanescent white dot syndrome: multimodal imaging and correlation with proposed pathophysiology," *Ophthalmic Surgery, Lasers and Imaging Retina*, vol. 44, no. 6, pp. 584–587, 2013.

[58] D. Li and S. Kishi, "Restored photoreceptor outer segment damage in multiple evanescent white dot syndrome," *Ophthalmology*, vol. 116, no. 4, pp. 762–770, 2009.

[59] R. Aoyagi, T. Hayashi, A. Masai et al., "Subfoveal choroidal thickness in multiple evanescent white dot syndrome," *Clinical and Experimental Optometry*, vol. 95, no. 2, pp. 212–217, 2012.

[60] R. Dell'Omo, A. Mantovani, R. Wong et al., "Natural evolution of fundus autofluorescence findings in multiple evanescent white dot syndrome: a long-term follow-up," *Retina*, vol. 30, no. 9, pp. 1479–1487, 2010.

[61] J. D. Gass, A. Agarwal, and I. U. Scott, "Acute zonal occult outer retinopathy: a long-term follow-up study," *American Journal of Ophthalmology*, vol. 134, no. 3, pp. 329–339, 2002.

[62] Q. V. Hoang, R. Gallego-Pinazo, and L. A. Yannuzzi, "Long-term follow-up of acute zonal occult outer retinopathy," *Retina*, vol. 33, no. 7, pp. 1325–1327, 2013.

[63] T. Wakazono, S. Ooto, M. Hangai, and N. Yoshimura, "Photoreceptor outer segment abnormalities and retinal sensitivity in acute zonal occult outer retinopathy," *Retina*, vol. 33, no. 3, pp. 642–648, 2013.

[64] R. F. Spaide and C. A. Curcio, "Anatomical correlates to the bands seen in the outer retina by optical coherence tomography: literature review and model," *Retina*, vol. 31, no. 8, pp. 1609–1619, 2011.

[65] M. Mkrtchyan, B. J. Lujan, D. Merino et al., "Outer retinal structure in patients with acute zonal occult outer retinopathy," *American Journal of Ophthalmology*, vol. 153, no. 4, pp. 757–68.e1, 2012.

[66] K. Bumsted and A. Hendrickson, "Distribution and development of short-wavelength cones differ between Macaca monkey and human fovea," *Journal of Comparative Neurology*, vol. 403, no. 4, pp. 502–516, 1999.

[67] P. R. Martin and U. Grünert, "Analysis of the short wavelength-sensitive ("blue") cone mosaic in the primate retina: comparison of New World and Old World monkeys," *Journal of Comparative Neurology*, vol. 406, no. 1, pp. 1–14, 1999.

[68] C. A. Curcio, K. A. Allen, K. R. Sloan et al., "Distribution and morphology of human cone photoreceptors stained with anti-blue opsin," *Journal of Comparative Neurology*, vol. 312, no. 4, pp. 610–624, 1991.

18

Emerging Therapeutic Strategies for Limbal Stem Cell Deficiency

Ying Dong ⓘ,[1,2] Han Peng,[2] and Robert M. Lavker[2]

[1]*Department of Ophthalmology, The First Affiliated Hospital, Chinese PLA General Hospital, Beijing 100048, China*
[2]*Department of Dermatology, Northwestern University, Chicago, IL 60611, USA*

Correspondence should be addressed to Ying Dong; dongying304@qq.com

Academic Editor: Karim Mohamed-Noriega

Identification and characterization of the limbal epithelial stem cells (LESCs) has proven to be a major accomplishment in anterior ocular surface biology. These cells have been shown to be a subpopulation of limbal epithelial basal cells, which serve as the progenitor population of the corneal epithelium. LESCs have been demonstrated to play an important role in maintaining corneal epithelium homeostasis. Many ocular surface diseases, including intrinsic (e.g., Sjogren's syndrome) or extrinsic (e.g., alkali or thermal burns) insults, which impair LESCs, can lead to limbal stem cell deficiency (LSCD). LSCD is characterized by an overgrowth of conjunctival-derived epithelial cells, corneal neovascularization, and chronic inflammation, eventually leading to blindness. Treatment of LSCD has been challenging, especially in bilateral total LSCD. Recently, advances in LESC research have led to novel therapeutic approaches for treating LSCD, such as transplantation of the cultured limbal epithelium. These novel therapeutic approaches have demonstrated efficacy for ocular surface reconstruction and restoration of vision in patients with LSCD. However, they all have their own limitations. Here, we describe the current status of LSCD treatment and discuss the advantages and disadvantages of the available therapeutic modalities.

1. Introduction

The functions of cornea include protecting the delicate internal parts of the eye and allowing proper transmission of light. The corneal epithelium is the outermost layer of cornea, which is a crucial barrier against mechanical, chemical, and pathogenic insults. In fulfilling its barrier function, this self-renewing stratified epithelium turns over every 5–7 days. The self-renewal of the corneal epithelium is governed by the stem cells that reside in the basal layer of the limbal epithelium, adjacent to the corneal epithelium [1]. The first observation that the limbal epithelium might be involved in replenishing the corneal epithelium came from Davanger and Evensen who noted "streaking" of the pigmented limbal epithelium into the corneal epithelium following an insult [2]; however, they did not suggest the involvement of stem cells in this process. In 1986, Schermer et al. proposed that the corneal epithelial stem cells resided in the limbal epithelial basal cells [3]. It was the landmark paper. In 1989, Cotsarelis et al. for the first time proved this hypothesis by demonstrating that label-retaining cells (a marker of slow-cycling cells, which is a characteristic of stem cells) were preferentially located in the basal layer of the limbal epithelium and not in the corneal epithelium [1]. Since then, the biology of limbal epithelial stem cells (LESCs) has attracted many attentions.

2. Characteristics of Limbal Epithelial Stem Cells

LESCs are morphologically small, have a high nuclear-to-cytoplasm ratio, and are relatively undifferentiated cells with rare cycling and high proliferative capacity [4, 5]. The difference of the limbal epithelial stem cells and corneal epithelium is shown in Table 1. More importantly, LESCs have the capability to regenerate the entire corneal epithelium [6]. Similar to other somatic stem cells, LESCs highly express stem cell markers, including transporters (e.g., ABCG2 and ABCB5) [7, 8], transcription factors (e.g., C/EBPδ, Bmi-1, ΔNp63α, and Pax6) [9–11], cell adhesion molecules and receptors (e.g., N-cadherin, integrins α9 and β1, and Frizzled (Fz)7), and cytokeratins (e.g., CK15, CK14, and CK19) [12–14] [15].

2.1. Low Differentiation. Limbal epithelial basal cells are relatively undifferentiated and thus lack the expression of

TABLE 1: The features of corneal epithelial cells and limbal epithelial stem cells.

	Limbal epithelial stem cells (LESCs)	Corneal epithelium (CE)
Morphology	High nucleus-to-cytoplasm ratio; smaller than CE ($10.1 \pm 0.8 \, \mu m$)	Lower nucleus-to-cytoplasm ratio; column cell ($17.1 \pm 0.8 \, \mu m$)
Blood supply	High vascularization	Avascular
Clonogenicity	Holoclones	Paraclones
Pigmentation	Intrinsic melanogenesis	Absent pigment, transparency
Epithelial cell marker	K5 and K14	K3, K12, and Cx43
Putative stem cell marker	ABCG2, K19, vimentin, integrin α9 and so on	—
Metabolic activity	Low	High
Cell cycling	Slow cycling	Fast cycling

differentiation markers such as keratin 3, keratin 12 [16], and connexin 43, which is associated with a more differentiated cell [17].

2.2. Infrequent Cycling. Stem cells are commonly believed to cycle infrequently [18]. This characteristic has been postulated to enable stem cells to preserve their proliferative capacity and to minimize DNA replication-associated errors [19, 20]. Utilizing this characteristic of infrequent cycling, LESCs were identified using the "label-retaining cells" (LRCs) technique. First, all of the dividing cells (including stem cells) are labeled by continuous exposure to either tritiated thymidine (^{3}H-Tdr) or bromodeoxyuridine (BrdU). After a chasing period (usually 4–8 weeks), the labeling signal in the rapidly dividing TA cells is diminished due to dilution or by transiting out of the tissue due to differentiation, whereas the slow-cycling stem cells still retain their labeling. Application of this labeling technique to mouse limbal/corneal epithelia revealed that the LRCs were exclusively localized in the basal layer of the limbal epithelium. In contrast, the peripheral and central corneal epithelia contained no LRC, which was compelling evidence that the corneal epithelial stem cells were located in the limbal epithelium [1, 19].

2.3. High Capacity for Self-Renewal and Proliferation. LESCs have high proliferative capacity, which is demonstrated in vitro by an ability to generate holoclone colonies [21]. On the contrary, in the transit-amplifying (TA) cells, only the progeny of LESCs are able to produce meroclone and paraclone colonies [21]. Holoclone, meroclone, and paraclone colonies represent three different proliferative capacity clonogenicity. Holoclone colonies are believed to be derived from stem cells and have the greatest proliferative capacity. Meroclone colonies are believed to be derived primarily from TA cells and have less cellular division potential. Finally, paraclone colonies are thought to be derived from mature TA cells and have the least proliferative potential. Cells from the stem cell-enriched limbal epithelium can undergo 80 to 100 cell division cycles and are capable to form holoclone colonies, whereas cells from the central corneal epithelium undergo 15 cell divisions maximally and only form paraclone colonies [21].

2.4. Limbal Niche. The limbal stem cell niche is a specific and highly regulated microenvironment, which is required for harboring and maintaining LESCs [22–26]. It has been suggested that the human limbal stem cell niche is located in the palisades of Vogt (recently termed "crypts") [27–30]. Limbal epithelial crypts (LECs) have been demonstrated to extend from the peripheral aspects of an interpalisade rete ridge and further into the conjunctival stroma as a solid chord of cells measuring up to $120 \, \mu m$ [27]. It is generally believed that the niche consists of three components: (i) cell-cell interactions between stem cells and TA cells, (ii) the basement membrane, and (iii) the extracellular matrix and mesenchymal cells directly adjacent to and beneath the basement membrane. Disruption of the limbal niche by various pathological conditions (e.g., severe immune response and wounding) can lead to LSCD.

3. Limbal Stem Cell Deficiency

Clinically, LSCD is caused by the depletion or dysfunction of LESCs, which leads to the inability to sustain corneal epithelial homeostasis [31–35]. Patients often present with pain, photophobia, and decreased vision in the acute stages of LSCD. Biomicroscopy shows conjunctival hyperemia, loss of the palisades of Vogt, and a "whorled-like" corneal epithelium [36, 37]. LSCD is also associated with poor epithelial adhesion, resulting in recurrent erosions and persistent corneal epithelial defects. At the chronic stage, the ocular surface is scarred and extensively neovascularized.

4. Clinical Treatments of LSCD

Clinical treatment of the LSCD varies based on the severity and extent of involvement. For those patients with mild and moderate LSCD, treatments involve the control of the symptoms and causes. For patients with severe LSCD, it is necessary to undergo ocular surface reconstruction (OSR). OSR is a series of procedures to reconstitute the anatomic and physiologic ocular surface, including amniotic membrane transplantation (AMT), conjunctival limbal grafting, simple limbal epithelial transplantation (SLET), and cultivated limbal epithelial transplantation (CLET) [33, 38–41]. The recent progress in understanding limbal epithelial stem cell biology has formed foundations for novel cell-based therapeutic strategies.

4.1. Amniotic Membrane Transplantation. Amniotic membrane transplantation (AMT) is a method to help recreate the integrity of the ocular surface. The amniotic membrane (AM) consists of an overlying basement membrane with a rich extracellular matrix, including heparin sulfate proteoglycans, laminin, and collagens. These components act as a scaffold for the epithelial cells [38, 42, 43]. The AM also contains various growth factors, protease inhibitors, and anti-inflammatory and antiangiogenic factors and thus exerts potent anti-inflammatory and antiscarring effects [44]. The AM mimics the natural stem cell niche and therefore has the potential to enhance the self-renewal of limbal epithelial stem cells [45]. For the past decade, the amniotic membrane has become an ideal substrate for various transplantation procedures on the ocular surface [46, 47].

4.2. Autologous Conjunctival Limbal Transplant. Traditional autologous limbal transplantation has a long history. In 1989, Kenyon and Tseng described a large series (26 consecutive cases) of conjunctival limbal autograft (CLAU) in patients with unilateral ocular surface diseases [48]. A six-month follow-up study showed that the CLAU resulted in the improvement in visual acuity, rapid surface healing, and stable epithelial adhesion without recurrent erosion or persistent epithelial defect, as well as a regression of corneal neovascularization. This pioneer work identified that the transplanted limbal tissue can rehabilitate the corneal surface [48]. However, traditional autologous limbal transplantation requires a large limbal epithelial biopsy from a healthy eye, which increased the potential of damaging the donor eye [49].

4.3. Allograft Limbal Stem Cell Transplant. For patients with a total bilateral LSCD, allograft limbal stem cell transplant is one of the approaches to reconstruct the ocular surface [6]. The conjunctiva and limbus, presumably including stem cells, can come from living relative (parent or sibling) or cadaveric limbal tissues. Allograft limbal stem cell transplant can provide immediate postoperative epithelialization and rapidly reconstruct the ocular surface. However, to avoid rejection of the allograft, systemic immunosuppression is required. Adverse effects related to long-term immunosuppression are common, including anemia, hyperglycemia, elevated creatinine, and elevated levels of liver function markers [50, 51]. Interestingly, a long-term study showed that eventually, only recipient DNAs were detectable in the regenerated epithelium of the majority of the successful cases. This suggests that the allografted limbal epithelium promotes regeneration of the corneal epithelium in patients with LSCD, at least in part, by activating residual stem cells and enhancing their self-renewal [52]. It is possible that allografted limbal stem cells secrete factors that are necessary for maintaining stem cell homeostasis. It is very important to elucidate what these factors are and whether direct application of such factors onto the ocular surface can restore the corneal epithelium.

4.4. Simple Limbal Epithelial Transplantation (SLET). In 2012, Sangwan et al. introduced a simple limbal epithelial transplantation (SLET) [53]. In this technique, a fresh amniotic membrane had been attached on the cornea by a fibrin glue; a small (2 × 2 mm) donor limbal graft from the unaffected eye

was harvested and divided into tiny pieces and then seeded on the AM. This technique provides a simple approach that makes the LESCs expand in vivo [54–60].

A multicenter study on 68 eyes from patients who underwent SLET for unilateral LSCD reported promising results [61]. Clinical success was achieved in 57 (84%) cases. With a median follow-up of 12 months, the survival probability exceeded 80%. Recently, long-term clinical outcomes of a large cohort of patients (125 cases) with unilateral LSCD occurring after ocular burns showed that 76% patients maintained a successful outcome. In addition to surface restoration, most patients undergoing SLET reported a significant improvement in visual acuity. Immunohistochemistry revealed successful regeneration of the normal corneal epithelium (CK3(+)/12(+)) without admixture of conjunctival cells (Muc5AC(−)/CK19 (−)) and replenishment of the limbal stem cell (ΔNp63α (+)/ABCG2(+)) reserve [62]. The SLET has a similar success rate to the traditional autologous limbal transplantation. Better yet, different from conjunctival limbal grafting, autologous SLET requires only a tiny limbal tissue from the unaffected eye carrying minimal risk to the donor eye. Additionally, in comparison with ex vivo cultivated limbal epithelial transplantation, SLET does not need clinical-grade laboratory support, which has the advantage of low cost and is easily replicable by practicing corneal surgeons [63].

5. Cell-Based Therapy

Cell therapy involves tissue engineering techniques and the idea of stem cell plasticity for achieving corneal epithelial regeneration. This approach represents new potential therapeutic modalities. The underlying principal is to use the least amount of tissue to ex vivo expand cells into an epithelial sheet on carriers and to reconstruct severely damaged ocular surfaces.

5.1. Cultivated Limbal Epithelial Transplantation (CLET). Transplantation of autologous cultures of limbal epithelial stem cells was first reported by Pellegrini et al. [64]. Two patients with unilateral LSCD at the severe chronic stage of alkali burns received CLET. Limbal epithelial cells from a 1-2 mm² limbal biopsy sample were expanded in vitro on a feeder layer consisting of nonproliferating 3T3-J2 feeder cells and a polymerized fibrin matrix. Confluent cultured limbal epithelial sheet was placed on a corneal wound bed. Two-year follow-up showed that the regenerated corneal epithelium was stable. In 2010, Pellegrini et al. reported a long-term clinical investigation of CLET with the large samples (112 LSCD patients) [65]. In this study, 76.6% eyes showed permanent restoration of a transparent, renewing the corneal epithelium. This suggests that CLET is an effective method to reconstruct the ocular surface [66, 67]. Interestingly, the failure of transplantation of the limbal epithelial cultures is significantly associated with the lack of holoclone-forming cells (stem cells) in limbal epithelial cultures. Therefore, it is of clinical significance to identify regulators that could be pharmacologically targeted to enhance the stem cell number.

5.2. New Approaches to Maximize Ex Vivo Expansion of Limbal Epithelial Cells. A major challenge for CLET-based therapies is to maintain LESC homeostasis and enhance the self-renewal of LESCs in limbal epithelial cultures during ex vivo expansion. MicroRNAs (miRNAs) are emerging as important controllers of stem cell potency, proliferation, and differentiation [68–74]. For example, miR-205 plays a potentially important role in regulating cell proliferation and survival, via targeting the PI3K/Akt pathway [75, 76]. Such a regulation could impact effective expansion of limbal epithelial cells. Another critical miRNA family is miR-103/107 that is preferentially expressed in the stem cell-enriched limbal epithelium and targets novel proteins involved in processes related to stem cell behavior [77]. miR-103/107 targets p90RSK2, a kinase that regulates G0/G1 progression, and this helps to maintain a slow-cycling phenotype [78]. miRs-103/107 also promote increased holoclone colony formation by regulating MAP3K7 signaling and JNK activation through noncanonical Wnt signaling. By targeting NEDD9 (HEF1), miR-103/107 ensures maintenance of the essential stem cell niche molecule, E-cadherin (E-cad) in limbal keratinocytes [78]. By targeting protein tyrosine phosphatase, receptor type M (PTPRM), miR-103/107 maintains low levels of Cx43, which is a feature of several stem cell-enriched epithelia [78]. Collectively, miR-103/107 plays critical roles in the regulation of stem cell proliferation and the interaction of stem cells with their surrounding cells [79]. These findings form a foundation for development of a novel approach to improve the preservation of limbal stem cells in ex vivo cultures prior to CLET. It has been demonstrated that microRNAs can be topically delivered into limbal/corneal epithelia [78]. Thus, it has a clinical potential to topically administer miR-103/107 into limbal/corneal epithelia, which may activate and preserve the remaining limbal stem cells of patients with LSCD.

It is well established that autophagy is required for stem cell homeostasis in various tissues [80]. Consistent with this idea, we have demonstrated that the autophagy activity is significantly higher in the basal layer of the limbal epithelium compared with the corneal epithelium. More interestingly, the holoclone colony-forming ability was markedly diminished in limbal epithelial cells when autophagy was blocked [81]. These new findings suggest that autophagy is a positive process for maintaining stem cells [82]. The signaling pathways that regulate autophagy specifically in the limbal basal layer need to be elucidated.

5.3. Cultivated Oral Mucosal Epithelial Transplantation (COMET). Bilateral LSCD patients who have no remaining LESCs can turn to autologous cultivated oral mucosal epithelial transplantation (COMET). It has been shown that COMET is a feasible substitute for allogenic limbal stem cell transplantation without the need for long-term systemic immunosuppression [83–89].

The cultivated oral epithelial cells formed a stratified tissue. The tissue-engineered oral epithelium expressed proliferation and progenitor markers Ki-67 and p63 in the basal layer of the cell sheets, suggesting that the epithelium had regenerative capacity [90]. The transplanted epithelium also expressed K3, K19, Ki-67, p63, p75, and the cornea-specific PAX6 and K12 [90]. This study confirms that the oral cells, transplanted to the corneal surface, can survive and stably reconstruct the ocular surface. They acquire some of the corneal epithelial-like characters at the ectopic site. However, compared with cultured limbal epithelial cells, COMET has significantly higher angiogenic potential. In addition, the underlying mechanisms involved in the transformation of the oral mucosal epithelial cells into the differentiated corneal epithelium remains unclear.

5.4. Mesenchymal Stem Cells. Mesenchymal stem cells (MSCs) are a group of fibroblast-like multipotent mesenchymal stromal cells [91]. MSC can be isolated from a wide range of tissues, including bone marrow, umbilical cord, adipose tissue [92], and corneal stroma [93]. Because of an urgent need for alternative autologous stem cell sources for bilateral LSCD, MSC has been tested in the treatment of LSCD. Holan et al. demonstrated that bone marrow MSCs (BM-MSCs) had similar therapeutic effects in the experimental LSCD model of alkali-injured rabbit eyes compared with LESCs [94]. Some studies suggested the differentiation of MSCs into corneal epithelial cells. However, the precise mechanism by which MSCs differentiate into corneal epithelial cells remains elusive. It has also been suggested that MSCs produce growth factors that can support the growth of residual corneal epithelial cells and LESCs [95]. Recent researches by Shaharuddin et al. found that cultured limbal MSCs expressed the common putative limbal stem cell markers, which demonstrated limbal-derived MSC-exhibited plasticity [96].

6. Conclusion

Basic science has contributed greatly to our understanding of the location, function, regulation of proliferation, and differentiation of limbal epithelial stem cells. Conventional autogenic and allogenic conjunctival limbal transplantation is an effective method but is limited by tissue availability. To overcome the shortage of donor-based tissues, scientists now focus their attention on cell-based therapy. With the refinement of in vitro culture and expansion techniques, and improved scaffolds and matrices, it is anticipated that a new generation of regenerative procedures will be available for use in the clinic to ultimately resolve the problem of LSCD. Finally, an emerging idea that supplies factors in vivo to activate and preserve the remaining limbal stem cells may lead to a pharmacological therapy which will ultimately replace surgery for treatment of corneal diseases with limbal stem cell deficiency.

Conflicts of Interest

The authors declare that there are no conflicts of interest regarding the publication of this paper.

Acknowledgments

This study was supported by the National Nature Science Foundation of China (nos. 31300814, 81670830, and 81770887), the National Key R&D Program of China (Project no. 2017YFA0103204), and the Technology Innovation Fund by The First Affiliated Hospital, Chinese PLA General Hospital (Project no. 2016FC-304Z-TSYS-02). This work was also supported by the National Institutes of Health grants EY06769, EY017539, and EY019463 (to R.M.L.), Dermatology Foundation Research Grant and Career Development Award (to H. P.), and a Midwest Eye Bank Research Grant (to H. P.).

References

[1] G. Cotsarelis, S. Z. Cheng, G. Dong, T. T. Sun, and R. M. Lavker, "Existence of slow-cycling limbal epithelial basal cells that can be preferentially stimulated to proliferate: implications on epithelial stem cells," *Cell*, vol. 57, no. 2, pp. 201–209, 1989.

[2] M. Davanger and A. Evensen, "Role of the pericorneal papillary structure in renewal of corneal epithelium," *Nature*, vol. 229, no. 5286, pp. 560-561, 1971.

[3] A. Schermer, S. Galvin, and T. T. Sun, "Differentiation-related expression of a major 64K corneal keratin in vivo and in culture suggests limbal location of corneal epithelial stem cells," *Journal of Cell Biology*, vol. 103, no. 1, pp. 49–62, 1986.

[4] C. G. Priya, T. Prasad, N. V. Prajna, and V. Muthukkaruppan, "Identification of human corneal epithelial stem cells on the basis of high ABCG2 expression combined with a large N/C ratio," *Microscopy Research and Technique*, vol. 76, no. 3, pp. 242–248, 2013.

[5] R. A. Thoft, L. A. Wiley, and N. Sundarraj, "The multipotential cells of the limbus," *Eye*, vol. 3, no. 2, pp. 109–113, 1989.

[6] R. J. Tsai and S. C. Tseng, "Human allograft limbal transplantation for corneal surface reconstruction," *Cornea*, vol. 13, no. 5, pp. 389–400, 1994.

[7] C. S. de Paiva, Z. Chen, R. M. Corrales, S. C. Pflugfelder, and D. Q. Li, "ABCG2 transporter identifies a population of clonogenic human limbal epithelial cells," *Stem Cells*, vol. 23, no. 1, pp. 63–73, 2005.

[8] B. R. Ksander, P. E. Kolovou, B. J. Wilson et al., "ABCB5 is a limbal stem cell gene required for corneal development and repair," *Nature*, vol. 511, no. 7509, pp. 353–357, 2014.

[9] V. Barbaro, A. Testa, E. Di Lorio, F. Mavilio, G. Pellegrini, and M. De Luca, "C/EBPdelta regulates cell cycle and self-renewal of human limbal stem cells," *Journal of Cell Biology*, vol. 177, no. 6, pp. 1037–1049, 2007.

[10] G. Pellegrini, E. Dellambra, O. Golisano et al., "p63 identifies keratinocyte stem cells," *Proceedings of the National Academy of Sciences of the United States of America*, vol. 98, no. 6, pp. 3156–3161, 2001.

[11] H. Ouyang, Y. Xue, Y. Lin et al., "WNT7A and PAX6 define corneal epithelium homeostasis and pathogenesis," *Nature*, vol. 511, no. 7509, pp. 358–361, 2014.

[12] K. Higa, N. Kato, S. Yoshida et al., "Aquaporin 1-positive stromal niche-like cells directly interact with N-cadherin-positive clusters in the basal limbal epithelium," *Stem Cell Research*, vol. 10, no. 2, pp. 147–155, 2013.

[13] K. Y. Chee, A. Kicic, and S. J. Wiffen, "Limbal stem cells: the search for a marker," *Clinical & Experimental Ophthalmology*, vol. 34, no. 1, pp. 64–73, 2006.

[14] P. B. Thomas, Y. H. Liu, F. F. Zhuang et al., "Identification of Notch-1 expression in the limbal basal epithelium," *Molecular Vision*, vol. 13, pp. 337–344, 2007.

[15] U. Schlotzer-Schrehardt and F. E. Kruse, "Identification and characterization of limbal stem cells," *Experimental Eye Research*, vol. 81, no. 3, pp. 247–264, 2005.

[16] M. Rodrigues, A. Ben-Zvi, J. Krachmer, A. Schermer, and T. T. Sun, "Suprabasal expression of a 64-kilodalton keratin (no. 3) in developing human corneal epithelium," *Differentiation*, vol. 34, no. 1, pp. 60–67, 1987.

[17] M. A. Kurpakus, M. T. Maniaci, and M. Esco, "Expression of keratins K12, K4 and K14 during development of ocular surface epithelium," *Current Eye Research*, vol. 13, no. 11, pp. 805–814, 1994.

[18] M. Boulton and J. Albon, "Stem cells in the eye," *International Journal of Biochemistry & Cell Biology*, vol. 36, no. 4, pp. 643–657, 2004.

[19] R. M. Lavker, G. Dong, S. Z. Cheng, K. Kudoh, G. Cotsarelis, and T. T. Sun, "Relative proliferative rates of limbal and corneal epithelia. Implications of corneal epithelial migration, circadian rhythm, and suprabasally located DNA-synthesizing keratinocytes," *Investigative Ophthalmology & Visual Science*, vol. 32, no. 6, pp. 1864–1875, 1991.

[20] R. M. Lavker, S. C. Tseng, and T. T. Sun, "Corneal epithelial stem cells at the limbus: looking at some old problems from a new angle," *Experimental Eye Research*, vol. 78, no. 3, pp. 433–446, 2004.

[21] Y. Barrandon and H. Green, "Three clonal types of keratinocyte with different capacities for multiplication," *Proceedings of the National Academy of Sciences of the United States of America*, vol. 84, no. 8, pp. 2302–2306, 1987.

[22] P. Eberwein and T. Reinhard, "Concise reviews: the role of biomechanics in the limbal stem cell niche: new insights for our understanding of this structure," *Stem Cells*, vol. 33, no. 3, pp. 916–924, 2015.

[23] S. C. Tseng, H. He, S. Zhang, and S. Y. Chen, "Niche regulation of limbal epithelial stem cells: relationship between inflammation and regeneration," *Ocular Surface*, vol. 14, no. 2, pp. 100–112, 2016.

[24] G. Yazdanpanah, S. Jabbehdari, and A. R. Djalilian, "Limbal and corneal epithelial homeostasis," *Current Opinion in Ophthalmology*, vol. 28, no. 4, pp. 348–354, 2017.

[25] J. Li, S. Y. Chen, X. Y. Zhao, M. C. Zhang, and H. T. Xie, "Rat limbal niche cells prevent epithelial stem/progenitor cells from differentiation and proliferation by inhibiting notch signaling pathway in vitro," *Investigative Ophthalmology & Visual Science*, vol. 58, no. 7, pp. 2968–2976, 2017.

[26] M. A. Dziasko, S. J. Tuft, and J. T. Daniels, "Limbal melanocytes support limbal epithelial stem cells in 2D and 3D microenvironments," *Experimental Eye Research*, vol. 138, pp. 70–79, 2015.

[27] H. S. Dua, V. A. Shanmuganathan, A. O. Powell-Richards, P. J. Tighe, and A. Joseph, "Limbal epithelial crypts: a novel anatomical structure and a putative limbal stem cell niche," *British Journal of Ophthalmology*, vol. 89, no. 5, pp. 529–532, 2005.

[28] A. M. Yeung, U. Schlotzer-Schrehardt, B. Kulkarni, N. L. Tint, A. Hopkinson, and H. S. Dua, "Limbal epithelial crypt: a model for corneal epithelial maintenance and novel limbal regional variations," *Archives of Ophthalmology*, vol. 126, no. 5, pp. 665–669, 2008.

[29] K. Grieve, D. Ghoubay, C. Georgeon et al., "Three-dimensional structure of the mammalian limbal stem cell niche," *Experimental Eye Research*, vol. 140, pp. 75–84, 2015.

[30] R. J. Tsai and R. Y. Tsai, "From stem cell niche environments to engineering of corneal epithelium tissue," *Japanese Journal of Ophthalmology*, vol. 58, no. 2, pp. 111–119, 2014.

[31] K. Sejpal, M. H. Ali, S. Maddileti et al., "Cultivated limbal epithelial transplantation in children with ocular surface burns," *JAMA Ophthalmology*, vol. 131, no. 6, pp. 731–736, 2013.

[32] M. Nubile, M. Lanzini, A. Miri et al., "In vivo confocal microscopy in diagnosis of limbal stem cell deficiency," *American Journal of Ophthalmology*, vol. 155, no. 2, pp. 220–232, 2013.

[33] J. Rossen, A. Amram, B. Milani et al., "Contact lens-induced limbal stem cell deficiency," *Ocular Surface*, vol. 14, no. 4, pp. 419–434, 2016.

[34] E. Chan, Q. Le, A. Codriansky, J. Hong, J. Xu, and S. X. Deng, "Existence of normal limbal epithelium in eyes with clinical signs of total limbal stem cell deficiency," *Cornea*, vol. 35, no. 11, pp. 1483–1487, 2016.

[35] K. H. Kim and S. I. Mian, "Diagnosis of corneal limbal stem cell deficiency," *Current Opinion in Ophthalmology*, vol. 28, no. 4, pp. 355–362, 2017.

[36] M. A. Lemp and W. D. Mathers, "Corneal epithelial cell movement in humans," *Eye*, vol. 3, no. 4, pp. 438–445, 1989.

[37] E. H. Chan, L. Chen, F. Yu, and S. X. Deng, "Epithelial thinning in limbal stem cell deficiency," *American Journal of Ophthalmology*, vol. 160, no. 4, pp. 669–677, 2015.

[38] S. C. Tseng, P. Prabhasawat, K. Barton, T. Gray, and D. Meller, "Amniotic membrane transplantation with or without limbal allografts for corneal surface reconstruction in patients with limbal stem cell deficiency," *Archives of Ophthalmology*, vol. 116, no. 4, pp. 431–441, 1998.

[39] T. P. Barreiro, M. S. Santos, A. C. Vieira, J. de Nadai Barros, R. M. Hazarbassanov, and J. A. Gomes, "Comparative study of conjunctival limbal transplantation not associated with the use of amniotic membrane transplantation for treatment of total limbal deficiency secondary to chemical injury," *Cornea*, vol. 33, no. 7, pp. 716–720, 2014.

[40] L. Liang, H. Sheha, J. Li, and S. C. Tseng, "Limbal stem cell transplantation: new progresses and challenges," *Eye*, vol. 23, no. 10, pp. 1946–1953, 2009.

[41] A. Kheirkhah, D. A. Johnson, D. R. Paranjpe, V. K. Raju, V. Casas, and S. C. Tseng, "Temporary sutureless amniotic membrane patch for acute alkaline burns," *Archives of Ophthalmology*, vol. 126, no. 8, pp. 1059–1066, 2008.

[42] H. Westekemper, F. C. Figueiredo, W. F. Siah, N. Wagner, K. P. Steuhl, and D. Meller, "Clinical outcomes of amniotic membrane transplantation in the management of acute ocular chemical injury," *British Journal of Ophthalmology*, vol. 101, no. 2, pp. 103–107, 2017.

[43] V. S. Sangwan, S. Burman, S. Tejwani, S. P. Mahesh, and R. Murthy, "Amniotic membrane transplantation: a review of current indications in the management of ophthalmic disorders," *Indian Journal of Ophthalmology*, vol. 55, no. 4, pp. 251–260, 2007.

[44] S. K. Sahu, P. Govindswamy, V. S. Sangwan, and R. Thomas, "Midterm results on ocular surface reconstruction using cultivated autologous oral mucosal epithelial transplantation," *American Journal of Ophthalmology*, vol. 143, no. 1, p. 189, 2007.

[45] M. A. Meallet, E. M. Espana, M. Grueterich, S. E. Ti, E. Goto, and S. C. Tseng, "Amniotic membrane transplantation with conjunctival limbal autograft for total limbal stem cell deficiency," *Ophthalmology*, vol. 110, no. 8, pp. 1585–1592, 2003.

[46] K. Dhamodaran, M. Subramani, H. Matalia, C. Jayadev, R. Shetty, and D. Das, "One for all: a standardized protocol for ex vivo culture of limbal, conjunctival and oral mucosal epithelial cells into corneal lineage," *Cytotherapy*, vol. 18, no. 4, pp. 546–561, 2016.

[47] Y. Feng, M. Borrelli, S. Reichl, S. Schrader, and G. Geerling, "Review of alternative carrier materials for ocular surface reconstruction," *Current Eye Research*, vol. 39, no. 6, pp. 541–552, 2014.

[48] K. R. Kenyon and S. C. Tseng, "Limbal autograft transplantation for ocular surface disorders," *Ophthalmology*, vol. 96, no. 5, pp. 709–722, 1989.

[49] J. Frucht-Pery, C. S. Siganos, A. Solomon, L. Scheman, C. Brautbar, and H. Zauberman, "Limbal cell autograft transplantation for severe ocular surface disorders," *Graefe's Archive for Clinical and Experimental Ophthalmolog*, vol. 236, no. 8, pp. 582–587, 1998.

[50] M. Krakauer, J. D. Welder, H. K. Pandya, N. Nassiri, and A. R. Djalilian, "Adverse effects of systemic immunosuppression in keratolimbal allograft," *Journal of Ophthalmology*, vol. 2012, Article ID 576712, 5 pages, 2012.

[51] E. J. Holland, G. Mogilishetty, H. M. Skeens et al., "Systemic immunosuppression in ocular surface stem cell transplantation: results of a 10-year experience," *Cornea*, vol. 31, no. 6, pp. 655–661, 2012.

[52] S. M. Daya, A. Watson, J. R. Sharpe et al., "Outcomes and DNA analysis of ex vivo expanded stem cell allograft for ocular surface reconstruction," *Ophthalmology*, vol. 112, no. 3, pp. 470–477, 2005.

[53] V. S. Sangwan, S. Basu, S. MacNeil, and D. Balasubramanian, "Simple limbal epithelial transplantation (SLET): a novel surgical technique for the treatment of unilateral limbal stem cell deficiency," *British Journal of Ophthalmology*, vol. 96, no. 7, pp. 931–934, 2012.

[54] G. Amescua, M. Atallah, N. Nikpoor, A. Galor, and V. L. Perez, "Modified simple limbal epithelial transplantation using cryopreserved amniotic membrane for unilateral limbal stem cell deficiency," *American Journal of Ophthalmology*, vol. 158, no. 3, pp. 469.e2–475.e2, 2014.

[55] S. K. Arya, A. Bhatti, A. Raj, and R. K. Bamotra, "Simple limbal epithelial transplantation in acid injury and severe dry eye," *Journal of Clinical and Diagnostic Research*, vol. 10, no. 6, p. ND06-07, 2016.

[56] S. Bhalekar, S. Basu, I. Lal, and V. S. Sangwan, "Successful autologous simple limbal epithelial transplantation (SLET) in previously failed paediatric limbal transplantation for ocular surface burns," *BMJ Case Reports*, vol. 2013, pii: bcr2013009888, 2013.

[57] E. Hernandez-Bogantes, G. Amescua, A. Navas et al., "Minor ipsilateral simple limbal epithelial transplantation (mini-SLET) for pterygium treatment," *British Journal of Ophthalmology*, vol. 99, no. 12, pp. 1598–1600, 2015.

[58] V. Mittal, R. Jain, R. Mittal, U. Vashist, and P. Narang, "Successful management of severe unilateral chemical burns in children using simple limbal epithelial transplantation (SLET)," *British Journal of Ophthalmology*, vol. 100, no. 8, pp. 1102–1108, 2016.

[59] J. Vazirani, M. H. Ali, N. Sharma et al., "Autologous simple limbal epithelial transplantation for unilateral limbal stem cell deficiency: multicentre results," *British Journal of Ophthalmology*, vol. 100, no. 10, pp. 1416–1420, 2016.

[60] J. Vazirani, S. Basu, H. Kenia et al., "Unilateral partial limbal stem cell deficiency: contralateral versus ipsilateral autologous cultivated limbal epithelial transplantation," *American Journal of Ophthalmology*, vol. 157, no. 3, pp. 584.e2–590.e2, 2014.

[61] S. Basu, H. Ali, and V. S. Sangwan, "Clinical outcomes of repeat autologous cultivated limbal epithelial transplantation for ocular surface burns," *American Journal of Ophthalmology*, vol. 153, no. 4, pp. 643–650, 2012.

[62] S. Basu, S. P. Sureka, S. S. Shanbhag, A. R. Kethiri, V. Singh, and V. S. Sangwan, "Simple limbal epithelial transplantation: long-term clinical outcomes in 125 cases of unilateral chronic ocular surface burns," *Ophthalmology*, vol. 123, no. 5, pp. 1000–1010, 2016.

[63] N. Gupta, J. Joshi, J. H. Farooqui, and U. Mathur, "Results of simple limbal epithelial transplantation in unilateral ocular

surface burn," *Indian Journal of Ophthalmology*, vol. 66, no. 1, pp. 45–52, 2018.

[64] G. Pellegrini, C. E. Traverso, A. T. Franzi, M. Zingirian, R. Cancedda, and M. De Luca, "Long-term restoration of damaged corneal surfaces with autologous cultivated corneal epithelium," *The Lancet*, vol. 349, no. 9057, pp. 990–993, 1997.

[65] P. Rama, S. Matuska, G. Paganoni, A. Spinelli, M. De Luca, and G. Pellegrini, "Limbal stem-cell therapy and long-term corneal regeneration," *New England journal of medicine*, vol. 363, no. 2, pp. 147–155, 2010.

[66] J. Cheng, H. Zhai, J. Wang, H. Duan, and Q. Zhou, "Long-term outcome of allogeneic cultivated limbal epithelial transplantation for symblepharon caused by severe ocular burns," *BMC Ophthalmology*, vol. 17, no. 1, p. 8, 2017.

[67] M. Kawashima, T. Kawakita, Y. Satake, K. Higa, and J. Shimazaki, "Phenotypic study after cultivated limbal epithelial transplantation for limbal stem cell deficiency," *Archives of Ophthalmology*, vol. 125, no. 10, pp. 1337–1344, 2007.

[68] V. K. Gangaraju and H. Lin, "MicroRNAs: key regulators of stem cells," *Nature Reviews Molecular Cell Biology*, vol. 10, no. 2, pp. 116–125, 2009.

[69] G. Tiscornia and G. C. Izpisua Belmonte, "MicroRNAs in embryonic stem cell function and fate," *Genes & Development*, vol. 24, no. 24, pp. 2732–2741, 2010.

[70] R. Yi, M. N. Poy, M. Stoffel, and E. Fuchs, "A skin microRNA promotes differentiation by repressing "stemness"," *Nature*, vol. 452, no. 7184, pp. 225–229, 2008.

[71] Z. Liu, W. Zhan, M. Zeng, J. Chen, H. Zou, and Z. Min, "Enhanced functional properties of human limbal stem cells by inhibition of the miR-31/FIH-1/P21 axis," *Acta Ophthalmologica*, vol. 95, no. 6, pp. e495–e502, 2017.

[72] H. Peng, R. B. Hamanaka, J. Katsnelson et al., "MicroRNA-31 targets FIH-1 to positively regulate corneal epithelial glycogen metabolism," *FASEB Journal*, vol. 26, no. 8, pp. 3140–3147, 2012.

[73] H. Peng, N. Kaplan, R. B. Hamanaka et al., "microRNA-31/factor-inhibiting hypoxia-inducible factor 1 nexus regulates keratinocyte differentiation," *Proceedings of the National Academy of Sciences of the United States of America*, vol. 109, no. 35, pp. 14030–14034, 2012.

[74] H. Peng, N. Kaplan, W. Yang, S. Getsios, and R. M. Lavker, "FIH-1 disrupts an LRRK1/EGFR complex to positively regulate keratinocyte migration," *American Journal of Pathology*, vol. 184, no. 12, pp. 3262–3271, 2014.

[75] R. M. Lavker, Y. Jia, and D. G. Ryan, "The tiny world of microRNAs in the cross hairs of the mammalian eye," *Human Genomics*, vol. 3, no. 4, pp. 332–348, 2009.

[76] D. Lin, A. Halilovic, P. Yue et al., "Inhibition of miR-205 impairs the wound-healing process in human corneal epithelial cells by targeting KIR4.1 (KCNJ10)," *Investigative Ophthalmology & Visual Science*, vol. 54, no. 9, pp. 6167–6178, 2013.

[77] C. C. Hsu, C. H. Peng, K. H. Hung et al., "Stem cell therapy for corneal regeneration medicine and contemporary nanomedicine for corneal disorders," *Cell Transplantation*, vol. 24, no. 10, pp. 1915–1930, 2015.

[78] H. Peng, J. K. Park, J. Katsnelson et al., "microRNA-103/107 family regulates multiple epithelial stem cell characteristics," *Stem Cells*, vol. 33, no. 5, pp. 1642–1656, 2015.

[79] J. K. Park, W. Yang, J. Katsnelson, R. M. Lavker, and H. Peng, "MicroRNAs enhance keratinocyte proliferative capacity in a stem cell-enriched epithelium," *PLoS One*, vol. 10, no. 8, article e0134853, 2015.

[80] D. J. Klionsky, K. Abdelmohsen, A. Abe et al., "Guidelines for the use and interpretation of assays for monitoring autophagy (3rd edition)," *Autophagy*, vol. 12, no. 1, pp. 1–222, 2016.

[81] H. Peng, J. K. Park, and R. M. Lavker, "Eyeing autophagy and macropinocytosis in the corneal/limbal epithelia," *Autophagy*, vol. 13, no. 5, pp. 975–977, 2017.

[82] H. Peng, J. K. Park, and R. M. Lavker, "Autophagy and macropinocytosis: keeping an eye on the corneal/limbal epithelia," *Investigative Ophthalmology & Visual Science*, vol. 58, no. 1, pp. 416–423, 2017.

[83] M. Eslani, A. Baradaran-Rafii, and S. Ahmad, "Cultivated limbal and oral mucosal epithelial transplantation," *Seminars in Ophthalmology*, vol. 27, no. 3-4, pp. 80–93, 2012.

[84] T. Nakamura, T. Inatomi, C. Sotozono, T. Amemiya, N. Kanamura, and S. Kinoshita, "Transplantation of cultivated autologous oral mucosal epithelial cells in patients with severe ocular surface disorders," *British Journal of Ophthalmology*, vol. 88, no. 10, pp. 1280–1284, 2004.

[85] T. Nakamura and S. Kinoshita, "New hopes and strategies for the treatment of severe ocular surface disease," *Current Opinion in Ophthalmology*, vol. 22, no. 4, pp. 274–278, 2011.

[86] P. Prabhasawat, P. Ekpo, M. Uiprasertkul et al., "Long-term result of autologous cultivated oral mucosal epithelial transplantation for severe ocular surface disease," *Cell and Tissue Banking*, vol. 17, no. 3, pp. 491–503, 2016.

[87] C. Sotozono, T. Inatomi, T. Nakamura et al., "Cultivated oral mucosal epithelial transplantation for persistent epithelial defect in severe ocular surface diseases with acute inflammatory activity," *Acta Ophthalmologica*, vol. 92, no. 6, pp. e447–e453, 2014.

[88] C. Sotozono, T. Inatomi, T. Nakamura et al., "Visual improvement after cultivated oral mucosal epithelial transplantation," *Ophthalmology*, vol. 120, no. 1, pp. 193–200, 2013.

[89] T. Nakamura, K. Takeda, T. Inatomi, C. Sotozono, and S. Kinoshita, "Long-term results of autologous cultivated oral mucosal epithelial transplantation in the scar phase of severe ocular surface disorders," *British Journal of Ophthalmology*, vol. 95, no. 7, pp. 942–946, 2011.

[90] S. Gaddipati, R. Muralidhar, V. S. Sangwan, I. Mariappan, G. K. Vemuganti, and D. Balasubramanian, "Oral epithelial cells transplanted on to corneal surface tend to adapt to the ocular phenotype," *Indian Journal of Ophthalmology*, vol. 62, no. 5, pp. 644–648, 2014.

[91] N. K. Satija, G. U. Gurudutta, S. Sharma et al., "Mesenchymal stem cells: molecular targets for tissue engineering," *Stem Cells and Development*, vol. 16, no. 1, pp. 7–23, 2007.

[92] A. C. Zannettino, S. Paton, A. Arthur et al., "Multipotential human adipose-derived stromal stem cells exhibit a perivascular phenotype in vitro and in vivo," *Journal of Cellular Physiology*, vol. 214, no. 2, pp. 413–421, 2008.

[93] J. L. Funderburgh, M. L. Funderburgh, and Y. Du, "Stem cells in the limbal stroma," *Ocular Surface*, vol. 14, no. 2, pp. 113–120, 2016.

[94] V. Holan, P. Trosan, C. Cejka et al., "A comparative study of the therapeutic potential of mesenchymal stem cells and limbal epithelial stem cells for ocular surface reconstruction," *Stem Cells Translational Medicine*, vol. 4, no. 9, pp. 1052–1063, 2015.

[95] D. Almaliotis, G. Koliakos, E. Papakonstantinou et al., "Mesenchymal stem cells improve healing of the cornea after alkali injury," *Graefe's Archive for Clinical and Experimental Ophthalmolog*, vol. 253, no. 7, pp. 1121–1135, 2015.

[96] B. Shaharuddin, C. Osei-Bempong, S. Ahmad et al., "Human limbal mesenchymal stem cells express ABCB5 and can grow on amniotic membrane," *Regenerative medicine*, vol. 11, no. 3, pp. 273–286, 2016.

19

Prevalence of Myopia among Children Attending Pediatrics Ophthalmology Clinic at Ohud Hospital, Medina, Saudi Arabia

Aisha Mohammed Alemam ⓘ,[1] **Mohammed Hamad Aldebasi** ⓘ,[2] **Abdulkarem Rehmatullah,**[3] **Rami Alsaidi,**[4] **and Ishraq Tashkandi**[5]

[1]*College of Medicine, Taiba University, Medina, Saudi Arabia*
[2]*College of Medicine, Al Imam Mohammad Ibn Saud Islamic University (IMSIU), Riyadh, Saudi Arabia*
[3]*MCPS, FICO(Lond), FRCSG, Paediatric Ophthalmologist, Ohud Hospital, Medina, Saudi Arabia*
[4]*Msc, Ohud Hospital Medina, Saudi Arabia*
[5]*MD, FRCSEdn, Consultant Pediatric Ophthalmologist, RTPD Ophthalmology Program, Ohud Hospital, Madina, Saudi Arabia*

Correspondence should be addressed to Aisha Mohammed Alemam; aisha.alemam@gmail.com

Academic Editor: Toshihide Kurihara

Introduction. Around half of the visually impaired population has uncorrected refractive errors (URE), and myopia constitutes a high proportion of them. URE should be screened and treated early to prevent long-term complications. The aim of this study was to determine the prevalence of myopia among all patients attending a pediatric outpatient clinic at Ohud Hospital in Medina, Saudi Arabia (KSA). *Method.* This study was conducted using a convenience sample of all patients attending the clinic (1500 patients) aged between 3 and 14 years, and they were enrolled in the study during the period from May 2017 until September 2017. *Result.* Of 1215 subjects, only 43 (3.54%) were diagnosed with myopia. Out of the study participants, 56.8% were female and the mean age was 9.7 ± 3.6. Myopia was more prevalent in male participants than female participants ($n = 525$, 4%, $n = 690$, 3.1%, $p = 0.5$). Low myopia was the most common form among the screened individuals. The level of myopia was associated with the degree of the strabismus angle. Approximately 22% of patients with myopia had >25° strabismus angle. There was a statistically significant association with both near work indoor and outdoor activities on weekends and the level of myopia. *Conclusion.* The prevalence of myopia among pediatrics patients in Medina is 3.54%. We hope that the results of this study will contribute to a better understanding of this public health issue in Saudi Arabia in order to implant a strict screening program for early detection and interventions to reduce the risk of further progression of visual impairment.

1. Introduction

Refractive errors (RE) are common health issue worldwide affecting a large proportion of the population, regardless of the sex, age, or race [1]. Fortunately, it can be easily measured, diagnosed, and managed either by spectacles or other refractive correction methods. If the RE is corrected inadequately or did not get treated at all, it may become a major cause of impaired vision or even blindness [2]. Uncorrected refractive errors (URE) represent almost half of the visually impaired population worldwide. Of those errors, myopia is the most commonly occurring [3]. Uncorrected

vision should be screened early and treated immediately to minimize long-term complications on both children and adults. These long-term complications might include diminished quality of life and learning obstacles that might affect the educational level and the economic attainment.

Early diagnosis and treatment of RE are one of the easiest ways to reduce impaired vision or even blindness [4]. The World Health Organization (WHO) recently has issued a strategy to eliminate the avoidable visual disability and blindness which includes the correction of refractive errors [5].

The prevalence of myopia is attracting researchers around the world recently as many recent studies have reported dramatic increases over the last two decades. Worldwide, the prevalence of myopia reveals that more than 22% of the current total world population or 1.5 billion individuals are myopic [6]. Onset of the myopia commonly starts from the primary schoolchildren aged between 8 and 12 years [7]. It is typically progressing until the age of twenty due to the continuation of the eye growth.

The estimation of the prevalence of myopia is important for both health-care professionals and policy makers. This reflects the importance of the early screening and prompt management in order to avoid further visual impairment. Unfortunately, this public health issue has not been well defined in Saudi Arabia.

During the early childhood, the eye grows in a way that reserve the balance of the change in the corneal power, lens power, anterior chamber depth (ACD), and the axial length (AL) which keeps the refractive state towards emmetropia [8, 9]. Several earlier studies have shown that the ocular axial length (AL) increases parallel to the overall growth and development of the child [10, 11]. The AL and its interaction with the corneal radius of curvature play a key role in the emmetropization of the vision, and it has been found to be one of the major variables used to assess the refractive status of the eye [12, 13].

The purpose of this clinic-based study is to determine the prevalence of myopia among all patients attending the pediatrics outpatient clinic at Ohud hospital, Medina, Saudi Arabia, to contribute in providing a strong background to regulate the clinic for prevention of progression of the condition and raise awareness about early detection of myopia and guide the intervention in Medina.

2. Methodology

2.1. Study Design, Setting, and Sampling. This is a cross-sectional clinic-based study to estimate the prevalence of myopia in the pediatrics ophthalmology clinic in Ohud Hospital, Medina, Saudi Arabia, from May 2017 until September 2017. All patients who have attended the clinic (1500 patients) aged between 3 and 14 years were enrolled in the study. After initial examination, children (82 patients) presented with organic defects in the eye such as corneal opacity, lens opacity, and choroid and retinal disorders were excluded. A total number of 1215 of subjects between the ages of 3 and 14 years undergoes further examination.

2.2. Study Tool. Patients' demographics and full medical history were documented. Every child underwent a complete initial ophthalmic examination by a qualified optometrist, including slit lamp examinations and ophthalmoscopes (Figure 1).

Subsequently, children were allocated into three groups according to their ages (less than 4 years, 5-6 years, and 7–14 years). For those who were 4 years old or younger, a cycloplegic refraction was performed by instilling 2 drops of 1% cyclopentolate with 10 minutes apart for each eye separately followed by a retinoscopy. For those who were 5-6 years old, a cycloplegic refraction was performed followed by

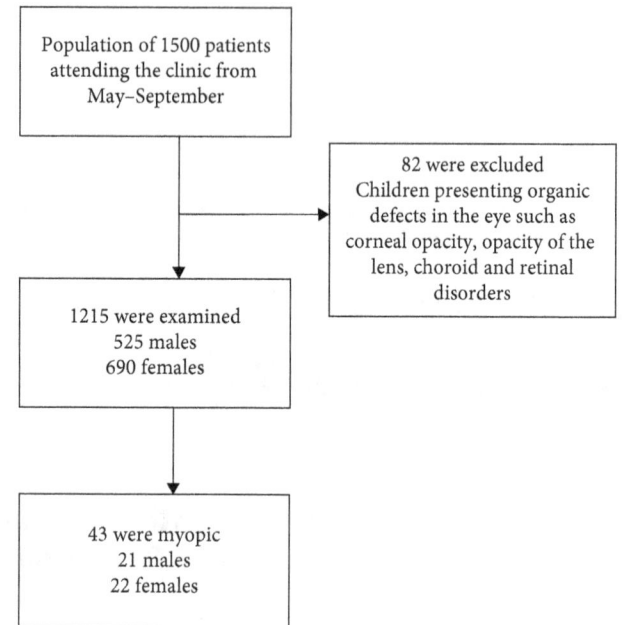

FIGURE 1: Flow diagram of the study population.

a subjective refraction after three days. Cyclopentolate drops were used to dilate the pupil of the eye and relaxing the ciliary muscles and the refractive status was measured after 1 hour by a retinoscope and after 3 days when the mydriasis effect released, we perform the subjective refraction based on retinoscopy results. The Allen's chart picture was used to assess the visual acuity.

The older age group underwent visual acuity testing using a Snellen eye chart for each eye separately, according to the standard protocol, and underwent subjective refraction testing for each individual eye. The binocular balance test was used to determine the subjective refraction endpoint. The IOLMaster 700 was used to measure the axial length for both eyes for each myopic subject.

In this study, we have classified the patients according to the refractive errors by the spherical equivalent (SE): myopia was defined as an SE of −0.5 diopters (D) or less and hyperopia as an SE of 0.5 D or more. Further classifications included low, moderate, and high myopia as an SE of −0.5 to −3.0 D, −3.1 to −6.0 D, and less than −6.0 D, respectively. Ocular deviation was assessed using the cover-uncover test, with the correction, if any, both at 3 m and at 40 cm. The participants were asked to look straight ahead at a fixed target at near (40 cm) and distance (3.0 m) letter at 3 m. The test started with occluding the left eye for 3 seconds. The observer looked for any correcting movement of the uncovered eye. After testing the right eye, the left eye was tested in a similar manner. If there was no manifest misalignment of either eye, the cover was moved back and forth between both eyes, with 1-2 seconds between movements. Ocular alignment was assessed using the cover and uncover test. Cover testing was performed using fixation targets at near (0.5 m) and distance (4.0 m). The degree of tropia was measured using the Hirschberg corneal light reflex.

2.3. Statistical Analysis. Data were analyzed using Statistical Package for the Social Sciences (SPSS) software. The analysis compared the means and standard deviation for the continuous variables and proportions for the categorical variables. The chi-squared test was used to examine the differences among categorical variables, and the student t-test was used for continuous variables. The prevalence was calculated in percentage along with 95% confidence interval. A P value of 0.05 or lower was considered as a cutoff point for statistical significance.

2.4. Ethical Consideration. Official approval was obtained from the research regulatory authority at the hospital prior to the data collection. The parents or guardians provided a written informed consent assent prior to the study and were asked to fill the questionnaire about the eye health of their children.

3. Results

Among the 1215 included subjects, only 43 (3.54%) were having myopia. Of the study participants, 56.8% were female, and the mean age for them was 9.7 ± 3.6. The majority were Saudis and living in Madinah (95%) and (90%), respectively. Around 90% of the participants were eyeglass wearers, and 90% of them had been wearing them for more than one year (Table 1).

Table 2 shows the association between the eye position and the strabismus angle with the degree of myopia. More than half of the myopic patients have had normal eye position (62.8%). Low myopia was the most common form among the screened individuals. The level of myopia was associated with the degree of the strabismus angle ($P < 0.002$). Approximately, the overall proportion of patients with myopia having $>25°$ strabismus angle was 25%.

Table 3 illustrates the amount of time spent doing indoor and outdoor activities and its association with the presence of myopia. There was a statistically significant association with near work-indoor and outdoor activities on the weekdays ($P < 0.001^*$) and ($P < 0.0125^*$), respectively. However, in the weekend, there was no association between either the near-indoor or outdoor activities and myopia.

Table 4 shows the relationship between the presence of myopia and other variables of interest. The visual acuity was associated with the level of myopia ($P < 0.003$). The level of myopia was associated with the axial length as well ($P < 0.001$). However, there was no relation between the level of myopia and the anterior chamber depth.

We found that 27.9% of the patients have paternal myopia ($P = 0.534$) and 32.6% of the patients have maternal myopia ($P = 0.564$).

Table 5 illustrates the amount of time that study participants spent doing outdoor activities on the weekdays and weekends and its association with the axial length and anterior chamber depth. There was a statistically significant association in both weekdays and weekend outdoor activities with the axial length and anterior chamber depth ($P = 0.010^*$) and ($P < 0.018^*$), respectively, for weekdays

and ($P = 0.046^*$) and ($P < 0.035^*$), respectively, for weekends.

4. Discussion

This is a clinic-based cross-sectional study of patients attending a pediatric ophthalmology clinic at Ohud Hospital in Medina, Saudi Arabia, between 3 and 14 years of age.

In this study, the prevalence of myopia was 3.5% out of 1215 respondents. It was more prevalent in males than in females (4% and 3.1%, respectively), which differs from other studies. A study conducted in 1995 of schoolchildren in Taiwan reported a lower prevalence and lesser degree of myopia among boys [14]. Other researchers in Finland reported a lower prevalence in boys compared to girls [15], and the possible explanation might be that girls at the primary school level tend to read and write more than boys. The subsequent increase in near-indoor work predisposes them to develop myopia. Further studies are needed to clarify such propositions.

Taking into consideration the difference in the definition of myopia, the prevalence of myopia found in this study is slightly similar to other studies conducted in different regions of Saudi Arabia. The prevalence was previously reported to be 5.8% in Qassim [16] and 2.5% in Riyadh [17].

In comparison with other countries, the prevalence of myopia in our study population is considered to be comparable to the prevalence in Australia 2% [18], Iran 4.3% [19], Ethiopia 2.6% [20], Macedonia 1.6% [21], and Nigeria 2.7% [22]. However, it was significantly lower than the prevalence in north India 79.5% [23], US 41.9% [24], and South Korea 47% [25]. The difference was slightly lower than the prevalence in Morocco 6.1% [26] and China 8% [27], as shown in Table 6.

The differences can be partially attributed to the differences in the study setting. It might also be attributed to the genetic susceptibility to myopia that varies across different races and cultural settings.

Previous studies [28–31] showed an increase in the prevalence of myopia parallel to the increase of age. In our study, the prevalence of myopia was not significantly higher in the range between 11 and 14 years than other younger age groups ($n = 31.3$, 4.7%, $P = 0.3$).

In regard to physical activities, indoor activities, such as watching TV, reading, playing video games, and doing homework, have been proposed to be in charge of the remarkable increment in the prevalence of myopia [32]. A study conducted in Australia among school children demonstrated that myopic children performed significantly more near work [33]. Our study demonstrated a statistically significant association with outdoor activities and axial length and anterior chamber depth in both weekdays and weekends ($P = 0.010^*$) and ($P < 0.018^*$), respectively, for the weekdays and ($P = 0.046^*$) and ($P < 0.035^*$), respectively, for the weekends, which contradict the result of other studies [18, 34, 35].

However, the association between outdoor activities and prevention of the onset and the progression of myopia is still not fully clear [36]. Several studies have recently suggested

TABLE 1: Demographic characteristics of the children included in the screening.

Variables		N (%)	No. of myopic patients	Prevalence of myopia	Chi-square	
					X^2	P value
Sex	Male	525 (43.2)	21	4.00		
	Female	690 (56.8)	22	3.19	0.331	0.565
Age	3–6	327 (26.9)	9	2.75		
	7–10	507 (41.7)	16	3.16	2.205	0.332
	11–14	381 (31.3)	18	4.72		
	Total	1215 (100%)	43			

TABLE 2: The association between severity of myopia with eye position and strabismus angle.

Variables			Myopia			Total	Chi-square	
			Low	Moderate	High		X^2	P value
Eye position	Normal	N	21	13	20	54		
		%	63.6	54.2	69.0	62.8		
	Exophoria	N	9	8	3	20		
		%	27.3	33.3	10.3	23.3	8.912	0.179
	Exotropia	N	3	3	4	10		
		%	9.1%	12.5%	13.8%	11.6%		
	Esotropia	N	0	0	2	2		
		%	0.0	0.0	6.9	2.3		
Strabismus angle	5°	N	8	2	0	10		
		%	66.7	18.2	0.0	31.3		
	10°	N	1	3	0	4		
		%	8.3	27.3	0.0	12.5		
	15°	N	0	1	5	6	24.999	0.002*
		%	0.0	9.1	55.6	18.8		
	20°	N	1	1	2	4		
		%	8.3	9.1	22.2	12.5		
	>25°	N	2	4	2	8		
		%	16.7	36.4	22.2	25.0		

*Significant at P value less than 0.05.

TABLE 3: Near work-indoor and outdoor activities and its association with the presence of myopia.

Variables	On school weekdays		On weekends	
	N	%	N	%
Near work-indoor activities (reading, watching TV, playing video games, and/or writing homework)				
<1 hour	11	25.6	6	13.9
1-2 hours	14	32.6	8	18.6
≥3 hours	18	41.9	29	67.4
P value	0.42		<0.001*	
Outdoor activities (football, running, and/or swimming)				
Not at all	14	32.5	12	27.9
<1 hour	11	25.6	7	16.3
1-2 hours	10	23.3	5	11.6
≥3 hours	8	18.6	19	44.2
P value	0.62		0.0125*	

that greater time spent in outdoor activities might be associated with the reduction in myopia prevalence [18, 37]. While the exact mechanism of this association is not well recognized, some theories have been proposed, as "light-dopamine theory," which stated that the exposure to the sunlight during outdoor activities stimulate the release of dopamine neurotransmitter from the retina which has been suggested to have the ability to inhibit elongation of the axial length of the eye [18, 34, 35]. Some studies showed that exposure to high light intensities can retard myopia in animals as chicks [38, 39] and monkeys [40]. Studies showed that the exposure to a light level of 15,000 lux for 5 hours per day produced significantly lower myopia and shorter axial length, whilst exposure to 500 lux did not retard eye growth and myopia in chicks [39]. The degree of protection was directly proportional to the increasing light levels [38]. The protective effect was more evident when exposed to a light intensity of about 10,000 lux, and this was significantly associated with higher vitreous dopamine concentration and lesser myopia development in chicks [41]. Moreover, the

TABLE 4: The relation between myopia and other variables of interest.

Variables	Low Mean ± SD	Moderate Mean ± SD	High Mean ± SD	P value
Age	9.5 ± 3.5	9.5 ± 3.3	10.1 ± 4.0	0.7
Visual acuity in logMAR	.25 ± 0.25	.49 ± 0.3	0.46 ± 0.3	0.003*
Axial length in mm	24.3 ± 2.2	24.3 ± 1.5	26.2 ± 1.7	0.000*
Anterior chamber depth in mm	3.48 ± 0.3	3.5 ± 0.4	3.5 ± 0.3	0.9

*Significant at P value less than 0.05.

TABLE 5: Outdoor activities and its association with the axial length and anterior chamber depth in weekdays and weekends.

	Not at all Mean	SD	<1 hour Mean	SD	1-2 hours Mean	SD	≥3 hours Mean	SD	P value
Outdoor activities (football, running, and swimming) on school weekdays									
Axial length	24.3	1.2	24.6	2.2	25.4	2.6	26.3	1.6	0.01*
Anterior chamber depth	3.4	0.3	3.4	0.4	3.6	0.2	3.6	0.2	0.01*
Outdoor activities (football, running, and swimming) on weekends									
Axial length	24.4	1.3	24.5	2.5	26.3	3.1	25.2	1.8	0.046*
Anterior chamber depth	3.4	0.3	3.4	0.5	3.5	0.2	3.6	0.2	0.035*

TABLE 6: Prevalence of myopia in different regions worldwide.

Country	Sample size	Studied age group (years)	Prevalence of myopia (%)
Saudi Arabia-Qassim (Aldebasi Yousef H)	5176	6–13	5.8%
Saudi Arabia-Riyadh (Al-Rowaily Mohammad A)	1319	4–8	2.5%
Nigeria-Aba (Atowa UC et al.)	1197	8–15	2.7%
Macedonia-Tetovo (Mahmudi E. et al.)	119	3–9	1.6%
Ethiopia-Addis Ababa (Jafer K et al.)	570	7–15	2.6%
Morocco (Anera et al.)	545	6–16	6.1%
Iran-Shiraz (Yekta et al.)	2130	5–15	4.3%
India-North India (Saxena Rohit et al.)	9884	5–15	79.5%
China-Guangzhou (He M et al.)	**5053**	**5–15**	**8%**
Australia-Sydney (Rose KA et al.)	**1735**	**6–12**	**2%**
US-California (Theophanous et al.)	60,789	**5–19**	**41.9%**
South Korea (Jang JU et al.)	1079	**8–13**	**47%**

sunlight in the outdoor area would lead to pupil constriction resulting in the increased depth of focus and decrease image blur [41, 42].

A previous study showed that myopia appeared to be more frequently seen in children with myopic parents [43]. In this study, the parental myopia was assessed to test the hypothesis of inherited susceptibility to develop myopia, and no significant evidence was found to prove this hypothesis. We found the axial length to be associated with the degree of myopia ($P < 0.0001$); however, there was no relation between the level of myopia and the anterior chamber depth. Previous studies found that eyes with higher myopia tend to have a deeper anterior chamber [44, 45]. Other studies found that individuals with hyperopia tend to have a shorter AL and myopia tend to have a longer AL [46]. Zadnik et al. found that hyperopic eyes (22.62 + 0.76 mm) have significantly ($P < .001$) shorter axial length than myopic eyes 25.16 + 1.23 mm [47]. Numerous studies [48, 49] showed a significant association between myopia and exotropia; however, our result showed no major association between them. Most of the patients were having normal eye position 62.8%

($P = 0.179$). Although low myopia was the most common form among the screened individuals, the level of myopia was associated with the degree of the strabismus angle ($P < 0.002$). The exact mechanism of the association between myopia and exotropia is not fully understood. Further studies are needed to prove this association and to clarify the link between them.

4.1. Limitation and Recommendation. Our study had some limitations. First, it was a clinic-based study; therefore, not all children in Medina city were included in the sample. We cannot generalize the results on the population of Medina. Second, the study was performed only within five months' duration, a longer duration would provide better knowledge on the prevalence of myopia, and we would have been able to follow the patient in order to study the impact of the growth of the eyeball and the progression of myopia.

Professional-based screening programs are recommended to address the issue of uncorrected refractive error in children in order to provide an early detection and to begin prompt treatment.

5. Conclusion

The prevalence of myopia among pediatrics patients in Medina is 3.5%. We believe that estimating the prevalence of myopia is important because it opens a new ground for policy making, program planning, and the establishment of health promotion interventions regarding ocular-related complications. We hope that the results of this study will contribute to a better understanding of this public health issue in KSA and help to highlight the need for screening, early detection, and subsequent interventions to reduce the risk of further progression of visual impairment.

Disclosure

These authors contributed equally to this work.

Conflicts of Interest

All of the authors declared no potential conflicts of interest with respect to the research, authorship, and/or publication of this article.

Acknowledgments

The authors gratefully acknowledge Tahani Muhil Alharbi, Razan Abdulraheem Almuzaini, Aseel Khalaf Alharbi, and Raha Abduljalil Alahmdi for collecting the data of this research. We extend our gratitude to the patients who volunteered and participated in this study.

References

[1] D. Pascolini and S. P. Mariotti, "Global estimates of visual impairment: 2010," British Journal of Ophthalmology, vol. 96, no. 5, pp. 614–618, 2012.

[2] S. Resnikoff, D. Pascolini, S. P. Mariotti, and G. P. Pokharel, "Global magnitude of visual impairment caused by uncorrected refractive errors in 2004," Bulletin of the World Health Organization, vol. 86, no. 1, pp. 63–70, 2008.

[3] E. H. Myrowitz, "Juvenile myopia progression, risk factors and interventions," Saudi Journal of Ophthalmology, vol. 26, no. 3, pp. 293–297, 2012.

[4] R. Baltussen, J. Naus, and H. Limburg, "Cost-effectiveness of screening and correcting refractive errors in school children in Africa, Asia, America and Europe," Health Policy (New York), vol. 89, no. 2, pp. 201–215, 2009.

[5] R. R. Berger, "The international agency for the prevention of blindness," American Journal of Ophthalmology, vol. 118, no. 3, pp. 406-407, 1994.

[6] B. Holden, P. Sankaridurg, E. Smith, T. Aller, M. Jong, and M. He, "Myopia, an underrated global challenge to vision: where the current data takes us on myopia control," Eye, vol. 28, no. 2, pp. 142–146, 2014.

[7] K. Rajendran, M. Haneef, K. Chandrabhanu, M. Muhammed, and R. T. Pillai, "A prevalence study on myopia among school going children in a rural area of South India," Indian Journal of Clinical Practice, vol. 25, no. 4, pp. 374–380, 2014.

[8] M. J. Hirsch and F. W. Weymouth, "Notes on ametropia—a further analysis of stenstrom's data," Optometry and Vision Science, vol. 24, no. 12, pp. 601–608, 1947.

[9] D. Troilo, "Neonatal eye growth and emmetropisation—a literature review," Eye, vol. 6, no. 2, pp. 154–160, 1992.

[10] R. A. Gordon and P. B. Donzis, "Refractive development of the human eye," Archives of Ophthalmology, vol. 103, no. 6, pp. 785–789, 1985.

[11] P. J. Foster, D. C. Broadway, S. Hayat et al., "Refractive error, axial length and anterior chamber depth of the eye in British adults: the EPIC-Norfolk Eye Study," British Journal of Ophthalmology, vol. 94, no. 7, pp. 827–830, 2010.

[12] T. Grosvenor and R. Scott, "Role of the axial length/corneal radius ratio in determining the refractive state of the eye," Optometry and Vision Science, vol. 71, no. 9, 1994.

[13] J. S. Ng, "Adler's physiology of the eye (11th ed.)," Optometry and Vision Science, vol. 89, no. 4, p. E513, 2012.

[14] L. L. K. Lin, Y. F. Shih, C. B. Tsai et al., "Epidemiologic study of ocular refraction among schoolchildren in Taiwan in 1995," Optometry and Vision Science, vol. 76, no. 5, pp. 275–281, 1999.

[15] E. Goldschmidt, "On the etiology of myopia. An epidemiological study," Acta ophthalmologica, p. 1, 1968.

[16] Y. H. Aldebasi, "Prevalence of correctable visual impairment in primary school children in Qassim Province , Saudi Arabia," Journal of Optometry, vol. 7, no. 3, pp. 168–176, 2014.

[17] M. A. Al-rowaily, "Prevalence of refractive errors among preschool children at king abdulaziz medical city , Riyadh , Saudi Arabia," Saudi Journal of Ophthalmology, vol. 24, no. 2, pp. 45–48, 2010.

[18] K. A. Rose, I. G. Morgan, J. Ip et al., "Outdoor activity reduces the prevalence of myopia in children," Ophthalmology, vol. 115, no. 8, pp. 1279–1285, 2008.

[19] A. Yekta, A. Fotouhi, H. Hashemi et al., "Prevalence of refractive errors among schoolchildren in Shiraz, Iran," Clinical and Experimental Ophthalmology, vol. 38, no. 3, pp. 242–248, 2010.

[20] J. Kedir and A. Girma, "Prevalence Of Refractive Error And Visual Impairment Among Rural School-Age Children Of Goro District, Gurage Zone, Ethiopia," Ethiopian Journal of Health Sciences, vol. 24, no. 4, pp. 3–8, 2008.

[21] E. Mahmudi, V. Mema, N. Burda, B. Selimi, and S. Zhugli, "Incidence of the refractive errors in children 3 to 9 years of age , in the city of Tetovo , Macedonia," Journal of Acute Disease, vol. 2, no. 1, pp. 52–55, 2013.

[22] U. C. Atowa, A. J. Munsamy, and S. O. Wajuihian, "Prevalence and risk factors for myopia among school children in Aba, Nigeria," African Vision and Eye Health, vol. 76, no. 1, 2017.

[23] R. Saxena, P. Vashist, R. Tandon et al., "Prevalence of myopia and its risk factors in urban school children in Delhi: the North India myopia study (NIM study)," PLoS One, vol. 10, no. 2, Article ID e0117349, 2015.

[24] C. Theophanous, B. Modjtahedi, M. Batech, D. Marlin, T. Luong, and D. Fong, "Myopia prevalence and risk factors in children," Clinical Ophthalmology, vol. 12, pp. 1581–1587, 2018.

[25] J. U. Jang and I.-J. Park, "The status of refractive errors in elementary school children in South Jeolla Province, South Korea," Clinical Optometry, p. 45, 2015.

[26] R. G. Anera, M. Soler, J. De, C. Cardona, and C. Salas, "Prevalence of refractive errors in school-age children in Morocco," *Clinical and Experimental Ophthalmology*, vol. 37, no. 2, pp. 191–196, 2009.

[27] M. He, J. Zeng, Y. Liu, J. Xu, G. P. Pokharel, and L. B. Ellwein, "Refractive error and visual impairment in urban children in southern China," *Investigative Opthalmology and Visual Science*, vol. 45, no. 3, pp. 793–799, 2004.

[28] P. Paudel, P. Ramson, T. Naduvilath et al., "Prevalence of vision impairment and refractive error in school children in Ba Ria - vung Tau province, Vietnam," *Clinical and Experimental Ophthalmology*, vol. 42, no. 3, pp. 217–226, 2014.

[29] K. S. Naidoo, A. Raghunandan, K. P. Mashige et al., "Refractive error and visual impairment in African children in South Africa," *Investigative Opthalmology and Visual Science*, vol. 44, no. 9, pp. 3764–3770, 2003.

[30] B. D. Kumah, A. Ebri, M. Abdul-Kabir et al., "Refractive error and visual impairment in private school children in Ghana," *Optometry and Vision Science*, vol. 90, no. 12, pp. 1456–1461, 2013.

[31] M. He, W. Huang, Y. Zheng, L. Huang, and L. B. Ellwein, "Refractive error and visual impairment in school children in rural southern China," *Ophthalmology*, vol. 114, no. 2, pp. 374–382, 2007.

[32] J. M. Ip, S. C. Huynh, D. Robaei et al., "Ethnic differences in the impact of parental myopia: findings from a population-based study of 12-year-old Australian children," *Investigative Opthalmology and Visual Science*, vol. 48, no. 6, pp. 2520–2528, 2007.

[33] A. N. French, I. G. Morgan, P. Mitchell, and K. A. Rose, "Risk factors for incident myopia in australian schoolchildren: the sydney adolescent vascular and eye study," *Ophthalmology*, vol. 120, no. 10, pp. 2100–2108, 2013.

[34] P. L. Megaw, M. G. Boelen, I. G. Morgan, and M. K. Boelen, "Diurnal patterns of dopamine release in chicken retina," *Neurochemistry International*, vol. 48, no. 1, pp. 17–23, 2006.

[35] D. McCarthy, P. Lueras, and P. G. Bhide, "Elevated dopamine levels during gestation produce region-specific decreases in neurogenesis and subtle deficits in neuronal numbers," *Brain Research*, vol. 1182, no. 1, pp. 11–25, 2007.

[36] F. Xiang, M. He, and I. G. Morgan, "The impact of parental myopia on myopia in Chinese children: population-based evidence," *Optometry and Vision Science*, vol. 89, no. 10, pp. 1487–1496, 2012.

[37] J. C. Sherwin, M. H. Reacher, R. H. Keogh, A. P. Khawaja, D. A. Mackey, and P. J. Foster, "The association between time spent outdoors and myopia in children and adolescents: a systematic review and meta-analysis," *Ophthalmology*, vol. 119, no. 10, pp. 2141–2151, 2012.

[38] C. Karouta and R. S. Ashby, "Correlation between light levels and the development of deprivation myopia," *Investigative Opthalmology and Visual Science*, vol. 56, no. 1, pp. 299–309, 2014.

[39] R. S. Ashby and F. Schaeffel, "The Effect of Bright Light on Lens Compensation in Chicks," *Investigative Opthalmology and Visual Science*, vol. 51, no. 10, p. 5247, 2018.

[40] E. L. Smith 3rd, L.-F. Hung, and J. Huang, "Protective effects of high ambient lighting on the development of form-deprivation myopia in rhesus monkeys," *Investigative Opthalmology and Visual Science*, vol. 53, no. 1, pp. 421–428, 2012.

[41] Y. Cohen, E. Peleg, M. Belkin, U. Polat, and A. S. Solomon, "Ambient illuminance, retinal dopamine release and refractive development in chicks," *Experimental Eye Researchs*, vol. 103, pp. 33–40, 2012.

[42] J. A. Guggenheim, C. Williams, K. Northstone et al., "Does vitamin D mediate the protective effects of time outdoors on myopia? Findings from a prospective birth cohort," *Investigative Ophthalmology and Visual Science*, vol. 55, no. 12, pp. 8550–8558, 2014.

[43] D. O. Mutti, G. L. Mitchell, M. L. Moeschberger, L. A. Jones, and K. Zadnik, "Parental myopia, near work, school achievement, and children's refractive error," *Investigative Ophthalmology and Visual Science*, vol. 43, no. 12, pp. 3633–3640, 2002.

[44] M. J. Chen, Y. T. Liu, C. C. Tsai, Y. C. Chen, C. K. Chou, and S. M. Lee, "Relationship between central corneal thickness, refractive error, corneal curvature, anterior chamber depth and axial length," *Journal of the Chinese Medical Association*, vol. 72, no. 3, pp. 133–137, 2009.

[45] E. P. Osuobeni, "Ocular components values and their intercorrelations in Saudi Arabians," *Ophthalmic and Physiological Optics*, vol. 19, no. 6, pp. 489–497, 1999.

[46] V. Bhardwaj and G. P. Rajeshbhai, "Axial length, anterior chamber depth-a study in different age groups and refractive errors," *Journal of Clinical and Diagnostic Research*, vol. 7, no. 10, pp. 2211-2212, 2013.

[47] K. Zadnik, R. E. Manny, J. A. Yu et al., "Ocular component data in schoolchildren as a function of age and gender," *Optometry and Vision Science*, vol. 80, no. 3, pp. 226–236, 2003.

[48] H. Zhu, J. J. Yu, R. B. Yu et al., "Association between childhood strabismus and refractive error in Chinese pre-school children," *PLoS One*, vol. 10, no. 3, Article ID e0120720, 2015.

[49] S. M. Tang, R. Y. T. Chan, S. Bin Lin et al., "Refractive errors and concomitant strabismus: a systematic review and meta-analysis," *Scientific Reports*, vol. 6, no. 1, 2016.

20

Evaluation of Navigated Laser Photocoagulation (Navilas 577+) for the Treatment of Refractory Diabetic Macular Edema

Fusae Kato, Miho Nozaki ⓘ, Aki Kato, Norio Hasegawa, Hiroshi Morita, Munenori Yoshida, and Yuichiro Ogura

Department of Ophthalmology and Visual Science, Nagoya City University Graduate School of Medical Sciences, 1-Kawasumi, Mizuho-ku, Nagoya 467-8601, Japan

Correspondence should be addressed to Miho Nozaki; miho.nozaki@gmail.com

Academic Editor: Dirk Sandner

Purpose. To evaluate navigated laser photocoagulation for the treatment of refractory diabetic macular edema (DME). *Methods*. Retrospective study of 25 eyes (21 patients) treated with Navilas 577+ focal laser system. Best-corrected visual acuity (BCVA) and spectral-domain optical coherence tomography (OCT) parameters were measured at baseline, 1, 3, and 6 months, and final visit. *Results*. The mean follow-up period was 12.8 ± 2.4 (7–16 months). All subjects had history of previous treatment which was injection of triamcinolone acetonide or antivascular endothelial growth factor (VEGF) agents. The navigated laser photocoagulation was delivered to the microaneurysms on indocyanine green angiography (ICGA) in 21 of 25 eyes (84%), fluorescein angiography (FA) guided in 3 eyes, and OCT angiography guided in 1 eye. After initial navigated laser treatment, 16 of 25 eyes (64%) were needed additional navigated laser photocoagulation, injection of triamcinolone acetonide, and/or injection of VEGF agents. Although median BCVA remained stable, the central retinal thickness and macular volume were significantly decreased over 6 months ($p < 0.05$). All patients were treated without complications. *Conclusions*. Focal photocoagulation using Navilas 577+ showed to be effective in treating DME with improvement in macular edema on OCT over 6 months. Navilas 577+ was beneficial to perform navigated laser photocoagulation based on three modalities (ICGA, FA, and OCT angiography).

1. Introduction

Diabetic macular edema (DME) occurs due to a malfunction of the blood-retinal barrier and death of endothelial cells leading to leakage of fluid and subsequent photoreceptor dysfunction [1, 2]. Focal laser treatment leads to the occlusion of these leaking microaneurysms (MAs), pathologic vessels, or subretinal sites of leakage [3]. As the Early Treatment Diabetic Retinopathy Study (ETDRS) research group showed, focal laser therapy can reduce moderate to severe vision loss, but the major effects were not seen till after 3 years of follow-up [4]. On the other hand, the advent of antivascular endothelial growth factor (VEGF) agents showed rapid and prominent effects on vision improvement in numerous multicenter trials [5–9]. Anti-VEGF agents have become the first-line treatment for DME. However, this treatment requires repeated intravitreous injections for an indefinite period, and safety concerns regarding to long-term systemic suppression of VEGF, which is a serious risk of cerebrovascular accidents especially in elderly patients, are emerging [10]. Recent meta-analysis has shown type 2 diabetic patients with DME or proliferative diabetic retinopathy (PDR) were associated with a twofold higher risk of fatal cardiovascular accidents compared with those without DME or PDR [11]. Therefore, a new optical treatment modality should be developed to improve the cost-effectiveness, safety, and visual outcomes. Liegl et al. reported the efficacy of a standardized combination therapy regimen (three ranibizumab injections followed by navigated focal laser) [12]. In their analysis, combination therapy regimen was significantly lower compared to ranibizumab monotherapy in terms of retreatment rate and number of injections among 12 months.

The navigated laser photocoagulator, also known as the Navilas laser system (OD-OS GmbH, Teltow, Germany), is computer-based system combined with wide-angle imaging camera. The Navilas has eye-tracking laser delivery system and allows more accurate for focal laser photocoagulation than conventional focal laser therapy for DME [13, 14]. The Navilas laser photocoagulation is performed based on preplanned treatment locations with the real-time fundus image. Navilas 577+ laser system is the new model of navigated laser system and has been approved in Japan in 2016. The preplanned treatment can be made based on color image, fluorescein angiography (FA), indocyanine green angiography (ICGA), optical coherence tomography (OCT), and/or OCT-angiography.

The aim of this study is to evaluate navigation laser photocoagulation (Navilas 577+ laser system) for the treatment of refractory DME patients.

2. Materials and Methods

This study was a retrospective, noncomparative case series performed at the eye center of Nagoya City University Graduate School of Medical Sciences. Institutional Review Board (IRB) approval (#60-17-0108) was obtained for the study protocol and procedures. The study adhered to the tenets of the Declaration of Helsinki.

Twenty-five eyes of 21 patients (14 men and 7women) with DME were included in this study between April 2016 and October 2016. The mean age was 68.3 ± 9.2 years (range 42–80 years). The mean follow-up period was 12.8 ± 2.4 (7–16 months). Before navigated laser treatment, 13 of 25 eyes (52%) had received sub-Tenon's injections of triamcinolone acetonide (TA) (Kenacort; Bristol-Myeres Squibb, Tokyo, Japan) and 12 or 25 eyes (48%) had received ranibizumab and/or aflibercept injections. Four eyes had received subthreshold laser using PASCAL Streamline (Topcon Medical Laser Systems, Santa Clara, CA, USA), and three eyes had received manual focal laser. One eye had received vitrectomy. There were some that overlapped in treatment history (Table 1).

All participants underwent a complete ophthalmologic examination, including the best-corrected visual acuity (BCVA), intraocular pressure, slit-lamp and indirect ophthalmoscopy, and OCT. The BCVA was measured with a Japanese standard decimal visual acuity chart, and decimal BCVA was calculated using the logarithm of the minimum angle of resolution (LogMAR) scale. Spectral-domain OCT (Cirrus HD-OCT; Carl Zeiss Meditec, Dublin, CA) was performed to evaluate morphological retinal changes, central retinal thickness (CRT), and macular volume (MV). FA and ICGA using the Heidelberg Spectralis HRA II (Heidelberg Engineering, Heidelberg, Germany) were performed to detect the leakage of MAs. DME type was classified as focal or diffuse based on the features below. The characteristics

TABLE 1: Baseline characteristics of patients.

Characteristic	Value
Number of eyes/patients	25 eyes/21 patients
Sex, n (%)	
Male	14 (64%)
Female	7 (36%)
Age (years)	
Range	42–80
Mean $\pm$ SD	68.3 ± 9.2
HbA1C (%)	
Mean $\pm$ SD	7.1 ± 1.2
Previous treatments, n	
STTA	13*
Anti-VEGF (ranibizumab, aflibercept)	12*
Subthreshold laser	4*
Conventional focal laser	3*
Vitrectomy	1*

*Including the overlap; VEGF: vascular endothelial growth factor; STTA: sub-Tenon's injections of triamcinolone acetonide.

of focal macular edema are (1) location outside the foveal center with or without center involvement; (2) asymmetric increases in retinal thickness on OCT scan; and (3) accumulation of pin-point leakage in early phase. The characteristics of diffuse macular edema are (1) increased retinal thickness with center involvement on the OCT macular thickness map; (2) symmetrically increased retinal thickness on B-scan OCT; and (3) fluorescein leakage starting from early phase and continuously increasing to late phase [2]. Fifteen eyes (60%) were classified as focal and 10 eyes (40%) were classified as diffuse edema.

A yellow wavelength (577 nm) photocoagulation was planned to target the leaking MAs and performed by the Navilas laser system. Briefly, treatment plan was made by physicians on a static image from FA, ICGA, and/or OCTA. The image which registered and overlaid onto the live retinal image in real time was on placing laser spot marks. After photocoagulation, a color image of the fundus was acquired to confirm that all laser applications accurately hit the preplanned points. In follow-up examinations, the patients received additional photocoagulation or medications if there were persistent of MAs or there were no findings of reduction in CRT.

Statistical analyses were performed with SPSS statistics 22 (IBM Corp., Armonk, NY, USA). In evaluating BCVA, CRT, and MV, changes (1, 3, 6 months and final visit) from baseline were analyzed using one-way repeated measures ANOVA and Bonferroni correction as post hoc test. A p value of <0.05 was considered statistically significant.

3. Results

The initial navigated laser photocoagulation was delivered to the MAs on ICGA in 21 of 25 eyes (84%). Three eyes underwent FA-guided photocoagulation. One eye had the allergy of dye injection and had undergone navigated photocoagulation on OCT angiography (Avanti OCT; Optovue, Fremont, CA, USA). The mean laser parameters were a spot size of 50–100 μm, duration between 20–100 milliseconds (ms), and power between 50–100 milliwatts (mW). Each patient received an average of 22 ± 17 burns for successful treatment. The initial laser application was performed without a contact lens in 12 of 25 eyes (48%).

After initial Navilas laser treatment, 9 of 25 eyes (36%) did not need any retreatments due to resolution of DME, although 4 eyes received sub-Tenon's injections of TA simultaneously. In other subjects, macular edema remained. Two eyes received intravitreal aflibercept (IVA) prior to navigated laser treatment within 4 weeks and 9 eyes were received IVA after navigated laser treatment. The average number of IVA is 1.55 ± 1.00 between 6 months. Some eyes received sub-Tenon' injections of TA and/or intravitreous injection of TA (MaQaid; Wakamoto Pharmaceutical Co., Ltd., Tokyo, Japan). Eleven eyes (44%) carried out additional Navilas laser photocoagulation. Three eyes were performed subthreshold laser, and 2 eyes were performed focal laser treatment by the slit-lamp delivery laser system (PASCAL Streamline) (Table 2).

Changes of mean visual acuity and parameters of OCT were showed in Figure 1. Mean logMAR BCVA, CRT, and MV at baseline were 0.21 ± 0.32, $417.7 \pm 108.3 \mu$m, and 12.3 ± 1.9 mm^3, respectively. Mean CRT at 6 months and the final visit decreased significantly compared with baseline (month 6; $346.4 \pm 110.4 \mu$m, the final visit; $322.3 \pm 78.6 \mu$m, $p < 0.05$). Mean MV at 6 months and the final visit also decreased significantly compared with baseline (month 6; 11.5 ± 1.8 mm^3, final visit; 11.3 ± 1.3 mm^3, $p < 0.01$). There were no remarkable changes in mean LogMAR BCVA after the navigated laser treatment (month 6; 0.25 ± 0.34, final visit; 0.23 ± 0.33). Eight eyes (89%) of nonretreated group were focal DME, whereas seven eyes (44%) of retreated group were focal edema. The difference in the morphology of DME between the nonretreated and retreated groups was significant ($p < 0.05$, fisher's exact test). There were no complications related to laser treatment.

3.1. Representative Cases of ICGA-Guided Navilas 577+ Laser Photocoagulation. A 77-year-old man presented with vision deterioration of the right eye due to DME. OCT macular map image revealed fovea-involving macular edema, and leaking MAs were detected on FA and ICGA corresponding with the OCT thickness map findings. Although combined therapy with sub-Tenon's capsular injection of TA and ICGA-guided manual focal laser photocoagulation using PASCAL had been applied in March 2016, the macular edema remained a month later. The navigated laser photocoagulation was planned and performed based on ICGA in April 2016. There was resolution of DME in 3 months after the navigated laser treatment (Figures 2(a)–2(e)).

A 42-year-old female consulted to our hospital with a complaint of vision deterioration in the right eye, which was affected with DME developed after panretinal photocoagulation. The eye had the history of steroid-induced glaucoma. ICGA-guided Navilas laser photocoagulation was planned and underwent in April 2016. One month after the

TABLE 2: The details of additional treatment after initial navigated laser photocoagulation.

No retreatment, n (%)	9 (36%)
Single navigated laser	5 (20%)
Navigated laser + STTA	4 (16%)
Additional treatment	16 (64%)
IVA	11*
STTA	6*
IVTA	5*
Navigated laser	11*
Subthreshold laser	3*
Manual focal laser	2*

*Including the overlap; STTA: sub-Tenon's injections of triamcinolone acetonide; IVA: intravitreal aflibercept; IVTA: intravitreal triamcinolone acetonide.

navigated laser photocoagulation, OCT findings on macular map and cross-sectional images became thinner and decimal visual acuity was remarkably improved from 0.5 to 0.8 (Figures 3(a)–3(e)).

4. Discussion

This retrospective case series of eyes with DME treated by Navilas 577+ laser system demonstrated reduction in CRT and MV at 6 months and final visit but no significant difference in logMAR BCVA. Moreover, other recent studies related to combination therapy of navigated laser and anti-VEGF agent have been published [12, 15, 16]. Their results indicate combination therapy is effective for visual gain and retinal stabilization, which can reduce number of injections. In our study, 11 eyes received injection of aflibercept following initial navigated laser, and their number of injection for 6 months were 1.55 ± 1.0, which was fewer than patients in major clinical trials [17]. As references, DME patients (23 eyes) treated anti-VEGF monotherapy in our institution received 2.52 ± 1.0 injections for the same duration of time. We considered there were two reasons why significant visual gain was not found in our study. One reason was many subjects had received several treatment histories before navigated focal laser was applied. The other was baseline BCVA in the current study was better than in those previous studies.

A randomized trial with navigated laser therapy (TREX-DME) for DME did not detect therapeutic benefits for navigated laser photocoagulation in visual gain and the CRT improved. The number of injections was not also significantly reduced at one year in combination therapy with anti-VEGF and navigated laser photocoagulation [18]. Although there was no significant difference in the mean maximal treatment interval with or without navigated laser photocoagulation, 38% of eyes with navigated laser photocoagulation were able to be maximally extended to 12 weeks, the benefit of adding navigated laser photocoagulation might be obvious with longer-term follow-up [18].

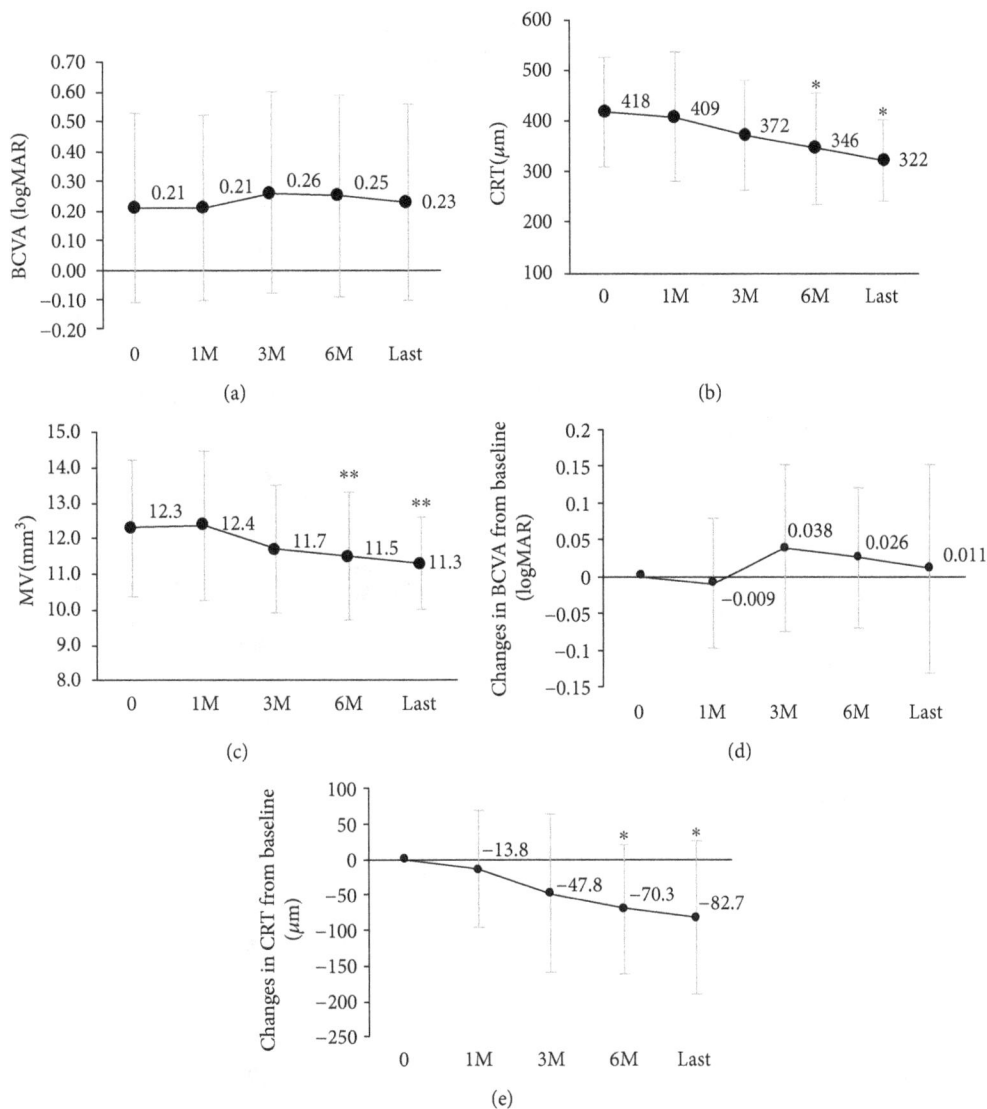

FIGURE 1: Comparison of pretreatment and posttreatment of the BCVA (a, d), CRT (b, e), and MV (c). The mean VA (± standard deviation) was unchanged from baseline to final visit; CRT and MV improved significantly ($*p < 0.05$, $**p < 0.05$). The comparison with baseline was evaluated by means of Bonferroni adjustment.

Predominantly, focal leakage from MAs showed less responsive to anti-VEGF therapy [19]. In our study, especially in cases where leaking MAs are mainly localized outside of the perifoveal capillary network, navigated laser therapy was effective. Other studies demonstrated combined conventional focal laser treatment could reduce the number of anti-VEGF injections for focal DME [7, 20]. To detect efficacy of focal laser therapy, it might be important individualized treatment be classified with different leakage subtype.

To mention with distinctive features in our current study, ICGA-guide navigated laser was performed to most of study eyes (84%). Indocyanine green dye is 98% bound to lipoproteins in the blood. Therefore, the dye hardly leaks, ICGA defines the detailed retinal vascular abnormalities better than FA [21–24]. Previously, we have reported that middle-to late-phase ICGA images show responsible MAs adjacent retinal edema, resulting in more precise and less number of focal laser photocoagulation spots [25, 26], and other groups

also reported the clinical efficacy of ICGA-guided laser [27, 28]. However, it is difficult to identify the location of MAs on ICGA, due to lack of information of foveal avascular zone. So, the navigated laser system overlaid fundus image is suitable for treatment with ICGA-guided laser photocoagulation. The navigated photocoagulation seems to demonstrate a higher laser spot application accuracy in focal laser therapy of DME than conventional laser technique [13, 14]. However, in our study, 44% of eyes were required additional navigated laser photocoagulation. The result may mean that it takes time to become skilled in performing laser photocoagulation with navigation system. Navilas laser system enables physician to coagulate MA under observing the fundus directly. Especially conventional laser photocoagulation for MA, the aiming beam has been focused on forward to the retinal pigment epithelium (RPE). With Navilas, the location in the X-Y directions is accurate, but the focus in the z-axis is impossible to adjust. Boiko and Maltsev reported the larger

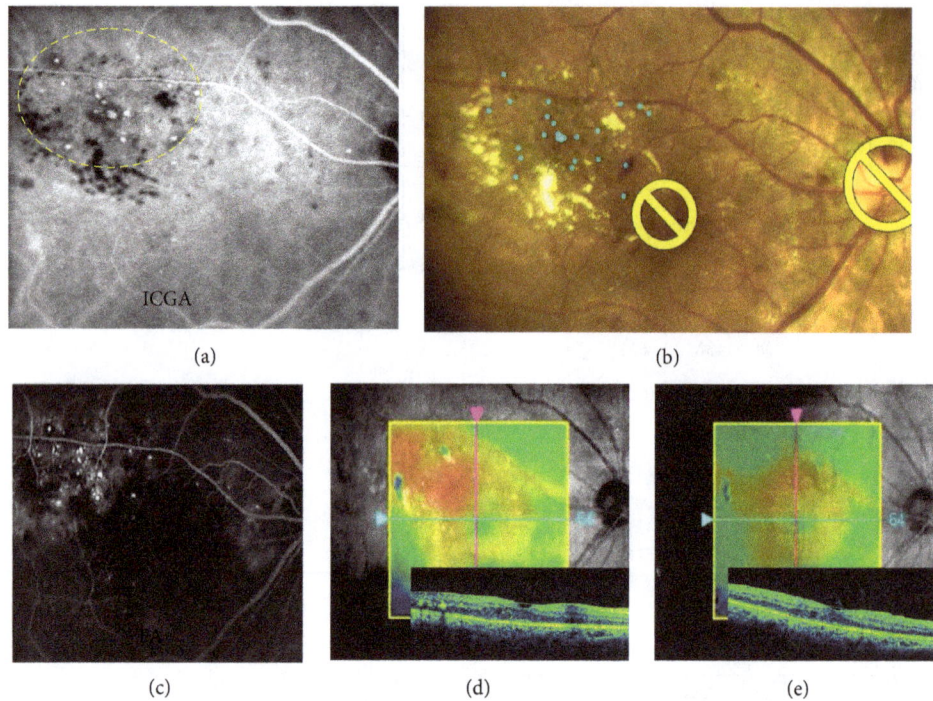

(a)

(b)

(c)

(d)

(e)

FIGURE 2: Representative case of ICGA-guided Navilas 577+ laser photocoagulation. A 77-year-old man underwent ICGA-guided navigated laser photocoagulation to treat DME which remained after focal laser using PASCAL (a–d). Image of treatment plan (blue dots) (b) was based on ICGA (a). After the navigated laser treatment, the macular edema was decreased in 3 months with no recurrences (e). The decimal visual acuity remained 0.9.

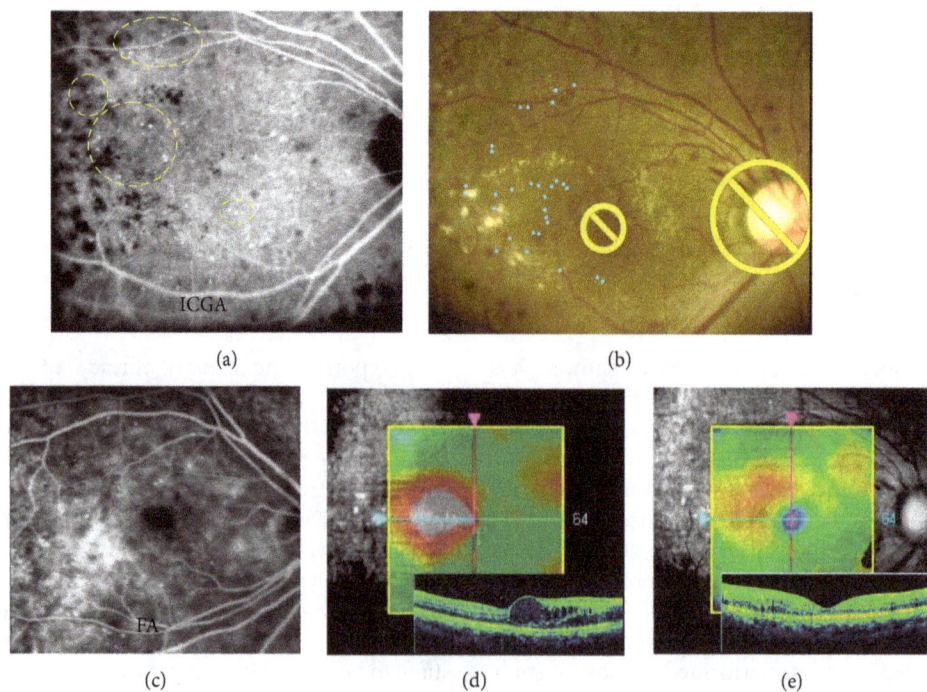

(a)

(b)

(c)

(d)

(e)

FIGURE 3: Representative case of ICGA-guided Navilas 577+ laser photocoagulation. A 42-year-old female underwent ICGA-guided navigated laser therapy (a–e). Some MAs were detected on late-phase ICGA indicated by yellow dashed line (a). Early-phase FA showed diffuse leakage from numerous MAs (c). Image of treatment plan (blue dots) (b) was based on ICGA (a). One month after the navigated laser photocoagulation, OCT findings on macular map and cross-sectional images became thinner and decimal visual acuity was remarkably improved from 0.5 to 0.8 (e).

diameter of laser burns and the more laser power needed following navigated focal laser in edematous retina compared with dry retina [29]. Therefore, it is recommended that navigated laser photocoagulation is performed under dry retinal conditions following a combination of intravitreal anti-VEGF or steroid injection with prompt or deferred focal laser treatment. In our study, 6 of 25 eyes (24%) received intravitreal anti-VEGF or steroid injection with prompt navigated focal laser treatment. Although there was no significant difference in retreatment rate of navigated laser photocoagulation with or without pretreatment of pharmacotherapy, it might be important to establish ideal protocol for treating thickened macular edema by Navilas laser system in future.

In addition, the MAs associated with DME were mainly found in deep capillary plexus of retina based on the OCT angiography (OCTA) [30]. Although OCTA cannot be used to visualize leakage, it is noninvasive, nondye imaging modality. In our study, only one eye was treated with OCTA-guided NAVILAS focal laser for the MAs located in deep capillary plexus, and we hope to study more number of eyes with OCTA-guided navigated focal laser in future.

There are several limitations to our current study. Because this study was a retrospective study, the additional intervention protocols, which were additional laser photocoagulation, anti-VEGF therapy, or steroid therapy, were not determined. This study was a nonrandomized study with no control groups and had relatively small number of patients and short follow-up period. Larger number and longer follow-up study would be warranted to study the efficacy of navigated focal laser photocoagulation for DME in future.

5. Conclusions

In conclusion, our study shows a significant decreasing of macular thickness using navigated laser photocoagulation based on multimodal imaging.

Conflicts of Interest

The authors declare that there is no conflict of interest regarding the publication of this paper.

References

[1] A. Das, P. G. McGuire, and S. Rangasamy, "Diabetic macular edema: pathophysiology and novel therapeutic targets," *Ophthalmology*, vol. 122, no. 7, pp. 1375–1394, 2015.

[2] H. Terasaki, Y. Ogura, S. Kitano et al., "Management of diabetic macular edema in Japan: a review and expert opinion," *Japanese Journal of Ophthalmology*, vol. 62, no. 1, pp. 1–23, 2018.

[3] J. Schulman, L. M. Jampol, and M. F. Goldberg, "Large capillary aneurysms secondary to retinal venous obstruction," *British Journal of Ophthalmology*, vol. 65, no. 1, pp. 36–41, 1981.

[4] "Photocoagulation for diabetic macular edema: Early Treatment Diabetic Retinopathy Study Report Number 1 Early Treatment Diabetic Retinopathy Study Research Group," *Archives of Ophthalmology*, vol. 103, no. 12, pp. 1796–1806, 1985.

[5] P. Mitchell, F. Bandello, U. Schmidt-Erfurth et al., "The RESTORE study: ranibizumab monotherapy or combined with laser versus laser monotherapy for diabetic macular edema," *Ophthalmology*, vol. 118, no. 4, pp. 615–625, 2011.

[6] Q. D. Nguyen, D. M. Brown, D. M. Marcus et al., "Ranibizumab for diabetic macular edema: results from 2 phase III randomized trials: RISE and RIDE," *Ophthalmology*, vol. 119, no. 4, pp. 789–801, 2012.

[7] T. Ishibashi, X. Li, A. Koh et al., "The REVEAL study: ranibizumab monotherapy or combined with laser versus laser monotherapy in Asian patients with diabetic macular edema," *Ophthalmology*, vol. 122, no. 7, pp. 1402–1415, 2015.

[8] J. F. Korobelnik, D. V. Do, U. Schmidt-Erfurth et al., "Intravitreal aflibercept for diabetic macular edema," *Ophthalmology*, vol. 121, no. 11, pp. 2247–2254, 2014.

[9] Diabetic Retinopathy Clinical Research Network, M. J. Elman, L. P. Aiello et al., "Randomized trial evaluating ranibizumab plus prompt or deferred laser or triamcinolone plus prompt laser for diabetic macular edema," *Ophthalmology*, vol. 117, no. 6, pp. 1064–1077.e35, 2010.

[10] R. L. Avery and G. M. Gordon, "Systemic safety of prolonged monthly anti-vascular endothelial growth factor therapy for diabetic macular edema: a systematic review and meta-analysis," *JAMA Ophthalmology*, vol. 134, no. 1, pp. 21–29, 2016.

[11] J. Xie, M. K. Ikram, M. F. Cotch et al., "Association of diabetic macular edema and proliferative diabetic retinopathy with cardiovascular disease: a systematic review and meta-analysis," *JAMA Ophthalmology*, vol. 135, no. 6, pp. 586–593, 2017.

[12] R. Liegl, J. Langer, F. Seidensticker et al., "Comparative evaluation of combined navigated laser photocoagulation and intravitreal ranibizumab in the treatment of diabetic macular edema," *PLoS One*, vol. 9, no. 12, article e113981, 2014.

[13] I. Kozak, S. F. Oster, M. A. Cortes et al., "Clinical evaluation and treatment accuracy in diabetic macular edema using navigated laser photocoagulator NAVILAS," *Ophthalmology*, vol. 118, no. 6, pp. 1119–1124, 2011.

[14] M. Kernt, R. E. Cheuteu, S. Cserhati et al., "Pain and accuracy of focal laser treatment for diabetic macular edema using a retinal navigated laser (Navilas®)," *Clinical Ophthalmology*, vol. 6, pp. 289–296, 2012.

[15] G. Barteselli, I. Kozak, S. el-Emam, J. Chhablani, M. A. Cortes, and W. R. Freeman, "12-month results of the standardised combination therapy for diabetic macular oedema: intravitreal bevacizumab and navigated retinal photocoagulation," *British Journal of Ophthalmology*, vol. 98, no. 8, pp. 1036–1041, 2014.

[16] J. J. Jung, R. Gallego-Pinazo, A. Lleó-Pérez, J. I. Huz, and I. A. Barbazetto, "NAVILAS laser system focal laser treatment for diabetic macular edema - one year results of a case series," *The Open Ophthalmology Journal*, vol. 7, no. 1, pp. 48–53, 2013.

[17] D. M. Brown, U. Schmidt-Erfurth, D. V. Do et al., "Intravitreal aflibercept for diabetic macular edema: 100-week results from the VISTA and VIVID studies," *Ophthalmology*, vol. 122, no. 10, pp. 2044–2052, 2015.

[18] J. F. Payne, C. C. Wykoff, W. L. Clark et al., "Randomized trial of treat and extend ranibizumab with and without navigated laser for diabetic macular edema: TREX-DME 1 year outcomes," *Ophthalmology*, vol. 124, no. 1, pp. 74–81, 2017.

[19] M. J. Allingham, D. Mukherjee, E. B. Lally et al., "A quantitative approach to predict differential effects of anti-VEGF treatment on diffuse and focal leakage in patients with diabetic

macular edema: a pilot study," *Translational Vision Science & Technology*, vol. 6, no. 2, p. 7, 2017.

[20] T. Hirano, Y. Toriyama, Y. Iesato et al., "Effect of leaking peri-foveal microaneurysms on resolution of diabetic macular edema treated by combination therapy using anti-vascular endothelial growth factor and short pulse focal/grid laser photocoagulation," *Japanese Journal of Ophthalmology*, vol. 61, no. 1, pp. 51–60, 2017.

[21] M. B. Parodi and G. Ravalico, "Detection of retinal arterial macroaneurysms with indocyanine green videoangiography," *Graefe's Archive for Clinical and Experimental Ophthalmology*, vol. 233, no. 2, pp. 119–121, 1995.

[22] W. A. Townsend-Pico, S. M. Meyers, and H. Lewis, "Indocyanine green angiography in the diagnosis of retinal arterial macroaneurysms associated with submacular and preretinal hemorrhages: a case series," *American Journal of Ophthalmology*, vol. 129, no. 1, pp. 33–37, 2000.

[23] H. Fujita, K. Ohno-Matsui, S. Futagami, and T. Tokoro, "Case report: indocyanine green dye leakage from retinal artery in branch retinal vein occlusion," *Japanese Journal of Ophthalmology*, vol. 44, no. 3, pp. 277–282, 2000.

[24] S. Harino, Y. Oshima, K. Tsujikawa, K. Ogawa, and J. E. Grunwald, "Indocyanine green and fluorescein hyperfluorescence at the site of occlusion in branch retinal vein occlusion," *Graefe's Archive for Clinical and Experimental Ophthalmology*, vol. 239, no. 1, pp. 18–24, 2001.

[25] Y. Hirano, T. Yasukawa, Y. Usui, M. Nozaki, and Y. Ogura, "Indocyanine green angiography-guided laser photocoagulation combined with sub-Tenon's capsule injection of triamcinolone acetonide for idiopathic macular telangiectasia," *British Journal of Ophthalmology*, vol. 94, no. 5, pp. 600–605, 2010.

[26] S. Ogura, T. Yasukawa, A. Kato et al., "Indocyanine green angiography-guided focal laser photocoagulation for diabetic macular edema," *Ophthalmologica*, vol. 234, no. 3, pp. 139–150, 2015.

[27] T. Ueda, F. Gomi, M. Suzuki et al., "Usefulness of indocyanine green angiography to depict the distant retinal vascular anomalies associated with branch retinal vein occlusion causing serous macular detachment," *Retina*, vol. 32, no. 2, pp. 308–313, 2012.

[28] M. Paques, E. Philippakis, C. Bonnet et al., "Indocyanine-green-guided targeted laser photocoagulation of capillary macroaneurysms in macular oedema: a pilot study," *British Journal of Ophthalmology*, vol. 101, no. 2, pp. 170–174, 2017.

[29] E. V. Boiko and D. S. Maltsev, "Combination of navigated macular laser photocoagulation and anti-VEGF therapy: precise treatment for macular edema under dry retinal conditions," *Journal of Ophthalmology*, vol. 2017, Article ID 7656418, 9 pages, 2017.

[30] N. Hasegawa, M. Nozaki, N. Takase, M. Yoshida, and Y. Ogura, "New insights into microaneurysms in the deep capillary plexus detected by optical coherence tomography angiography in diabetic macular edema," *Investigative Ophthalmology & Visual Science*, vol. 57, no. 9, pp. OCT348–OCT355, 2016.

21

Efficacy and Safety of Bevacizumab in the Treatment of Pterygium

Yi Sun [ID],[1] Bowen Zhang [ID],[2] Xiuhua Jia,[1] Shiqi Ling,[1] and Juan Deng [ID][1]

[1]*Department of Ophthalmology, Third Affiliated Hospital of Sun Yat-Sen University, Guangzhou 510630, China*
[2]*Surgical Department, The First Affiliated Hospital of Guangzhou Medical University, Guangzhou 510120, China*

Correspondence should be addressed to Juan Deng; viviadeng@163.com

Academic Editor: Lisa Toto

Purpose. Studies investigating efficacy and safety of bevacizumab in pterygium have increased and reported controversial results. Thus, we updated this meta-analysis to clarify the issue. *Methods.* Studies were selected through search of the databases Embase, PubMed, Web of Science, and the Cochrane Central Register of Controlled Trials (CENTRAL) from their inception up until June 2017. The pooled risk ratio (RR) and 95% confidence interval (CI) were calculated for recurrence and complication rates by using random effects model. *Results.* 1045 eyes in 18 randomized controlled trials (RCTs) enrolled. Overall, the pooled estimate showed a statistically significant effect of bevacizumab on the reduction of recurrence (RR 0.74, 95% CI 0.56–0.97, $P = 0.03$). Subgroup analyses presented significant results beneficial to bevacizumab (primary pterygium group, RR 0.53, 95% CI 0.33–0.83, $P = 0.006$; conjunctival autograft group, RR 0.48, 95% CI 0.25–0.91, $P = 0.02$; and follow-up longer than 12 months group, RR 0.36, 95% CI 0.13–0.99, $P = 0.05$). No statistically significant difference was observed in complication rates. *Conclusions.* Application of bevacizumab showed a statistically significant decrease in recurrence rate following removal of primary pterygia, or in cases with conjunctival autograft, or with follow-up longer than 12 months, while complications were not increased.

1. Introduction

Pterygium is one of the most common ocular surface diseases, which is characterized by the fibrovascular conjunctiva tissue proceeding from the bulbar conjunctiva towards the cornea. It limits eye movements and causes dry eye, irritation, foreign body sensation, and even decrease of visual acuity [1]. The primary treatment for pterygium is surgery, and the major problem of the treatment is the high recurrence rate, varying between 38% and 88% in bare sclera, 5%–30% in conjunctival autograft, and 0%–15% in limbal conjunctival autograft [2]. Many adjuvant therapies have been developed to reduce recurrence including mitomycin C [3, 4], 5-FU [5–7], and radiotherapy [8, 9].

In 2001, expression of vascular endothelial growth factor (VEGF) was firstly demonstrated in pterygia [10]. Pterygia present higher levels of VEGF compared with normal conjunctiva [11–16]. This brings about speculation that anti-VEGF drugs may be useful for pterygia patients. Bevacizumab is a recombinant human monoclonal antibody against VEGF, which is approved by FDA treating neoplasms. Many randomized controlled trials (RCTs) were performed to assess the safety and efficacy of bevacizumab in management of pterygium, showing conflicting conclusions [17–34]. A meta-analysis of 9 RCTs was conducted in 2014 [35], and the result showed that topical or subconjunctival bevacizumab had no statistically significant effect on preventing pterygium recurrence. However, the result was not been consistently supported by another 9 new RCTs published after 2014 [26–34]. The conclusion might be altered by the addition of 9 new studies. Therefore, we performed an additional meta-analysis to further evaluate the impact of bevacizumab on the recurrence and complication rates in the treatment of pterygium.

2. Methods

2.1. Search Strategy. The databases of Embase, PubMed, Web of Science, and the Cochrane Central Register of Controlled Trials (CENTRAL) were searched from their inception up until June 2017. Details of the search strategies were described in the Search Strategy file. Endnote software was used to exclude the duplications. Titles and abstracts were scrutinized to deduct apparently irrelevant studies. Full texts were retrieved and assessed for qualification. A manual search was executed by checking the reference lists of all retrieved studies and reviewing articles to distinguish studies not found by the electronic searches. Language was not restricted.

2.2. Inclusion and Exclusion Criteria. The articles were considered qualified if the studies fulfilled the following inclusion criteria: (1) participants: pterygium patients (including primary pterygium, impending recurrent pterygium, and recurrent pterygium); (2) intervention: topical or subconjunctival bevacizumab, regardless of operation or not. The dose of bevacizumab, follow-up periods, or length of fibrovascular growth passing the corneal limbus were not confined; (3) comparison: bevacizumab and control; (4) outcomes: recurrence and/or complication rates; and (5) publication type: RCT. RCTs without exact raw data available for extraction were excluded.

2.3. Outcome Measurements. The primary outcome measurements were recurrence and complication rates. Recurrence was diagnosed when any fibrovascular growth crossed the limbus and extended over the cornea to any distance by slit-lamp examination. The number of recurrences was estimated at the endpoint of the follow-up in each study. Complications such as lacrimation, inflammation, photophobia, conjunctival erythema, conjunctival flap edema, conjunctival graft loss, subconjunctival hemorrhage, corneal dellen, severe conjunctival or corneal scarring, and systemic complications were counted. The number of complications at the last documenting time during the follow-up in each study was calculated.

2.4. Data Extraction. The data were extracted by two reviewers (Yi Sun and Bowen Zhang) independently. Discrepancies were resolved by discussion to reach a consensus between the investigators. The information collected from each study included the first author's last name, year of publication, study design, location and duration of the study, sample size including sex, age, and diagnoses, type of treatment and control, route of administration, and dose of bevacizumab.

2.5. Risk of Bias Assessment. Two reviewers (Yi Sun and Bowen Zhang) separately evaluated the risk of bias in each study according to the methods described in the Cochrane Handbook for Systematic Reviews of Interventions 5.3. The authors reviewed the studies and assigned a value of "high,"

"low," or "unclear" to the following items: (1) selection bias (Was there sufficient generation of the randomization sequence and allocation concealment?); (2) performance and detection bias (Was there blinding of participants, personnel, and outcome assessors?); (3) attrition bias (Were there incomplete outcome data and how to deal with this?); (4) reporting bias (Was there evidence of reporting outcome selectively?); and (5) other sources of bias (Were there any other potential threats to validity?). Any disagreement was discussed until a consensus was reached.

2.6. Statistical Analysis. The recurrence and complication rates were handled as dichotomous variables measured as the risk ratio (RR) with a 95% confidence interval (CI). Due to the diversity in sample size and the differences in clinical characteristics among the studies, it was presumed that heterogeneity existed even when no statistical significance was observed. Therefore, the data were pooled using a random effects model. Statistical heterogeneity among the studies was assessed by calculating a Cochran Q statistic and an I^2 statistic. Subgroup analysis and sensitivity analysis for the recurrence rate were carried out to evaluate the impact of the following factors on the results: (a) participants: primary pterygium, impending recurrent pterygium, and recurrent pterygium; (b) intervention: topical use or subconjunctival injection of bevacizumab; type of operation or not; and (c) follow-up periods: ≤6 months, 6 ~ 12 months, and ≥12 months. We explored asymmetry in funnel plots to detect publication biases. The analysis was performed using RevMan 5.3 (The Cochrane Collaboration, Copenhagen, Denmark).

3. Results

3.1. Literature Search. Literature search and selection process are summarized in Figure 1. A total of 99 articles were initially enrolled. After removing duplications, the abstracts of the remaining studies were inspected, and 29 articles with possibly relevant trials were further identified in full texts. Eighteen randomized controlled trials (RCTs) were deemed eligible after a full text screening and were finally included in this meta-analysis.

3.2. Characteristics and Quality Assessment of the Included Studies. Characteristics of included studies are summarized in Table 1. In total, 18 RCTs were included in this review [17–34]. 17 studies were published in English and 1 in Chinese. 1045 eyes were enrolled: 561 in the bevacizumab group and 484 in the control group. Quality assessment was conducted according to Cochrane Handbook for Systematic Reviews of Interventions 5.3. The risks of biases in these studies are shown in supplementary data file (available here).

3.3. Meta-Analysis. 15 studies reported recurrences. Definitions of pterygium recurrence of the included randomized clinical trials are shown in Table 2. Overall recurrence rate of this meta-analysis was summarized in supplementary data file. The pooled results demonstrated that bevacizumab significantly reduced the pterygium recurrence (RR 0.74,

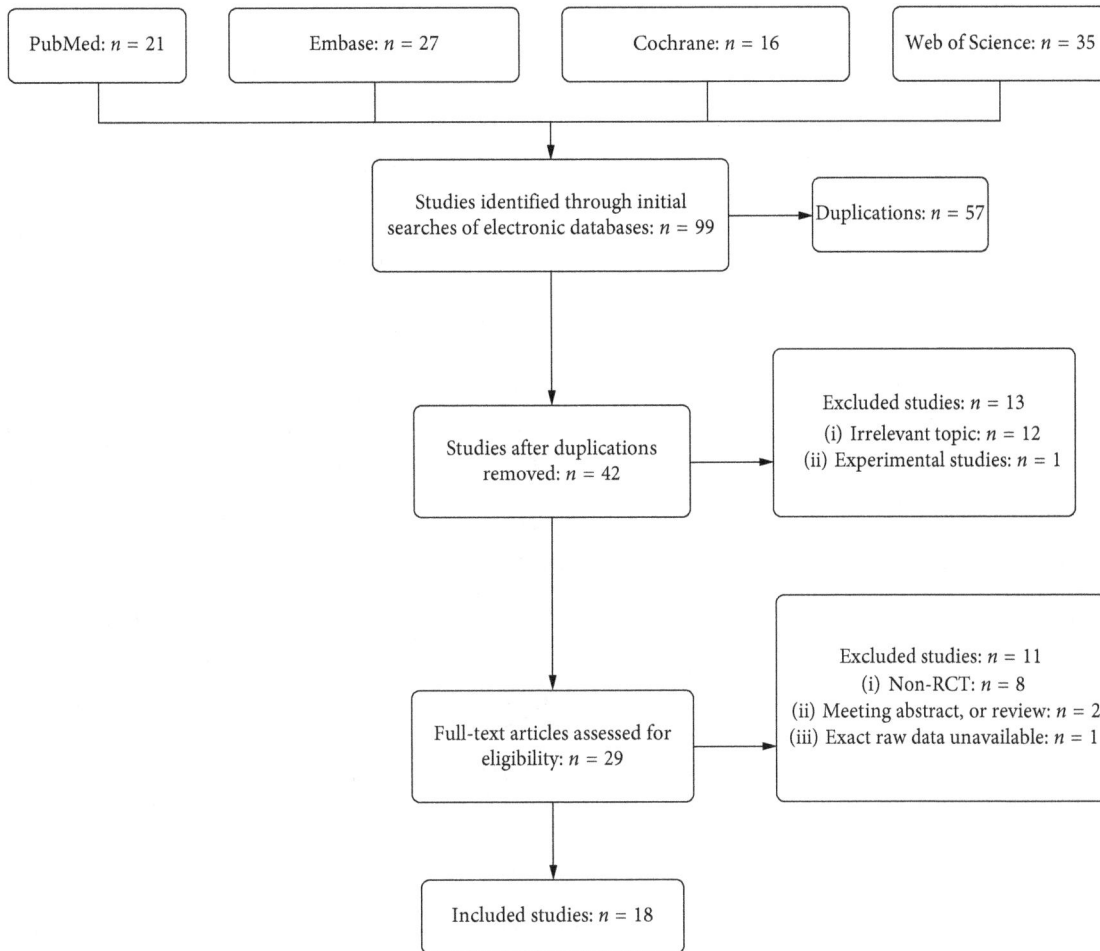

FIGURE 1: Flow diagram for the literature search and selection process.

95% CI 0.56–0.97, $P = 0.03$; $P_{\text{heterogeneity}} = 0.03$, $I^2 = 46\%$). Subgroup analysis for the recurrence rate based on the pterygium types showed a statistically significant decrease in recurrence rate in the primary pterygium group (RR 0.53, 95% CI 0.33–0.83, $P = 0.006$; $P_{\text{heterogeneity}} = 0.21$, $I^2 = 25\%$), while not in the recurrent pterygium group (RR 1.00, 95% CI 0.93–1.07, $P = 0.91$; $P_{\text{heterogeneity}} = 0.55$, $I^2 = 0\%$) (Figure 2). Similarly, significant results in favor of bevacizumab were found in the conjunctival autograft group (RR 0.48, 95% CI 0.25–0.91, $P = 0.022$; $P_{\text{heterogeneity}} = 0.87$, $I^2 = 0\%$) (Figure 3) and the follow-up longer than 12 months group (RR 0.36, 95% CI 0.13–0.99, $P = 0.05$; $P_{\text{heterogeneity}} = 0.15$, $I^2 = 41\%$) (Figure 4). There was no statistically significant difference between the topical bevacizumab group (RR 0.38, 95% CI 0.12–1.23, $P = 0.11$; $P_{\text{heterogeneity}} = 0.002$, $I^2 = 76\%$) and the subconjunctival bevacizumab group (RR 0.87, 95% CI 0.70–1.07, $P = 0.18$; $P_{\text{heterogeneity}} = 0.64$, $I^2 = 0\%$) (supplementary data file).

17 studies reporting complications were analyzed. There was no statistically significant difference between bevacizumab group and control group (RR 0.87, 95% CI 0.66–1.13, $P = 0.30$; $P_{\text{heterogeneity}} = 0.52$, $I^2 = 0\%$) (supplementary data file). Further analysis of the subconjunctival hemorrhage rate showed that a statistically significant difference was not found

between groups (RR 1.50, 95% CI 0.63–3.59, $P = 0.36$; $P_{\text{heterogeneity}} = 0.69$, $I^2 = 0\%$) (supplementary data file).

Publication bias for recurrence rates and complications was checked by evaluating funnel plots (supplementary data file).

4. Discussion

This meta-analysis, updated with 1045 eyes in 18 RCTs showed that bevacizumab would significantly reduce pterygium recurrence rate after surgery in either case of primary pterygium or use of conjunctival autograft or follow-up longer than 12 months. Complications of bevacizumab were not increased compared with the control.

An earlier meta-analysis performed by Hu indicated that bevacizumab had no statistically significant effect on preventing pterygium recurrence [35]. Hu included 9 RCTs, of which 7 reported recurrence and 8 reported complications, whereas in our current meta-analysis, we report raw data on recurrences in 15 and complications in 17 studies. The inclusion of more trials and more cases renders our analysis more statistically significant.

According to Prabhasawat [36], corneal recurrence with fibrovascular tissue covering the excision area and invading the cornea (grade 4) was the true recurrence. However, the

TABLE 1: Characteristics of the included randomized clinical trials.

Author (year)	Location	No. of eyes (Bev/Con)	Administration route of bevacizumab	Mean age (Bev/Con, y)	Type of pterygium	Follow-up (m)	Treatment method
Fallah (2010)	Iran	26/28	Topical	49.96/51.61	Impending recurrent	3 ~ 6	Nonsurgery
Razeghinejad (2010)	Iran	15/15	Subconjunctival	45.8/41.6	Primary	8 vs 7.4	Conjunctival autograft
Banifatemi (2011)	Iran	22/22	Subconjunctival	41.95/44.13	Primary	1	Conjunctival autograft
Enkvetchakul (2011)	Thailand	34/40	Subconjunctival	51.5/49	Primary	6	Nonsurgery
Shenasi (2011)	Iran	33/33	Subconjunctival	58.67/55.94	Primary	9	Bare sclera
Shahin (2012)	Egypt	20/21	Subconjunctival	58.40/57.58	Primary	8	Conjunctivolimbal autograft
Lekhanont (2012)	Thailand	60/20	Subconjunctival	48.98/48.27	Impending recurrent	3	Nonsurgery
Ozgurhan (2013)	Turkey	22/22	Topical	48.4/50.5	Recurrent	6	Conjunctival autograft
Xu (2013)	China	40/40	Subconjunctival	44/41	Primary	12	Conjunctivolimbal autograft
Nava-Castaneda, A (2014)	Mexico	33/16	Subconjunctival	48.75/47.8	Primary	12	Conjunctival autograft
Karalezli (2014)	Turkey	42/46	Topical	58.82/53.04	Primary	29.3 VS 28.5	Conjunctival autograft
Razeghinejad(2014)	Iran	20/21	Subconjunctival	41.95/44.13	Primary	6	Conjunctival autograft
Ozsutcu(2014)	Turkey	30/30	Subconjunctival	43.25/41.68	Primary	9	Conjunctival autograft
Kasetsuwan(2015)	Thailand	12/10	Topical	50.7/59.3	Primary	3	Bare sclera
Hwang(2015)	Korea	36/33	Topical	71.3/73.4	Primary	6	Bare sclera
Singh(2015)	India	30/30	Subconjunctival	37.33	Primary	3	Conjunctival autograft
Bekibele(2016)	Nigeria	26/27	Subconjunctival	49.2/52.0	Primary	18.35	Conjunctiva autograft
Motarjemizadeh (2016)	Iran	60/30	Topical	39.47/40.97	Primary	12	Bare sclera

Bev: bevacizumab; Con, control; y, year; m, month.

TABLE 2: Definition of pterygium recurrence of the included randomized clinical trials.

Author (year)	Definition of recurrence
Fallah (2010)	Fibrovascular tissue stretching onto cornea
Razeghinejad (2010)	Fibrovascular tissue extending more than 1.5 mm across limbus
Shenasi (2011)	Fibrovascular growth crossing limbus and extending over the cornea to any distance
Shahin (2012)	4 grades classified
Lekhanont (2012)	Fibrovascular tissue invading cornea or when the lesion was categorized as grade 4
Ozgurhan (2013)	No specific definition
Xu (2013)	Fibrovascular tissue invading cornea
Nava-Castaneda, A (2014)	4 grades classified
Karalezli (2014)	Fibrovascular growth passing the corneal limbus by more than 1mm
Razeghinejad (2014)	More than 1.5 mm of fibrovascular tissue overgrowth on cornea and any fibrovascular tissue crossing limbus
Ozsutcu (2014)	Any fibrovascular growth of conjunctival tissue extending more than 1.5 mm across limbus
Kasetsuwan (2015)	4 grades classified
Singh (2015)	4 grades classified
Bekibele (2016)	Growth of fibrovascular tissue 1 mm or more into cornea
Motarjemizadeh (2016)	New vessels or fibrovascular connective tissues crossing corneal limbus

| Study or subgroup | Bevacizumab | | Control | | | Risk ratio | Risk ratio |
	Events	Total	Events	Total	Weight	IV, random, 95% CI	IV, random, 95% CI
1.5.1 Primary pterygium group							
Bekibele 2016	1	26	1	27	1.0%	1.04 [0.07, 15.75]	
Karalezli 2014	1	42	2	46	1.3%	0.55 [0.05, 5.82]	
Kasetsuwan 2015	1	12	3	10	1.6%	0.28 [0.03, 2.27]	
Motarjemizadeh 2016	4	60	14	30	5.9%	0.14 [0.05, 0.40]	
Nava-Castaneda 2014	0	33	2	16	0.8%	0.10 [0.01, 1.97]	
Ozsutcu 2014	3	30	8	30	4.3%	0.38 [0.11, 1.28]	
Razeghinejad 2010	2	15	2	15	2.1%	1.00 [0.16, 6.20]	
Razeghinejad 2014	4	20	8	21	5.8%	0.53 [0.19, 1.47]	
Shahin 2012	2	20	1	21	1.3%	2.10 [0.21, 21.39]	
Shenasi 2011	15	33	19	33	16.0%	0.79 [0.49, 1.27]	
Singh 2015	0	30	0	30		Not estimable	
Xu 2013	5	40	6	40	5.2%	0.83 [0.28, 2.51]	
Subtotal (95% CI)		361		319	45.4%	0.53 [0.33, 0.83]	
Total events	38		66				

Heterogeneity: tau^2 = 0.13; chi^2 = 13.30, df = 10 (P = 0.21); I^2 = 25%

Test for overall effect: Z = 2.74 (P = 0.006)

1.5.2 Recurrent pterygium group							
Fallah 2010	26	26	28	28	29.9%	1.00 [0.93, 1.07]	
Lekhanont 2012	46	60	16	20	24.0%	0.96 [0.74, 1.24]	
Ozgurhan 2013	0	22	2	22	0.8%	0.20 [0.01, 3.94]	
Subtotal (95% CI)		108		70	54.6%	1.00 [0.93, 1.07]	
Total events	72		46				

Heterogeneity: tau^2 = 0.00; chi^2 = 1.21, df = 2 (P = 0.55); I^2 = 0%

Test for overall effect: Z = 0.11 (P = 0.91)

Total (95% CI)		469		389	100.0%	0.74 [0.56, 0.97]	
Total events	110		112				

Heterogeneity: tau^2 = 0.06; chi^2 = 24.00, df = 13 (P = 0.03); I^2 = 46%

Test for overall effect: Z = 2.15 (P = 0.03)

Test for subgroup differences: chi^2 = 7.26, df = 1 (P = 0.007), I^2 = 86.2%

0.002　0.1　1　10　500
Favours [Bevacizumab]　Favours [control]

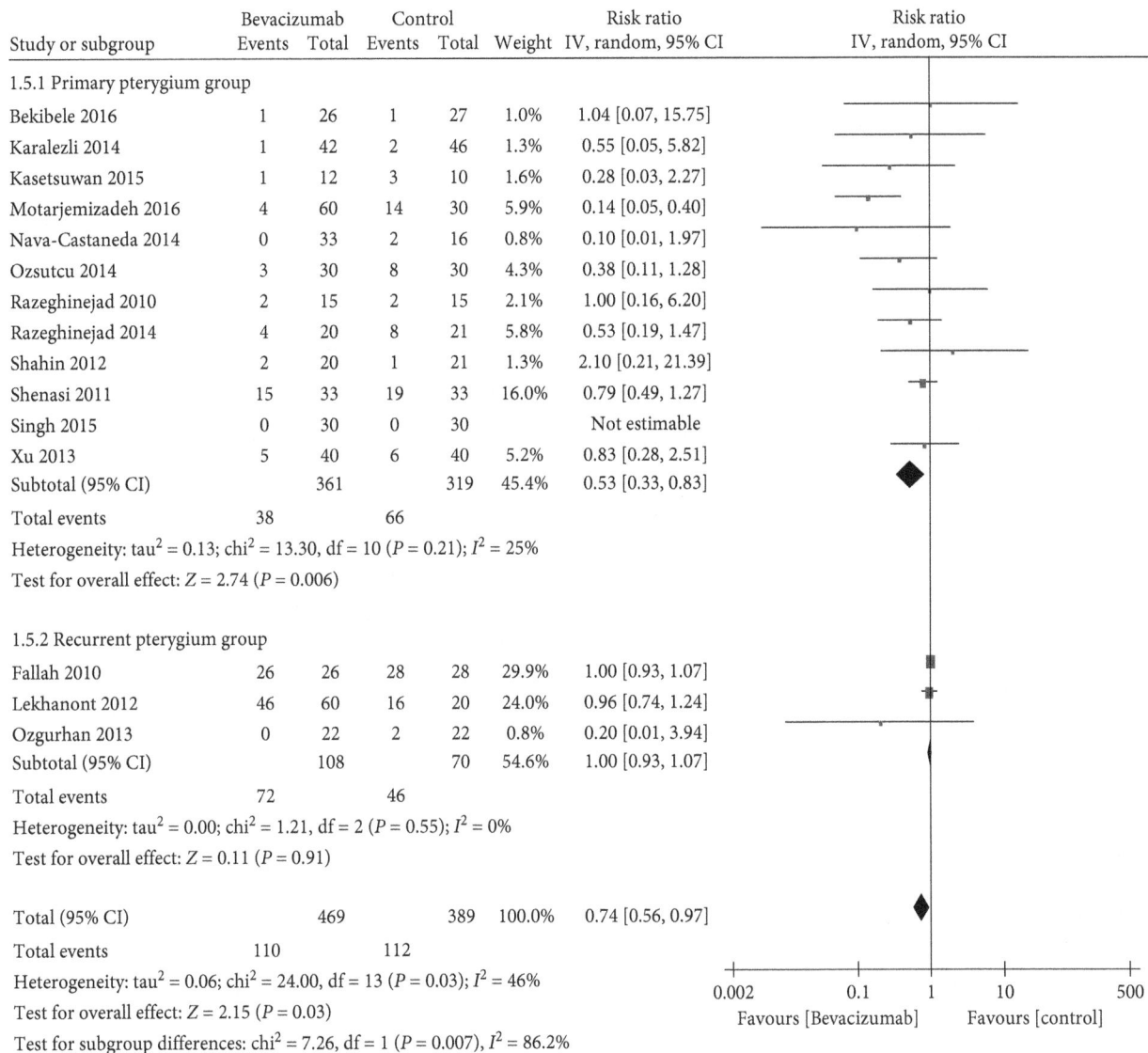

FIGURE 2: Subgroup analysis for the recurrence rates according to types of pterygium (n = 15, the remainder 3 studies without recurrence).

definition of recurrence adopted in literatures varied. The inconsistent definition of pterygium recurrence in the included studies (Table 2) implied that the conclusion of the meta-analysis should be interpreted prudently. Study by Razeghinejad defined recurrence as any fibrovascular growth of conjunctival tissue extending more than 1.5 mm across the limbus [37]. In addition, data of recurrence in table 3 of the literature were found incorrect. Thus, the study was excluded. Moreover, the significant effect of bevacizumab on decreasing recurrence in the follow-up longer than 12 months group would suggest that longer follow-up in the future studies could further favor the effect.

RR for the overall recurrence rate was 0.74, with 95% CI [0.56, 0.97]. After removal of the study by Motarjemizadeh [31], I^2 decreased to 0% and RR was 0.98, with 95% CI [0.92, 1.05], but it did not affect the conclusive result in subgroup analysis on the pterygium type or administration route of

bevacizumab. Therefore, sensitivity analysis was unstable and the heterogeneity was mainly caused by this study. However, there was no reason to exclude the study after comprehensive reading of the full text.

There was no statistically significant difference in overall complications and subconjunctival hemorrhage between bevacizumab group and control group, showing the safety of bevacizumab. The sensitivity analysis for the complication was stable. It is different from the previous meta-analysis by Hu [35], who reported the bevacizumab group was associated with a higher risk of developing subconjunctival hemorrhage.

The funnel plot for the recurrence and complication rates displayed asymmetry. This could be due to factors other than publication bias, including poor methodological quality, true heterogeneity, artefactual variation, and chance.

Study or subgroup	Bevacizumab Events	Total	Control Events	Total	Weight	Risk ratio IV, random, 95% CI
1.4.1 Nonsurgery						
Fallah 2010	26	26	28	28	29.9%	1.00 [0.93, 1.07]
Lekhanont 2012	46	60	16	20	24.0%	0.96 [0.74, 1.24]
Subtotal (95% CI)		86		48	53.8%	1.00 [0.93, 1.07]
Total events	72		44			

Heterogeneity: tau^2 = 0.00; chi^2 = 0.10, df = 1 (P = 0.76); I^2 = 0%

Test for overall effect: Z = 0.08 (P = 0.93)

1.4.2 Bare sclera						
Kasetsuwan 2015	1	12	3	10	1.6%	0.28 [0.03, 2.27]
Motarjemizadeh 2016	4	60	14	30	5.9%	0.14 [0.05, 0.40]
Shenasi 2011	15	33	19	33	16.0%	0.79 [0.49, 1.27]
Subtotal (95% CI)		105		73	23.5%	0.34 [0.09, 1.27]
Total events	20		36			

Heterogeneity: tau^2 = 0.98; chi^2 = 9.31, df = 2 (P = 0.010); I^2 = 79%

Test for overall effect: Z = 1.60 (P = 0.11)

1.4.3 Conjunctival autograft						
Bekibele 2016	1	26	1	27	1.0%	1.04 [0.07, 15.75]
Karalezli 2014	1	42	2	46	1.3%	0.55 [0.05, 5.82]
Nava-Castaneda 2014	0	33	2	16	0.8%	0.10 [0.01, 1.97]
Ozgurhan 2013	0	22	2	22	0.8%	0.20 [0.01, 3.94]
Ozsutcu 2014	3	30	8	30	4.3%	0.38 [0.11, 1.28]
Razeghinejad 2010	2	15	2	15	2.1%	1.00 [0.16, 6.20]
Razeghinejad 2014	4	20	8	21	5.8%	0.53 [0.19, 1.47]
Singh 2015	0	30	0	30		Not estimable
Subtotal (95% CI)		218		207	16.2%	0.48 [0.25, 0.91]
Total events	11		25			

Heterogeneity: tau^2 = 0.00; chi^2 = 2.52, df = 6 (P = 0.87); I^2 = 0%

Test for overall effect: Z = 2.26 (P = 0.02)

1.4.4 Conjunctivolimbal autograft						
Shahin 2012	2	20	1	21	1.3%	2.10 [0.21, 21.39]
Xu 2013	5	40	6	40	5.2%	0.83 [0.28, 2.51]
Subtotal (95% CI)		60		61	6.5%	0.99 [0.36, 2.68]
Total events	7		7			

Heterogeneity: tau^2 = 0.00; chi^2 = 0.50, df = 1 (P = 0.48); I^2 = 0%

Test for overall effect: Z = 0.02 (P = 0.98)

Total (95% CI)		469		389	100.0%	0.74 [0.56, 0.97]
Total events	110		112			

Heterogeneity: tau^2 = 0.06; chi^2 = 24.00, df = 13 (P = 0.03); I^2 = 46%

Test for overall effect: Z = 2.15 (P = 0.03)

Test for subgroup differences: chi^2 = 7.49, df = 3 (P = 0.06), I^2 = 59.9%

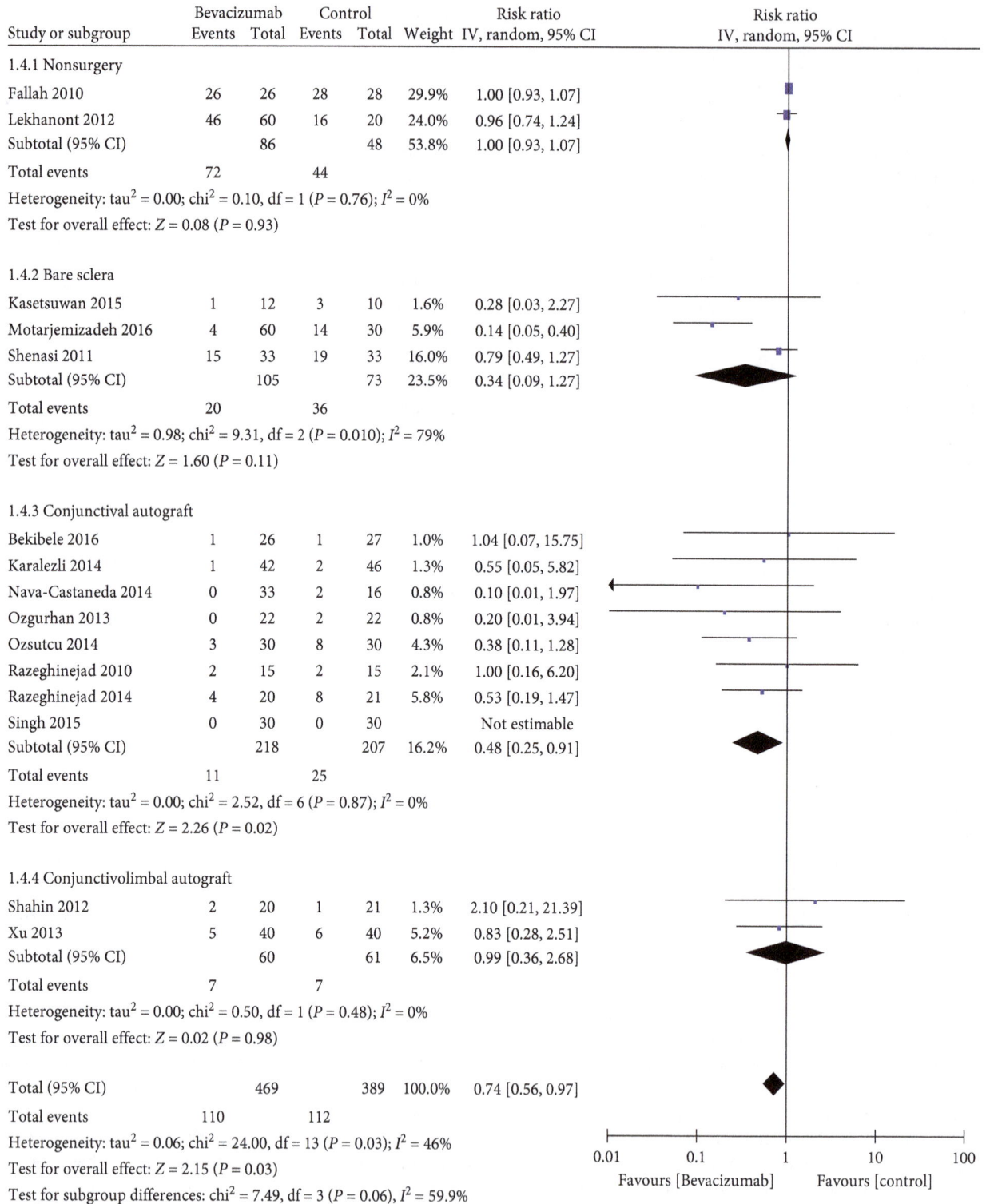

FIGURE 3: Subgroup analysis for the recurrence rates according to the treatment (n = 15, the remainder 3 studies without recurrence).

Study or subgroup	Bevacizumab Events	Bevacizumab Total	Control Events	Control Total	Weight	Risk ratio IV, random, 95% CI	Risk ratio IV, random, 95% CI
1.7.1 ≤ 6 months							
Fallah 2010	26	26	28	28	29.9%	1.00 [0.93, 1.07]	
Kasetsuwan 2015	1	12	3	10	1.6%	0.28 [0.03, 2.27]	
Lekhanont 2012	46	60	16	20	24.0%	0.96 [0.74, 1.24]	
Ozgurhan 2013	0	22	2	22	0.8%	0.20 [0.01, 3.94]	
Razeghinejad 2014	4	20	8	21	5.8%	0.53 [0.19, 1.47]	
Singh 2015	0	30	0	30		Not estimable	
Subtotal (95% CI)		170		131	62.0%	0.99 [0.91, 1.08]	
Total events	77		57				

Heterogeneity: tau^2 = 0.00; chi^2 = 4.09, df = 4 (P = 0.39); I^2 = 2%

Test for overall effect: Z = 0.28 (P = 0.78)

Study or subgroup	Bevacizumab Events	Bevacizumab Total	Control Events	Control Total	Weight	Risk ratio IV, random, 95% CI	Risk ratio IV, random, 95% CI
1.7.2 6–12 months							
Ozsutcu 2014	3	30	8	30	4.3%	0.38 [0.11, 1.28]	
Razeghinejad 2010	2	15	2	15	2.1%	1.00 [0.16, 6.20]	
Shahin 2012	2	20	1	21	1.3%	2.10 [0.21, 21.39]	
Shenasi 2011	15	33	19	33	16.0%	0.79 [0.49, 1.27]	
Subtotal (95% CI)		98		99	23.8%	0.76 [0.50, 1.15]	
Total events	22		30				

Heterogeneity: tau^2 = 0.00; chi^2 = 2.12, df = 3 (P = 0.55); I^2 = 0%

Test for overall effect: Z = 1.30 (P = 0.20)

Study or subgroup	Bevacizumab Events	Bevacizumab Total	Control Events	Control Total	Weight	Risk ratio IV, random, 95% CI	Risk ratio IV, random, 95% CI
1.7.3 ≥ 12 months							
Bekibele 2016	1	26	1	27	1.0%	1.04 [0.07, 15.75]	
Karalezli 2014	1	42	2	46	1.3%	0.55 [0.05, 5.82]	
Motarjemizadeh 2016	4	60	14	30	5.9%	0.14 [0.05, 0.40]	
Nava-Castaneda 2014	0	33	2	16	0.8%	0.10 [0.01, 1.97]	
Xu 2013	5	40	6	40	5.2%	0.83 [0.28, 2.51]	
Subtotal (95% CI)		201		159	14.2%	0.36 [0.13, 0.99]	
Total events	11		25				

Heterogeneity: tau^2 = 0.49; chi^2 = 6.76, df = 4 (P = 0.15); I^2 = 41%

Test for overall effect: Z = 1.99 (P = 0.05)

Study or subgroup	Bevacizumab Events	Bevacizumab Total	Control Events	Control Total	Weight	Risk ratio IV, random, 95% CI	Risk ratio IV, random, 95% CI
Total (95% CI)		469		389	100.0%	0.74 [0.56, 0.97]	
Total events	110		112				

Heterogeneity: tau^2 = 0.06; chi^2 = 24.00, df = 13 (P = 0.03); I^2 = 46%

Test for overall effect: Z = 2.15 (P = 0.03)

Test for subgroup differences: chi^2 = 5.22, df = 2 (P = 0.07), I^2 = 61.7%

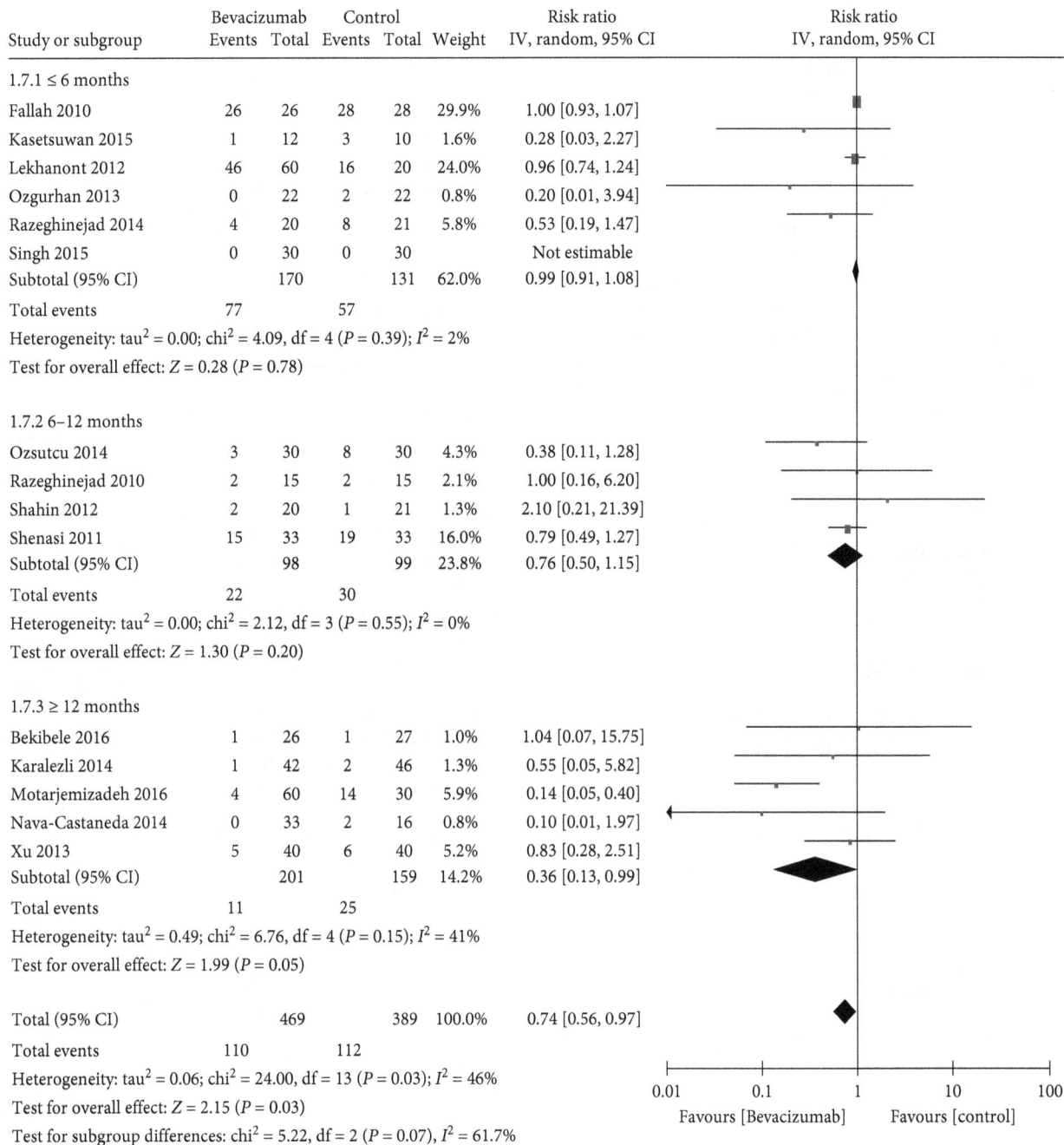

FIGURE 4: Subgroup analysis for the recurrence rates according to the follow-up time (n = 15, the remainder 3 studies without recurrence).

Our study had several potential limitations. First, the heterogeneity may result from different administration route of bevacizumab, different type of pterygium, surgeon's experience, and follow-up duration. Second, sensitivity analyses of the recurrence rate were not stable. Therefore, caution is required in their interpretation and more research is still needed.

Despite these limitations, the evidence from the updated meta-analysis shows that bevacizumab application following pterygium surgery provides a statistically significant decrease in recurrence rate in cases of primary pterygium, or use of conjunctival autograft, or follow-up longer than 12 months without an increase in complications. Further study of the long-term efficacy of bevacizumab on reducing pterygium recurrence based on the definition of true recurrence (grade 4) will be needed.

Disclosure

The funding organization played no role in the design or conduct of this study.

Conflicts of Interest

The authors declare that there are no conflicts of interest regarding the publication of this paper.

Authors' Contributions

Yi Sun and Bowen Zhang contributed equally.

Acknowledgments

The study was supported by Guangdong Natural Science Foundation (2016A030313208).

References

[1] J. Chui, N. Di Girolamo, D. Wakefield, and M. T. Coroneo, "The pathogenesis of pterygium: current concepts and their therapeutic implications," *Ocular Surface*, vol. 6, pp. 24–43, 2008.

[2] D. Hacıoğlu and H. Erdöl, "Developments and current approaches in the treatment of pterygium," *International Ophthalmology*, vol. 37, pp. 1073–1081, 2017.

[3] N. Verma, J. A. Garap, R. Maris, and A. Kerek, "Intraoperative use of mitomycin C in the treatment of recurrent pterygium," *Papua and New Guinea Medical Journal*, vol. 41, pp. 37–42, 1998.

[4] L. Mastropasqua, P. Carpineto, M. Ciancaglini, and P. Enrico Gallenga, "Long term results of intraoperative mitomycin C in the treatment of recurrent pterygium," *British Journal of Ophthalmology*, vol. 80, pp. 288–291, 1996.

[5] C. O. Bekibele, A. M. Baiyeroju, B. A. Olusanya, A. O. Ashaye, and T. S. Oluleye, "Pterygium treatment using 5-FU as adjuvant treatment compared to conjunctiva autograft," *Eye*, vol. 22, pp. 31–34, 2008.

[6] C. Akarsu, P. Taner, and A. Ergin, "5-fluorouracil as chemoadjuvant for primary pterygium surgery: preliminary report," *Cornea*, vol. 22, pp. 522–526, 2003.

[7] J. Pikkel, Y. Porges, and A. Ophir, "Halting pterygium recurrence by postoperative 5-fluorouracil," *Cornea*, vol. 20, pp. 168–171, 2001.

[8] T. Simşek, I. Günalp, and H. Atilla, "Comparative efficacy of β-irradiation and mitomycin-C in primary and recurrent pterygium," *European Journal of Ophthalmology*, vol. 11, pp. 126–132, 2001.

[9] B. G. Ajayi and C. O. Bekibele, "Evaluation of the effectiveness of post-operative beta-irradiation in the management of pterygium," *African Journal of Medicine and Medical Sciences*, vol. 31, pp. 9–11, 2002.

[10] D. H. Lee, H. J. Cho, J. T. Kim, J. S. Choi, and C. K. Joo, "Expression of vascular endothelial growth factor and inducible nitric oxide synthase in pterygia," *Cornea*, vol. 20, pp. 738–742, 2001.

[11] K. Gumus, S. Karakucuk, G. E. Mirza, H. Akgun, H. Arda, and A. O. Oner, "Overexpression of vascular endothelial growth factor receptor 2 in pterygia may have a predictive value for a higher postoperative recurrence rate," *British Journal of Ophthalmology*, vol. 98, pp. 796–800, 2014.

[12] J. Fukuhara, S. Kase, T. Ohashi et al., "Expression of vascular endothelial growth factor C in human pterygium," *Histochemistry and Cell Biology*, vol. 139, pp. 381–389, 2013.

[13] N. Di Girolamo, M. T. Coroneo, and D. Wakefield, "Active matrilysin (MMP-7) in human pterygia: potential role in angiogenesis," *Investigative Ophthalmology & Visual Science*, vol. 42, pp. 1963–1968, 2001.

[14] N. Di Girolamo, J. Chui, M. T. Coroneo, and D. Wakefield, "Pathogenesis of pterygia: role of cytokines, growth factors, and matrix metalloproteinases," *Progress in Retinal and Eye Research*, vol. 23, pp. 195–228, 2004.

[15] J. Jin, M. Guan, J. Sima et al., "Decreased pigment epithelium-derived factor and increased vascular endothelial growth factor levels in pterygia," *Cornea*, vol. 22, pp. 473–477, 2003.

[16] M. Aspiotis, E. Tsanou, S. Gorezis et al., "Angiogenesis in pterygium: study of microvessel density, vascular endothelial growth factor, and thrombospondin-1," *Eye*, vol. 21, pp. 1095–1101, 2007.

[17] M. R. Razeghinejad, H. Hosseini, F. Ahmadi, F. Rahat, and H. Eghbal, "Preliminary results of subconjunctival bevacizumab in primary pterygium excision," *Ophthalmic Research*, vol. 43, pp. 134–138, 2010.

[18] A. Shenasi, F. Mousavi, S. Shoa-Ahari, B. Rahimi-Ardabili, and R. F. Fouladi, "Subconjunctival bevacizumab immediately after excision of primary pterygium: the first clinical trial," *Cornea*, vol. 30, pp. 1219–1222, 2011.

[19] E. B. Ozgurhan, A. Agca, N. Kara, K. Yuksel, A. Demircan, and A. Demirok, "Topical application of bevacizumab as an adjunct to recurrent pterygium surgery," *Cornea*, vol. 32, pp. 835–838, 2013.

[20] A. Nava-Castañeda, O. Olvera-Morales, C. Ramos-Castellon, L. Garnica-Hayashi, and Y. Garfias, "Randomized controlled trial of conjunctival autografting combined with subconjunctival bevacizumab for primary pterygium treatment: one

year follow-up," *Clinical & Experimental Ophthalmology*, vol. 42, pp. 235–241, 2014.

[21] K. Lekhanont, T. Patarakittam, P. Thongphiew, O. Suwan-apichon, and P. Hanutsaha, "Randomized controlled trial of subconjunctival bevacizumab injection in impending recurrent pterygium: a pilot study," *Cornea*, vol. 31, pp. 155–161, 2012.

[22] M. R. Fallah, K. Khosravi, M. N. Hashemian, A. H. Beheshtnezhad, M. T. Rajabi, and M. Gohari, "Efficacy of topical bevacizumab for inhibiting growth of impending recurrent pterygium," *Current Eye Research*, vol. 35, pp. 17–22, 2010.

[23] M. M. Shahin, A. M. Elbendary, and M. M. Elwan, "Intraoperative subconjunctival bevacizumab as an adjunctive treatment in primary pterygium: a preliminary report," *Ophthalmic Surgery, Lasers, and Imaging*, vol. 43, pp. 459–466, 2012.

[24] M. Banifatemi, M. R. Razeghinejad, H. Hosseini, and A. Gholampour, "Bevacizumab and ocular wound healing after primary pterygium excision," *Journal of Ocular Pharmacology and Therapeutics*, vol. 27, pp. 17–21, 2011.

[25] O. Enkvetchakul, O. Thanathanee, R. Rangsin, K. Lekhanont, and O. Suwan-Apichon, "A randomized controlled trial of intralesional bevacizumab injection on primary pterygium: preliminary results," *Cornea*, vol. 30, pp. 1213–1218, 2011.

[26] M. R. Razeghinejad and M. Banifatemi, "Subconjunctival bevacizumab for primary pterygium excision;a randomized clinical trial," *Journal of Ophthalmic & Vision Research*, vol. 9, pp. 22–30, 2014.

[27] M. Ozsutcu, E. Ayintap, J. C. Akkan, A. Koytak, and C. Aras, "Repeated bevacizumab injections versus mitomycin C in rotational conjunctival flap for prevention of pterygium recurrence," *Indian Journal of Ophthalmology*, vol. 62, pp. 407–411, 2014.

[28] P. Singh, L. Sarkar, H. S. Sethi, and V. S. Gupta, "A randomized controlled prospective study to assess the role of subconjunctival bevacizumab in primary pterygium surgery in Indian patients," *Indian Journal of Ophthalmology*, vol. 63, pp. 779–784, 2015.

[29] N. Kasetsuwan, U. Reinprayoon, and V. Satitpitakul, "Prevention of recurrent pterygium with topical bevacizumab 0.05% eye drops: a randomized controlled trial," *Clinical Therapeutics*, vol. 37, pp. 2347–2351, 2015.

[30] S. Hwang and S. Choi, "A comparative study of topical mitomycin C, cyclosporine, and bevacizumab after primary pterygium surgery," *Korean Journal of Ophthalmology*, vol. 29, pp. 375–381, 2015.

[31] Q. Motarjemizadeh, N. S. Aidenloo, and S. Sepehri, "A comparative study of different concentrations of topical bevacizumab on the recurrence rate of excised primary pterygium: a short-term follow-up study," *International Ophthalmology*, vol. 36, pp. 63–71, 2016.

[32] C. O. Bekibele, T. F. Sarimiye, A. Ogundipe, and S. Olaniyan, "5-fluorouracil vs avastin as adjunct to conjunctival autograft in the surgical treatment of pterygium," *Eye*, vol. 30, pp. 515–521, 2016.

[33] Q. B. Xu, L. W. Zhu, and G. Z. Xu, "Comparative study of pterygium surgery combined with bevacizumab or mitomycin C," *International Eye Science*, vol. 13, pp. 2532–2534, 2013.

[34] A. Karalezli, C. Kucukerdonmez, Y. A. Akova, and B. E. Koktekir, "Does topical bevacizumab prevent postoperative recurrence after pterygium surgery with conjunctival autografting?," *International Journal of Ophthalmology*, vol. 7, pp. 512–516, 2014.

[35] Q. Hu, Y. Qiao, X. Nie, X. Cheng, and Y. Ma, "Bevacizumab in the treatment of pterygium: a meta-analysis," *Cornea*, vol. 33, pp. 154–160, 2014.

[36] P. Prabhasawat, K. Barton, G. Burkett, and S. C. Tseng, "Comparison of conjunctival autografts, amniotic membrane grafts, and primary closure for pterygium excision," *Ophthalmology*, vol. 104, pp. 974–985, 1997.

[37] R. Razeghinejad, M. Banifatemi, and H. Hosseini, "The effect of different doses of subconjunctival bevacizumab on the recurrence rate of excised primary pterygium," *Bulletin of the Belgian Societies of Ophthalmology*, vol. 322, pp. 13–20, 2013.

22

Changes and Diurnal Variation of Visual Quality after Orthokeratology in Myopic Children

Hao-Chen Guo ⓘ, **Wan-Qing Jin** ⓘ, **An-Peng Pan, Qin-Mei Wang, Jia Qu, and A-Yong Yu**

The Eye Hospital of Wenzhou Medical University, Wenzhou, Zhejiang, China

Correspondence should be addressed to A-Yong Yu; yaybetter@hotmail.com

Academic Editor: José M. Gonzalez-Méijome

Purpose. To assess the changes and the diurnal variation of visual quality after orthokeratology in myopic children. *Methods.* Forty-four eyes of 22 subjects with a mean age of 10.55 ± 1.53 years (8 to 14 years) were enrolled in this prospective study. Their spherical equivalent ranged from -1.25 to -4.25 diopters (D) and astigmatism was less than 1.00 D. Parameters including corneal curvature, ocular objective scatter index (OSI), the modulation transfer function (MTF), root mean square of ocular and corneal wavefront aberrations, and contrast sensitivity function (CSF) were measured before and at two time points during the same day after 1 month of orthokeratology. *Results.* After orthokeratology, uncorrected visual acuity (UCVA) and spherical equivalent were significantly improved from baseline ($P < 0.001$), and their diurnal variation was not significant ($P = 0.083, 0.568$). OSI increased from 0.29 ± 0.15 to 0.65 ± 0.31 ($P < 0.001$). MTF decreased significantly ($P < 0.01$). Corneal curvature and ocular total aberration decreased ($P < 0.001$), while the ocular and corneal higher-order aberration increased significantly ($P < 0.01$). The CSF under photopic condition decreased at 3 cpd ($P = 0.006$) and increased at 18 cpd ($P = 0.012$). The diurnal variation of CSF at 18 cpd under mesopic and high glare conditions and at 12 cpd under photopic condition was significant ($P = 0.002, 0.01, 0.017$). *Conclusions.* Orthokeratology can effectively improve UCVA and high spatial frequency CSF by decreasing the low-order aberrations. However, MTF and CSF at low spatial frequency decreased because of the increase of intraocular scattering and high-order aberrations. Meanwhile, CSF at high spatial frequency fluctuates significantly at two times during the same day after 1 month orthokeratology.

1. Introduction

Orthokeratology involves wearing of specially designed gas-permeable contact lenses which temporarily reshape corneal contour [1]. This procedure can offer patients useful vision during waking hours without involving additional corrective devices, such as spectacles or daily wear contact lenses. However, unstable vision during waking hours, transient light distortion under low-light condition, and dissatisfied night vision were reported by certain patients [2]. Several studies have demonstrated that overnight orthokeratology may increase corneal and ocular higher order aberrations [3–5] and decrease contrast sensitivity function (CSF) [4–6]. Furthermore, several short-term studies have reported that the influence of orthokeratology on refraction and visual acuity gradually diminished during the day once the lens was removed [7–10], which may cause uncomfortable visual experience as mentioned above. These studies focus mostly

on wavefront aberration, visual acuity, and refraction. However, these assessments are insufficient to fully understand the effects of orthokeratology on visual quality because retinal image is affected not only by ocular aberration but also by intraocular scattering [11, 12].

Research based on double-pass technique have revealed that the retinal image quality may be overestimated by aberrometric techniques which often failed to take the effect of diffuse light (dispersion or scattering) into account, and the double-pass system has been proven to be a useful tool for comprehensive evaluation of optical quality of the eye because it can provide parameters that included intraocular scattering [12–14]. There were few studies using double-pass technique to evaluate the visual quality after orthokeratology. Jeon et al. [15] used the double-pass system in 13 patients (24 eyes) and found that the intraocular scattering increased after 1 month of orthokeratology lenses wear. However, that study did not involve the diurnal variation of visual quality. Recent studies suggested that the combined effect of ocular aberration and intraocular scattering on the visual quality was not a simple summation, and the peripheral aberration could compromise partial effect of scattering [16]. The study on contact lenses using the double-pass technique found that corneal swelling caused increased intraocular scattering, resulting in a significant impact on the optical quality of the eye [17]. Currently, limited data were available on the changes and diurnal variation of comprehensive visual quality after orthokeratology in myopic children. This study aimed to provide information on changes and diurnal variation of visual quality after orthokeratology by analyzing the data of refraction, intraocular scattering, corneal topography, wavefront aberration, CSF, and subjective questionnaire. The comprehensive measurements of these changes are essential for a better understanding of the impact of orthokeratology on vision, especially in children.

2. Methods

In this prospective study, 44 eyes of 22 myopic patients (9 boys, 13 girls) with a mean age of 10.55 ± 1.53 yrs (mean ± standard deviation, range: 8 to 14 yrs) were enrolled. Spherical equivalent ranged from -1.25 to -4.25 D (-2.81 ± 0.87 D), and astigmatism was less than 1.00 D (0.48 ± 0.21 D). The best corrected visual acuity (BCVA) was 20/20 or better. After 1 month of orthokeratology, only eyes with an uncorrected visual acuity (UCVA) of 20/20 or better were included. Subjects with a history of contact lens wear or any current ocular or systemic disease such as a significant dry eye, papillary conjunctivitis, keratoconus, corneal dystrophies, and corneal opacities that could affect ocular physiology were excluded. This study was in accordance with the tenets of the Declaration of Helsinki and approved by the Ethics Committee at the Eye Hospital of Wenzhou Medical University. Informed consent was obtained from each subject and patient.

The baseline measurements were taken in both eyes before orthokeratology lens fitting in the morning at the initial visit, including visual acuity (logarithmic visual acuity chart, GB 11533—1989), manifest refraction (Phoroptor, Phorovist 200), corneal curvature (Keratometer, OM-4), noncontact tonometer (Nidek NT-2000), corneal topography (E300 Corneal Topographer), corneal endothelial count (Topcon, SP-2000P), and axial length (IOL-MASTER, Zeiss). For each subject, the best suitable orthokeratology lens was chosen from three brands (Table 1) according to the different fitting situations. The subjects were recommended to wear the lenses 7 nights a week and at least 8 hours per night to ensure the best situation of UCVA. All the subjects were monitored by the same experienced doctor. One month after orthokeratology, the measurements were taken immediately following lens removal in the morning and 8 hours later in the afternoon during the same day. At every visit, all the measurements were taken within 30 minutes to minimize the fluctuation of each parameter.

2.1. Double-Pass Measurements. The objective parameters of optical quality were measured by a double-pass optical quality

analysis system (OQAS II, Visiometrics S.L., Tarrasa, Spain). A single light source produced by a 780 nm laser beam adequately filtered and collimated was used as a starting point. The beam image was projected onto the eye retina. When it reflects on the retina, the light crosses the ocular medium twice and OQAS II analyses the size and shape of the reflected point of light [14]. Room illumination was kept low during the measurement to ensure a natural pupil diameter larger than 5 mm without dilation. The measurements were taken with artificial pupil diameters of 3, 4, and 5 mm, respectively. Astigmatism >0.50 D was corrected by using external ophthalmic cylindrical lenses. The main parameters provided by the double-pass system were the modulation transfer function (MTF) cut-off frequency in cycles per degree (cpd), Strehl ratio (SR), OQAS values (OVs) 100%, 20%, and 9%, objective scatter index (OSI), and tear film mean OSI (TFM-OSI). Three consecutive measurements were obtained for each eye and the mean value was calculated.

2.2. Wavefront Aberration Measurements. Wavefront aberrations and treatment zone after orthokeratology were measured with Nidek OPD-Scan III (Nidek Technologies, Gamagori, Japan) (based on automatic retinoscopy; provides integrated corneal topography and wavefront measurement in one device) [18]. Ocular and corneal wavefront aberrations for a 3, 4, or 5 mm optical zone across the undilated pupil were measured. Data were expanded with the normalized Zernike polynomials up to the eighth order. Magnitudes of the coefficients of the Zernike polynomials were represented as the root mean square (RMS). Total aberration, higher-order aberration, third- to eighth-order coefficient, astigmatism, spherical aberration, coma, trefoil, and tetrafoil were measured and analyzed separately. Horizontal and vertical diameters across the center of treatment zone (corneal refractive power within 45.0 D) were measured from the instantaneous map of cornea provided by OPD-Scan III (Figure 1) and the average was used. Measurements were repeated at least five times for each eye, and the three best-focused images were selected. The average values were used for subsequent analysis.

2.3. Contrast Sensitivity Function. CSF was measured under mesopic (2.7 cd/m^2) and photopic (85 cd/m^2) conditions, with and without high glare (CSV-1000E, VectorVision, Greenville Ohio, USA). CSF under mesopic conditions was measured in dark room and first tested without glare and then with glare. The combination of contrast and glare test was performed with halogen glare lights positioned at the sides of the console. The glare lights did not alter the illumination of the console. Monocular measurements were taken at 2.5 m distance with the best spectacle correction before orthokeratology and without correction after orthokeratology. The contrast threshold in logarithmic values for 3, 6, 12, and 18 cpd and the area under the log CSF (AULCSF) were used for subsequent analysis [19].

2.4. Subjective Questionnaire. Quality of Life Impact of Refractive Correction (QIRC) [20] was used to evaluate the

TABLE 1: The orthokeratology lens parameters in this study.

Brand	E&E	Euclid	Lucid
Origin	China	USA	Korea
Material	Boston XO	Boston equalens II	Boston XO
Dk (cm^2/sec) ($mL \cdot O_2$/mL·mmHg) (ISO/fatt)	$100 * 10^{-11}$	$90 * 10^{-11}$	$140 * 10^{-11}$
The overall diameter (mm)	10.6	10.6	10.6
The optic zone diameter (mm)	6	6.2	6.2
The reverse curve (mm)	0.6	0.5	0.9
The anchor curve (mm)	1.3	1.2	0.8
The peripheral curve (mm)	0.4	0.5	0.5
The central thickness (mm)	0.22	0.22	0.23

subjective vision experience by the same ophthalmologist. Each subject was tested twice separately before and 1 month after orthokeratology.

2.5. Statistical Analysis. All statistical analyses were performed using SPSS 18.0 (SPSS Inc, Chicago, Illinois, USA). All continuous variables were expressed as the mean ± standard deviations (Mean ± SD). The normality of each variable was checked with the 1-sample Kolmogorov-Smirnov test. Comparisons of the parameters before and after orthokeratology and between morning and afternoon on the same day were performed by using a paired t-test. The level of significance was P less than 0.05.

3. Results

Among the 22 children who were enrolled at baseline, 3 of them dropped out of the study because their UCVA did not achieve 20/20 due to the decentration of orthokeratology lens. Among the 19 children, 4 subjects finished partial measurements due to poor cooperation.

One month after orthokeratology, LogMAR UCVA in the morning (−0.066 ± 0.09) was significantly improved from baseline (0.557 ± 0.23, $P < 0.001$) and did not differ from that in the afternoon (0.049 ± 0.05, $P = 0.083$).

Table 2 showed manifest sphere refraction and corneal curvature significantly reduced after orthokeratology ($P < 0.001$). Regular astigmatism did not change significantly ($P = 0.155$). The diurnal variation of corneal curvature was statistically significant ($P < 0.001$), but sphere refraction was not ($P = 0.568$).

One month after orthokeratology, OSI significantly increased from 0.295 ±0.15 to 0.652 ± 0.31 ($P < 0.001$), TFM-OSI increased from 0.572 ± 0.29 to 1.212 ± 0.97 ($P < 0.002$), MTF cut-off, SR, and OVs decreased significantly ($P < 0.033$). The diurnal variation of these parameters was not significant (Table 3).

Tables 4 and 5 showed ocular and corneal aberrations respectively. One month after orthokeratology, ocular total aberration decreased significantly ($P < 0.001$). Ocular higher-order aberration, corneal total aberration, and corneal higher-order aberration increased significantly ($P < 0.01$) (Figures 2 and 3). Ocular and corneal coma, trefoil, tetrafoil, and spherical aberrations for 3, 4, and 5 mm optical zone increased significantly, except the ocular sixth- to eighth-order aberrations for 3 mm optical zone. The

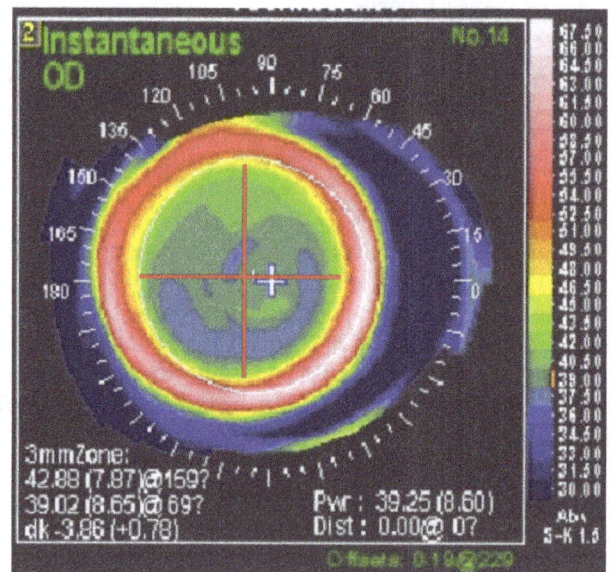

FIGURE 1: Instantaneous map. *The instantaneous map calculates the corneal curvature radiuses from the shape between the infinitesimal intervals along meridians reflecting more local corneal curvatures (shapes).

TABLE 2: Effects of orthokeratology on refraction and corneal curvature ($n = 22$ eyes, mean ± SD).

Time	Sphere (D)	Cylinder (D)	K1 (D)	K2 (D)
AM baseline	−3.83 ± 0.97	−0.47 ± 0.43	42.05 ± 1.26	43.19 ± 1.37
AM 1 month	−1.03 ± 0.85	−0.69 ± 0.57	39.75 ± 0.97	40.64 ± 1.27
PM 1 month	−1.10 ± 0.68	−0.66 ± 0.52	40.02 ± 1.05	40.95 ± 1.27
P1	<0.001	0.155	<0.001	<0.001
P2	0.568	0.500	<0.001	<0.001

Paired t-test. P1: comparison between AM baseline and AM 1 month after orthokeratology; P2: comparison between AM and PM during the same day 1 month after orthokeratology; K1: flat keratometric value; K2: steep keratometric value.

diurnal variation of aberrations was not significant, except ocular spherical aberration for 3 mm optical zone ($P = 0.03$). Treatment zone diameters (TZD) decreased from 4.12 ± 0.18 mm to 3.95 ± 0.23 mm ($P = 0.001$), and the average change was 0.16 ± 0.13 mm.

TABLE 3: Effects of orthokeratology on OSI, TFM-OSI, MTF cut-off, SR, and OVs (n = 22 eyes, mean ± SD).

Time	OSI	TFM-OSI	MTF	SR	OVs-100%	OVs-20%	OVs-9%
3 mm optical zone							
AM baseline	—	—	48.332 ± 8.10	0.309 ± 0.07	1.611 ± 0.27	1.778 ± 0.40	1.922 ± 0.49
AM 1 month	—	—	38.812 ± 9.58	0.225 ± 0.07	1.294 ± 0.32	1.292 ± 0.41	1.316 ± 0.46
PM 1 month	—	—	42.225 ± 8.93	0.250 ± 0.07	1.408 ± 0.30	1.448 ± 0.42	1.489 ± 0.48
P1	—	—	<0.001	<0.001	<0.001	<0.001	<0.001
P2	—	—	0.067	0.064	0.068	0.053	0.068
4 mm optical zone							
AM baseline	0.295 ± 0.15	0.572 ± 0.29	46.089 ± 7.26	0.280 ± 0.05	1.537 ± 0.24	1.652 ± 0.35	1.733 ± 0.38
AM 1 month	0.652 ± 0.31	1.212 ± 0.97	37.312 ± 8.16	0.211 ± 0.05	1.244 ± 0.27	1.216 ± 0.33	1.233 ± 0.35
PM 1 month	0.712 ± 0.43	1.128 ± 0.59	38.856 ± 9.55	0.223 ± 0.06	1.295 ± 0.32	1.300 ± 0.41	1.325 ± 0.45
P1	<0.001	0.002	<0.001	<0.001	<0.001	<0.001	<0.001
P2	0.239	0.63	0.32	0.169	0.326	0.204	0.189
5 mm optical zone							
AM baseline	—	—	44.812 ± 8.87	0.275 ± 0.06	1.494 ± 0.30	1.602 ± 0.40	1.687 ± 0.46
AM 1 month	—	—	37.174 ± 7.96	0.215 ± 0.05	1.239 ± 0.27	1.209 ± 0.32	1.243 ± 0.36
PM 1 month	—	—	39.124 ± 10.37	0.224 ± 0.06	1.304 ± 0.35	1.322 ± 0.44	1.339 ± 0.44
P1	—	—	0.003	0.001	0.003	0.001	0.001
P2	—	—	0.177	0.294	0.178	0.051	0.109

Paired *t*-test. P1: comparison between AM baseline and AM 1 month after orthokeratology; P2: comparison between AM and PM during the same day 1 month after orthokeratology.

TABLE 4: Effects of orthokeratology on ocular aberrations (n = 22 eyes, mean ± SD).

Time	Coma	Trefoil	Tetrafoil	Sph	S3	S4	S5	S6	S7	S8
3 mm optical zone										
Baseline AM	0.019 ± 0.01	0.044 ± 0.02	0.023 ± 0.01	−0.004 ± 0.01	0.050 ± 0.02	0.028 ± 0.01	0.017 ± 0.01	0.017 ± 0.01	0.013 ± 0.01	0.011 ± 0.01
1 month AM	0.049 ± 0.03	0.077 ± 0.04	0.037 ± 0.02	0.019 ± 0.02	0.099 ± 0.04	0.050 ± 0.02	0.029 ± 0.02	0.025 ± 0.02	0.018 ± 0.01	0.015 ± 0.01
1 month PM	0.052 ± 0.03	0.081 ± 0.05	0.030 ± 0.03	0.023 ± 0.01	0.101 ± 0.06	0.046 ± 0.03	0.027 ± 0.02	0.019 ± 0.01	0.015 ± 0.01	0.013 ± 0.01
P1	<0.001	0.002	0.005	<0.001	<0.001	<0.001	<0.001	0.11	0.081	0.235
P2	0.618	0.665	0.216	0.03	0.799	0.331	0.752	0.233	0.409	0.428
4 mm optical zone										
Baseline AM	0.043 ± 0.02	0.081 ± 0.03	0.035 ± 0.02	−0.010 ± 0.02	0.095 ± 0.03	0.047 ± 0.02	0.033 ± 0.01	0.028 ± 0.01	0.022 ± 0.01	0.018 ± 0.01
1 month AM	0.196 ± 0.09	0.136 ± 0.08	0.072 ± 0.03	0.099 ± 0.06	0.256 ± 0.10	0.143 ± 0.06	0.087 ± 0.04	0.060 ± 0.03	0.039 ± 0.03	0.033 ± 0.03
1 month PM	0.210 ± 0.08	0.145 ± 0.08	0.062 ± 0.05	0.108 ± 0.04	0.264 ± 0.10	0.141 ± 0.06	0.083 ± 0.05	0.046 ± 0.02	0.031 ± 0.02	0.026 ± 0.02
P1	<0.001	0.005	<0.001	<0.001	<0.001	<0.001	<0.001	0.001	0.007	0.017
P2	0.158	0.634	0.417	0.14	0.587	0.839	0.672	0.116	0.282	0.329
5 mm optical zone										
Baseline AM	0.091 ± 0.05	0.129 ± 0.04	0.059 ± 0.03	−0.019 ± 0.05	0.166 ± 0.05	0.091 ± 0.04	0.064 ± 0.03	0.047 ± 0.03	0.039 ± 0.02	0.032 ± 0.02
1 month AM	0.532 ± 0.26	0.223 ± 0.10	0.120 ± 0.06	0.333 ± 0.16	0.603 ± 0.26	0.393 ± 0.15	0.181 ± 0.09	0.112 ± 0.05	0.082 ± 0.05	0.065 ± 0.04
1 month PM	0.540 ± 0.24	0.222 ± 0.10	0.093 ± 0.07	0.328 ± 0.14	0.602 ± 0.24	0.373 ± 0.14	0.157 ± 0.08	0.095 ± 0.05	0.074 ± 0.04	0.051 ± 0.03
P1	<0.001	<0.001	<0.001	<0.001	<0.001	<0.001	<0.001	<0.001	0.001	0.002
P2	0.762	0.969	0.181	0.73	0.968	0.224	0.238	0.233	0.536	0.213

Paired *t*-test. P1: comparison between AM baseline and AM 1 month after orthokeratology; P2: comparison between AM and PM during the same day 1 month after orthokeratology.

Changes in AULCSF under mesopic, photopic, and high glare conditions were not statistically significant before and after orthokeratology. The log CSF under photopic condition increased at 18 cpd (P = 0.012), but decreased at 3 cpd (P = 0.006). AULCSF under high glare and photopic conditions, log CSF at 18 cpd under mesopic and high glare conditions, log CSF at 12 cpd under photopic condition all increased significantly in the

TABLE 5: Effects of orthokeratology on corneal aberrations ($n = 22$ eyes, mean ± SD).

Time	Coma	Trefoil	Tetrafoil	Sph	S3	S4	S5	S6	S7	S8
3 mm optical zone										
Baseline AM	0.048 ± 0.02	0.143 ± 0.05	0.105 ± 0.05	0.009 ± 0.01	0.155 ± 0.05	0.140 ± 0.05	0.091 ± 0.03	0.102 ± 0.03	0.063 ± 0.02	0.071 ± 0.02
1 month AM	0.120 ± 0.09	0.210 ± 0.14	0.171 ± 0.10	0.026 ± 0.03	0.251 ± 0.16	0.243 ± 0.16	0.162 ± 0.10	0.184 ± 0.12	0.104 ± 0.06	0.129 ± 0.09
1 month PM	0.109 ± 0.11	0.202 ± 0.14	0.170 ± 0.09	0.027 ± 0.02	0.242 ± 0.17	0.235 ± 0.15	0.149 ± 0.10	0.176 ± 0.12	0.097 ± 0.07	0.123 ± 0.09
P1	0.002	0.047	0.011	0.003	0.015	0.005	0.005	0.003	0.01	0.004
P2	0.663	0.836	0.946	0.924	0.825	0.81	0.616	0.77	0.666	0.761
4 mm optical zone										
Baseline AM	0.121 ± 0.05	0.452 ± 0.21	0.310 ± 0.11	0.038 ± 0.02	0.482 ± 0.19	0.413 ± 0.12	0.335 ± 0.11	0.314 ± 0.09	0.278 ± 0.12	0.221 ± 0.06
1 month AM	0.534 ± 0.39	0.673 ± 0.42	0.604 ± 0.35	0.198 ± 0.17	0.903 ± 0.53	0.820 ± 0.46	0.657 ± 0.32	0.641 ± 0.35	0.468 ± 0.26	0.440 ± 0.24
1 month PM	0.409 ± 0.40	0.561 ± 0.31	0.494 ± 0.34	0.200 ± 0.10	0.733 ± 0.49	0.696 ± 0.43	0.555 ± 0.30	0.533 ± 0.38	0.365 ± 0.25	0.357 ± 0.21
P1	<0.001	0.036	<0.001	<0.001	0.002	<0.001	<0.001	<0.001	0.004	<0.001
P2	0.056	0.192	0.181	0.923	0.101	0.237	0.12	0.192	0.055	0.149
5 mm optical zone										
Baseline AM	0.411 ± 0.37	0.439 ± 0.39	0.330 ± 0.32	0.099 ± 0.15	0.668 ± 0.46	0.490 ± 0.45	0.645 ± 0.45	0.366 ± 0.30	0.497 ± 0.27	0.253 ± 0.20
1 month AM	1.016 ± 0.42	1.175 ± 0.66	0.858 ± 0.53	0.451 ± 0.33	1.644 ± 0.62	1.454 ± 0.67	1.412 ± 0.69	1.266 ± 0.84	1.205 ± 0.83	1.042 ± 0.59
1 month PM	1.231 ± 1.39	0.956 ± 1.12	0.738 ± 0.71	0.408 ± 0.37	1.629 ± 1.77	1.388 ± 1.38	1.182 ± 1.28	0.993 ± 0.99	0.918 ± 0.92	0.823 ± 0.89
P1	<0.001	<0.001	<0.001	<0.001	<0.001	<0.001	<0.001	<0.001	0.001	<0.001
P2	0.474	0.443	0.528	0.636	0.971	0.844	0.485	0.346	0.296	0.292

Paired *t*-test. P1: comparison between AM baseline and AM 1 month after orthokeratology; P2: comparison between AM and PM during the same day 1 month after orthokeratology.

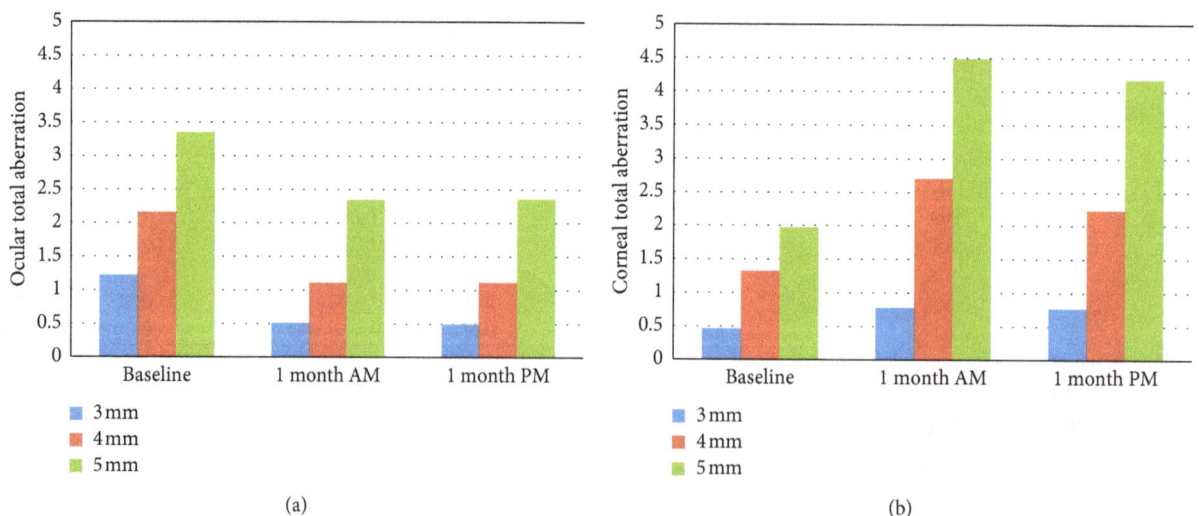

FIGURE 2: Effects of orthokeratology on ocular and corneal total aberrations ($n = 22$ eyes).

afternoon compared to the parameters in the morning at 1 month. Besides the above mentioned, no significant diurnal variation was found for other parameters of CSF (Table 6).

The survey of the subjective questionnaire showed that the dry eye symptom was more remarkable after orthokeratology ($P = 0.03$), nevertheless the feeling of asthenopia was relieved ($P = 0.01$). The mean score of satisfaction to orthokeratology was 92.25. During the whole day and night, self-reported vision was stable in 10 children (45%), 1 subject (5%) had a fluctuating vision, and 11 children (50%) reported that the vision in the morning was better than that in the evening.

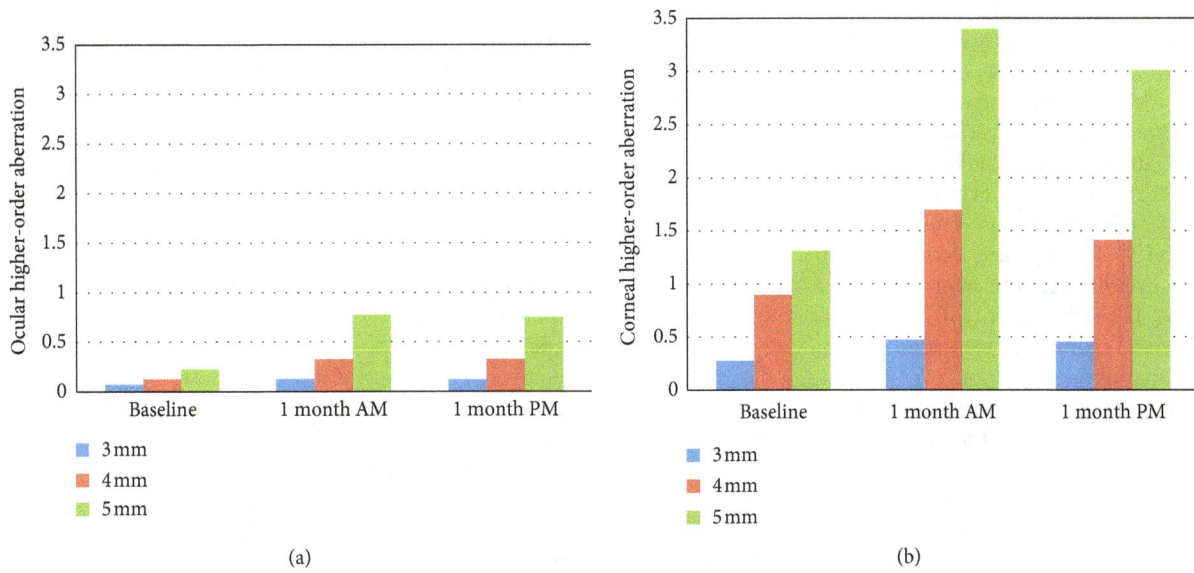

FIGURE 3: Effects of orthokeratology on ocular and corneal higher-order aberrations ($n = 22$ eyes).

TABLE 6: Effects of orthokeratology on contrast sensitive function ($n = 22$ eyes, mean ± SD).

Time	3 cpd	6 cpd	12 cpd	18 cpd	AULCSF
			Mesopic		
AM baseline	1.620 ± 0.19	1.677 ± 0.17	1.552 ± 0.21	1.266 ± 0.37	1.245 ± 0.10
AM 1 month	1.606 ± 0.16	1.700 ± 0.26	1.573 ± 0.29	1.272 ± 0.36	1.257 ± 0.16
PM 1 month	1.632 ± 0.12	1.706 ± 0.21	1.551 ± 0.34	1.408 ± 0.38	1.267 ± 0.15
P1	0.706	0.634	0.7	0.913	0.659
P2	0.342	0.87	0.654	0.002	0.655
			High glare		
AM baseline	1.636 ± 0.25	1.686 ± 0.24	1.483 ± 0.25	1.267 ± 0.37	1.235 ± 0.13
AM 1 month	1.577 ± 0.20	1.669 ± 0.32	1.517 ± 0.28	1.338 ± 0.35	1.235 ± 0.19
PM 1 month	1.613 ± 0.18	1.746 ± 0.22	1.562 ± 0.31	1.431 ± 0.38	1.285 ± 0.14
P1	0.19	0.787	0.514	0.233	0.992
P2	0.387	0.086	0.226	0.01	0.018
			Photopic		
AM baseline	1.722 ± 0.17	1.657 ± 0.21	1.57 ± 0.29	1.266 ± 0.36	1.251 ± 0.13
AM 1 month	1.631 ± 0.14	1.716 ± 0.28	1.59 ± 0.27	1.397 ± 0.37	1.279 ± 0.17
PM 1 month	1.678 ± 0.14	1.775 ± 0.19	1.67 ± 0.22	1.430 ± 0.38	1.326 ± 0.11
P1	0.006	0.317	0.746	0.012	0.431
P2	0.115	0.129	0.017	0.371	0.01

Paired t-test. P1: comparison between AM baseline and AM 1 month after orthokeratology; P2: comparison between AM and PM during the same day 1 month after orthokeratology.

4. Discussion

Orthokeratology can reduce the refractive error by remodeling the anterior surface of cornea temporarily [21]. With the improvement of refraction, the low-order aberrations, which constituted 80%~85% of the ocular total aberration, reduced. Therefore, UCVA could be 20/20 or better after orthokeratology, as demonstrated in this study that most children whose best corrected visual acuity were 20/20 with spectacles before orthokeratology achieved 20/20 or better UCVA after 1 month of orthokeratology. Some research [22–24] indicated that orthokeratology could improve UCVA effectively. In addition, the increase of high

spatial frequency CSF may be due to the improvement of UCVA after 1 month of orthokeratology because the high spatial frequency CSF mainly reflected the central macular vision. Furthermore, the improvement of vision and self-confidence after removal of spectacles as psychological and physiological factors may play a role. Nichols et al. [25] discovered that the changes of visual and refractive outcomes became stable around 1 month after orthokeratology. Soni et al. [23] even indicated that full effect of orthokeratology was achieved by the end of 1 week and remain stable for all waking hours of the day. Kang et al. [26] demonstrated that cornea experienced regression of correcting effects in the initial period of orthokeratology. This regression caused decline of visual acuity in the afternoon as corneal asphericity returns. However, the diurnal variation stabilized by 1 month. According to our results, the area of treatment zone at PM was smaller than that at AM, suggesting that the cornea had shape regression. Also, the diurnal variation of corneal curvature was statistically significant. However, the mean diurnal variation of flat and steep corneal curvature within 8 hours after lens removal was 0.27 D and 0.31 D, respectively. Taking into account that the axial length of normal eyes in the afternoon is shorter than that in the morning [27], the extent of diurnal variation of corneal shape after 1 month of orthokeratology had no influence on either manifest refraction or UCVA, indicating that orthokeratology was effective to improve UCVA and the effect was stable after 1 month of lens wear in myopic children.

However, the objective measurements revealed that the optical quality declined after orthokeratology. The value of MTF cut-off, SR, and OVs decreased. Overnight orthokeratology may cause midperipheral stromal thickening [28]. De Juan et al. [17] demonstrated that corneal swelling had a significant impact on the optical quality of the eye. The OSI significantly increased after orthokeratology. Jeon et al. [15] found that OSI increased after orthokeratology but still less than 1.0 on average, which is within the normal range [29]. This was consistent with our results and indicated that the visual quality can remain relatively good despite the slight increasing of intraocular scattering after orthokeratology. In our study, the mean value of OSI for all the myopic children was 0.29 ± 0.15 before orthokeratology, which was better than the result reported by Martínez-Roda et al. (0.38 ± 0.19) [29]. This may be due to the discrepancy of age distribution between the two studies. The intraocular scatter usually increased with age [30]. Furthermore, the TFM-OSI increased, illustrating that the stability of tear film decreased after orthokeratology. The results of subjective questionnaire survey also demonstrated that orthokeratology increases dry eye symptoms (photophobia, dryness, etc.). The stability of tear film also influenced the visual quality.

Ocular higher-order aberration, corneal total aberration, and corneal higher-order aberration increased after orthokeratology in this study. This was consistent with the previously published studies [4, 6, 31]. Corneal refractive therapy significantly increased spherical aberration in the positive direction with an impact on visual quality [32], which was also consistent with our results. It was reported that contrast sensitivity function after orthokeratology deteriorated in proportion to the increases in higher-order aberration [4]. As a consequence, the low spatial frequency CSF decreased, especially the decrease of log CSF at 3 cpd had statistical significance. The decrease of low spatial frequency CSF may be due to the midperipheral corneal steepening in the process of wearing orthokeratology, which affected the imaging function of peripheral retina. Hiraoka et al. [4] researched a group of myopic adults (46 eyes of 23 patients) undergoing overnight orthokeratology and evaluated the change of CSF. They found that orthokeratology treatment resulted in statistically significant decrease of CSF at all spatial frequencies, and AULCSF was significantly

reduced from 1.451 ± 0.120 to 1.291 ± 0.177 ($P < 0.0001$). In the present study, the decrease of low spatial frequency CSF was consistent with the result of Hiraoka et al., but we found that AULCSF increased after orthokeratology and the high spatial frequency CSF increased in accordance with the improved UCVA [33]. Hiraoka et al. [34] mentioned that decentered orthokeratology lens could result in decreased CSF after treatment. All the subjects in our study who finished the follow-up were well fitted without obvious decentration of orthokeratology lenses, and this maybe the reason why the AULCSF did not decrease in this study. This indicated that orthokeratology influenced the low spatial frequency CSF, but did not compromise and even improve the high spatial frequency CSF. Lee et al. [35] reported that there were no statistically proved correlations between higher order aberrations and optical quality parameters (MTF cut-off and SR) for adults after refractive surgery. Whether the parameters of the myopic children with orthokeratology have the same outcomes needs further investigations.

In previous research, the corneal thickness [36], axial length, and intraocular pressure [37] showed diurnal changes in human eyes without orthokeratology treatment. Chakraborty et al. [38] indicated that ocular spherical aberration underwent statistically significant diurnal variation, i.e., spherical aberration was positive during the day and gradually became more negative toward the later afternoon/evening. They also found that the anterior corneal curvature was the flattest in the morning and gradually became steeper throughout the day, which led to a significant myopic refractive shift in spherical equivalent refraction later in the day, but it had an apparent paradoxical relationship with the fluctuation in axial length [27] (the longest axial length during the day and the shortest at night). All these physiological fluctuations may result in a compounded effect of visual quality in myopic children with orthokeratology treatment. In our study, the diurnal changes of objective parameters that already included the compounded influence of physiological fluctuations were stable. For 3 mm optical zone at 1 month, though the diurnal variation of ocular spherical aberration was significant (0.019 ± 0.016 μm AM and 0.023 ± 0.011 μm PM, $P = 0.03$), corneal spherical aberration had no significant difference between the two time points. This indicated that the change of ocular spherical aberration was not induced by cornea. Furthermore, the corneal higher-order aberration had no change between the two time points. However, the parameter of the range beyond 5 mm was not measured, so the slight change in the central 3 mm optical zone could not exclude the effect of the change of corneal shape beyond 5 mm range. Berntsen et al. [6] studied 20 myopic adults and found that the change of spherical aberration did not play an important role in the increasing of higher-order aberration for a 3 mm pupil. So we inferred that the diurnal change of spherical aberration might have no clinical significance. The CSF at 1 month PM was slightly better than that at 1 month AM, especially the high spatial frequency CSF increased significantly. This may be due to the quick disappearance of corneal edema after lens removal [10, 17], while the refractive regression was not significant in the afternoon.

The change of optical quality of orthokeratology was a combination of the reduced refraction, the increased intraocular scattering, and the change of ocular and corneal aberrations. Any of the factors was independent and also interrelated to influence the different spatial frequency of CSF and UCVA. David et al. [39] suggested that LASIK provided better visual quality outcomes than orthokeratology for the treatment of low-to-moderate myopia. For myopic adults, considering exclusively the visual quality results, LASIK was a better treatment option than orthokeratology. However, the ablation procedure of refractive surgery may increase ocular scattering [35] and the procedure was irreversible. For myopic children, whose eyes had not yet stopped growing, orthokeratology would be the better choice because the effect of orthokeratology was reversible with regard to optical quality of the eye [40] and the corneal morphology [41]. Furthermore, orthokeratology was a safe option for myopia retardation [42]. Queiros et al. [43] found that orthokeratology achieved the best score among the four treatments (LASIK, spectacle, soft contact lens, and orthokeratology) in the satisfaction for correction and appearance. In the present study, the subjective questionnaire survey on myopic children after orthokeratology indicated that the satisfaction was relatively high, and only three of the children had a transient complaint of light distortion. Santolaria Sanz et al. [44] reported that light distortion tends to return to baseline after one week of treatment, suggesting that neural adaptation is capable of overcoming optical quality degradation. However, still 50% of children consciously thought night vision was worse compared to the vision in the morning and 1 subject (5%) had a fluctuating vision. According to our results, the value of MTF cut-off, SR, and OVs decreased and the high-order aberrations increased with the expanding of pupil diameter. This indicated that visual quality descends under dark environment with larger pupil. The poor night vision may due to the combined effects of more refractive regression and larger pupil diameter at night. More aberration and scattering also resulted in the decrease of the nighttime visual quality. This study did not involve the visual quality at night and the continuous change within the 8 hours during the day was not assessed. Further research was needed to investigate the relationship between the dynamic change of cornea and the change of visual quality after orthokeratology. As the visual quality after orthokeratology was a result of multiple factors, we should not only see the advantage that it can improve UCVA and control the progress of myopia but also consider the declined visual quality and the discomfort complained by children after orthokeratology. Scientific and objective attitude toward the popularity of orthokeratology could serve the clinical practice better.

5. Conclusions

Orthokeratology can effectively improve UCVA and high spatial frequency CSF by decreasing the low-order aberrations. However, MTF and CSF at low spatial frequency decreased because of the increase of intraocular scattering and high-order aberrations. Meanwhile, CSF at high spatial frequency fluctuates significantly at two times during the same day after 1 month orthokeratology. All these significant influence on children's vision provided valuable clues for future lens design and clinical practice.

Disclosure

Drs. Hao-Chen Guo and Wan-Qing Jin are co-first authors of the article. Portions of the data were previously presented in a poster form at the 120th Annual AOA Congress and 47th Annual AOSA Conference: Optometry's Meeting, Washington, DC, June 21–25, 2017 (http://docplayer. net/53226091-poster-presentations-120th-annual-aoa-congress-47th-annual-aosa-conference-optometry-s-meeting.html).

Conflicts of Interest

The authors report no conflicts of interest and have no proprietary interest in any of the materials mentioned in this article.

Acknowledgments

This study is based on the work funded by Zhejiang Provincial Foundation of China for Distinguished Young Talents in Medicine and Health under Grant No. 2010QNA018 and Zhejiang Provincial Natural Science Foundation of China under Grant No. LY14H120007.

References

[1] H. A. Swarbrick, "Orthokeratology review and update," *Clinical and Experimental Optometry*, vol. 89, no. 3, pp. 124–143, 2006.

[2] E. Santolaria, A. Cervino, A. Queiros, R. Brautaset, and J. M. Gonzalez-Meijome, "Subjective satisfaction in long-term orthokeratology patients," *Eye & Contact Lens: Science & Clinical Practice*, vol. 39, no. 6, pp. 388–393, 2013.

[3] T. Hiraoka, A. Furuya, Y. Matsumoto et al., "Quantitative evaluation of regular and irregular corneal astigmatism in patients having overnight orthokeratology," *Journal of Cataract & Refractive Surgery*, vol. 30, no. 7, pp. 1425–1429, 2004.

[4] T. Hiraoka, C. Okamoto, Y. Ishii, T. Kakita, and T. Oshika, "Contrast sensitivity function and ocular higher-order aberrations following overnight orthokeratology," *Investigative Opthalmology & Visual Science*, vol. 48, no. 2, pp. 550–556, 2007.

[5] P. Gifford, M. Li, H. Lu, J. Miu, M. Panjaya, and H. A. Swarbrick, "Corneal versus ocular aberrations after overnight orthokeratology," *Optometry and Vision Science*, vol. 90, no. 5, pp. 439–447, 2013.

[6] D. A. Berntsen, J. T. Barr, and G. L. Mitchell, "The effect of overnight contact lens corneal reshaping on higher-order aberrations and best-corrected visual acuity," *Optometry and Vision Science*, vol. 82, no. 6, pp. 490–497, 2005.

[7] L. Sorbara, D. Fonn, T. Simpson, F. Lu, and R. Kort, "Reduction of myopia from corneal refractive therapy," *Optometry and Vision Science*, vol. 82, no. 6, pp. 512–518, 2005.

[8] J. T. Barr, M. J. Rah, W. Meyers, and J. Legerton, "Recovery of refractive error after corneal refractive therapy," *Eye &*

Contact Lens: Science & Clinical Practice, vol. 30, no. 4, pp. 247–251, 2004.

[9] P. S. Soni, T. T. Nguyen, and J. A. Bonanno, "Overnight orthokeratology: refractive and corneal recovery after discontinuation of reverse-geometry lenses," *Eye & Contact Lens: Science & Clinical Practice*, vol. 30, no. 4, pp. 254–262, 2004.

[10] S. Haque, D. Fonn, T. Simpson, and L. Jones, "Corneal and epithelial thickness changes after 4 weeks of overnight corneal refractive therapy lens wear, measured with optical coherence tomography," *Eye & Contact Lens: Science & Clinical Practice*, vol. 30, no. 4, pp. 189–193, 2004.

[11] P. Artal, "Understanding aberrations by using double-pass techniques," *Journal of Refractive Surgery*, vol. 16, no. 5, pp. S560–S562, 2000.

[12] F. Diaz-Douton, A. Benito, J. Pujol, M. Arjona, J. L. Gu¨ell, and P. Artal, "Comparison of the retinal image quality with a Hartmann-Shack wavefront sensor and a double-pass instrument," *Investigative Opthalmology & Visual Science*, vol. 47, no. 4, pp. 1710–1716, 2006.

[13] J. Santamaria, P. Artal, and J. Bescos, "Determination of the point-spread function of human eyes using a hybrid optical-digital method," *Journal of the Optical Society of America A*, vol. 4, no. 6, pp. 1109–1114, 1987.

[14] C. C. Xu, T. Xue, Q. M. Wang, Y.-N. Zhou, J.-H. Huang, and A.-Y. Yu, "Repeatability and reproducibility of a double-pass optical quality analysis device," *PLoS One*, vol. 10, no. 2, Article ID e0117587, 2015.

[15] H. M. Jeon, D. S. Ahn, D. J. Lee, S. J. Moon, and K. H. Lee, "The effects of overnight orthokeratology lens wear on ocular scatter," *Journal of the Korean Ophthalmological Society*, vol. 55, no. 11, p. 1595, 2014.

[16] G. M. Perez, S. Manzanera, and P. Artal, "Impact of scattering and spherical aberration in contrast sensitivity," *Journal of Vision*, vol. 9, no. 3, p. 19, 2009.

[17] V. De Juan, M. Aldaba, R. Martin, M. Vilaseca, J. M. Herreras, and J. Pujol, "Optical quality and intraocular scattering assessed with a double-pass system in eyes with contact lens induced corneal swelling," *Contact Lens and Anterior Eye*, vol. 37, no. 4, pp. 278–284, 2014.

[18] J. B. Won, S. W. Kim, E. K. Kim, B. J. Ha, and T.-I. Kim, "Comparison of internal and total optical aberrations for 2 aberrometers: iTrace and OPD scan," *Korean Journal of Ophthalmology*, vol. 22, no. 4, p. 210, 2008.

[19] R. A. Applegate, H. C. Howland, R. P. Sharp, A. J. Cottingham, and R. W. Yee, "Corneal aberrations and visual performance after radial keratotomy," *Journal of Refractive Surgery*, vol. 14, no. 4, pp. 397–407, 1998.

[20] K. Pesudovs, E. Garamendi, and D. B. Elliott, "The quality of life impact of refractive correction (QIRC) questionnaire: development and validation," *Optometry and Vision Science*, vol. 81, no. 10, pp. 769–777, 2004.

[21] A. Alharbi and H. A. Swarbrick, "The effects of overnight orthokeratology lens wear on corneal thickness," *Investigative Opthalmology & Visual Science*, vol. 44, no. 6, pp. 2518–2523, 2003.

[22] I. G. Stillitano, M. R. Chalita, P. Schor et al., "Corneal changes and wavefront analysis after orthokeratology fitting test," *American Journal of Ophthalmology*, vol. 144, no. 3, pp. 378–386, 2007.

[23] P. S. Soni, T. T. Nguyen, and J. A. Bonanno, "Overnight orthokeratology: visual and corneal changes," *Eye & Contact Lens: Science & Clinical Practice*, vol. 29, no. 3, pp. 137–145, 2003.

[24] K. L. Johnson, L. G. Carney, J. A. Mountford, M. J. Collins, S. Cluff, and P. K. Collins, "Visual performance after overnight orthokeratology," *Contact Lens and Anterior Eye*, vol. 30, no. 1, pp. 29–36, 2007.

[25] J. J. Nichols, M. M. Marsich, M. Nguyen, J. T. Barr, and M. A. Bullimore, "Overnight orthokeratology," *Optometry and Vision Science*, vol. 77, no. 5, pp. 252–259, 2000.

[26] S. Y. Kang, B. K. Kim, and Y. J. Byun, "Sustainability of orthokeratology as demonstrated by corneal topography," *Korean Journal of Ophthalmology*, vol. 21, no. 2, pp. 74–78, 2007.

[27] R. Chakraborty, S. A. Read, and M. J. Collins, "Diurnal variations in axial length, choroidal thickness, intraocular pressure, and ocular biometrics," *Investigative Opthalmology & Visual Science*, vol. 52, no. 8, pp. 5121–5129, 2011.

[28] A. Alharbi, D. La Hood, and H. A. Swarbrick, "Overnight orthokeratology lens wear can inhibit the central stromal edema response," *Investigative Opthalmology & Visual Science*, vol. 46, no. 7, pp. 2334–2340, 2005.

[29] J. A. Martinez-Roda, M. Vilaseca, J. C. Ondategui et al., "Optical quality and intraocular scattering in a healthy young population," *Clinical and Experimental Optometry*, vol. 94, no. 2, pp. 223–229, 2011.

[30] K. Kamiya, K. Umeda, H. Kobashi, K. Shimizu, T. Kawamorita, and H. Uozato, "Effect of aging on optical quality and intraocular scattering using the double-pass instrument," *Current Eye Research*, vol. 37, no. 10, pp. 884–888, 2012.

[31] T. Hiraoka, Y. Matsumoto, F. Okamoto et al., "Corneal higher-order aberrations induced by overnight orthokeratology," *American Journal of Ophthalmology*, vol. 139, no. 3, pp. 429–436, 2005.

[32] A. Queiros, C. Villa-Collar, J. M. Gonzalez-Meijome, J. Jorge, and A. R. Gutierrez, "Effect of pupil size on corneal aberrations before and after standard laser in situ keratomileusis, custom laser in situ keratomileusis, and corneal refractive therapy," *American Journal of Ophthalmology*, vol. 150, no. 1, pp. 97e1–109e1, 2010.

[33] R. Montes-Mico and W. N. Charman, "Choice of spatial frequency for contrast sensitivity evaluation after corneal refractive surgery," *Journal of Refractive Surgery*, vol. 17, no. 6, pp. 646–651, 2001.

[34] T. Hiraoka, T. Mihashi, C. Okamoto, F. Okamoto, Y. Hirohara, and T. Oshika, "Influence of induced decentered orthokeratology lens on ocular higher-order wavefront aberrations and contrast sensitivity function," *Journal of Cataract & Refractive Surgery*, vol. 35, no. 11, pp. 1918–1926, 2009.

[35] K. Lee, J. M. Ahn, E. K. Kim, and T. I. Kim, "Comparison of optical quality parameters and ocular aberrations after wavefront-guided laser in-situ keratomileusis versus wavefront-guided laser epithelial keratomileusis for myopia," *Graefe's Archive for Clinical and Experimental Ophthalmology*, vol. 251, no. 9, pp. 2163–2169, 2013.

[36] C. L. Harper, M. E. Boulton, D. Bennett et al., "Diurnal variations in human corneal thickness," *British Journal of Ophthalmology*, vol. 80, no. 12, pp. 1068–1072, 1996.

[37] S. A. Read, M. J. Collins, and D. R. Iskander, "Diurnal variation of axial length, intraocular pressure, and anterior eye biometrics," *Investigative Opthalmology & Visual Science*, vol. 49, no. 7, pp. 2911–2918, 2008.

[38] R. Chakraborty, S. A. Read, and M. J. Collins, "Diurnal variations in ocular aberrations of human eyes," *Current Eye Research*, vol. 39, no. 3, pp. 271–281, 2014.

[39] M. C. David, G. Santiago, A. D. Cesar, F. B. Teresa, and M. M. Robert, "Visual quality differences between orthokeratology and LASIK to compensate low-moderate myopia," *Cornea*, vol. 32, no. 8, pp. 1137–1141, 2013.

[40] T. Hiraoka, C. Okamoto, Y. Ishii, F. Okamoto, and T. Oshika, "Recovery of corneal irregular astigmatism, ocular higher-order aberrations, and contrast sensitivity after discontinuation of overnight orthokeratology," *British Journal of Ophthalmology*, vol. 93, no. 2, pp. 203–208, 2009.

[41] L. Yang, X. Guo, and P. Xie, "Observation of orthokeratology discontinuation," *Chinese Journal of Ophthalmology*, vol. 51, no. 3, pp. 178–182, 2015.

[42] Y. M. Liu and P. Xie, "The safety of orthokeratology-a systematic review," *Eye & Contact Lens: Science & Clinical Practice*, vol. 42, no. 1, pp. 35–42, 2016.

[43] A. Queiros, C. Villa-Collar, A. R. Gutierrez, J. Jorge, and J. M. Gonzalez-Meijome, "Quality of life of myopic subjects with different methods of visual correction using the NEI RQL-42 questionnaire," *Eye & Contact Lens: Science & Clinical Practice*, vol. 38, no. 2, pp. 116–121, 2012.

[44] E. S. Sanz, A. Cervino, A. Queiros, C. Villa-Collar, D. Lopes-Ferreira, and J. M. González-Méijome, "Short-term changes in light distortion in orthokeratology subjects," *BioMed Research International*, vol. 2015, Article ID 278425, 7 pages, 2015.

23

Efficacy and Safety of an Aflibercept Treat-and-Extend Regimen in Treatment-Naïve Patients with Macular Oedema Secondary to Central Retinal Vein Occlusion (CRVO)

Jose Garcia-Arumi [ID],[1] Francisco Gómez-Ulla,[2] Navea Amparo [ID],[3] Enrique Cervera,[4] Alex Fonollosa,[5] Luis Arias [ID],[6] Javier Araiz,[7] Juan Donate,[8] Marta Suárez de Figueroa,[9] Lucia Manzanas,[10] Jaume Crespí,[11] and Roberto Gallego[12]

[1]Hospital Universitari Vall d'Hebron, Barcelona, Spain
[2]Instituto Oftalmológico Gómez-Ulla, Complejo Hospitalario Universitario de Santiago de Compostela, A Coruña, Spain
[3]FISABIO-Oftalmología Médica, Valencia, Spain
[4]Hospital General de Valencia, Valencia, Spain
[5]Hospital Universitario de Cruces, Barakaldo, Spain
[6]Hospital Universitari de Bellvitge, Barcelona, Spain
[7]Instituto Clínico Quirúrgico de Oftalmología, Bilbo, Bizkaia, Spain
[8]Hospital Clínico San Carlos, Madrid, Spain
[9]VISSUM, Madrid, Spain
[10]Hospital Clínico Universitario de Valladolid, Valladolid, Spain
[11]Hospital de la Santa Creu i Sant Pau, Barcelona, Spain
[12]Unidad de Mácula, Clínica OFTALVIST, Valencia, Spain

Correspondence should be addressed to Jose Garcia-Arumi; jgarcia.arumi@gmail.com

Academic Editor: Pierluigi Iacono

Objectives. To evaluate efficacy and safety of an aflibercept treat-and-extend (TAE) regimen in patients with macular oedema (MO) secondary to central retinal vein occlusion (CRVO). *Design, Setting, and Patients.* Phase IV, prospective, open-label, single-arm trial in 11 Spanish hospitals. Treatment-naïve patients with <6 month diagnosis of MO secondary to CRVO and best-corrected visual acuity (BCVA) of 73-24 ETDRS letters were included between 23 January 2015 and 17 March 2016. *Intervention.* Intravitreal aflibercept 2 mg monthly (3 months) followed by proactive individualized dosing. *Main Outcomes.* Mean change in BCVA after 12 months. *Results.* 24 eyes (24 patients) were included; mean (SD) age: 62.8 (15.0) years; 54.2% male; median (IQR) time since diagnosis: 7.6 (3.0, 15.2) days. Mean BCVA scores significantly improved between baseline (56.0 (16.5)) and Month 12 (74.1 (17.6)); mean (95% CI) change: 14.8 (8.2, 21.4); $P = 0.0001$. Twelve (50.0%) patients gained ≥15 ETDRS letters. Foveal thickness improved between baseline (mean: 569.4 (216.8) μm) and Month 12 (mean 257.4 (48.4) μm); $P < 0.0001$. At Month 12, 8.3% patients had MO. The mean (SD) number of injections: 8.3 (3.0). No treatment-related AEs were reported. Five (20.8%) patients experienced ocular AEs. Two nonocular serious AEs were reported. *Conclusions.* An aflibercept TAE regimen improves visual acuity in patients with MO secondary to CRVO over 12 months with good tolerability.

1. Introduction

Retinal vein occlusion (RVO) is thought to result from a thrombotic event or vessel wall pathology that can severely impact visual acuity [1, 2]. Macular oedema (MO) secondary to RVO is the second-most common retinal vascular disease after diabetic retinopathy and is subdivided into central retinal vein occlusion (CRVO) and branch retinal vein occlusion (BRVO) based on the location of the occlusion [3].

Central retinal vein occlusion is estimated to affect between 0.3% and 2.1% of the global population with no significant variation in prevalence due to ethnicity or gender [4]. Like BRVO, clinical features of CRVO include dilated and tortuous retinal veins, deep and superficial retinal haemorrhages, cotton wool spots, and retinal oedema [5]. However, unlike BRVO, these features are found in all quadrants of the retina in CRVO. Visual loss after CRVO commonly occurs as a result of MO, ischemia, or in more advanced stages, occurs as a result of vitreous haemorrhage or neovascularisation.

Current therapeutic options for the treatment of MO secondary to CRVO include laser photocoagulation, vascular endothelial growth factor (VEGF) inhibitors, and intraocular steroids [6]. Several recent meta-analyses have shown treatment of MO secondary to CRVO with anti-VEGF agents resulted in improved best-corrected visual acuity (BCVA) over time and fewer adverse events compared to placebo, corticosteroids, or laser photocoagulation [7–9]. An assessment of clinical evidence by the American Academy of Ophthalmology concluded that anti-VEGF pharmacotherapy was safe and effective over two years for MO secondary to CRVO [10]. Network meta-analysis of drug treatments to manage MO secondary to CRVO found no evidence of differences in efficacy between the anti-VEGF agents: ranibizumab, aflibercept, bevacizumab, or corticosteroid triamcinolone [11].

The recombinant fusion protein aflibercept (Eylea; Regeneron Pharmaceuticals), a fusion protein of key domains from human VEGF receptors 1 and 2, was approved by the US Food and Drug Administration (FDA) in 2011 and by the European Medicines Agency in 2012 for the treatment of patients with neovascular age-related macular degeneration (nAMD) [12, 13]. A higher VEGF affinity and a longer half-life compared to older anti-VEGF agents reduce the frequency of intravitreal (IVT) injections needed to maintain therapeutic effect, thus potentially reducing the clinical burden placed on patients by reducing the number of treatment visits [14–18].

The findings of the sister confirmatory phase III randomised controlled GALILEO and COPERNICUS trials showed IVT aflibercept improved 12-month visual and anatomical outcomes when administered pro re nata (PRN) following six monthly injections in patients with MO secondary to CRVO, provided that the patients were administered aflibercept following the initial event [5, 19, 20].

The treat-and-extend (TAE) regimen is a proactive individualized treatment regimen designed to maximize the benefit to risk ratio of anti-VEGF agents. It is frequently used for the treatment of nAMD [21–23]. Compared to fixed dose and PRN regimens, the TAE regimen reduces treatment burden and does not require disease reactivation for continued treatment [23]. Under this regimen, anti-VEGF agents are administered as fixed loading doses until clinical remission, followed by increasing treatment intervals until a maximal safe interval is reached (usually 10–12 weeks). Treatment intervals are shortened by two weeks if there are any negative changes in clinical parameters. Recent studies of ranibizumab or bevacizumab have shown the TAE regimen to be suitable for the treatment of diabetic MO and MO secondary to CRVO over one year [24, 25].

The objective of this study was to prospectively evaluate the 12-month efficacy and safety of an aflibercept TAE regimen in patients with MO secondary to CRVO.

2. Methods

2.1. Trial Design. This phase IV, prospective, open-label, single-arm, multicentre trial was conducted in 11 trial sites (tertiary healthcare facilities located in the Basque Country, Castille and León, Catalonia, Madrid, and Valencia autonomous communities) in Spain (NEUTON Trial (RET-AFLI-2014-01); EudraCT Number: 2014-000975-21). The trial was conducted in accordance with the ethical principles of the declaration of Helsinki and Good Clinical Practice guidelines. All ethics committees approved the trial protocol and its amendments.

2.2. Patients. The main inclusion criteria were as follows: willingness to provide informed consent; aged ≥18 years; a diagnosis of MO secondary to RCVO within the last six months with mean central subfield thickness of ≥250 μm (spectral-domain optical coherence tomography (SD-OCT)); a baseline BCVA score in the study eye of between 73 and 24 early treatment diabetic retinopathy study (ETDRS) letters (inclusive) measured using the ETDRS chart at four meters (Snellen equivalent: 20/40 to 20/320); a baseline BCVA score of greater ≥20/400 in the Snellen optotype (0.05 decimal, 1 line of sight) in the contralateral eye; the absence of cataracts or other eye diseases that may affect visual acuity.

The main exclusion criteria (in the study eye) were as follows: prior anti-VEGF treatment, photodynamic therapy, corticosteroid treatment or thermal laser treatment; intraocular surgery (including cataract surgery) within three months prior to first aflibercept administration; scarring, fibrosis or atrophy that affects the centre of the fovea; ruptures/tears in the pigmentary retinal epithelial that affect the fovea; severe proliferative macular ischemia or iris rubeosis; prior vitrectomy, submacular surgery or any other surgical procedure for nAMD; or active intraocular inflammation in the study eye.

2.3. Trial Interventions. During the loading phase (first three months), IVT aflibercept 2 mg (40 mg/ml) was given once monthly (Week 0, 4, and 8). If the patient improved or showed signs of BCVA stability (no change or a decrease of <5 EDTRS letters during three consecutive evaluations) and/or visual and morphological outcomes (an increase of ≥50 μm central retinal thickness with the absence of new cystic alterations or subretinal fluid or the absence of persistent or recurrent exudation (intraretinal/subretinal) by SD-OCT) after three consecutive visits (Week 4, 8, and 12), the TAE phase began six weeks thereafter (at Week 18). The treatment window was extended by two weeks per visit if no evidence of disease activity was observed (in relation to the period since the last visit) for a maximum of 12 weeks. If there were signs of disease, the patient was retreated and the next visit was scheduled for four weeks later. The trial concluded at the end-of-trial (EOT) visit at Month 12.

2.4. Trial Procedures. At baseline eligibility criteria, demographic data, medical history, physical examination, concomitant medication, pregnancy test (if applicable), intraocular pressure (IOP), BCVA score, SD-OCT, fundus fluorescein angiography (FA), retinography, eye fundus photography, and adverse events (AEs) were assessed or reported. During the loading phase (Month 0–2; Week 0–8), TAE phase (Month 3–12; Weeks 12–48), and EOT visit (Month 12; Week 52) concomitant medication, IOP, BCVA, SD-OCT, FA imaging, and AEs were assessed or reported. All FA images and retinographies were sent to the Instituto Oftalmológico Gómez-Ulla reading centre (Responsible reader: Francisco Gómez-Ulla). Optical coherence tomography assessments were performed using Zeiss® (Cirrus version 4.0 or higher), Topcon® (3D, 2000 or 2000 plus), or Heidelberg® (Spectralis version 5.1 or higher) SD-OCT imaging devices, dependent on availability at each trial site. Patients were evaluated with the same device for the duration of the trial.

2.5. Trial Outcomes. The primary outcome was mean change in BCVA (ETDRS letters) between baseline and Month 12 (EOT) visit. Secondary outcomes included proportion of patients gaining ≥15 ETDRS letters at Month 12; mean change in BCVA at Month 3 (Week 12–14, after loading doses) versus baseline; mean changes in foveal thicknesses (SD-OCT) at months 3 and 12 versus baseline; proportion of patients free of MO (SD-OCT; central foveal thickness < 200 μm) at Months 3 and 12; mean number of injections; and proportion of patients not requiring additional TAE injections. Safety outcomes included ocular and nonocular AEs and serious AEs (SAEs). Key nonocular adverse events were considered to be those defined by the Antiplatelet Trialists' Collaboration as Arteriothrombolic Events (APTC ATE) [26].

2.6. Sample Size and Statistical Analysis. Based on the 1-year results from the GALILEO trial (mean change in BCVA of 16.9 ETDRS letters in patients with MO secondary to CRVO receiving aflibercept every month for 20 weeks followed by PRN thereafter) [19], a total of 43 patients was estimated to detect a significant mean change in BCVA at 12 months with 95% power, a significance level (alpha) of 0.01, and

a standard deviation of 25 letters. Estimating a 15% loss to follow-up, a sample size of 50 patients was planned.

The intention-to-treat (ITT) population used for all efficacy analyses included all patients enrolled in the trial who had received at least one dose of aflibercept and who had undergone at least one postbaseline BCVA assessment. The safety population used for all safety analyses included all patients who had received at least one dose of aflibercept.

All data were descriptively analysed. Continuous variables were presented with the number of observations, mean, 95% confidence interval (CI) for the mean, median, standard deviation (SD), and interquartile range (IQR). Categorical variables, however, were described in terms of frequencies and percentages. Changes from baseline were analysed using McNemar's tests for categorical variables and parametric (Student's *t*-test for paired data) or nonparametric (Wilcoxon signed-rank test) tests for continuous variables, as applicable. The level of significance used for all tests was 0.05 (two-tailed). No imputation for missing data was performed.

Data analysis was performed using the SAS® statistical package for Windows (version 9.4, SAS Institute Inc., Cary, U.S.).

3. Results

3.1. Patient Disposition and Baseline Characteristics. A total of 31 eyes from 31 patients were screened for trial inclusion, and 24 eyes from 24 patients were enrolled in the trial between 23 January 2015 and 17 March 2016. Eighteen (58.6%) patients completed the 12 months of follow-up; two (8.3%) patients discontinued due to a withdrawal of consent, one (4.2%) due to a protocol deviation, one (4.2%) due to a loss of visual acuity without MO, one (4.2%) lost to follow-up, and one (4.2%) withdrawn due to not meeting all eligibility criteria.

Baseline characteristics are shown in Table 1. The mean ± SD age at trial inclusion was 62.8 ± 15.0 years, and 54.2% were male. Median (IQR) time since diagnosis was 7.6 (3.0, 15.2) days with a mean ± SD intraocular pressure (IOP) of 15.7 ± 3.0 mmHg. Arterial hypertension and dyslipidaemia were the most common medical history or concomitant pathologies.

3.2. BCVA at Month 12. The mean ± SD baseline BCVAs in the study and contralateral eye were 56.0 ± 16.5 and 81.0 ± 9.3 ETDRS letters, respectively (Tables 1 and 2). At Month 12, mean ± SD BCVA in the study eye was 74.1 ± 17.6, corresponding to a mean (95% CI) increase of 14.8 (8.2, 21.4) ETDRS letters ($P = 0.0001$) (Table 2).

3.3. Secondary Endpoints. The mean ± SD BCVA after the three monthly aflibercept IVT loading doses was 70.8 ± 19.6, a mean (95% CI) increase of 14.0 (7.8, 20.2) ETDRS letters ($P = 0.0001$) (Table 2). Analysis of BCVA over time showed a relatively stable improvement in BCVA after three months that was maintained over follow-up until Month 12

TABLE 1: Baseline characteristics.

Baseline characteristics	ITT population (N = 24)
Age (years), mean (SD)	62.8 (15.0)
Male, N (%)	13 (54.2)
Caucasian ethnicity, N (%)	24 (100.0)
Time from MO secondary to CRVO diagnosis (days), median (IQR)	7.6 (3.0, 15.2)
IOP in study eye (mmHg), mean (SD)	15.7 (3.0)
Baseline BCVA score (ETDRS) in contralateral eye, letters, mean (SD)	81.0 (9.3)
Patients with any relevant medical history/concomitant pathology	23 (95.8)
Arterial hypertension	17 (70.8)
Dyslipidaemia	8 (33.3)
Cataracts	5 (20.8)
Anxiety	3 (12.5)
Diabetes mellitus	3 (12.5)
Obesity	3 (12.5)
Others*	17 (70.8)

BCVA: best-corrected visual acuity; CRVO: central retinal vein occlusion; ETDRS: early treatment diabetic retinopathy study; IOP: intraocular pressure; IQR: interquartile range; ITT: intention-to-treat; MO: macular oedema; SD: standard deviation. *Conditions experienced by <10% of the patient population.

(Table 2). Twelve (50.0%) patients gained ≥15 ETDRS letters by Month 12.

Mean ± SD foveal thickness decreased from 569.4 ± 216.8 μm at baseline to a mean (95% CI) of 291.9 (223.1, 360.7) at Month 3, a significant reduction of 272.2 (167.0, 377.4) μm (P < 0.0001) (Table 2). At Month 12, the reduction in foveal thickness was 296.0 (196.8, 395.1) μm (P < 0.0001).

Nineteen (79.2%) patients did not exhibit signs of MO at Month 3 or Month 12 (Table 2). One (4.2%) patient continued to exhibit MO for the duration of the study, one (4.2%) patient resolved during the TAE phase, and one (4.2%) patient temporarily resolved during the loading phase but relapsed during the TAE phase.

3.4. Exposure to Aflibercept. Twenty-two (91.7%) patients completed the loading phase (three aflibercept injections); one (4.2%) patient was withdrawn after receiving one injection, and one (4.2%) patient was lost to follow-up after receiving two injections. A mean ± SD of 8.3 ± 3.0 aflibercept injections were received by patients during the trial (Table 2) with 14 (58.3%) receiving ≤8 injections (Figure 1).

3.5. Safety. Overall, one (4.2%) patient experienced a nonfatal APTC ATE event (stroke) of moderate severity that was unrelated to study treatment, required hospitalisation prolongation, and was resolved by the end of the study (Table 3). The same patient also experienced a SAE (lung neoplasm surgery) that was of moderate severity, unrelated to study treatment, but required hospitalisation prolongation. Nonserious ocular AEs were experienced by five (20.8%)

TABLE 2: BCVA and secondary endpoints after loading doses (month 3), at end of trial (month 12), and aflibercept exposure.

	ITT population (N = 24)	P value*
BCVA score (ETDRS letters)		
Week 0 (baseline), N	24	
Mean (SD) score	56.0 (16.5)	
Month 3, N	21	
Mean (SD) score	70.8 (19.6)	
95% CI	61.9, 79.7	
Mean (95% CI) change from baseline	14.0 (7.8, 20.2)	0.0001
Month 12 (EOT), N	21	
Mean (SD) score	74.1 (17.6)	
95% CI	66.1, 82.1	
Mean (95% CI) change from baseline	14.8 (8.2, 21.4)	0.0001
Proportion gaining ≥15 ETDRS letters at EOT, N (%)		
Yes	12 (50.0)	
No	9 (37.5)	
Not available	3 (12.5)	
Retinal (foveal) thickness by SD-OCT (μm)		
Week 0 (baseline), N	24	
Mean (SD) score	569.4 (216.8)	
Month 3, N	21	
Mean (SD) score	291.9 (151.2)	
95% CI	223.1, 360.7	
Mean (95% CI) change from baseline	−272.2 (−377.4, −167.0)	<0.0001
Month 12 (EOT), N	21	
Mean (SD) score	257.4 (48.4)	
95% CI	235.4, 279.5	
Mean (SD) change from baseline	−296.0 (−395.1, −196.8)	<0.0001
Proportion with MO (SD-OCT), N (%)		
Week 0 (baseline), N	24	
Yes	24 (100.0)	
Month 3, N	21	
Yes	2 (8.3)	
No	19 (79.2)	
Month 12 (EOT), N	21	
Yes	2 (8.3)	
No	19 (79.2)	
Exposure: number of aflibercept injections		
Number of injections		
Mean (SD)	8.3 (3.0)	
Median (IQR)	8.0 (8.0, 10.5)	
TAE injection interval (weeks)		
Mean (SD)	7.0 (2.2)	
Median (IQR)	6.1 (5.2, 9.1)	

BCVA: best-corrected visual acuity; ETDRS: early treatment diabetic retinopathy study; EOT: end of trial; IQR: interquartile range; ITT: intention-to-treat; MO: macular oedema; SD: standard deviation; SD-OCT: spectral-domain optical coherence tomography. TAE: treat-and-extend. *All values compared to baseline using Student's t-test for paired samples.

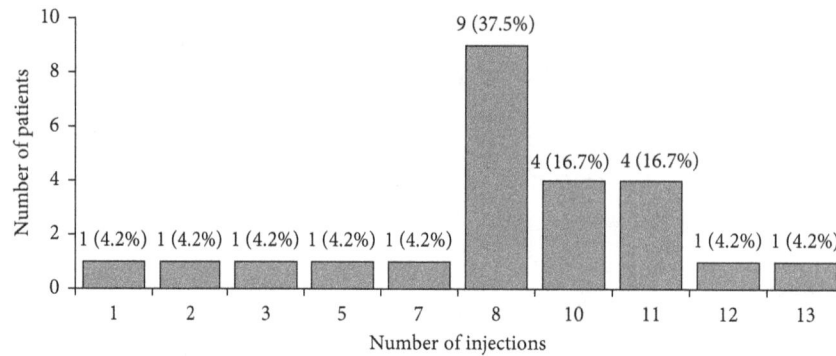

FIGURE 1: Number of aflibercept injections received by patients during the trial.

TABLE 3: Summary of adverse events.

	Safety population (N = 24) N (%)
Serious adverse events (SAEs)	
Nonfatal APTC ATE events (not related to trial treatment)	1 (4.2)
Stroke	1 (4.2)
Other nonfatal SAEs	1 (4.2)
Systemic (nonocular; not related to trial treatment)	
Lung neoplasm surgery	1 (4.2)
Adverse events (AEs)	
Nonserious ocular AEs (not related to trial treatment)	5 (20.8)
Keratitis	2 (8.3)
Vitreous detachment	2 (8.3)
Aggravated cataract	1 (4.2)
Epiretinal membrane	1 (4.2)
Hyposphagma	1 (4.2)
Increased intraocular pressure	1 (4.2)
Nonserious systemic (nonocular) AEs (not related to trial treatment)*	9 (37.5)
Bronchitis	2 (8.3)

APTC ATE: antiplatelet trialists' collaboration arteriothrombolic event.
*AEs experienced by >1 patient presented.

patients; the most severe AE was vitreous detachment of moderate severity that had not resolved at the end of the study. One (4.2%) patient experienced two ocular AEs (aggravated cataracts and epiretinal membrane), both of mild severity and both not resolved at the end of the study. With regard to systemic AEs, nine (37.5%) patients experienced at least one AE; only one AE (bronchitis) was reported for over one patient—both patients experienced bronchitis of mild severity that was resolved by the end of the study.

4. Discussion

Currently, TAE regimens are increasingly used in daily practice for the management of exudative macular diseases to the detriment of fixed and PRN regimens. On one hand, the main advantages of TAE are: (1) proactive treatment that avoids further retinal cells damage derived from disease recurrence, (2) reduction in the number of monitoring visits,

(3) predictability of the treatment administration both for the patient and the ophthalmologist, (4) customized treatment for every patient enabling to know the time of the reactivation of the disease. In addition, TAE offers better anatomical and visual results in comparison with PRN regimens and equivalent results with fixed either monthly or bimonthly treatment regimens [21, 27]. However, one of the main concerns that has been raised is that a prolonged TAE could induce an overtreatment with potential unknown side effects if a dry macula is repeatedly injected over time. Likewise, it has not been clearly defined the optimal moment to interrupt the TAE treatment.

The most recommended TAE regimen is based on a gradual two-week extension interval in the absence of disease activity with a maximal extension of 12 weeks [21]. The extension should be initiated after a loading phase consisting of three consecutive monthly injections. Nevertheless, there is no total consensus about this since some ophthalmologists prefer to initiate the extension after the first injection or after a loading phase of two injections. In the present study, we decided to use a loading phase of three injections to try to maximize an initial visual gain that could be maintained with the subsequent TAE during all the study duration.

Confirmatory phase III randomised, controlled trials have shown monthly followed by PRN IVT aflibercept resulting in improved visual and anatomical outcomes in patients with MO secondary to CRVO; however, it remains unknown whether similar improvements could be maintained under a TAE regimen [4, 19, 20]. In this trial, a significant mean 14 ETDRS letter improvement in BCVA was recorded at the end of the loading phase (Month 3) that was followed by a peak BCVA improvement of 14.8 ETDRS letters at the end of the TAE regimen (Month 12). These findings are consistent with the results from the GALILEO (N = 103) and COPERNICUS (N = 115) trials which observed peak BCVA improvements of 18.0 and 17.3 ETDRS letters, respectively, after the six monthly aflibercept doses (primary endpoint) that were maintained at 12 months following a PRN regimen (16.9 and 16.2 ETDRS letter improvement, respectively) [19, 20]. Further similarity can be found in the retrospective study by Rahimy et al. where initial gains in BCVA at three months were maintained at 12 months in patients with MO secondary to CRVO treated with IVT bevacizumab or ranibizumab under a TAE regimen [25].

Despite comparable improvements in BCVA, the proportion of patients in whom a vision gain of ≥15 letters was exhibited at Month 12 ($N = 12$, 50%) was less than the proportions reported in the GALILEO ($N = 62$, 60.2%) and COPERNICUS trials ($N = 115$; 55.3%) [19, 20]. Given the small sample size in the present study, it is unclear whether this disparity is significant and clinically relevant. Differences in study design, such as loading phase duration or data analysis (last observation carried forward approach used for data analysis in the two phase III trials vs. no imputation in this study), may account for or contribute to the observed difference.

Anatomical changes in retinal thickness showed a similar pattern of improvement as BCVA, with a significant reduction in foveal thickness occurring after the loading phase that was maintained at Month 12. The mean reduction in central retinal (foveal) thickness at Month 3 (mean: 272.2 μm reduction) was less than the overall 448.6 μm and 457.2 μm reductions observed at the end of the six monthly injections in the GALILEO and COPERNICUS studies, respectively [19, 20]. While the magnitude of the reduction was smaller in the present study, most likely due to the fewer monthly aflibercept injections, in all trials, these anatomical improvements were maintained at Month 12. Further contrast can be observed compared to TAE bevacizumab or ranibizumab, where reductions in central retinal thickness were continual over the course of 12 months, albeit with a final reduction similar to that presented here at Month 3 [25].

Overall, the proportion of patients with MO decreased by 90.5% ($N = 19$) by Month 3, with a similar proportion reported at Month 12; one patient exhibited recurrent MO while another resolved during the TAE phase. As only two patients had unresolved MO by the EOT visit, no comparison of baseline characteristics yield insight into possible contributing factors for this observation.

Exposure to aflibercept was measured by the number of injections, duration of treatment, and the proportion of patients requiring further treatment after receiving the loading doses. The mean (SD) injection interval during the TAE phase was 7.0 (2.2) weeks. The overall mean number of injections was similar to the mean number of bevacizumab or ranibizumab injections when administered on a TAE regimen [25]. This contrasts with the GALILEO and COPERNICUS trials where a respective mean number of 11.8 and 9.9 injections were administered during the first year; however, this is likely attributable to the treatment regimen (six monthly doses followed by PRN) [19, 20].

In terms of safety, two SAEs were reported during the study in one patient. The patient experienced a stroke and lung neoplasm surgery, neither of which were related to trial treatment. The absence of ocular SAEs was in contrast to both the GALILEO and COPERNICUS trials, which reported a respective 1.9% ($N = 2$) and 3.5% ($N = 4$) of patients experienced ocular SAEs when aflibercept was injected monthly (weeks 0–24) and 8.2% ($N = 8$) and 2.7% ($N = 3$) of patients when aflibercept was injected PRN (weeks 24–52)

[19, 20]. Furthermore, no nonserious AEs related to treatment were reported, either systemic or ocular AEs. The proportion of patients who experienced nonserious ocular AEs in this trial was lower than that reported in the GALILEO trial where 54.8% (between weeks 0–24) and 69.1% (weeks 24–52) of patients receiving aflibercept reported at least one ocular AE [19].

The shortcomings of this trial include the small number of patients enrolled and the absence of a control group, which limit any conclusions being drawn.

5. Conclusion

The present trial suggests that aflibercept is efficacious in patients with MO secondary to CRVO when treated with a TAE regimen. The low incidence of ocular AEs suggests the TAE regimen may be preferable over other treatment regimens. Studies in larger cohorts of patients with MO secondary to CRVO should be carried out in order to confirm the results of this trial.

Conflicts of Interest

Jose Garcia-Arumi serves as a member of the Advisory board of Bayer and Novartis. Francisco Gómez-Ulla serves as a member of the Advisory board of Bayer. Luis Arias is a consultor of Allergan, Bayer, and Novartis. Javier Araiz is a consultant of Alcon, Bayer, and Novartis. Marta S. Figueroa is a consultant of Novartis, Bayer, Allergan, Roche, Alcon, Zeiss, and Baush & Lomb. Roberto Gallego is a consultor of Novartis and Roche and speaker of Carl Zeiss Meditec, Heidelberg Engineering, and Novartis. The other authors declare no conflicts of interest.

Acknowledgments

The authors would like to thank the NEUTON trial participants for their participation in this trial. Writing support was provided by Jonathan Mackinnon, PhD, from TFS Develop with financial support provided by Bayer Hispania S.L. The trial was sponsored by Fundación RETINAPLUS+ and financially supported by Bayer Hispania S.L. *NEUTON Trial Investigators (alphabetical order)*: Alejandro Fonollosa, Amparo Navea, Enrique Cervera, Jaume Crespí, Javier Araiz, José García Arumí, Juan Donate, Lucia Manzanas Leal, Luis Arias, Marta S. de Figueroa, and Roberto Gallego.

References

[1] K. Hatz and M. Martinez, "Retinal vein occlusion: an interdisciplinary approach," *Therapeutische Umschau*, vol. 73, no. 2, pp. 85–89, 2016.

[2] S. S. Hayreh, M. B. Zimmerman, and P. Podhajsky, "Incidence of various types of retinal vein occlusion and their recurrence

and demographic characteristics," *American Journal of Ophthalmology*, vol. 117, no. 4, pp. 429–441, 1994.

[3] S. Rogers, R. L. McIntosh, N. Cheung et al., "The prevalence of retinal vein occlusion: pooled data from population studies from the United States, Europe, Asia, and Australia," *Ophthalmology*, vol. 117, no. 2, pp. 313.e1–319.e1, 2010.

[4] W. Rhoades, D. Dickson, Q. D. Nguyen, and D. Do, "Management of macular edema due to central retinal vein occlusion–the role of aflibercept," *Taiwan Journal of Ophthalmology*, vol. 7, no. 2, pp. 70–76, 2017.

[5] A. A. Aref and I. U. Scott, "Management of macular edema secondary to central retinal vein occlusion: an evidence-based update," *Advances in Therapy*, vol. 28, no. 1, pp. 40–50, 2011.

[6] R. Channa, M. Smith, and P. A. Campochiaro, "Treatment of macular edema due to retinal vein occlusions," *Clinical Ophthalmology*, vol. 5, pp. 705–713, 2011.

[7] W. Song and X. Xia, "Ranibizumab for macular edema secondary to retinal vein occlusion: a meta-analysis of dose effects and comparison with no anti-VEGF treatment," *BMC Ophthalmology*, vol. 15, no. 1, 2015.

[8] T. Qian, M. Zhao, and X. Xu, "Comparison between anti-VEGF therapy and corticosteroid or laser therapy for macular oedema secondary to retinal vein occlusion: a meta-analysis," *Journal of Clinical Pharmacy and Therapeutics*, vol. 42, no. 5, pp. 519–529, 2017.

[9] P. Huang, W. Niu, Z. Ni, R. Wang, and X. Sun, "A meta-analysis of anti-vascular endothelial growth factor remedy for macular edema secondary to central retinal vein occlusion," *PLoS One*, vol. 8, no. 12, Article ID e82454, 2013.

[10] S. Yeh, S. J. Kim, A. C. Ho et al., "Therapies for macular edema associated with central retinal vein occlusion: a report by the american academy of ophthalmology," *Ophthalmology*, vol. 122, no. 4, pp. 769–778, 2015.

[11] J. A. Ford, D. Shyangdan, O. A. Uthman, N. Lois, and N. Waugh, "Drug treatment of macular oedema secondary to central retinal vein occlusion: a network meta-analysis," *BMJ Open*, vol. 4, no. 7, article e005292, 2014.

[12] M. W. Stewart, S. Grippon, and P. Kirkpatrick, "Aflibercept," *Nature Reviews Drug Discovery*, vol. 11, no. 4, pp. 269-270, 2012.

[13] A. Ferreira, A. Sagkriotis, M. Olson, J. Lu, C. Makin, and F. Milnes, "Treatment frequency and dosing interval of ranibizumab and aflibercept for neovascular age-related macular degeneration in routine clinical practice in the USA," *PLoS One*, vol. 10, no. 7, Article ID e0133968, 2015.

[14] M. W. Stewart and P. J. Rosenfeld, "Predicted biological activity of intravitreal VEGF Trap," *British Journal of Ophthalmology*, vol. 92, no. 5, pp. 667-668, 2008.

[15] J. Holash, S. Davis, N. Papadopoulos et al., "VEGF-trap: a VEGF blocker with potent antitumor effects," *Proceedings of the National Academy of Sciences*, vol. 99, no. 17, pp. 11393–11398, 2002.

[16] D. M. Brown, J. S. Heier, T. Ciulla et al., "Primary endpoint results of a phase II study of vascular endothelial growth factor trap-eye in wet age-related macular degeneration," *Ophthalmology*, vol. 118, no. 6, pp. 1089–1097, 2011.

[17] J. S. Heier, D. Boyer, Q. D. Nguyen et al., "The 1-year results of CLEAR-IT 2, a phase 2 study of vascular endothelial growth factor trap-eye dosed as-needed after 12-week fixed dosing," *Ophthalmology*, vol. 118, no. 6, pp. 1098–1106, 2011.

[18] J. S. Heier, D. M. Brown, V. Chong et al., "Intravitreal aflibercept (VEGF trap-eye) in wet age-related macular degeneration," *Ophthalmology*, vol. 119, no. 12, pp. 2537–2548, 2012.

[19] J.-F. Korobelnik, F. G. Holz, J. Roider et al., "Intravitreal aflibercept injection for macular edema resulting from central retinal vein occlusion: one-year results of the phase 3 GALILEO study," *Ophthalmology*, vol. 121, no. 1, pp. 202–208, 2014.

[20] D. M. Brown, J. S. Heier, W. L. Clark et al., "Intravitreal aflibercept injection for macular edema secondary to central retinal vein occlusion: 1-year results from the phase 3 COPERNICUS study," *American Journal of Ophthalmology*, vol. 155, no. 3, pp. 429.e7–437.e7, 2013.

[21] K. B. Freund, J.-F. Korobelnik, R. Devenyi et al., "Treat-and-extend regimens with anti-VEGF agents in retinal diseases: a literature review and consensus recommendations," *Retina*, vol. 35, no. 8, pp. 1489–1506, 2015.

[22] S. Mrejen, J. J. Jung, C. Chen et al., "Long-term visual outcomes for a treat and extend anti-vascular endothelial growth factor regimen in eyes with neovascular age-related macular degeneration," *Journal of Clinical Medicine*, vol. 4, no. 7, pp. 1380–1402, 2015.

[23] S. R. Rufai, H. Almuhtaseb, R. M. Paul et al., "A systematic review to assess the "treat-and-extend" dosing regimen for neovascular age-related macular degeneration using ranibizumab," *Eye*, vol. 31, no. 9, pp. 1337–1344, 2017.

[24] J. F. Payne, C. C. Wykoff, W. L. Clark, B. B. Bruce, D. S. Boyer, and D. M. Brown, "Randomized trial of treat and extend ranibizumab with and without navigated laser for diabetic macular edema: TREX-DME 1 year outcomes," *Ophthalmology*, vol. 124, no. 1, pp. 74–81, 2017.

[25] E. Rahimy, N. Rayess, C. J. Brady et al., "Treat-and-extend regimen for macular edema secondary to central retinal vein occlusion: 12-month results," *Ophthalmology Retina*, vol. 1, no. 2, pp. 118–123, 2017.

[26] Antiplatelet Trialists' Collaboration, "Collaborative overview of randomised trials of antiplatelet therapy Prevention of death, myocardial infarction, and stroke by prolonged antiplatelet therapy in various categories of patients," *BMJ*, vol. 308, no. 6921, pp. 81–106, 1994.

[27] C. C. Wykoff, D. E. Croft, D. M. Brown et al., "Prospective trial of treat-and-extend versus monthly dosing for neovascular age-related macular degeneration: TREX-AMD 1-year results," *Ophthalmology*, vol. 122, no. 12, pp. 2514–2522, 2015.

24

Comparison of Intravitreal Aflibercept and Ranibizumab following Initial Treatment with Ranibizumab in Persistent Diabetic Macular Edema

Ali Demircan ⓘ**, Zeynep Alkin** ⓘ**, Ceren Yesilkaya** ⓘ**, Gokhan Demir, and Burcu Kemer**

Beyoglu Eye Research and Training Hospital, Istanbul, Turkey

Correspondence should be addressed to Ali Demircan; alidemircanctf@yahoo.com

Academic Editor: Yoshihiro Takamura

Purpose. To compare the visual and anatomic outcomes in patients with persistent diabetic macular edema (DME) who switched from ranibizumab to aflibercept with those who continued with previous ranibizumab therapy. *Methods.* In this retrospective comparative study, medical records of consecutive patients with center-involved DME $\geq 350 \mu m$ who had at least three recent consecutive monthly ranibizumab injections followed by as-needed therapy with either aflibercept or ranibizumab were reviewed. Data were collected at presentation (preinjection), at the intermediary visit, and at the last visit (at the end of the follow-up period). *Results.* Forty-three eyes of 43 patients were divided into two groups: the switch group ($n = 20$) and the ranibizumab group ($n = 23$). Though no significant improvement was found in the mean BCVA from the intermediary visit to the last visit, there was a difference in the mean CMT in the switch group and the ranibizumab group ($p < 0.001$ and $p = 0.03$, resp.). The mean CMT decreased after the intermediary visit by $188.6 \pm 120.5 \mu m$ in the switch group and by $60.3 \pm 117.1 \mu m$ in the ranibizumab group ($p = 0.003$). *Conclusions.* Both aflibercept and ranibizumab decreased CMT in patients with persistent DME who showed a poor response to ranibizumab injections. However, switching to aflibercept provided only morphologic improvement.

1. Introduction

Diabetic retinopathy is the leading cause of visual impairment among working-age people aged <45 years around the world and is rising in prevalence [1, 2]. Diabetic macular edema (DME) leads to visual impairment in diabetic retinopathy, and its prevalence has been estimated as 6.8% in the diabetic population [3]. Currently, clinical trials providing level 1 evidence have revealed that antivascular endothelial growth factor (VEGF) agents, United States Food and Drug Administration-approved ranibizumab and aflibercept, as well as off-label bevacizumab, are the most effective treatment options for improvement of visual acuity and macular morphology for center-involving DME compared with laser [4–6]. The RISE-RIDE trials for ranibizumab, VIVID-VISTA trials for aflibercept, and numerous studies with level 2 and 3 evidence for bevacizumab demonstrated that almost 40% of patients gained 15 letters or more

on Snellen eye charts at two years of follow-up [4–8]. Although a significant proportion of patients had visual and anatomic improvement in prospective multicenter studies with regular treatment and follow-up schedules, a considerable amount of patients showed poor response to current anti-VEGF treatment. Hence, it is logical to switch anti-VEGF agents between each other if the previous treatment is not sufficient to resolve macular edema. However, few studies have assessed the results of switching anti-VEGF therapies in patients with poor response to DME [9–12]. In light of these findings, there is still a question that remains to be answered regarding whether macular edema resolves when previous treatment is continued. To date, there are limited data about switching anti-VEGF agents regarding their effectiveness in DME. The aim of this study was to address the outcomes of aflibercept use in patients who did not respond to previous ranibizumab treatment. Therefore, the visual and anatomic outcomes of switching therapy from ranibizumab to aflibercept were compared with those of patients treated with ranibizumab only in persistent/nonresolving macular edema secondary to diabetes.

2. Methods

In this retrospective, observational, comparative case series, data were collected from the records of sequential patients who were followed up for DME. To identify eligible patients who were both treated with ranibizumab injections (0.5 mg/0.05 mL) continuously and previously treated with ranibizumab and were subsequently switched to aflibercept (2 mg/0.05 mL), electronic medical records of patients with DME between August 2015 and May 2017 were reviewed. Written informed consent was obtained from all patients before the injections, and the protocol of the study adhered to the tenets of the Declaration of Helsinki.

To be included in the study, each patient was required to meet all of the following criteria: patients with type 2 diabetes aged ≥ 18 years, center-involving DME (central macular thickness (CMT) $\geq 350 \,\mu$m), and best corrected visual acuity (BCVA) of $\geq 20/400$. Patients were excluded if they had any of the following treatments within 6 months prior to study entry: intravitreal or sub-Tenon's injections of steroids, intravitreal dexamethasone implant, intravitreal anti-VEGF injections, focal/grid macular laser photocoagulation, panretinal photocoagulation, cataract surgery, or pars plana vitrectomy. Patients who had macular edema secondary to a cause other than diabetes or any concomitant ocular pathologies aside from diabetic retinopathy or vitreoretinal surface disorders were also excluded.

Afterwards, the patients ($n = 43$) were divided into two groups: the switch group ($n = 20$) consisted of patients who demonstrated poor response or an increase in CMT after the last three monthly ranibizumab injections following former ranibizumab treatment and then switched to aflibercept and the ranibizumab group ($n = 23$) comprised patients who demonstrated a poor response (decrease in CMT < 10%) after the last three monthly ranibizumab injections following former ranibizumab treatment and then continued to receive ranibizumab injections.

In the presence of persisting subretinal or intraretinal fluid, treatment with ranibizumab or aflibercept was continued using an as-needed regimen until no improvement in CMT was seen.

The decision to treat using an as-needed regimen, which followed an optical coherence tomography- (OCT-) guided treatment protocol, was made by a retina specialist. If no center-involved macular edema was seen, monthly monitoring visits were arranged and further injections of ranibizumab or aflibercept were withheld. In case of newly formed or persistent macular edema or increase in CMT $\geq 50 \,\mu$m compared with the previous visit, retreatment with either intravitreal ranibizumab or aflibercept was applied.

At each visit, a complete ophthalmologic examination including measurement of BCVA using Snellen charts, slit-lamp biomicroscopy, intraocular pressure measurement using applanation tonometry, and dilated biomicroscopic fundus examination was conducted and OCT imaging using

a SPECTRALIS OCT (SPECTRALIS; Heidelberg Engineering, Heidelberg, Germany) was performed. Data were collected at presentation (preinjection), at the intermediary visit (preswitch visit in the switch group and 4–6 weeks after the last injection of three monthly ranibizumab injections in the ranibizumab group), and at the last visit (at the end of the follow-up period). Only data of patients who completed a minimum 6-month follow-up period after the intermediary visit were collected for analysis.

CMT, which is defined as the mean thickness of the neurosensory retina in the central 1 mm diameter, was computed through OCT mapping software provided by the device. OCT characteristics of DME were classified as cystoid macular edema (CME), serous retinal detachment (SRD), and sponge-like retinal swelling [13]. CME associated with or without sponge-like retinal swelling was classified as CME. The presence of disorganization of inner retinal layers (DRIL) and disruption of the ellipsoid zone (EZ) (formerly termed inner segment/outer segment photoreceptor junction) were evaluated on the central B scan which was identified as the central scan passing through the central foveal area on the infrared image. DRIL was defined as any irregularity obscuring the well-delineated boundaries between the inner retinal layers (the ganglion cell-inner plexiform layer complex, inner nuclear layer, and outer plexiform layer). Foveal 1 mm zone was evaluated for the presence of DRIL and disruption of EZ. If $\geq 50\%$ of the central foveal 1 mm zone was affected by DRIL, then DRIL was considered as present according to a previous study [14]. If EZ was disrupted within the 1 mm foveal area, EZ was graded as not intact [15]. B scans were evaluated by two independent specialists (Ali Demircan and Zeynep Alkin). The observed agreement between the 2 graders was 92.7%. All disagreement scans were resolved by mutual agreement.

The demographic features of patients at baseline, BCVA and CMT values obtained at all visits, and the mean number of anti-VEGF injections at the first and last visits were recorded. The mean changes in CMT and BCVA from baseline at the last visit were the primary outcomes and were used to compare the efficacy of both treatments. The percentage of patients who gained ≥ 1 line in BCVA, with CMT < 350 μm at the last visit, and with $\geq 10\%$ reduction in CMT were secondary outcomes.

2.1. Statistical Analysis. Data were analyzed using SPSS 22.0 program (SPSS Chicago, Illinois, USA). Snellen BCVA was converted into logarithm of the minimal angle of resolution (logMAR) for statistical analysis. Continuous variables are expressed as mean $\pm$ standard deviation (SD). Categorical variables are expressed as numbers (n) and percentages (%). The distribution of the variables was measured using the Kolmogorov–Smirnov test. The Mann–Whitney U test was used for the analysis of independent quantitative data. The Wilcoxon test was used for the analysis of dependent quantitative data. The chi-square test was used to analyze independent qualitative data, and Fisher's exact test was used when chi-square test conditions were not met. Spearman's correlation analysis was used for correlation analyses.

3. Results

A total of 43 eyes of 43 patients were included; these comprised both patients who switched from ranibizumab to aflibercept (switch group, $n = 20$) and those treated with ranibizumab only (ranibizumab group, $n = 23$). The mean age was 62.1 ± 7.5 years in the switch group and 63.4 ± 6.5 years in the ranibizumab group. No significant difference was found between the groups ($p = 0.37$). The demographics and clinical characteristics of the patients in both groups are shown in Table 1.

The mean BCVA (logMAR) in the switch and ranibizumab groups was 0.67 ± 0.38 (range: 1.3–0.2) and 0.73 ± 0.34 (range: 1.3–0.15), respectively, at presentation. No statistically significant difference was found between the groups ($p = 0.55$). In the switch group, the mean BCVA (logMAR) improved from 0.68 ± 0.40 at the intermediary visit to 0.58 ± 0.38 at the last visit. Compared with the intermediary visit, there was no statistically significant improvement at the last visit ($p = 0.08$). In the ranibizumab group, the mean BCVA (logMAR) improved from 0.71 ± 0.37 at the intermediary visit to 0.67 ± 0.37 at the last visit; no significant difference was found at the last visit compared with the intermediary visit ($p = 0.12$).

The changes in the mean CMT of the two groups are shown in Figure 1. The mean CMT in the switch and ranibizumab groups was $506.9 \pm 102.2\,\mu m$ (range: 360–707 μm) and $487.3 \pm 82.6\,\mu m$ (range: 387–692 μm) at presentation and $530.7 \pm 91.8\,\mu m$ and $473.5 \pm 78.4\,\mu m$ at the intermediary visit. No statistically significant difference was found between the groups ($p = 0.53$, $p = 0.07$, resp.).

The mean CMT decreased from $530.7 \pm 91.8\,\mu m$ and $473.5 \pm 78.4\,\mu m$ at the intermediary visit to $342.1 \pm 87.5\,\mu m$ and $413.2 \pm 123.8\,\mu m$ at the last visit in the switch and ranibizumab groups, respectively. Compared with the intermediary visit, there was a significant decrease at the last visit in the switch and ranibizumab groups ($p < 0.001$ and $p = 0.03$ resp.). The mean CMT decreased after the intermediary visit by $188.6 \pm 120.5\,\mu m$ in the switch group and by $60.3 \pm 117.1\,\mu m$ in the ranibizumab group. A significant difference was found in CMT reduction between the switch group and the ranibizumab group ($p = 0.003$).

At the last visit, 5 of 20 eyes (25%) in the switch group and 4 of 23 eyes (17.3%) in the ranibizumab group showed a ≥1 line improvement in BCVA. The number of eyes with ≥10% reduction in CMT at the last visit was 18 of 20 eyes (90%) in the switch group and 11 of 23 eyes (47.8%) in the ranibizumab group. There were 12 of 20 eyes (60%) in the switch group and 7 of 23 eyes (34.7%) in the ranibizumab group in which CMT was <350 μm at the last visit.

At the intermediary visit, 20 of the 20 eyes (100%) in the switch group and 23 of the 23 eyes (100%) in the ranibizumab group had CME on OCT. SRD was present in 8 eyes (40%) in the switch group and 5 eyes (21.7%) in the ranibizumab group. Eight eyes (40%) in the switch group and 6 eyes (26%) in the ranibizumab group had the presence of DRIL. EZ disruption was present in 9 eyes (45%) in the switch group and 7 eyes (30.4%) in the ranibizumab group.

TABLE 1: Demographics and number of ranibizumab injections in both groups.

	Switch group $n = 20$	Ranibizumab group $n = 23$	p
Age (years)			0.37
Mean (±SD)	62.1 ± 7.5	63.4 ± 6.5	
Median (min–max)	60 (50–76)	64 (53–72)	
Gender			0.09
Male	9 (45%)	13 (56.5%)	
Female	11 (55%)	10 (43.4%)	
Number of ranibizumab injections before intermediary visit			0.64
Mean (±SD)	5.3 ± 1.2	5.5 ± 0.9	
Median (min–max)	5 (3–5)	5 (3–5)	

n: number; SD: standard deviation.

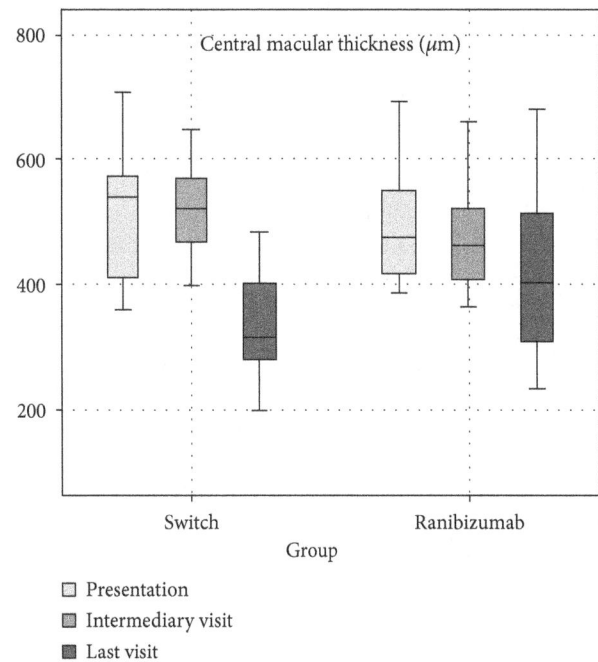

FIGURE 1

The mean number of ranibizumab injections was 5.3 ± 1.2 (range: 4–9) in the switch group and 5.5 ± 0.9 (range: 4–7) in the ranibizumab group before the intermediary visit in a mean period of 12 months. No statistically significant difference was found between the groups ($p = 0.64$). Eyes in the switch and ranibizumab groups received a mean number of 3.5 ± 0.7 (range: 3–5) and 3.7 ± 0.6 (range: 3–5) injections from the intermediary visit and the last visit, respectively, with a mean duration of 6.7 ± 0.8 months. There was no significant difference between the switch group and the ranibizumab group in the mean number of injections after the intermediary visit ($p = 0.32$).

4. Discussion

Vascular endothelial growth factor is an important mediator in the pathogenesis of DME. Intravitreal injections of anti-VEGFs have been established as the main treatment of DME in the last few years. In spite of regular treatment, there are a proportion of patients who incompletely respond to anti-VEGF agents. The Diabetic Retinopathy Clinical Research Network (DRCRnet) Protocol I showed that 52% of patients treated with ranibizumab failed to achieve ≥2 line improvement in BCVA and that 40% had no resolution of retinal thickening at the second year [16]. When treating DME with anti-VEGF agents, the physician has the option of trying other anti-VEGFs or corticosteroids in patients with poor response. Although there are no large randomized prospective clinical trials comparing treatment regimens for refractory DME, several smaller uncontrolled studies demonstrated visual and/or morphologic improvement after switching patients who showed poor response from aflibercept to ranibizumab injections [9–12].

Lim et al. reported visual and morphologic improvements after switching to aflibercept in 21 eyes of 19 patients with DME who had a poor response to multiple bevacizumab/ranibizumab injections [11]. A study by Bahrami et al. similarly demonstrated the beneficial effect of aflibercept on both visual improvement as well as morphologic improvement in patients with DME who had poor response to previous bevacizumab injections [17]. Wood et al. showed only morphologic improvement with aflibercept in patients with poor response to ranibizumab and/or bevacizumab injections in their prospective study [18]. However, the majority of patients (11 of 14) in their study were evaluated after only one aflibercept injection. Rahimy et al. also demonstrated only a morphologic response to aflibercept injections after previous bevacizumab/or ranibizumab therapy, and they explained this result by irreversible functional damage caused by long-standing DME [19]. Switching to aflibercept resulted in some anatomic improvement in the majority of patients in all studies.

In our study, both ranibizumab and aflibercept treatments provided only morphologic improvement in patients who have poor response to previous ranibizumab treatment. A greater decrease in macular thickness in the switch group than in the ranibizumab group in the current study might be explained by the blocking of all isoforms of VEGF-A, VEGF-B, and PlGF with aflibercept in contrast to inactivation of only VEGF-A with ranibizumab. Some studies showed that PlGF may have a place in the pathogenesis of DME. Increasing intravitreal concentrations of PlGF has been associated with progressively advancing degrees of diabetic retinopathy [20–23]. Blockade of this protein might play a role in such patients. Moreover, the greater improvement in macular morphology with aflibercept might be related to patients' inherent characteristics rather than features of aflibercept. In addition to all these possible explanations, patients treated with repetitive ranibizumab/bevacizumab injections may demonstrate tachyphylaxis or a diminished therapeutic response to these agents over time as suggested in a great number of studies [24, 25].

Additionally, there was a trend towards greater visual acuity improvement after switching to aflibercept, but it was not statistically significant. The discrepancy between morphologic and functional outcomes may be explained by irreversible functional damage caused by long-standing DME. Switching to intravitreal steroids with good functional and morphologic outcomes after ranibizumab failure in DME treatment has been shown in previous studies [26]. A switch to another pharmaceutical class such as corticosteroids is a logical option in case of failure of other therapies in DME.

All of the previous studies only reported outcomes of patients with a poor response to bevacizumab/ranibizumab who switched to aflibercept and had no comparison between the outcomes of switched patients and those of patients who continued with previous anti-VEGF treatment. It is not clear whether the visual and/or anatomic recovery in these patients originated from the new intravitreal anti-VEGF agent or from the total number of anti-VEGF injections applied because it was demonstrated that there was a delayed responder group treated with ranibizumab that showed some visual and anatomic improvement when treatment was continued with further ranibizumab injections.

The major limitations of this study were the relatively small sample size and short follow-up time as well as its retrospective design. Further prospective and randomized studies with larger sample sizes and longer duration are needed to evaluate the effectiveness of aflibercept injections in the visual and morphologic improvements following changing previous treatment in persistent DME.

In the current study, we compared a switch group that comprised patients who switched to aflibercept after showing a poor response to previous ranibizumab treatment with a ranibizumab group composed of patients who continued with ranibizumab injections despite the presence of poor response to this treatment. To the best of our knowledge, this is the first study in the literature to compare these treatments in persistent DME.

In conclusion, the results of our study showed that switching therapy from intravitreal ranibizumab to aflibercept in persistent DME provided only morphologic improvement. The discrepancy between morphologic and functional outcomes may be explained by irreversible functional damage caused by long-standing DME.

Conflicts of Interest

The authors declare that they have no conflicts of interest.

References

[1] R. N. Frank, "Diabetic retinopathy," *New England Journal of Medicine*, vol. 350, no. 1, pp. 48–58, 2004.

[2] J. W. Y. Yau, S. L. Rogers, R. Kawasaki et al., "Global prevalence and major risk factors of diabetic retinopathy," *Diabetes Care*, vol. 35, no. 3, pp. 556–564, 2012.

[3] R. Klein, B. E. K. Klein, S. E. Moss, M. D. Davis, and D. L. DeMets, "The Wisconsin epidemiologic study of diabetic

retinopathy. IV. Diabetic macular edema," *Ophthalmology*, vol. 91, no. 12, pp. 1464–1474, 1984.

[4] Q. D. Nguyen, D. M. Brown, D. M. Marcus et al., "Ranibizumab for diabetic macular edema: results from 2 phase III randomized trials: RISE and RIDE," *Ophthalmology*, vol. 119, no. 4, pp. 789–801, 2012.

[5] D. M. Brown, U. Schmidt-Erfurth, D. V. Do et al., "Intravitreal aflibercept for diabetic macular edema: 100-week results from the VISTA and VIVID studies," *Ophthalmology*, vol. 122, no. 10, pp. 2044–2052, 2015.

[6] R. Rajendram, S. Fraser-Bell, A. Kaines et al., "A 2-year prospective randomized controlled trial of intravitreal bevacizumab or laser therapy (BOLT) in the management of diabetic macular edema: 24-month data: report 3," *Archives of Ophthalmology*, vol. 130, no. 8, pp. 972–979, 2012.

[7] L. Wu, M. A. Martínez-Castellanos, H. Quiroz-Mercado et al., "Twelve-month safety of intravitreal injections of bevacizumab (Avastin®): results of the Pan-American Collaborative Retina Study Group (PACORES)," *Graefe's Archive for Clinical and Experimental Ophthalmology*, vol. 246, no. 1, pp. 81–87, 2008.

[8] Diabetic Retinopathy Clinical Research Network, "A phase II randomized clinical trial of intravitreal bevacizumab for diabetic macular edema," *Ophthalmology*, vol. 114, no. 10, pp. 1860–1867.e7, 2007.

[9] F. Mira, M. Paulo, F. Henriques, and J. Figueira, "Switch to aflibercept in diabetic macular edema patients unresponsive to previous anti-VEGF therapy," *Journal of Ophthalmology*, vol. 2017, Article ID 5632634, 4 pages, 2017.

[10] K. A. Klein, T. S. Cleary, and E. Reichel, "Effect of intravitreal aflibercept on recalcitrant diabetic macular edema," *International Journal of Retina and Vitreous*, vol. 3, no. 1, p. 16, 2017.

[11] L. S. Lim, W. Y. Ng, R. Mathur et al., "Conversion to aflibercept for diabetic macular edema unresponsive to ranibizumab or bevacizumab," *Clinical Ophthalmology*, vol. 9, pp. 1715–1718, 2015.

[12] Y. Y. Chen, P. Y. Chang, and J. K. Wang, "Intravitreal aflibercept for patients with diabetic macular edema refractory to bevacizumab or ranibizumab: analysis of response to aflibercept," *Asia-Pacific Journal of Ophthalmology*, vol. 6, no. 3, pp. 250–255, 2017.

[13] T. Otani, S. Kishi, and Y. Maruyama, "Patterns of diabetic macular edema with optical coherence tomography," *American Journal of Ophthalmology*, vol. 127, no. 6, pp. 688–693, 1999.

[14] J. K. Sun, S. H. Radwan, A. Z. Soliman et al., "Neural retinal disorganization as a robust marker of visual acuity in current and resolved diabetic macular edema," *Diabetes*, vol. 64, no. 7, pp. 2560–2570, 2015.

[15] U. Soiberman, M. Goldstein, P. Pianka, A. Loewenstein, and D. Goldenberg, "Preservation of the photoreceptor layer following subthreshold laser treatment for diabetic macular edema as demonstrated by SD-OCT," *Investigative Ophthalmology & Visual Science*, vol. 55, no. 5, pp. 3054–3059, 2014.

[16] Diabetic Retinopathy Clinical Research Network, M. J. Elman, L. P. Aiello et al., "Randomized trial evaluating Ranibizumab plus prompt or deferred laser or triamcinolone plus prompt laser for diabetic macular edema," *Ophthalmology*, vol. 117, no. 6, pp. 1064–1077.e35, 2010.

[17] B. Bahrami, T. Hong, M. Zhu, T. E. Schlub, and A. Chang, "Switching therapy from bevacizumab to aflibercept for the management of persistent diabetic macular edema,"

Graefe's Archive for Clinical and Experimental Ophthalmology, vol. 255, no. 6, pp. 1133–1140, 2017.

[18] E. H. Wood, P. A. Karth, D. M. Moshfeghi, and T. Leng, "Short-term outcomes of aflibercept therapy for diabetic macular edema in patients with incomplete response to ranibizumab and/or bevacizumab," *Ophthalmic Surgery, Lasers and Imaging Retina*, vol. 46, no. 9, pp. 950–954, 2015.

[19] E. Rahimy, A. Shahlaee, M. A. Khan et al., "Conversion to aflibercept after prior anti-VEGF therapy for persistent diabetic macular edema," *American Journal of Ophthalmology*, vol. 164, pp. 118–127.e2, 2016.

[20] N. Papadopoulos, J. Martin, Q. Ruan et al., "Binding and neutralization of vascular endothelial growth factor (VEGF) and related ligands by VEGF trap, ranibizumab and bevacizumab," *Angiogenesis*, vol. 15, no. 2, pp. 171–185, 2012.

[21] A. N. Witmer, G. F. J. M. Vrensen, C. J. F. Van Noorden, and R. O. Schlingemann, "Vascular endothelial growth factors and angiogenesis in eye disease," *Progress in Retinal and Eye Research*, vol. 22, no. 1, pp. 1–29, 2003.

[22] K. Kovacs, K. V. Marra, G. Yu et al., "Angiogenic and inflammatory vitreous biomarkers associated with increasing levels of retinal ischemia," *Investigative Ophthalmology & Visual Science*, vol. 56, no. 11, pp. 6523–6530, 2015.

[23] N. Miyamoto, Y. de Kozak, J. C. Jeanny et al., "Placental growth factor-1 and epithelial haemato–retinal barrier breakdown: potential implication in the pathogenesis of diabetic retinopathy," *Diabetologia*, vol. 50, no. 2, pp. 461–470, 2007.

[24] F. Forooghian, C. Cukras, C. B. Meyerle, E. Y. Chew, and W. T. Wong, "Tachyphylaxis after intravitreal bevacizumab for exudative age-related macular degeneration," *Retina*, vol. 29, no. 6, pp. 723–731, 2009.

[25] S. Schaal, H. J. Kaplan, and T. H. Tezel, "Is there tachyphylaxis to intravitreal anti-vascular endothelial growth factor pharmacotherapy in age-related macular degeneration?," *Ophthalmology*, vol. 115, no. 12, pp. 2199–2205, 2008.

[26] I. Zhioua, O. Semoun, F. Lalloum, and E. H. Souied, "Intravitreal dexamethasone implant in patients with ranibizumab persistent diabetic macular edema," *Retina*, vol. 35, no. 7, pp. 1429–1435, 2015.

25

Extended Injection Intervals after Switching from Ranibizumab to Aflibercept in Macular Edema due to Central Retinal Vein Occlusion

Sylvia Nghiem-Buffet ⓘ,[1,2] Agnès Glacet-Bernard,[3] Manar Addou-Regnard,[3]
Eric H. Souied ⓘ,[3] Salomon Y. Cohen,[1,3] and Audrey Giocanti-Auregan[2]

[1]Centre Ophtalmologique d'Imagerie et de Laser, 11 Rue Antoine Bourdelle, Paris, France
[2]Ophthalmology Department, DHU Vision and Handicaps, APHP, Avicenne Hospital, Paris 13 University,
125 Rue de Stalingrad, Bobigny, France
[3]Department of Ophthalmology, Centre Hospitalier Intercommunal, Université Paris-Est-Créteil, Paris 12 University,
40 Avenue de Verdun, 91000 Créteil, France

Correspondence should be addressed to Sylvia Nghiem-Buffet; buffet.nghiem@free.fr

Academic Editor: Manuel S. Falcão

Purpose. To assess treatment interval extension after switching from ranibizumab to aflibercept intravitreal injections in macular edema (ME) due to central retinal vein occlusion (CRVO) with an insufficient response or frequent recurrences to initial treatment. *Methods.* CRVO eyes treated with ranibizumab injections on a treat-and-extend (TAE) basis with an insufficient response or frequent recurrences were switched to aflibercept. Primary endpoint was the change in injection intervals before and after the switch. *Results.* Eleven eyes were included in this retrospective bicentric study. Before switching, patients received a mean number of 15.3 ranibizumab injections (range, 6-34) during a mean follow-up of 23.4 months (range, 6-57). After switching to aflibercept, patients received a mean number of 12.4 injections (range, 6-20) during a mean follow-up of 25.5 months (range, 16-38). Treatment interval could be extended from 6.1 (range, 4-8) to 11 weeks (range, 8-16) ($p = 0.001$) corresponding to a mean extension of injection interval of +4.9 weeks. *Conclusion.* In case of insufficient response or frequent recurrences of ME due to CRVO in patients treated with ranibizumab on a TAE basis, switching to aflibercept could allow extending treatment intervals, which could reduce the injection burden for these patients.

1. Introduction

Macular edema (ME) is the leading cause of vision loss in case of central retinal vein occlusion (CRVO). The prognosis of this disease has recently been considerably improved through the use of intravitreal injections of anti-VEGF agents [1–4] or corticosteroids [5, 6].

ME secondary to CRVO is mainly due to an abnormal vascular permeability involving the vascular endothelial growth factor (VEGF) [7]. Anti-VEGF therapy is one of the treatments available for ME since 2011: in 2011, ranibizumab (Lucentis) has been approved by the Food and Drug Administration

(FDA) following the CRUISE study [8], and then aflibercept (Eylea) has been approved for the treatment of ME due to CRVO in 2013 following the GALILEO [1] and COPERNICUS [3] phase 3 clinical trials. In France, both ranibizumab and aflibercept are covered by the healthcare system.

Thus, the first anti-VEGF treatment prescribed in our practice for ME secondary to CRVO was ranibizumab because of its earlier availability. The RETAIN study [9] has shown that among patients with ME due to CRVO well managed with ranibizumab, 56.2% of patients still required frequent retreatment for the third and the fourth year of follow-up. In these particular cases in which the response to ranibizumab seems insufficient or when an extension of treatment intervals is not possible, a switch to another drug may help to manage ME and to reduce treatment burden for patients. Clinicians may either change pharmaceutical class and use dexamethasone implant or switch to another anti-VEGF treatment. Some studies have reported results supporting the efficacy of switching to aflibercept after ranibizumab failure [10–14].

Unlike ranibizumab, aflibercept binds not only to VEGF-A but also to VEGF-B and placental growth factor (PlGF) [15]. This different mechanism of action may explain the possible efficacy of aflibercept after ranibizumab failure even if they belong to the same therapeutic class.

The aim of this study was to assess the extension of treatment intervals after switching from ranibizumab to aflibercept intravitreal injections in recurrent ME and in ME with insufficient response to initial treatment in CRVO.

2. Methods

A retrospective study was conducted in two tertiary centers specialized in imaging and treatment of retinal diseases (Centre Ophtalmologique d'Imagerie et de Laser in Paris and the Department of Ophthalmology of the Intercommunal Hospital Center in Créteil, France). All consecutive patients treated with ranibizumab on a TAE regimen for ME due to CRVO and switched to aflibercept between January 2014 and December 2015 were included. The TAE schedule consisted of an initial intravitreal ranibizumab loading dose of three consecutive monthly injections, followed by monthly injections until the macula was dry on SD-OCT. The interval between treatments was extended by fixed 2-week increments if no exudative changes were observed on SD-OCT. In case of fluid recurrence on SD-OCT, the interval was reduced back down by one or two weeks.

The decision to switch to aflibercept was at the discretion of one of the investigators (SNB and AGB) in case of frequent recurrences or insufficient response to ranibizumab defined in this study as follows:

> Frequent recurrences were defined by a maximum relapse-free interval of 8 weeks or less. The patients were considered to have frequent recurrences of ME due to CRVO, although it was controlled with ranibizumab, if the interval between injections was less than or equal to 8 weeks. The interval between injections was based on a TAE regimen. This interval was the maximum interval needed to prevent ME recurrence and to stabilize visual acuity.

> Insufficient response to ranibizumab treatment was defined by a reduction in central retinal thickness (CRT) but persistence of fluid or cystoid change in the central subfield despite at least 6 monthly ranibizumab injections with the impossibility to extend interval more than 4 weeks. Persistent ME was defined on SD-OCT (Cirrus 5000, ZEISS Meditec, Germany; Spectralis, Heidelberg, Germany) by a loss of the foveal pit and a CRT >300 μm.

This study was conducted in accordance with the tenets of the Declaration of Helsinki, and an informed consent was obtained from all patients. Approval was obtained from the Federation France Macula ethics committee.

Inclusion criteria were as follows:

(i) Patients aged at least 18 years

(ii) Patients with ME due to CRVO treated with ranibizumab on a TAE regimen with frequent recurrences or insufficient response to treatment

(iii) Patients with a minimum follow-up of twelve months after the switch to aflibercept.

Exclusion criteria were as follows: other ocular conditions impairing vision, fewer than six ranibizumab injections prior to the switch to aflibercept, and incomplete imaging or clinical data.

All patients underwent a complete ophthalmological examination before switching including medical history and comorbidities (high blood pressure), best-corrected visual acuity (BCVA) on the ETDRS chart, intraocular pressure, slit-lamp examination, and SD-OCT. Based on these examinations, one of the investigators (SNB and AGB) decided to switch to aflibercept. Visual acuity and SD-OCT were repeated on a TAE basis after switching to aflibercept.

The following data were collected: time interval between injections, number of injections, BCVA, and (CRT) assessed by SD-OCT.

The primary endpoint was the interval between aflibercept injections after switching and comparing the previous interval between ranibizumab injections.

Secondary endpoints were changes in BCVA and CRT after switching to aflibercept.

Statistical analysis was performed using a Wilcoxon test with GraphPad software (Statview® 1998, SAS Institute Inc.) A p value < 0.05 was considered statistically significant.

3. Results

3.1. Patients Demographic and Baseline Characteristics. Eleven eyes of 11 patients (2 women and 9 men) were included. Patient mean age was 67.1 years (range, 44 to 83 years). Eight out of the 11 patients had a well-perfused form of CRVO, while 3 patients had a mixed CRVO form with ME and peripheral ischemia requiring panretinal photocoagulation. Four eyes (36%) had previously been treated for open-angle glaucoma. Three patients (27%) had previously been diagnosed with high blood pressure, 3 (27%) with cardiac arrhythmia, and one (9%) with type 1 diabetes with mild nonproliferative diabetic retinopathy before CRVO occurrence.

Before switching to aflibercept, 3 patients had previously been switched to dexamethasone implant (Ozurdex) (1–3 injections), but they were rapidly switched back to ranibizumab because of raised intraocular pressure. They were then switched to aflibercept when it became available in France. The data are summarized in Table 1.

3.2. Interval between Injections. Before switching, patients received a mean number of 15.3 ± 9.8 ranibizumab injections (range, 6 to 34 injections) during a mean follow-up of 23.4 ± 15.9 months (range, 6 to 57 months). Related to the

TABLE 1: Demographics, baseline, and follow-up characteristics of patients with CRVO.

Demographics	
Patients (eyes)	11 (11)
Mean age, years (range)	67.1 (44–83)
Women, *n* (%)	2 (18)
Diabetes, *n* (%)	1 (9)
Diabetic retinopathy, *n* (%)	1 (9)
Preswitch follow-up in months, mean (range)	23.4 (6–57)
Patients previously switched to steroid implant injections, *n* (range of injections)	3 (1–3)
Scatter panretinal photocoagulation, *n* (%)	3 (27%)
Previous ranibizumab injections number, mean ± SD	15.3 ± 9.8
Aflibercept injections number after switch, mean ± SD	12.4 ± 4.2
Postswitch follow-up, in month, mean (range)	25.5 (16–38)

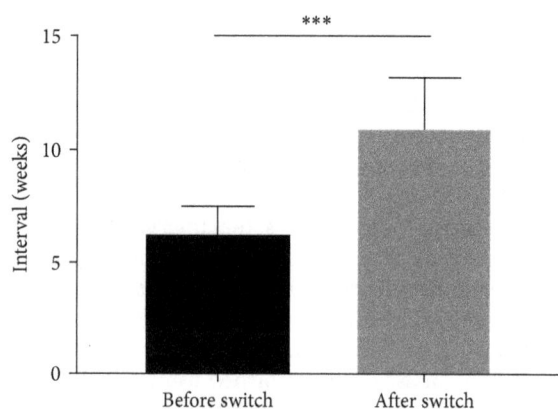

FIGURE 1: Injection interval before and after the switch to aflibercept. The error bars are interquartile range.

treatment duration and the TAE regimen, the mean ranibizumab injection interval acquired was 6.1 ± 1.4 weeks (range, 4 to 8 weeks) and remained stable for each patient but could not be more extended unless ME recurrence. Only one patient had a 4-week interval treatment and showed anatomic and functional improvement but with persistence of macular fluid. Thus, he was switched to aflibercept after 6 months and 6 ranibizumab injections. He showed a complete resolution of fluid in the macula with aflibercept and could be progressively extended to a 10-week interval treatment.

After switching to aflibercept, patients received a mean number of 12.4 ± 4.2 injections (range, 6 to 20 injections) during a mean follow-up of 25.5 ± 5.8 months (range, 16 to 38 months). Due to the switch to aflibercept, the treatment interval was extended from 6.1 ± 1.4 weeks (range, 4 to 8 weeks) to 11 ± 2.3 weeks (range, 8 to 16 weeks) ($p = 0.001$) corresponding to a treatment interval gain of 4.9 ± 1.9 weeks (range, 2 to 8 weeks) (Figure 1).

Among patients who were switched to aflibercept, 100% responded to ranibizumab, but 27% (3 patients) only partially responded with persistent fluid on SD-OCT. After switching to aflibercept, 100% of patients responded to

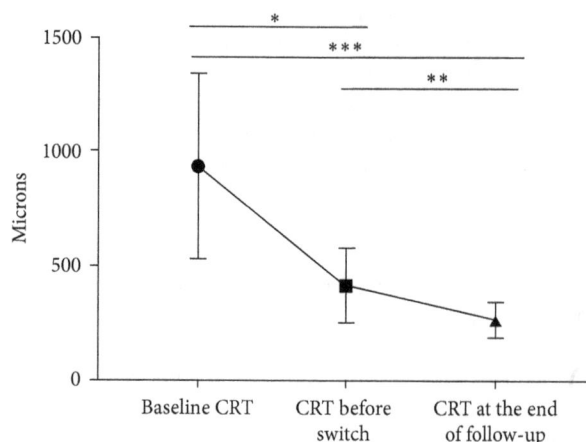

FIGURE 2: Change in central retinal thickness (CRT) before any injection (baseline), just before the switch to aflibercept, and after the switch at the end of follow-up.

aflibercept, and 90% (10 patients) experienced a complete fluid resorption seen on SD-OCT with restoration of a foveal pit. The only patient with persistent macular thickening also had a significant epimacular membrane but no persistent cystoid space left or serous detachment was observed, and the CRT was significantly decreased after the switch to aflibercept.

3.3. Functional Outcomes. The initial BCVA before any intravitreal injection was of 41.1 ± 20.9 letters (range, 2 to 65 letters). The mean BCVA before the switch was of 60.5 ± 13 letters (range, 35 to 75 letters), corresponding to a visual gain of +19.4 letters ($p = 0.033$). The mean BCVA at the end of follow-up after switching to aflibercept was of 62 ± 16.6 letters (range, 20 to 81 letters) corresponding to a visual gain of +1.5 letters due to the switch ($p = 0.84$).

3.4. Anatomical Outcomes. The mean initial CRT before any treatment was $936 \pm 402.5 \, \mu m$. The mean CRT before switching to aflibercept was $411.2 \pm 161.8 \, \mu m$, and it significantly decreased to $264.4 \pm 74.3 \, \mu m$ ($p = 0.002$) at the end of follow-up (Figure 2).

4. Discussion

In this retrospective study, we showed that, in selected cases of ME due to CRVO with frequent recurrences or insufficient anatomical response to ranibizumab with TAE regimen, switching to aflibercept could significantly improve anatomical outcomes ($-146.8 \, \mu m$) and extend the injection interval by 4.9 weeks with a sustained visual acuity gain after a mean follow-up of 25.5 ± 5.8 months (range, 16 to 38 months) after the switch.

Few studies in the literature have focused on visual and functional outcomes after switching from ranibizumab to aflibercept in ME due to CRVO. A retrospective study assessing 6 consecutive eyes with persistent ME despite intravitreal injections of ranibizumab or bevacizumab, conducted in 2014 [13] with a 7-month follow-up, has shown a complete fluid resolution after 1 or 2 aflibercept injections with a modest but sustained visual gain in 3 out of the 6 patients. Another retrospective study [14] assessing 13 eyes with CRVO with insufficient response to ranibizumab or bevacizumab injected every 6 weeks that were switched to aflibercept on a TAE basis has shown that the mean injection interval significantly increased by 0.51 months after 1-year follow-up and that the relapse-free interval also significantly increased by 3.02 weeks, with significantly improved functional and anatomical outcomes. Another retrospective study [10], assessing 17 eyes with ME due to CRVO resistant to bevacizumab or ranibizumab, has shown a significant functional and anatomical improvement after switch to aflibercept. In the later study, a treat-and-extend regimen was used before and after the switch, and the mean interval between intravitreal injections was not extended after the switch. A more recent study [12] assessing 42 eyes with persistent or recurrent ME due to CRVO that received at least 3 ranibizumab and/or bevacizumab intravitreal injections, and then switched to aflibercept, has reported a significant anatomical improvement without significant functional improvement and a significant extension of the interval between injections from 5.6 weeks before the switch to 7.6 weeks after the switch.

Taken together, all these studies and our findings seem to show that switching from ranibizumab/bevacizumab to aflibercept could allow extending the injection interval in a selected population of patients with insufficient anatomical response to ranibizumab or bevacizumab or with frequent recurrences. Despite anatomical improvement, these studies did not show systematic functional improvement. In our series, even CRT improved significantly after the switch, and no functional improvement (BCVA) was observed. This fact is probably caused by morphologic and macula changes in cases with chronic and recurrent ME.

Interestingly, to our knowledge, our study has the longest described follow-up after the switch to aflibercept with a mean of 25.5 ± 5.8 months. The RETAIN study [9] has estimated that, after 48 months of follow-up, 56.2% of patients still required frequent reinjections. Switching to aflibercept could in these selected cases allow reducing the frequency of injections and the treatment burden for both patients and caregivers.

To explain the extension of treatment intervals after switching to aflibercept, we could assume that (i) aflibercept could have a greater affinity for VEGF-A compared to ranibizumab or bevacizumab, (ii) the action of aflibercept not only on VEGF-A but also on PlGF and VEGF-B, could be involved in maintaining its efficacy, (iii) there could be a "switch effect" due to tachyphylaxis developed in response to the first molecule used before the switch, or (iv) the disease could improve by itself over time per se. The latter seems less likely since several studies in the literature have shown an increased treatment interval after switching to aflibercept despite variable follow-up durations before and after the switch. Concerning possible tachyphylaxis to ranibizumab, the treatment frequency did not change before switching to aflibercept in our patients. Ranibizumab treatment interval remained stable but could not be more extended unless ME recurrence. After the switch, the injection interval could be elongated in all our patients, and higher efficacy of the aflibercept treatment could be assumed.

However, to confirm the imputability of aflibercept in this extended relapse-free interval, further controlled studies comparing the efficacy and treatment intervals between ranibizumab and aflibercept are needed. A recent retrospective observational study [16], including 62 naive patients, has shown similar functional and anatomical outcomes after 18 months of follow-up with both treatments with a similar number of injections.

Our study has some limitations, including its retrospective design, a very limited number of eyes, and the absence of the controlled arm. However, our long follow-up after the switch of 25.5 ± 5.8 months (range, 16 to 38 months) confirms a sustained efficacy of aflibercept after the switch at least in terms of anatomical outcomes and treatment interval extension.

In conclusion, in case of insufficient response or frequent recurrences of ME due to CRVO treated with ranibizumab on a TAE basis, switching to aflibercept could allow extending treatment interval, which could reduce the injection burden for these patients. Moreover, after switching to aflibercept despite the absence of significant visual gain, VA stabilization could be expected with a significant anatomical improvement.

Conflicts of Interest

The authors declare that there are no conflicts of interest regarding the publication of this paper. Sylvia Nghiem-Buffet is a consultant for Allergan, Bayer, Novartis, and Zeiss outside of the submitted work. Agnès Glacet-Bernard is a consultant for Allergan, Bayer, and Novartis outside of the submitted work. Manar Addou-Regnard has nothing to disclose. Eric H. Souied is a consultant for Allergan, Bayer, Novartis, and Thea outside of the submitted work. Salomon Y. Cohen is a consultant for Alcon, Allergan, Bayer, Novartis, Roche, and Thea outside of the submitted work. Audrey Giocanti-Auregan is a consultant for Alimera, Allergan, Bayer, Novartis, and Optos Plc outside of the submitted work.

Acknowledgments

The authors thank AVOPH (Association for Vision in Ophthalmology) Avicenne Hospital, 125 rue de Stalingrad, 93000 Bobigny, France, and CIL-ASSOC (Association for Research—Centre d'Imagerie et de Laser, Paris, France).

References

[1] Y. Ogura, J. Roider, J. F. Korobelnik et al., "Intravitreal aflibercept for macular edema secondary to central retinal

vein occlusion: 18-month results of the phase 3 GALILEO study," *American Journal of Ophthalmology*, vol. 158, no. 5, pp. 1032.e2–1038.e2, 2014.

[2] M. Larsen, S. M. Waldstein, F. Boscia et al., "Individualized ranibizumab regimen driven by stabilization criteria for central retinal vein occlusion: twelve-month results of the CRYSTAL study," *Ophthalmology*, vol. 123, no. 5, pp. 1101–1111, 2016.

[3] J. S. Heier, W. L. Clark, D. S. Boyer et al., "Intravitreal aflibercept injection for macular edema due to central retinal vein occlusion: two-year results from the COPERNICUS study," *Ophthalmology*, vol. 121, no. 7, pp. 1414.e1–1420.e1, 2014.

[4] P. A. Campochiaro, D. M. Brown, C. C. Awh et al., "Sustained benefits from ranibizumab for macular edema following central retinal vein occlusion: twelve-month outcomes of a phase III study," *Ophthalmology*, vol. 118, no. 10, pp. 2041–2049, 2011.

[5] J. A. Haller, F. Bandello, R. Belfort Jr. et al., "Randomized, sham-controlled trial of dexamethasone intravitreal implant in patients with macular edema due to retinal vein occlusion," *Ophthalmology*, vol. 117, no. 6, pp. 1134.e3–1146.e3, 2010.

[6] H. Hoerauf, N. Feltgen, C. Weiss et al., "Clinical efficacy and safety of ranibizumab versus dexamethasone for central retinal vein occlusion (COMRADE C): a European label study," *American Journal of Ophthalmology*, vol. 169, pp. 258–267, 2016.

[7] H. Noma, H. Funatsu, T. Mimura, S. Harino, and S. Hori, "Vitreous levels of interleukin-6 and vascular endothelial growth factor in macular edema with central retinal vein occlusion," *Ophthalmology*, vol. 116, no. 1, pp. 87–93, 2009.

[8] D. M. Brown, P. A. Campochiaro, R. P. Singh et al., "Ranibizumab for macular edema following central retinal vein occlusion: six-month primary end point results of a phase III study," *Ophthalmology*, vol. 117, no. 6, pp. 1124.e1–1133.e1, 2010.

[9] P. A. Campochiaro, R. Sophie, J. Pearlman et al., "Long-term outcomes in patients with retinal vein occlusion treated with ranibizumab: the RETAIN study," *Ophthalmology*, vol. 121, no. 1, pp. 209–219, 2014.

[10] M. N. Cohen, S. K. Houston, A. Juhn et al., "Effect of aflibercept on refractory macular edema associated with central retinal vein occlusion," *Canadian Journal of Ophthalmology*, vol. 51, no. 5, pp. 342–347, 2016.

[11] L. Lehmann-Clarke, A. Dirani, I. Mantel, and A. Ambresin, "The effect of switching ranibizumab to aflibercept in refractory cases of macular edema secondary to ischemic central vein occlusion," *Klinische Monatsblätter für Augenheilkunde*, vol. 232, no. 4, pp. 552–555, 2015.

[12] T. D. Papakostas, L. Lim, T. van Zyl et al., "Intravitreal aflibercept for macular oedema secondary to central retinal vein occlusion in patients with prior treatment with bevacizumab or ranibizumab," *Eye*, vol. 30, no. 1, pp. 79–84, 2016.

[13] J. A. Eadie, M. S. Ip, and A. D. Kulkarni, "Response to aflibercept as secondary therapy in patients with persistent retinal edema due to central retinal vein occlusion initially treated with bevacizumab or ranibizumab," *Retina*, vol. 34, no. 12, pp. 2439–2443, 2014.

[14] M. Pfau, H. Fassnacht-Riederle, M. D. Becker, N. Graf, and S. Michels, "Clinical outcome after switching therapy from ranibizumab and/or bevacizumab to aflibercept in central retinal vein occlusion," *Ophthalmic Research*, vol. 54, no. 3, pp. 150–156, 2015.

[15] N. Papadopoulos, J. Martin, Q. Ruan et al., "Binding and neutralization of vascular endothelial growth factor (VEGF) and related ligands by VEGF Trap, ranibizumab and bevacizumab," *Angiogenesis*, vol. 15, no. 2, pp. 171–185, 2012.

[16] I. Chatziralli, G. Theodossiadis, M. M. Moschos, P. Mitropoulos, and P. Theodossiadis, "Ranibizumab versus aflibercept for macular edema due to central retinal vein occlusion: 18-month results in real-life data," *Graefe's Archive for Clinical and Experimental Ophthalmology*, vol. 255, no. 6, pp. 1093–1100, 2017.

26

Anterior Chamber Flare as an Objective and Quantitative Noninvasive Method for Oculopathy in Transthyretin V30M Amyloidosis Patients

João Beirão ⓘ,[1] Vasco Miranda,[2] Beatriz Pinheiro-Torres,[3] João Coelho ⓘ,[2] Maria-João Menéres,[2] and Pedro Menéres[1]

[1]Instituto de Ciências Biomédicas Abel Salazar, Universidade do Porto, Porto, Portugal
[2]Centro Hospitalar Porto, Porto, Portugal
[3]Alimera Sciences, Alpharetta, USA

Correspondence should be addressed to João Beirão; brandaobeirao@gmail.com

Academic Editor: Miguel Rechichi

Purpose. Assess the aqueous humor flare in transthyretin V30M amyloidosis patients (ATTRV30M). *Materials and Methods.* This is a retrospective, cross-sectional, noninterventional comparative study including 28 ATTRV30M patients with a unilateral scalloped iris. For comparative analysis, the fellow eye, the nonscalloped iris eye, from each patient was used as control. All patients underwent aqueous humor flare meter and intraocular pressure (IOP) measurements. *Results.* Mean aqueous humor flare was significantly higher in the eyes with the scalloped iris than the control group with the nonscalloped iris (14.1 ± 2.2 versus 6.5 ± 0.9 pc/ms, respectively). No significant differences in IOP were found in the scalloped iris eyes than those in the nonscalloped iris control group (17.1 ± 0.8 versus 16.8 ± 0.7 mmHg, respectively). No significant correlation was not found between the flare and the IOP value within groups. *Conclusions.* In this study, aqueous humor flare values in the scalloped iris eyes may be a valid marker for controlling the stage of the oculopathy in ATTRV30M patients.

1. Introduction

Hereditary transthyretin V30M amyloidosis (ATTRV30M) is an autosomal dominant disorder and is a very common form of hereditary amyloidosis caused by extracellular deposition of variants of transthyretin (TTR) in several tissues, including the eye [1, 2]. More than 100 amyloidogenic TTR mutations have been documented [3], but in the Portuguese type, the variant TTR has a substitution of methionine for valine at position 30. Despite the worldwide distribution of the disease, Portugal remains the main geographic focus of amyloidosis TTR V30M [4]. ATTRV30M patients are usually classified as presenting an early onset disease (onset before 50 years of age) or a late-onset disease (onset after 50 years of age). Early onset is associated with a more aggressive, rapidly progressing disease, especially if symptoms appear before 40 years of age [5]. Most Portuguese ATTRV30M patients are early-onset cases, with a worse prognosis regarding the severity of symptoms and an expected survival of 10 to 15 years without treatment. Liver transplantation is one of the treatments for ATTRV30M amyloidosis as it removes circulating mutant TTR and interrupts the progression of the disease and improve survival and quality of life [6]. Tafamidis, an oral, non-NSAID, highly specific TTR stabilizer has emerged as the new standard of care for ATTRV30M and remains the only medicine approved for the treatment of transthyretin amyloidosis in adult patients with stage 1 symptomatic polyneuropathy [7].

Nevertheless, the intraocular production of TTR V30M by the retinal and ciliary pigment epithelium remains unchanged, contributing to the progression of amyloid deposition-associated ocular manifestations such as abnormal conjunctival vessels, dry eye, scalloped pupils, deposition of amyloid on the anterior surface of the lens and on the pupil border, vitreous amyloidosis, glaucoma, and retinal angiopathy. Moreover, their prevalence increases over time [8].

Glaucoma is an ocular neurodegenerative disease and one of the most common causes of blindness worldwide [9]. It is characterized by retinal ganglion cell degeneration which can lead to optic atrophy and visual field defects [10]. Multiple factors play a role in the etiology and pathology of the disease, being intraocular pressure (IOP) the most important risk factor usually caused by abnormal aqueous humor outflow [11]. Extensive research over the last decade has shown that no amyloid secondary glaucomatous proteomics and oxidative damage can also lead to unfavourable effects on the trabecular meshwork and increased resistance to intraocular aqueous humor drainage [11–19]. Moreover, assessments of the involvement of ATTRV30M in ocular complications showed that glaucoma was strongly associated with the presence of scalloped iris [20]. Still, the nature of the interaction mechanism of iris deformation and aqueous humor flow was not evaluated and is not fully understood yet [8, 21].

However, the presence of scalloped iris before the onset of glaucoma was also observed [20]. Laser flare cell meter is an objective, sensitive, and noninvasive method for evaluating the aqueous flare and allows a quantitative assessment of anterior chamber inflammation and breakdown of the blood-aqueous barrier [22–24]. Several studies have shown altered flare values in glaucomatous eyes and speculated the role of the anterior chamber aqueous flare in predicting the risk of glaucoma [25–30]. Therefore, the aim of this analysis is to assess the blood-aqueous barrier (BAB) function with the use of a laser flare meter in ATTRV30M Portuguese patients with and without scalloped iris.

2. Materials and Methods

This was a retrospective, cross-sectional, noninterventional study conducted at the Ophthalmic Department from Centro Hospitalar do Porto, Porto. Written informed consent was obtained from all patients. This study was performed in accordance with the Declaration of Helsinki of the World Medical Association and was approved by the Ethics Committee of the Centro Hospitalar do Porto.

2.1. Patients. The study included a retrospective cohort of 28 consecutive patients (60.7% men; mean age: 46.5 (35–61) years) examined for ocular abnormalities at the Ophthalmology Service of Centro Hospitalar do Porto. All patients had the ATTR V30M mutation confirmed by genetic analysis and presented unilateral scalloped iris. These patients presented in both eyes no abnormalities in optic nerve and visual field nor ongoing treatment with ocular hypotensive eyedrops and/or previous glaucoma or ocular surgery. The only ocular treatment was artificial tears, and all eyes had best corrected visual acuity of 1.0 (Snellen equivalent). For comparative analysis, the fellow eye, the nonscalloped iris eye, from each patient was used as control. Data collection was from patients' medical records and included demographic data summarized in Table 1.

2.2. Measurement of Blood-Aqueous Barrier Function. To clarify the relationship between IOP increase and the blood-aqueous barrier function in both scalloped iris eyes and

TABLE 1: Demographic and clinical data of ATTRV30M patients.

Characteristics	ATTRV30M patients ($n = 28$)
Age, years	46.9 ± 5.6
Male/female	60.7%/39.3%
Time of ATTRV30M diagnosis, years	14.6 ± 3.9
Liver transplantation, %	96.4%
Time from liver transplantation, years	12.3 ± 3.4
Patients under tafamidis treatment, n	1

nonscalloped iris eyes (control), we measured the IOP values by using Goldmann applanation tonometry and the anterior chamber flare. Flare values were measured quantitatively by laser flare meter (LFM) (Kowa FM-700, Berkshire, UK) without pupil dilatation. On each occasion, 10 readings with a variation of less than 5% were taken. The highest and lowest values were discarded, and the remaining eight were averaged to obtain the flare measurement. Laser flare values were expressed in photon counts/millisecond (pc/ms) and standard deviation (SD) was calculated. Calibration of the laser flare meter was performed according to the manual.

2.3. Statistical Analysis. For continuous variables, such as IOP and anterior chamber flare, the observed values were summarized descriptively (mean ± SD). Student's two-group paired t-test was used to determine the significance of between-group differences in IOP and anterior chamber flare. Association between IOP and flare within each group was analyzed using Pearson's correlation coefficient. Statistical significance was declared at a type 1 error rate of 0.050. Statistical calculations and analyses were performed using SAS for PC, version 9.3 (SAS Inc, Cary, NC).

3. Results

Fifty-six eyes of 28 ATTRV30M patients participated in this analysis. Patients' characteristics are shown in Figure 1 and Table 1. In this study, highly statistical significant differences were found in the disorder in the BAB between the scalloped iris eyes and the nonscalloped iris eyes (control). The aqueous humor flare values in the eyes with a scalloped iris were significantly higher than those in the nonscalloped iris control group ($p < 0.001$), while there were no significant differences in IOP between groups ($p = 0.163$) (Table 2; Figures 2 and 3). There was no significant correlation between the flare and the IOP values within groups (scalloped iris eyes group, Spearman-rho $= -0.06$, $p = 0.749$; nonscalloped iris eyes group (control), Spearman-rho $= 0.28$, $p = 0.135$).

4. Discussion

The present study demonstrated that the aqueous humor flare values were significantly higher in the ATTRV30M scalloped iris eyes than those in the nonscalloped iris eyes (control group), and the IOP value was not significantly correlated with the increase in flare in both groups.

We previously reported a strong association between glaucoma and scalloped iris and advise to increase the frequency of IOP surveillance and look for glaucoma in these

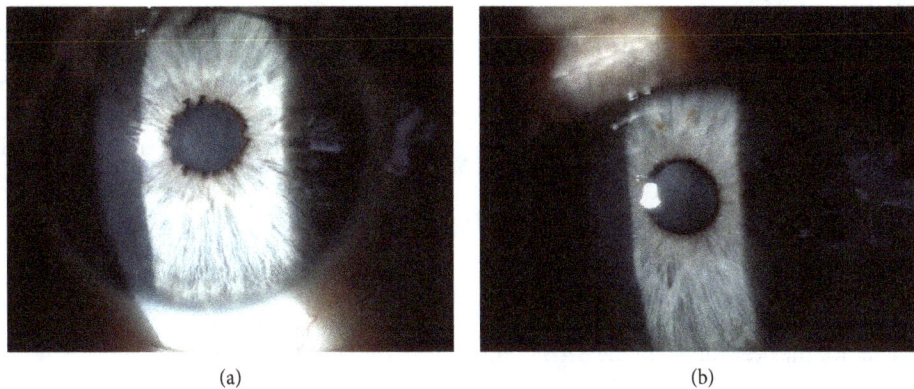

(a)   (b)

FIGURE 1: ATTRV30M scalloped iris eye (a) and the nonscalloped iris eye (control) (b) same patient.

TABLE 2: IOP and aqueous flare values.

Parameters	Scalloped iris	Nonscalloped iris (control group)	p value
Mean flare (pc/ms)	14.1 ± 2.2	6.5 ± 0.9	$p < 0.001$
Mean IOP (mmHg)	17.1 ± 0.8	16.8 ± 0.7	$p = 0.163$

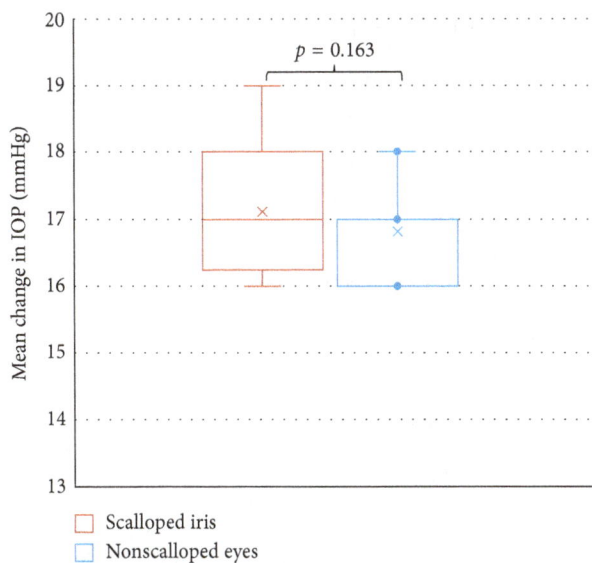

FIGURE 2: IOP distribution of ATTRV30M patients with scalloped iris and nonscalloped iris eyes (control).

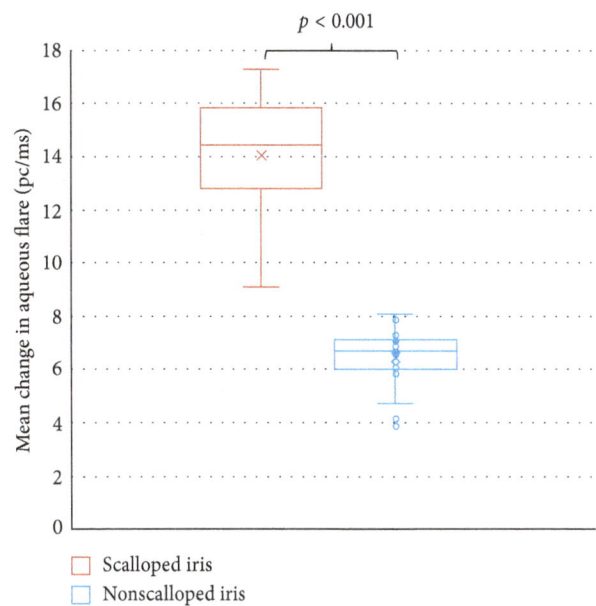

FIGURE 3: Aqueous flare distribution of ATTRVM30 patients with scalloped iris and nonscalloped iris eyes (control).

eyes [20, 28]. Nevertheless, our study showed no significant increase in IOP and na increased protein concentration in the aqueous humor in the scalloped iris eyes. These results may suggest the use of the flare meter method for predicting the risk of glaucoma in ATTRV30M scalloped iris eyes.

Several studies have addressed the changes to the aqueous humor proteome in glaucoma using other techniques with collection of aqueous humor samples after and/or during surgery [11, 13–19]. Inoue et al. reported higher levels of cytokines and growth factors in the aqueous humor of open-angle glaucoma eyes using multiplex bead immunoassay [13]. Imbalanced metabolism, lack of reactive oxygen species detoxification, low-grade, and chronic

inflammation in the aqueous humor of open-angle glaucoma eyes were also assessed by several groups by mass spectrometry [15–21].

The laser flare meter is a precise, objective, and noninvasive method that can reliably measure the function of the BAB and the level of inflammation [25, 31]. The increase in aqueous flare echoes a disruption of the BAB, which allows leakage of serum proteins, as well as inflammatory molecules and cells, into the anterior segment by causing a change in aqueous protein composition and concentration [13, 26].

Evaluation of the anterior aqueous flare in patients with glaucoma has also been addressed recently [27–29, 32]. Many groups have assessed the anterior chamber aqueous flare in glaucomatous eyes after treatment with anti-glaucomatous drugs. Interestingly, Kahloun et al. used the flare meter to evaluate the anterior chamber aqueous flare in patients with pseudoexfoliation syndrome with or without glaucoma and found that a high anterior aqueous flare could be a predictor for the development of glaucoma [27].

In our study, we observed an increased protein concentration in the aqueous humor of ATTRV30M patients with scalloped iris eyes without IOP increased values. An increase in protein concentration in the aqueous is the most straightforward evidence for the breakdown of the BAB [25].

Some authors hypothesize that the breakdown of BAB initially is due to endothelial injury caused by the mutant TTR [33, 34], but there must be another complementary mechanism since patients are transplanted and have no TTR mutant in circulation. The damage should be from outside the vessels were circulates the mutant TTR (aqueous humor and vitreous). As ATTR V30M patients have a proinflammatory state [35], we hypothesize that in response to this stimulation, the ciliary pigmented epithelium may release a large variety of cytokines and fibrin aggregates which may induce the breakdown of the BAB and outflow resistance in the anterior segment of the eye in ATTRV30M patients. As described previously, the intraocular production of TTR V30M by the retinal and ciliary pigment epithelium remains unchanged in these patients [8]. And the total aqueous humor TTR levels are almost the same in liver transplanted and nontransplanted ATTR V30M patients [10]. Thus, we hypothesize that an increased concentration of the unstable TTR V30M in patients' eyes could also contribute to the breakdown of the BAB and increased development of a mechanical barrier to the outflow of the aqueous humor, resulting in IOP elevation and worsening the prognostic for glaucoma development [30].

Therefore, anterior aqueous flare measurements should be considered in the staging and evaluation of the risk progression to glaucoma and be considered as a marker of ocular disease progression in ATTRV30M patients. The flare cell meter may help us to objectify the action of a possible treatment directed to the oculopathy and indirectly targeting the central nervous system [36, 37]. Further, longitudinal studies are warranted to assess the predictive value of aqueous flare for glaucoma development.

This study had some limitations. Further analysis is needed in order to determine which mediators are associated with the breakdown of the BAB function in these ATTRV30M patients. Furthermore, further histological or biochemical analysis to determine whether the source of increased aqueous flare values resulted from the breakdown of the BAB itself or simply from proteins diffusing from the posterior segment caused by the breakdown of the blood-retinal barrier.

5. Conclusions

In this study, we found that the aqueous humor flare value was significantly higher in the scalloped iris eyes than that in the nonscalloped eyes in ATTRV30M patients without significant differences in IOP between groups. As a marker for inflammation, and breakdown of the BAB, flare values suggest that controlling the stage and progression of glaucoma might be key in the surveillance scalloped iris eyes in ATTRV30M patients and may be considered as an evaluation method of future treatments.

Conflicts of Interest

The authors declare that there are no conflicts of interest.

References

[1] N. M. Beirão, V. Miranda, I. Beirão et al., "The use of intravitreal ranibizumab to treat neovascular glaucoma because of retinal amyloid angiopathy in familial amyloidosis transthyretin v30m related," *Retinal Cases & Brief Reports*, vol. 7, no. 1, pp. 114–116, 2013.

[2] A. Rousseau, G. Kaswin, D. Adams et al., "Ocular involvement in familial amyloid polyneuropathy," *Journal Français d'Ophtalmologie*, vol. 36, no. 9, pp. 779–788, 2013.

[3] L. H. Connors, A. M. Richardson, R. Théberge, and C. E. Costello, "Tabulation of transthyretin (TTR) variants as of 1/1/2000," *Amyloid*, vol. 7, no. 1, pp. 54–69, 2000.

[4] J. M. Beirão, J. Malheiro, C. Lemos et al., "Impact of liver transplantation on the natural history of oculopathy in Portuguese patients with transthyretin (V30M) amyloidosis," *Amyloid*, vol. 22, no. 1, pp. 31–35, 2015.

[5] C. Lemos, T. Coelho, M. Alves-Ferreira et al., "Overcoming artefact: anticipation in 284 Portuguese kindreds with familial amyloid polyneuropathy (FAP) ATTRV30M," *Journal of Neurology, Neurosurgery & Psychiatry*, vol. 85, no. 3, pp. 326–330, 2014.

[6] T. Yamashita, Y. Ando, S. Okamoto et al., "Long-term survival after liver transplantation in patients with familial amyloid polyneuropathy," *Neurology*, vol. 78, no. 9, pp. 637–643, 2012.

[7] Vyndaqel® Summary of Characteristics, http://www.ema.europa.eu/docs/en_gb/document_library/epar__product_information/human/002294/wc500117862.pdf, October 2017.

[8] J. M. Beirão, J. Malheiro, C. Lemos, I Beirão, P. Costa, and P. Torres, "Ophthalmological manifestations in hereditary transthyretin (ATTR V30M) carriers: a review of 513 cases," *Amyloid*, vol. 22, no. 2, pp. 117–122, 2015.

[9] M. Munar-Qués, L. Salva-Ladaria, P. Mulet-Perera, M. Solé, F. R. López-Andreu, and M. J. M. Saraiva, "Vitreous amyloidosis after liver transplantation in patients with familial amyloid polyneuropathy: ocular synthesis of mutant transthyretin," *Amyloid*, vol. 7, no. 4, pp. 266–269, 2000.

[10] K. Haraoka, Y. Ando, E. Ando et al., "Presence of variant transthyretin in aqueous humor of a patient with familial amyloidotic polyneuropathy after liver transplantation," *Amyloid*, vol. 9, no. 4, pp. 247–251, 2002.

[11] H. A. Quigley and A. T. Broman, "The number of people with glaucoma worldwide in 2010 and 2020," *British Journal of Ophthalmology*, vol. 90, no. 3, pp. 262–267, 2006.

[12] Y. H. Kwon, J. H. Fingert, M. H. Kuehn, and W. L. M. Alward, "Primary open-angle glaucoma," *New England Journal of Medicine*, vol. 360, no. 11, pp. 1113–1124, 2009.

[13] T. Inoue, T. Kawaji, and H. Tanihara, "Elevated levels of multiple biomarkers of Alzheimer's disease in the aqueous humor of eyes

with open-angle glaucoma," *Investigative Opthalmology & Visual Science*, vol. 54, no. 8, pp. 5353–5358, 2013.

[14] U. Roy Chowdhury, C. R. Hann, W. D. Stamer, and M. P. Fautsch, "Aqueous humor outflow: dynamics and disease," *Investigative Opthalmology & Visual Science*, vol. 56, no. 5, pp. 2993–3003, 2015.

[15] M. A. Kaeslin, H. E. Killer, C. A. Fuhrer, N. Zeleny, A. Robert Huber, and A. Neutzner, "Changes to the aqueous humor proteome during glaucoma," *PLoS One*, vol. 11, no. 10, Article ID e0165314, 2016.

[16] C. Benoist d'Azy, B. Pereira, F. Chiambaretta, and F. Dutheil, "Oxidative and anti-oxidative stress markers in chronic glaucoma: a systematic review and meta-analysis," *PLoS One*, vol. 11, no. 12, Article ID e0166915, 2016.

[17] E. Ergan, F. Ozturk, E. Beyazyildiz et al., "Oxidant/antioxidant balance in the aqueous humor of patients with glaucoma," *International Journal of Ophthalmology*, vol. 9, no. 2, pp. 249–252, 2016.

[18] S. Funke, N. Perumal, K. Bell, N. Pfeiffer, and F. H. Grus, "The potential impact of recent insights into proteomic changes associated with glaucoma," *Expert Review of Proteomics*, vol. 14, no. 4, pp. 311–334, 2017.

[19] J. Cabrerizo, J. A. Urcola, and E. Vecino, "Changes in the lipidomic profile of aqueous humor in open-angle glaucoma," *Journal of Glaucoma*, vol. 26, no. 4, pp. 349–355, 2017.

[20] A. Goyal, A. Srivastava, R. Sihota, and J. Kaur, "Evaluation of oxidative stress markers in aqueous humor of primary open angle glaucoma and primary angle closure glaucoma patients," *Current Eye Research*, vol. 39, no. 8, pp. 823–829, 2014.

[21] F. J. Hernández-Martínez, P. Piñas-García, A. V. Lleó-Pérez et al., "Biomarkers of lipid peroxidation in the aqueous humor of primary open-angle glaucoma patients," *Archivos de la Sociedad Española de Oftalmología*, vol. 91, no. 8, pp. 357–362, 2016.

[22] W. Wang, X. Quian, H. Song, M. Zhang, and Z. Liu, "Fluid and structure coupling analysis of the interaction between aqueous humor and iris," *BioMedical Engineering OnLine*, vol. 15, no. 2, p. 133, 2016.

[23] M. He, Y. Lu, X. Liu, T. Ye, and P. J. Foster, "Histologic changes of the iris in the development of angle closure in Chinese eyes," *Journal of Glaucoma*, vol. 17, no. 5, pp. 386–392, 2008.

[24] S. Schröder, P. S. Muether, A. Caramoy et al., "Anterior chamber aqueous flare is a strong predictor for proliferative vitreoretinopathy in patients with rhegmatogenous retinal detachment," *Retina*, vol. 32, no. 1, pp. 38–42, 2012.

[25] M. Sawa, Y. Tsurimaki, T. Tsuru, and H. Shimizu, "New quantitative method to determine protein concentration and cell number in aqueous in vivo," *Japanese Journal of Ophthalmology*, vol. 32, no. 2, pp. 132–142, 1988.

[26] M. Sawa, "Clinical application of laser flare-cell meter," *Japanese Journal of Ophthalmology*, vol. 34, no. 3, pp. 346–363, 1990.

[27] R. Kahloun, S. Attia, I. Ksiaa et al., "Anterior chamber aqueous flare, pseudoexfoliation syndrome, and glaucoma," *International Ophthalmology*, vol. 36, no. 5, pp. 671–674, 2016.

[28] F. Selen, O. Tekeli, and Ö. Yanık, "Assessment of the anterior chamber flare and macular thickness in patients treated with topical antiglaucomatous drugs," *Journal of Ocular Pharmacology and Therapeutics*, vol. 33, no. 3, pp. 170–175, 2017.

[29] K. Ishida, N. Moroto, K. Murata, and T. Yamamoto, "Effect of glaucoma implant surgery on intraocular pressure reduction, flare count, anterior chamber depth, and corneal endothelium in primary open-angle glaucoma," *Japanese Journal of Ophthalmology*, vol. 61, no. 4, pp. 334–346, 2017.

[30] M. Cellini, R. Caramazza, D. Bonsanto, B. Bernabini, and E. C. Campos, "Prostaglandin analogs and blood-aqueous barrier integrity: a flare cell meter study," *Ophthalmologica*, vol. 218, no. 5, pp. 312–317, 2004.

[31] C. Rosenfeld, M. O. Price, X. Lai et al., "Distinctive and pervasive alterations in aqueous humor protein composition following different types of glaucoma surgery," *Molecular Vision*, vol. 21, pp. 911–918, 2015.

[32] E. Strobbe, M. Cellini, M. Fresina, and E. C. Campos, "ET-1 plasma levels, aqueous flare, and choroidal thickness in patients with retinitis pigmentosa," *Journal of Ophthalmology*, vol. 2015, Article ID 292615, 6 pages, 2015.

[33] H. Koike, S. Ikeda, M. Takahashi et al., "Schwann cell and endothelial cell damage in transthyretin familial amyloid polyneuropathy," *Neurology*, vol. 87, no. 21, pp. 2220–2229, 2016.

[34] A. Rousseau, C. Terrada, S. Touhami et al., "Angiographic signatures of the predominant form of familial transthyretin amyloidosis (Val30Met mutation)," *American Journal of Ophthalmology*, vol. 192, pp. 169–177, 2018.

[35] M. L. Fiszman, M. Di Egidio, K. C. Ricart et al., "Evidence of oxidative stress in familial amyloidotic polyneuropathy type 1," *Archives of Neurology*, vol. 60, no. 4, pp. 593–597, 2003.

[36] A. C. Silva-Araújo, M. A. Tavares, J. S. Cotta, and J. F. Castro-Correia, "Aqueous outflow system in familial amyloidotic polyneuropathy, Portuguese type," *Graefe's Archive for Clinical and Experimental Ophthalmology*, vol. 231, no. 3, pp. 131–135, 1993.

[37] L. F. Maia, R. Magalhães, J. Freitas et al., "CNS involvement in V30M transthyretin amyloidosis: clinical, neuropathological and biochemical findings," *Journal of Neurology, Neurosurgery & Psychiatry*, vol. 86, no. 2, pp. 159–167, 2015.

27

Treatment of Diabetic Macular Edema with Intravitreal Antivascular Endothelial Growth Factor and Prompt versus Deferred Focal Laser during Long-Term Follow-Up and Identification of Prognostic Retinal Markers

Birgit Weingessel [ID],[1,2] Kata Mihaltz [ID],[1] Andreas Gleiss,[3] Florian Sulzbacher,[1,2] Christopher Schütze [ID],[1,2] and Pia V. Vécsei-Marlovits[1,2]

[1]*Department of Ophthalmology, Hietzing Hospital, Wolkersbergenstrasse 1, Vienna, Austria*
[2]*Karl Landsteiner Institute for Process Optimization and Quality Management in Cataract Surgery, Wolkersbergenstrasse 1, Vienna, Austria*
[3]*Center for Medical Statistics, Informatics and Intelligent Systems, Medical University of Vienna, Vienna, Austria*

Correspondence should be addressed to Christopher Schütze; christopher.schuetze@wienkav.at

Academic Editor: Lawrence S. Morse

Purpose. Long-term follow-up of patients with diabetic macular edema (DME) treated with intravitreal antivascular endothelial growth factor (anti-VEGF) combined focal laser and identification of prognostic morphological characteristics. *Methods.* Prospective clinical trial (50 treatment-naive eyes) with DME randomized 1 : 1 receiving intravitreal ranibizumab (0.5 mg/0.05 ml) and prompt grid laser compared with ranibizumab and deferred laser. Morphological characteristics potentially relevant for prognosis were assessed at baseline, month 6, month 9, and years 1, 2, 3, 4, and 5 of follow-up. *Results.* Although functional results were slightly higher in the prompt group at week 12 (0.5; 20/40 Snellen (SD = 0.04, 0.3 logMAR) versus 0.4; 20/50 Snellen (SD = 0.04, logMAR: 0.4), $p = 0.4$) and month 9 (prompt group: 0.5; 20/40 Snellen (SD = 0.03, 0.3 logMAR) versus deferred group: 0.4; 20/50 Snellen (SD = 0.04, 0.4 logMAR), $p = 0.4$), these were statistically insignificant. There was no significant benefit regarding functionality during long-term follow-up in the prompt group compared to the deferred group. BCVA in the eyes with clusters of hyperreflective foci in the central macular region was inferior compared with the eyes without these alterations at year 5 (0.39; 20/50 Snellen, (SD = 0.25, 0.4 logMAR) versus 0.63; 20/80 Snellen (SD = 0.22, 0.2 logMAR), $p < 0.01$). *Conclusion.* Grid laser and ranibizumab therapy are effective in DME management during the long-term follow-up. Intraretinal hyperreflective material in SD-OCT is negatively related to BCVA.

1. Introduction

Diabetic macular edema (DME) is the most common cause of visual impairment in diabetic patients [1]. More than four hundred million adults are affected by diabetes mellitus worldwide. Ninety percent of diabetic patients will have some form of retinopathy 25 years following diagnosis [2].

It is estimated that 25% of individuals with type 1 diabetes and 15% of patients with type 2 diabetes develop macular edema and that one half of these patients lose two or more lines of visual acuity (VA) during the disease course [2, 3].

Elevated levels of vascular endothelial growth factor (VEGF) have shown to promote permeability of retinal vasculature leading to macular edema in diabetic patients [4, 5].

Besides regulation of blood glucose level and blood pressure, DME has been treated with focal/grid laser until recently that reduced the risk of moderate vision loss (defined as a loss of more than 3 lines of VA) by 50% in 3 years. In patients with central macular edema with baseline VA of <0.5, 11% of the eyes gained more than 3 lines in one year and 16% more than 3 lines following 3 years [4–6].

With the introduction of anti-VEGF agents, a milestone in the management of DME has been achieved by lowering intraocular VEGF levels and thereby reducing macular edema resulting in restoration of visual function. In the Intravitreal Aflibercept for Diabetic Macular Edema (VIVID/VISTA) studies, randomized diabetic patients received aflibercept or focal/grid laser treatment. Mean VA improvement was lowest in the laser groups (+0.9 and +0.7) compared with that of the aflibercept arms for VIVID and VISTA, respectively [7].

The Ranibizumab for Diabetic Macular Edema (RISE/RIDE) studies showed that laser monotherapy was not as effective in improving VA compared with ranibizumab treatment that was effective in rapidly and sustainably improving VA and in reducing the risk of further vision loss and in improving macular edema in patients with DME [8].

The Ranibizumab Plus Prompt Or Deferred Laser Or Triamcinolone Plus Prompt Laser For Diabetic Macular Edema (DRCR.net Protocol I Study) indicated that nonetheless ranibizumab plus deferred laser reached best VA results; it is significant to note that ranibizumab plus prompt laser-treated eyes reached a similar 5-year VA with lower number of injections needed (median: 17 versus. 13, resp.) and a median of 3 focal/grid photocoagulation managements. Furthermore, the original laser group achieved best outcomes regarding central macular thickness (CMT) reduction [9].

Therefore, it has been shown that macular laser therapy may still play an important role as an adjuvant therapy because it is able to improve macular thickness outcomes and to reduce the number of intravitreal injections needed. However, the determination of morphological retinal features that are relevant for functional prognosis seems indispensable when aiming for the identification of more individualized treatment procedures for DME patients.

The study presented here provides additional information to functional/anatomical outcomes in eyes with DME treated with anti-VEGF combined with prompt compared to deferred laser therapy and identifies prognostically relevant morphological characteristics using high-resolution spectral domain optical coherence tomography (SD-OCT) during long-term follow-up.

2. Materials and Methods

This prospective longitudinal randomized interventional clinical trial included 50 treatment-naive patients (50 eyes) with diabetic macular edema (DME). Patients were recruited at the Department of Ophthalmology, Hietzing Hospital, Vienna, Austria. Signed informed consent was obtained from each patient, and the character of the study was explained in detail preceding patient inclusion. The local ethics committee approved the study protocol that followed the ethical tenets of the Declaration of Helsinki.

2.1. Inclusion and Exclusion Criteria. Patients underwent a comprehensive ophthalmological examination that included slit lamp biomicroscopy, funduscopy, tonometry (intraocular pressure-IOP), fluorescein angiography (FA), and SD-OCT (Spectralis HRA + OCT, Heidelberg

Engineering, Heidelberg, Germany). In case of DME that was detected clinically and on FA as well as in SD-OCT (diffuse macular edema with central retinal thickness (CRT) $\geq 300\,\mu m$ involving the center of the macular area), patients were included into the present study following informed consent. Inclusion criteria were further best-corrected visual acuity (BCVA) between 0.06; 6/120 (1.2 logMAR) and 0.63; 20/32 (0.20 logMAR). Data were analyzed every 6 weeks until month 6, followed by month 9 and years 1, 2, 3, 4, and 5.

Investigators who measured visual acuity were all masked to the respective study arm. The method used for measuring visual acuity was Snellen charts.

The eyes with other retinal diseases (i.e., age-related macular degeneration (AMD) and associated choroidal neovascularization (CNV), cystoid macular edema (CME) of other origin (e.g., uveitis, Irvine–Gass syndrome, and retinal vein occlusion), or retinal dystrophies) were excluded from the study. Further exclusion criteria were previous treatment of DME with laser and/or intravitreal injections with anti-VEGF or triamcinolone or panretinal photocoagulation at least 3 months prior to the baseline visit. Moreover, patients who had intraocular surgery at least 6 months prior to the first visit were excluded from the study. Myocardial infarction or stroke 6 months or less prior to baseline as well as hypertension >180/110 mmHg and unstable blood glucose levels (HbA1C $\geq 9.0\%$) were exclusion criteria. An upper limit of CRT of $\geq 600\,\mu m$ in SD-OCT was defined for study inclusion in order to eliminate presence of eyes with extensive structural damage.

2.2. Randomization and Treatment Methods. The eyes of eligible patients were randomized into 2 groups (ratio 1 : 1), and they either received ranibizumab and focal/grid laser on the same day ("prompt" group, 25 eyes, 50%) or ranibizumab one week prior to laser treatment ("deferred" group, 25 eyes, 50%). Randomization was performed with the Randomizer® software available at the Medical University of Vienna (http://www.meduniwien.ac.at/randomizer/).

When both the eyes of a patient were affected by diabetic retinopathy (DR) and met the inclusion criteria, the left eye was randomized to prompt laser treatment and anti-VEGF, and the right eye received deferred laser therapy in addition to intravitreal anti-VEGF.

Ranibizumab (0.5 mg/0.05 ml) was injected via pars plana using a 30-gauge needle following topical application of betadine solution and anesthesia with oxybuprocaine. Retreatment was performed on the same day of the clinical examination if retreatment criteria were met. These followed the DRCR.net protocol [10] that continued retreatment every 6 weeks until no further functional and morphological improvement was reached, which was defined as a decrease in CRT of <10% and an increase in BCVA of <5 letters compared with the last intravitreal anti-VEGF injection.

Focal laser treatment was performed using argon laser photocoagulation (VISULAS 532s®, Carl Zeiss Meditec) operating at 532 nm. Laser therapy was accomplished only once and not repeated during the observation period. Light was focused on the retina applying a Mainster Focal/Grid Laser contact lens (Ocular Instruments, Bellevue, WA, USA). Focal photocoagulation was used for treatment of macular edema as described by ETDRS [5]. No spots were applied closer to the foveal avascular zone than $500\,\mu m$. Duration used was 100 ms, and the treatment goal was to obtain burns as light as possible that were only barely visible at the level of the outer retina. Direct treatment of microaneurysms was performed. In case of development of proliferative DR (neovascularization on the optic disc (NVD) or elsewhere (NVE)) detected clinically or on FA, panretinal photocoagulation was initiated.

All patients who were primarily included into this study are and will be continuously followed and treated as needed at the Department of Ophthalmology, Hietzing Hospital, Vienna, Austria.

2.3. Imaging Procedures and Data Analyses.

High-resolution retinal imaging that acquires three-dimensional cross-sectional retinal datasets was performed using Spectralis OCT. The device obtains a variable quantity of B-scans and implements an eye tracker to minimize artifacts that are caused by eye motion. The system combines infrared (IR) fundus autofluorescence (FAF), FA, and a scanning laser ophthalmoscopy (SLO) unit. In the present study, macular raster scans measuring $6000\,\mu m$ in diameter were used. Macular volume scans were generated automatically using the software provided by Spectralis (version 6.3.2.0).

Accumulations of clusters of hyperreflective material in the central macular B-scans of an SD-OCT dataset (1 cluster = accumulation of a minimum of 3 adjacent hyperreflective foci) were analyzed and compared by 2 independent readers regarding frequency of occurrence in both treatment groups. Presence of intraretinal exudative foci was correlated to the functional outcome during follow-up.

2.4. Statistical Analyses.

CRT and BCVA were determined as primary outcome measures at designated time points. BCVA is specified in Snellen and logMAR units and standard deviation (SD) is given as Snellen equivalents. Prognostic relevant morphological parameters were identified qualitatively and quantitatively (%). BCVA is given in decimal, Snellen, and logMAR units.

Sample size calculation was based on a Wilcoxon ranksum test (nQuery-Version 6.01). For comparison analyses between BCVA, CRT, and frequency of intraretinal hyperreflective foci among treatment groups and between different points in time, the paired t-test and Mann–Whitney U test were used. Risk of retreatment was investigated in a logistic regression model. Excel 2014, MedCalc (version 13.3.3.0), and Past Project (version 3.06) were used to perform statistical analyses. Statistical significance was defined as $p < 0.05$.

3. Results

The mean age of patients was 66.2 (SD = 9.0 years, min = 49 years, and max = 84 years). There was no significant difference regarding age between treatment groups. Twenty patients were female, and 30 were male. Table 1 summarizes baseline characteristics of patients of each treatment group.

TABLE 1: Baseline parameters of patients with diabetic macular edema (DME) enrolled in the current study.

Prompt laser group	
Age (mean/SD)	65.3/8.3
Gender (male/female)	17/11
Visual acuity (Snellen/SD/logMAR)	0.32/0.03/0.50
Central retinal thickness (μm)	460.3/67.3
Deferred laser group	
Age (mean/SD)	67.2/9.7
Gender (male/female)	18/9
Visual acuity (Snellen/SD/logMAR)	0.32/0.03/0.50
Central retinal thickness (μm)	454.1/95.6

SD = standard deviation.

3.1. Functional and Morphological Parameters.

Figure 1 and Table 2 summarize results regarding BCVA and CRT outcomes. Overall, mean BCVA changed from 0.32; 20/63 Snellen (SD = 0.03, 0.5 logMAR) at baseline to 0.68; 20/32 Snellen (SD = 0.25, 0.2 logMAR) at year 5 of follow-up ($p > 0.1$). The mean BCVA changed from 0.32; 20/63 Snellen (SD = 0.03, 0.5 logMAR) at baseline to 0.58; 20/40 Snellen (SD = 0.31, 0.2 logMAR) at year 5 in the prompt group ($p < 0.001$) and from 0.32; 20/63 Snellen (SD = 0.03, 0.5 logMAR) at baseline to 0.61; 20/32 Snellen (SD = 0.31, 0.2 logMAR) at year 5 in the deferred treatment group ($p < 0.001$). Difference of BCVA between treatment groups was statistically insignificant at year 5 ($p = 0.3$). Although our results revealed slightly better functional results in the beginning of the treatment phase in the prompt group at week 12 (prompt group: 0.5; 20/40 Snellen (SD = 0.04, 0.3 logMAR) versus deferred group: 0.4; 20/50 Snellen (SD = 0.04, logMAR: 0.4), $p = 0.4$) and month 9 (prompt group: 0.5; 20/40 Snellen (SD = 0.03, 0.3 logMAR): versus deferred group: 0.4; 20/50 Snellen (SD = 0.04, 0.4 logMAR), $p = 0.4$) of follow-up, differences in visual acuity between both groups were insignificant during the long-term follow-up. There was no significant difference in CRT when comparing the prompt and deferred treatment group at week 12 ($p = 0.08$) and month 9 ($p = 0.3$) of follow-up. Average CRT values of the entire study population changed from $457.2\,\mu m$ (SD = $90.7\,\mu m$) at baseline to $348.3\,\mu m$ (SD = $62.0\,\mu m$) at the end of the observation period ($p < 0.01$). Mean CRT decreased from $460.3\,\mu m$ (SD = $87.4\,\mu m$) at baseline to $354.4\,\mu m$ (SD = $108.9\,\mu m$) in the prompt group ($p < 0.001$) and from $454.1\,\mu m$ (SD = $95.6\,\mu m$) at baseline to $327.6\,\mu m$ (SD = $69.7\,\mu m$, $p < 0.001$) in the deferred group at year 5.

In general, reduction of retinal edema was more distinct in the eyes of the prompt group (particularly at an early disease stage) as compared with the deferred group (Figure 2).

Until month 6 of follow-up (prompt treatment group: total of 49 intravitreal injections needed, potential maximum cumulative number of injections = 119; deferred treatment group: 47 injections needed, potential maximum cumulative number of injections = 111), there was a statistically insignificant likelihood of a lower retreatment rate in the deferred group compared with the prompt group (odds ratio: 0.43, 95% confidence interval (CI): 0.11–1.65), though statistically insignificant ($p = 0.21$).

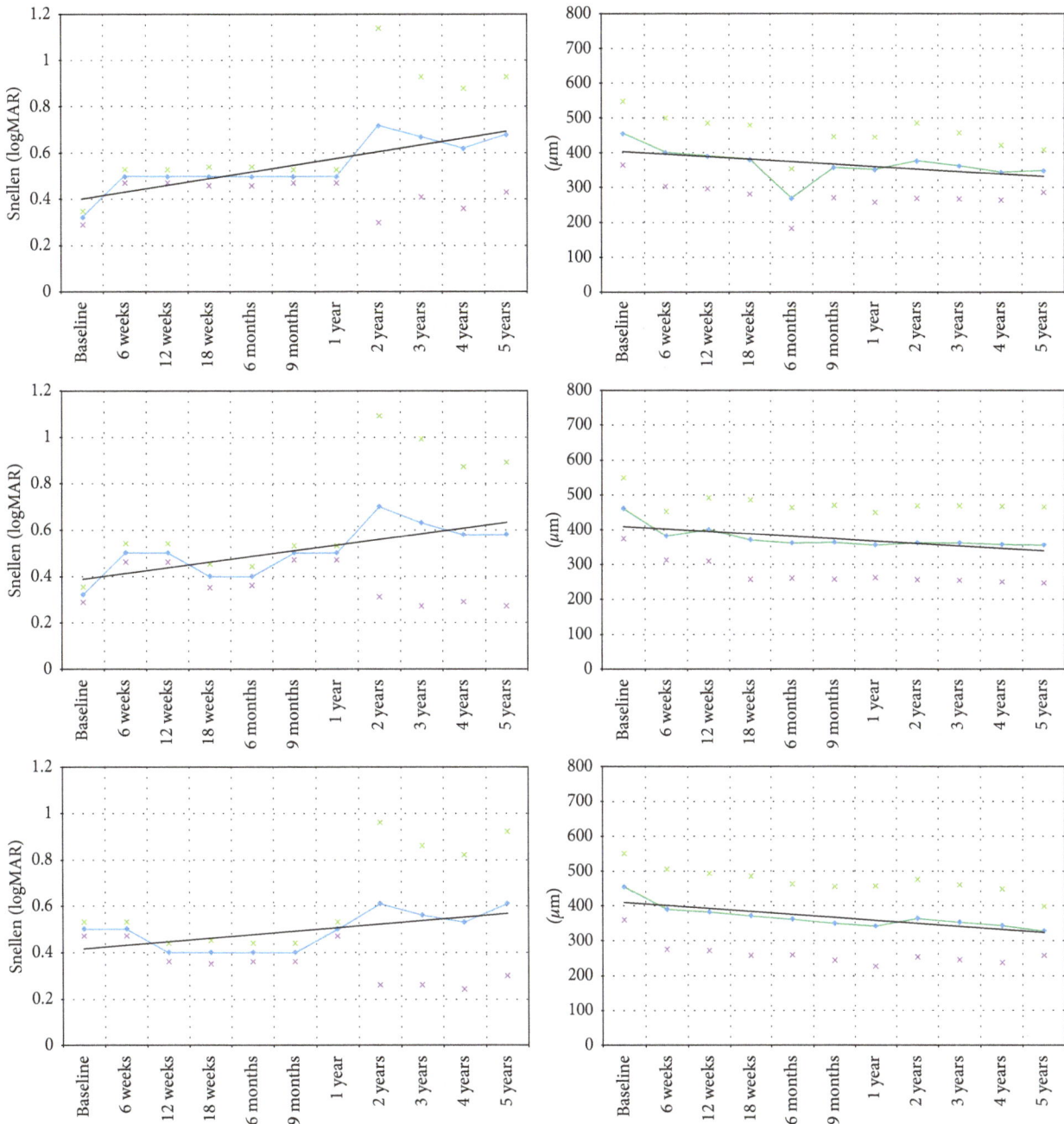

FIGURE 1: Best-corrected visual acuity (BCVA) and central retinal thickness (CRT) in eyes with diabetic macular edema (DME) treated with intravitreal antivascular endothelial growth factor (anti-VEGF) combined with prompt or deferred focal macular laser. Although functional results in eyes treated with immediate anti-VEGF therapy combined with laser at week 12 (prompt treatment group: 0.5; 20/40 Snellen (SD = 0.04, 0.3 logMAR) versus deferred treatment group: 0.4; 20/50 Snellen (SD = 0.04, logMAR: 0.4), $p = 0.4$) and month 9 (prompt group: 0.5; 20/40 Snellen (SD = 0.03, 0.3 logMAR) versus deferred group: 0.4; 20/50 Snellen (SD = 0.04, 0.4 logMAR), $p = 0.4$)) were slightly better; no meaningful functional benefit was observed in the prompt group during long-term follow-up. BCVA = best-corrected visual acuity. CRT = central retinal thickness. Black lines represent trend lines. Stars represent standard deviation. p values indicate change compared with baseline. (a) BCVA-entire study population (50 eyes). (b) CRT-entire study population (50 eyes). (c) BCVA-prompt/deferred (light blue line) group (25/25 eyes). (d) CRT-prompt/deferred (light green line) group (25/25 eyes).

Baseline BCVA ($p = 0.19$) and CRT ($p = 0.75$) values did not differ significantly between the prompt or deferred treatment groups.

No severe ocular adverse events (i.e., endophthalmitis or persistent arterial nonperfusion) occurred in this study.

Regarding clusters of intraretinal material detected in the central macular area by OCT imaging, these hyperreflective foci consistently correlated with lipid exudates seen on biomicroscopy. BCVA in the eyes with clusters of intra-retinal foci in the central macular area (one cluster depicts an

TABLE 2: Functional ((best-corrected visual acuity (BCVA)) and morphological (central retinal thickness (CRT)) results in eyes with diabetic macular edema (DME, 50 eyes, top) treated with intravitreal ranibizumab and immediate focal laser therapy (prompt group, 25 eyes, middle) and eyes treated with intravitreal ranibizumab and deferred laser (25 eyes, bottom).

	Baseline	6 weeks	12 weeks	18 weeks	6 months	9 months	1 year	2 years	3 years	4 years	5 years
Entire study population											
BCVA	0.32	0,50	0.50	0.50	0.50	0.50	0.50	0.72	0.67	0.62	0.68
SD	0.03	0,03	0.03	0.04	0.04	0.03	0.03	0.42	0.26	0.26	0.25
logMAR (Snellen)	0.50 (20/40)	0.30 (20/63)	0.30 (20/63)	0.30 (20/63)	0.30 (20/63)	0.30 (20/63)	0.30 (20/63)	0.20 (20/100)	0.25 (20/80)	0.30 (20/63)	0.20 (20/100)
CRT	457.20	401.6	391.3	381.10	269.60	358.90	351.90	377.40	363.00	343.80	348.30
SD	90.70	98.40	94.20	99.30	85.70	88.30	93.00	108.20	95.20	78.70	62.00
Prompt treatment group											
BCVA	0.32	0.50	0.50	0.40	0.04	0.50	0.50	0.70	0.63	0.58	0.58
SD	0.03	0.04	0.04	0.05	0.04	0.03	0.03	0.39	0.36	0.29	0.31
logMAR (Snellen)	0.50 (20/40)	0.30 (20/63)	0.30 (20/63)	0.40 (20/50)	0.40 (20/50)	0.30 (20/63)	0.30 (20/63)	0.20 (20/100)	0.20 (20/100)	0.30 (20/63)	0.30 (20/63)
CRT	460.30	381.60	399.40	370.20	360.70	362.80	354.70	360.70	360.70	357.00	354.40
SD	87.40	70.20	91.50	113.50	101.50	106.10	94.10	105.80	106.90	108.00	108.90
Deferred treatment group											
BCVA	0.32	0.50	0.40	0.40	0.40	0.40	0.50	0.61	0.56	0.53	0.61
SD	0.03	0.03	0.04	0.05	0.04	0.04	0.03	0.35	0.30	0.29	0.31
logMAR (Snellen)	0.50 (20/40)	0.30 (20/63)	0.40 (20/50)	0.40 (20/50)	0.40 (20/50)	0.40 (20/50)	0.30 (20/63)	0.30 (20/63)	0.30 (20/63)	0.30 (20/63)	0.30 (20/63)
CRT	454.10	389.70	382.00	370.20	360.70	348.80	340.90	363.40	352.40	342.10	327.60
SD	95.60	114.80	110.10	113.50	101.50	106.10	114.80	111.10	107.30	104.50	69.70

Note. BCVA = best-corrected visual acuity, SD = standard deviation, and CRT = central retinal thickness.

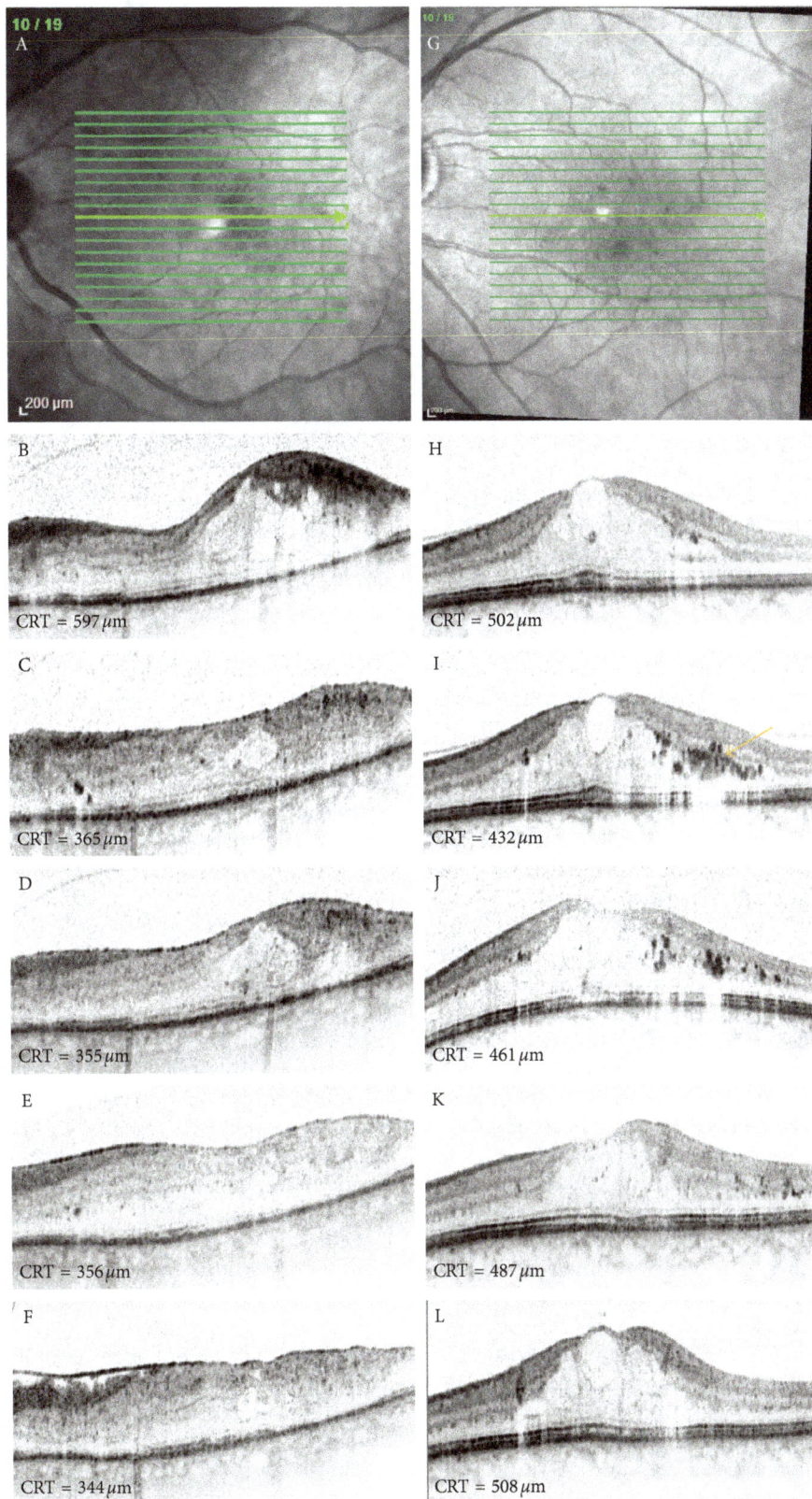

FIGURE 2: Spectral domain optical coherence tomography (SD-OCT) images of the left eye of 2 patients treated with ranibizumab and prompt focal laser therapy (A–F) or ranibizumab in addition to deferred laser (H–L) at baseline (B, H), 6 months (C, I), 1 year (D, J), 2 years (E, K), and 5 years (F, L) following baseline. SD-OCT images indicate a more rapid and consistent decrease of central retinal thickness (CRT) values in the eye treated with prompt laser therapy compared with the eye randomized for deferred focal laser treatment. In this example, the decrease in CRT is particularly evident in the eye that received prompt laser therapy in the beginning of the treatment phase (until month 6) compared with the eye that was scheduled for the deferred group. Note that the baseline CRT was similar in both eyes of the different treatment arms. The arrow indicates clusters of hyperreflective intraretinal material.

accumulation of a minimum of 3 adjacent hyperreflective foci as evident in SD-OCT B-scans (22 eyes, 44%, Figure 2)) was inferior compared with the eyes without (28 eyes) clusters of intraretinal hyperreflective material within retinal layers prior to treatment (0.20; 20/100 Snellen (SD = 0.03, 0.7 logMAR) versus 0.25; 20/80 Snellen (SD = 0.03, 0.6 logMAR), $p = 0.25$, Table 3). At 5 years of follow-up, this development of inferiority of visual function was maintained (0.39; 20/50 Snellen (SD = 0.25, 0.5 logMAR) versus 0.68; 20/32 Snellen (SD = 0.22, 0.2 logMAR), $p = 0.25$, Figure 3, Table 3). Frequency and intensity of hyperreflective foci in outer retinal layers decreased until year 5 of follow-up compared with baseline.

4. Discussion

Diabetic retinopathy (DR) is a retinal vascular disorder that occurs as a complication of diabetes mellitus (DM) and is the leading cause of blindness in the developed world [1, 10, 11]. The condition results in retinal ischemia (i.e., microaneurysms, hemorrhages, cotton wool spots, intraretinal microvascular abnormalities, or macular edema) and/or signs of increased retinal vascular permeability. Loss of vision is a consequence of various pathophysiological mechanisms including neovascularization that may cause vitreous hemorrhage, retinal detachment, or capillary nonperfusion. Retinopathy occurs in most patients with DM of longer duration, though its incidence can be reduced by aggressive control of hyperglycemia and hypertension [12].

The recent advent of antivascular endothelial growth factor (anti-VEGF) has revolutionized the management of DR with a significant improvement in the overall prognosis. In the management of diabetic macular edema (DME) intravitreally administered ranibizumab has been shown to achieve favorable treatment outcomes in various randomized prospective clinical trials, reaching significant functional and morphological improvements [9, 13]. However, the development towards more individualized treatment strategies in eyes with DME demands the identification of prognostically relevant morphological features that allow for a better understanding regarding treatment response during the long-term follow-up.

Hence, it was the aim of the current study to evaluate functional and morphological outcomes in the eyes with DME treated with ranibizumab and immediate focal laser therapy compared with eyes treated with intravitreal ranibizumab and deferred laser. This study showed that treatment with anti-VEGF in addition to focal laser is effective and safe in the management of DME during a long-term period of 5 years. Results revealed that the use of prompt laser in addition to intravitreal ranibizumab is not advantageous compared with anti-VEGF therapy during the long-term follow-up. However, as our findings revealed that functional results in the prompt group were slightly higher (though not statistically significant) compared with the deferred treatment group in an earlier treatment phase; this suggests that focal laser therapy in the eyes with DME is justified.

Previous findings [14–16] are in accordance with the results of our study, signifying consistency of the treatment regimen.

The analysis of Protocol I data presented by Gonzales et al. [14] determined whether early visual acuity (VA) response to ranibizumab in diabetic macular edema is associated with long-term outcome and showed that ranibizumab ± laser therapy resulted in similar rates (~40%) of BCVA improvement following 12 weeks of treatment. The eyes with suboptimal early BCVA response showed poorer long-term visual outcomes than eyes with pronounced early response [14].

Similar to the READ-2 study (Nguyen et al. [13]), the Ranibizumab Monotherapy or Combined with Laser versus Laser Monotherapy for Diabetic Macular Edema (RESTORE) study achieved favorable functional and morphological results using intravitreal ranibizumab combined with laser [15].

Furthermore, the effectivity of intravitreal anti-VEGF combined with laser has been shown in the Diabetic Retinopathy Clinical Research Network trial at the 1-year of follow-up. At 3 years, prompt laser was not better compared with deferring laser for 24 weeks or more [16].

The study presented here further showed that morphological features like center-involving intraretinal hyperreflective material detected by SD-OCT may represent a negative predictive factor in the eyes with DME because the initially observed inferior VA of the eyes revealing intraretinal hyperreflective foci at baseline remained until the end of the follow-up period (0.39; 20/50 Snellen (SD = 0.25) versus 0.68; 20/63 Snellen (SD = 0.22), $p = 25$, Table 3). Hyperreflective intraretinal spots define exudates as visible clinically and were described previously by Vujosevic et al. [17]. Hyperreflective structures seen in SD-OCT correlated to hard exudates observed in biomicroscopy in our study. The eyes that displayed hyperreflective structures in outer retinal layers in the present study showed a marked decrease of these alterations following treatment with anti-VEGF during follow-up. As BCVA generally improved as treatment with ranibizumab progressed, it may be suggested that a reduction of intraretinal hyperreflective foci followed by anti-VEGF therapy may at least partly represent a positive predictive morphological feature in the eyes with DME. This assumption has also been suggested previously [18], it and is supported by our findings during an observation period of 5 years.

Intraretinal hyperreflective foci were further less frequently present in the prompt treatment group compared with the deferred group as treatment progressed (57% versus 43% of cases with clusters of intraretinal hyperreflective structures at the end of the observation period), potentially signifying a therapeutic benefit as compared with deferred laser. However; this finding needs to be confirmed in larger prospective clinical trials.

Described hyperreflective intraretinal alterations may further be clinically relevant in an early stage of DR as it has been described previously that these hyperreflective spots are present in diabetic eyes even when retinopathy is undetectable clinically, increasing in number when DR progresses. This hypothesis is supported by the inferior VA in eyes with hyperreflective intraretinal alterations in our study. In addition, Niu et al. [18] showed that the area and

TABLE 3: Functional (best-corrected visual acuity (BCVA)) and morphological (central retinal thickness (CRT)) results in eyes with diabetic macular edema (DME) following treatment with intravitreal ranibizumab and focal laser therapy that reveal clusters of hyperreflective foci in the central macular area (27 eyes, 54%) and eyes without hyperreflective intraretinal foci (23 eyes, 46%). Results show that BCVA in eyes revealing clusters of hyperreflective foci in the central macular region detected by spectral domain optical coherence tomography (SD-OCT) was significantly inferior compared with eyes without clusters of hyperreflective intraretinal foci at year 5 (0.39 Snellen (SD = 0.25, 0.4 logMAR) versus 0.63 Snellen (SD = 0.22, 0.2 logMAR), $p < 0.01$)

	Baseline	6 weeks	12 weeks	18 weeks	6 months	9 months	1 year	2 years	3 years	4 years	5 years
Eyes revealing clusters of hyperreflective foci in the central macular area in SD-OCT											
BCVA	0.32	0.50	0.50	0.50	0.50	0.50	0.50	0.72	0.67	0.62	0.68
SD	0.03	0.03	0.03	0.04	0.04	0.03	0.03	0.42	0.26	0.26	0.25
logMAR (Snellen)	0.50 (20/40)	0.30 (20/63)	0.30 (20/63)	0.30 (20/63)	0.30 (20/63)	0.30 (20/63)	0.30 (20/63)	0.20 (20/100)	0.20 (20/100)	0.20 (20/100)	0.20 (20/100)
CRT	457.20	401.60	391.30	381.10	269.60	358.90	351.90	377.40	363.00	343.80	348.30
SD	90.70	98.40	94.20	99.30	85.70	88.30	93.00	108.20	95.20	78.70	62.00
Eyes without clusters of hyperreflective foci in the central macular area in SD-OCT											
BCVA	0.32	0.50	0.50	0.40	0.40	0.50	0.50	0.70	0.63	0.58	0.58
SD	0.03	0.04	0.04	0.05	0.04	0.03	0.03	0.39	0.36	0.29	0.31
logMAR (Snellen)	0.50 (20/40)	0.30 (20/63)	0.30 (20/63)	0.40 (20/50)	0.40 (20/50)	0.30 (20/63)	0.30 (20/63)	0.20 (20/100)	0.20 (20/100)	0.30 (20/63)	0.30 (20/63)
CRT	460.30	381.60	399.40	370.20	360.70	362.80	354.70	360.70	360.70	357.00	354.40
SD	87.40	70.20	91.50	113.50	101.50	106.10	94.10	105.80	106.90	108.00	108.90

Note. BCVA = best-corrected visual acuity, SD = standard deviation, and CRT = central retinal thickness.

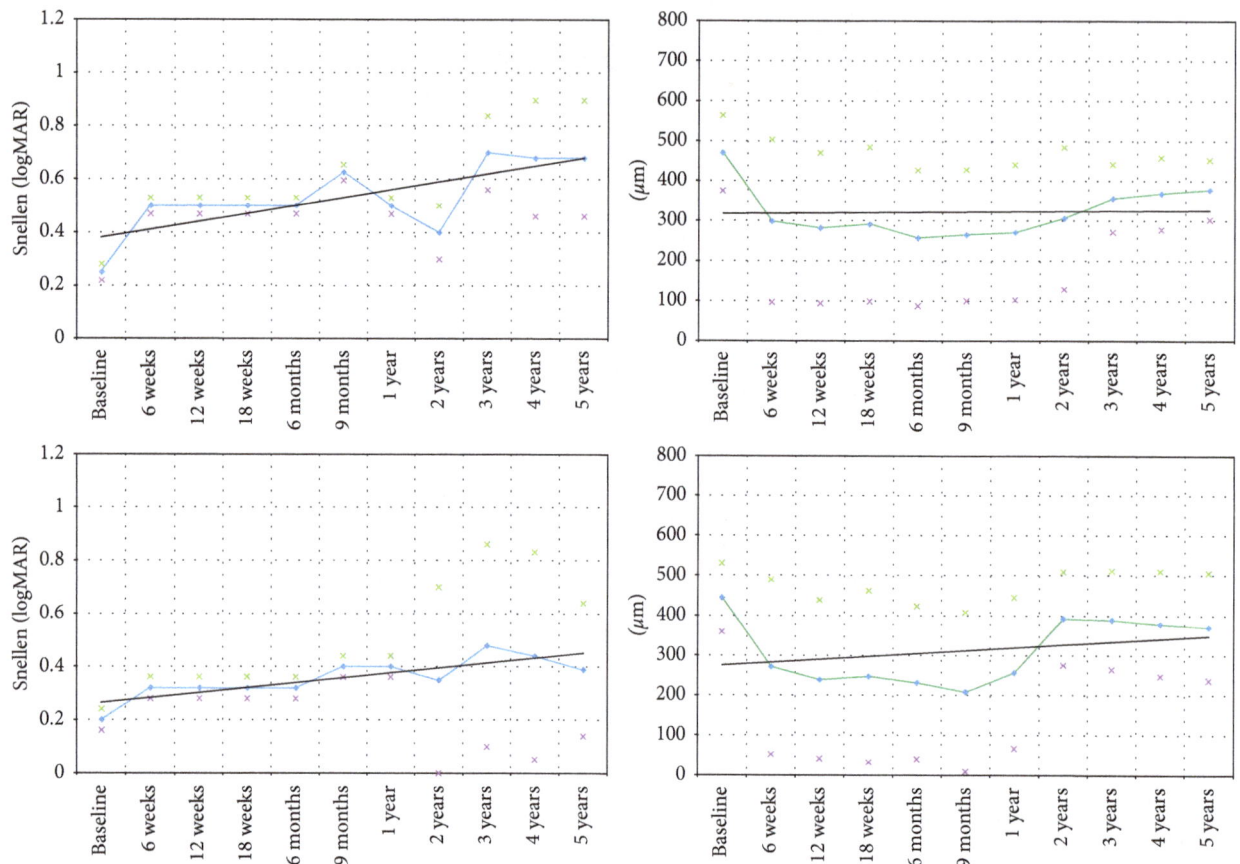

FIGURE 3: Best-corrected visual acuity (BCVA) and central retinal thickness (CRT) in eyes with diabetic macular edema (DME) treated with intravitreal antivascular endothelial growth factor (anti-VEGF) and focal macular laser. Data represent eyes revealing clusters of intraretinal hyperreflective material as detected on spectral domain optical coherence tomography (SD-OCT) and eyes without these morphological changes. BCVA in eyes with clusters of hyperreflective foci in the central macular region detected by SD-OCT was significantly inferior compared with eyes without intraretinal hyperreflective foci at year 5 of follow-up (0.39; 20/50 Snellen (SD = 0.25, 0.4 logMAR) versus 0.63; 20/32 Snellen (SD = 0.22, 0.2 logMAR), $p < 0.01$). BCVA = best-corrected visual acuity. CRT = central retinal thickness. Black lines represent trend lines. Stars indicate standard deviation. p values indicate change compared with baseline. (a) BCVA in eyes with (22 eyes) and without (20 eyes, light blue line) intraretinal hypherreflective foci in SD-OCT. (b) CRT in eyes with (22 eyes) and without (28 eyes, light green line) intraretinal hypherreflective foci in SD-OCT.

amount of hyperreflective spots can serve as a potential discriminant indicator for the severity of DR. The current study confirmed this hypothesis in a long-term clinical setting. Our findings regarding a clinically predictive value of hyperreflective intraretinal foci are further supported by Kang et al. [19] who demonstrated that the number of hyperreflective foci in outer retinal layers visible in SD-OCT at baseline might predict the final VA in DME.

Although it has been shown by Kang et al. [19] that higher total and low-density lipoprotein cholesterol levels were associated with presence of hyperreflective foci in SD-OCT, the precise origin of these hyperreflective foci remains to be shown in histopathological studies or by using tissue-specific retinal imaging modalities (i.e., polarization sensitive OCT (PS-OCT)) [20] that provide inherent tissue contrast visualization. Intraretinal exudative material may also contain intraretinal macrophages and represent the level of inflammatory activity in DME. This may explain the negative correlation between intraretinal hyperreflective foci and visual function.

It remains to be shown if the eyes with extensive exudative material in the central macular region and reduced BCVA in our study would profit from an individualized and more intense anti-VEGF treatment strategy, as has been suggested by others previously [21].

Limitations of the current study are the relatively low number of patients and the lack of identification of other morphological parameters in OCT (i.e., integrity of the retinal pigment epithelium (RPE) or the identification and segmentation of individual outer retinal layers in SD-OCT) that may serve as relevant prognostic markers in eyes with DME and will be addressed in future investigations. Furthermore, treating physicians were not masked according to the group of patients, which is considered as a study limitation.

Another drawback of this study is that patients with DME in addition to neovascularization on the disc (NVD) or elsewhere (NVE) were not analyzed separately or compared to the study population presented here. Regarding treatment with anti-VEGF in DME, only ranibizumab was assessed in our investigation; though evaluation of intraretinal morphological changes following treatment with bevacizumab, aflibercept, dexamethasone, or triamcinolone should be considered in future investigations (including the identification of functionally relevant morphological characteristics) in order to possibly implement individualized patient management strategies during a long-term follow-up period.

Although our study showed no severe ocular adverse events like endophthalmitis or arterial nonperfusion, enhanced investigation regarding ophthalmological or systemic adverse events would further have increased the validity of our study.

The lack of a comparison analysis between the eyes treated with anti-VEGF alone and the eyes receiving anti-VEGF in addition to focal laser is another drawback of the current study.

An automated segmentation analysis software algorithm used for quantification of intraretinal hyperreflective foci in all B-scans of dense volume SD-OCT datasets in this study would further have been advantageous.

It may be suggested that change in BCVA primarily resulted due to treatment with focal laser and anti-VEGF, as only 6 eyes (12%) of the current study received cataract surgery during the observation period.

To conclude, the study presented here showed that combined treatment with ranibizumab and focal laser effectively reduces visual loss due to DME, which is a major sight-threatening cause in diabetic patients. Our results regarding functional long-term development are in conjunction with those of several previous clinical trials [7–9,14–16] that evaluate the efficacy of anti-VEGF and laser treatment in DR, favoring anti-VEGF. Nevertheless, macular laser can still be applied and seems particularly favorable in the beginning of the treatment phase. Furthermore, the combined therapy with anti-VEGF and macular laser can exploit the synergistic effects of both therapies, leading to a simpler and more practical management of patients during the long-term follow-up. Our results suggest that anti-VEGF treatment in addition to prompt laser is favorable because of sparing an additional visit for patients. Moreover, the findings of our study may aid in the identification of prognostic morphological features that are clinically relevant for patients with DME and potentially significant for the development of prospective individualized therapeutic procedures in order to reduce the burden of frequent clinical management for affected patients.

5. Conclusions

The present study showed that grid laser and ranibizumab treatment are effective in DME management during the long-term follow-up. Overall, there was no meaningful functional benefit in the long run when comparing prompt versus deferred focal laser combined with anti-VEGF in the long run. Morphological characteristics like intraretinal hyperreflective material shown in SD-OCT are negatively related to functionality in DME patients.

Conflicts of Interest

Each of the authors warrants that he or she has no commercial associations that might pose a conflict of interest in context with the article.

References

[1] R. Klein, B. E. Klein, S. E. Moss, M. D. Davis, and D. L. DeMets, "The wisconsin epidemiologic study of diabetic retinopathy. IV: diabetic macular edema," *Ophthalmology*, vol. 91, no. 12, pp. 1464–1474, 1984.

[2] S. E. Moss, R. Klein, and B. E. Klein, "The 14-year incidence of visual loss in a diabetic population," *Ophthalmology*, vol. 105, no. 6, pp. 998–1003, 1998.

[3] M. W. Stewart, "A review of ranibizumab for the treatment of diabetic retinopathy," *Ophthalmology and Therapy*, vol. 6, no. 1, pp. 33–47, 2017.

[4] H. Funatsu, H. Yamashita, K. Sakata et al., "Vitreous levels of vascular endothelial growth factor and intracellular adhesion molecule 1 are related to diabetic macular edema," *Ophthalmology*, vol. 112, no. 5, pp. 806–816, 2005.

[5] D. M. Nathan, S. Genuth, J. Lachin et al., "Photocoagulation therapy for diabetic eye disease: Early Treatment Diabetic Retinopathy Study Research Group," *JAMA*, vol. 254, no. 21, pp. 3086-3087, 1985.

[6] D. M. Nathan, S. Genuth, J. Lachin et al., "The effect of intensive treatment of diabetes on the development and progression of long-term complications in insulin-dependent diabetes mellitus," *New England Journal of Medicine*, vol. 329, no. 14, pp. 977–986, 1993.

[7] D. M. Brown, U. Schmidt-Erfurth, D. V. Do et al., "Intravitreal aflibercept for diabetic macular edema: 100-week results from the VISTA and VIVID studies," *Ophthalmology*, vol. 122, no. 10, pp. 2044–2052, 2015.

[8] N. M. Bressler, R. Varma, I. J. Suñer et al., "Vision-related function after ranibizumab treatment for diabetic macular edema: results from RIDE and RISE," *Ophthalmology*, vol. 121, no. 12, pp. 2461–2472, 2014.

[9] A. Ophir, "Early and long-term responses to anti-vascular endothelial growth factor therapy in diabetic macular edema: analysis of protocol I data," *American Journal of Ophthalmology*, vol. 177, pp. 230-231, 2017.

[10] Diabetic Retinopathy Clinical Research Network, L. P. Aiello, R. W. Beck et al., "Rationale for the diabetic retinopathy clinical research network treatment protocol for center-involved diabetic macular edema," *Ophthalmology*, vol. 118, no. 12, pp. e5–e14, 2011.

[11] J. H. Kempen, B. J. O'Colmain, M. C. Leske et al., "The prevalence of diabetic retinopathy among adults in the United States," *Archives of Ophthalmology*, vol. 122, no. 4, pp. 552–563, 2004.

[12] E. Liu, J. E. Craig, and K. Burdon, "Diabetic macular oedema: clinical risk factors and emerging genetic influences," *Clinical and Experimental Optometry*, vol. 100, no. 6, pp. 569–576, 2017.

[13] Q. D. Nguyen, S. M. Shah, J. S. Heier et al., "Primary end point (six months) results of the ranibizumab for edema of the macula in diabetes (READ-2) study," *Ophthalmology*, vol. 116, no. 11, pp. 2175–2181.e1, 2009.

[14] V. H. Gonzalez, J. Campbell, N. M. Holekamp et al., "Early and long-term responses to anti-vascular endothelial growth factor therapy in diabetic macular edema: analysis of protocol

I data," *American Journal of Ophthalmology*, vol. 172, pp. 72–79, 2016.

[15] P. Mitchell, F. Bandello, U. Schmidt-Erfurth et al., "The RESTORE study: ranibizumab monotherapy or combined with laser versus laser monotherapy for diabetic macular edema," *Ophthalmology*, vol. 118, no. 4, pp. 615–625, 2011.

[16] I. Zucchiatti and F. Bandello, "Intravitreal ranibizumab in diabetic macular edema: long-term outcomes," *Developments in Ophthalmology*, vol. 60, pp. 63–70, 2017.

[17] S. Vujosevic, S. Bini, T. Torresin et al., "Hyperreflective retinal spots in normal and diabetic eyes: B-scan and en face spectral domain optical coherence tomography evaluation," *Retina*, vol. 37, no. 6, pp. 1092–1103, 2017.

[18] S. Niu, C. Yu, Q. Chen et al., "Multimodality analysis of hyper-reflective foci and hard exudates in patients with diabetic retinopathy," *Scientific Reports*, vol. 7, no. 1, p. 1568, 2017.

[19] J. W. Kang, H. Chung, and H. Chan Kim, "Correlation of optical coherence tomographic hyperreflective foci with visual outcomes in different patterns of diabetic macular edema," *Retina*, vol. 36, no. 9, pp. 1630–1639, 2016.

[20] J. Lammer, M. Bolz, B. Baumann et al., "Imaging retinal pigment epithelial proliferation secondary to PASCAL photocoagulation in vivo by polarization-sensitive optical coherence tomography," *American Journal of Ophthalmology*, vol. 155, no. 6, pp. 1058–1067.e1, 2013.

[21] H. Mehta, S. Fraser-Bell, A. Yeung et al., "Efficacy of dexamethasone versus bevacizumab on regression of hard exudates in diabetic maculopathy: data from the BEVORDEX randomised clinical trial," *British Journal of Ophthalmology*, vol. 10, no. 7, pp. 1000–1004, 2016.

28

Less Expansion of Short-Pulse Laser Scars in Panretinal Photocoagulation for Diabetic Retinopathy

Masahiko Higaki, Miho Nozaki ⓘ, Munenori Yoshida, and Yuichiro Ogura

Department of Ophthalmology and Visual Science, Nagoya City University Graduate School of Medical Sciences, Nagoya 467-8601, Japan

Correspondence should be addressed to Miho Nozaki; miho.nozaki@gmail.com

Academic Editor: Lawrence S. Morse

Purpose. To compare the expansion rates of laser photocoagulation scars between the conventional laser and short-pulse laser using fundus autofluorescence (FAF). *Methods.* Retrospective chart review. Conventional laser was performed on 6 eyes of 6 patients, and short-pulse laser was performed on 11 eyes of 8 patients with diabetic retinopathy. FAF images were obtained by Optos® 200Tx (Optos, Dunfermline, Scotland, UK) at 1, 3, 6, and 12 months after treatment. The average area of 20 photocoagulation scars was measured by using ImageJ software. The expansion rates were calculated from the proportion of the averaged area against the optic disc area. Regression of retinopathy and central macular thickness were also evaluated. *Results.* The expansion rates of the conventional laser scars compared with the size at 1 month after treatment were 1.12 ± 0.08 (3 M), 1.27 ± 0.12 (6 M), and 1.39 ± 0.11 (12 M). The expansion rates of the short-pulse laser scars were 1.04 ± 0.05 (3 M), 1.09 ± 0.04 (6 M), and 1.13 ± 0.05 (12 M). The expansion rates of the short-pulse laser were significantly lower than those of the conventional laser ($p < 0.01$). *Conclusion.* FAF images were useful to evaluate the changes in the photocoagulation scar sizes. The scars with the short-pulse laser showed lower expansion rates than those of the conventional laser.

1. Introduction

Diabetic retinopathy is the leading cause of blindness in the working population of the Western world [1]. Although panretinal photocoagulation (PRP) is the standard therapy for reducing the activity of diabetic retinopathy [2], PRP sometimes results in decreased visual acuity due to PRP-induced macular edema [3–5]. Recently, short-pulse pattern scan laser system (PASCAL® Streamline, Topcon Medical Laser systems, Santa Clara, CA, USA) has been developed [6, 7], and it is known that short-pulse laser treatment is quicker, generates less heat, and is less painful to eyes than the conventional laser treatment [6]. Moreover, some reports indicate that short-pulse laser treatment induces less inflammation, fewer inflammatory cytokines in the sensory retina, and less macular thickening in patients with diabetic retinopathy than the conventional pulse duration [2–4, 8, 9].

Despite these advantages of the short-pulse laser, some studies indicate that short-pulse laser is less effective than the conventional laser treatment in treatment for the high-risk proliferative diabetic retinopathy. They suggested that the reason for the differences was that the total area of PRP scars generated by the conventional laser exceeded that of short-pulse laser although both groups were treated with the same number of laser spots [5, 10]. The photocoagulation scars performed by the conventional laser have a tendency to expand after treatment [5, 8, 11–14]. However, some reports revealed that the expansion rate of photocoagulation scars performed by the short-pulse laser is lower than that of the conventional laser [8, 12, 15]. In these reports, the laser scars were evaluated by using examination including color fundus photographs, fluorescein angiograms, and infrared images [8, 12] or OCT [16].

FAF imaging is a noninvasive technique used to assess retinal pigment epithelial (RPE) cells and now widely used to evaluate age-related macular degeneration [17], retinitis pigmentosa [18], and other chorioretinal diseases. FAF signals increase with lipofuscin accumulation in RPE cells and decrease with RPE atrophy [19]. Analysis of FAF is an effective method to observe the functions of the RPE cells. Since retinal laser photocoagulation targets to RPE, FAF analysis after laser photocoagulation is thought to be an effective method to evaluate the RPE alterations and efficacy of laser photocoagulation. Although Muqit et al. already evaluated laser photocoagulation scars using FAF, they compared the FAF changes between the conventional laser and short-pulse laser only for 4 weeks [15], or they only followed FAF changes of 2 cases treated with short-pulse laser PRP [16].

In this study, we aimed to compare the FAF changes between the conventional laser and short-pulse laser in treatment of diabetic retinopathy, in terms of laser scar expansion rates and disease regression for 12 months.

2. Methods

This study was a retrospective cohort study. This study was approved by the Institutional Review Board of Nagoya City University Graduate School of Medical Science, conducted in accordance with the ethical standards stated in the 1964 Declaration of Helsinki.

All patients were treated at Nagoya City University Hospital between September 2013 and February 2015. All patients were followed for at least 12 months after laser photocoagulation. The patients with media opacities such as corneal opacity, cataract, and vitreous hemorrhage, which may influence the FAF images, were excluded.

We evaluated the best corrected visual acuity (BCVA), the central macular thickness (CMT) in OCT (Cirrus HD-OCT 4000, Carl Zeiss Meditec, Dublin, CA, Germany), the regressions of neovascularization, and the expansion of photocoagulation scars in 17 eyes of 12 patients with diabetic retinopathy (PDR; 5 eyes, NPDR; 12 eyes).

The BCVA was measured with a Japanese standard decimal visual acuity chart, and decimal BCVA was calculated using the logarithm of the minimum angle of resolution (logMAR) scale.

FAF images were taken by Optos 200Tx at 1, 3, 6, and 12 months after treatment. We measured the pixel sizes of an optic disc and 20 laser scars near the vascular arcade on each visit using the digital image analysis software ImageJ (developed by Wayne Rasband, National Institutes of Health, Bethesda, MD, USA; available at http://rsb.info.nih.gov/ij/index.html) (Figures 1 and 2) and calculated the expansion rates from the proportions of the average area of laser scars against the optic disc area. All the measurements were performed twice by one investigator (Masahiko Higaki's visual inspection on clopped magnified images). Results were obtained by analyzing the mean values of the two measurements. The intraclass correlation coefficient (ICC, %) was also calculated to evaluate reproducibility.

The regressions of neovascularization were evaluated by fluorescein angiography (FA). FA was performed 6 months and 12 months after treatment to evaluate the efficacy of photocoagulation, and if there were any residual nonperfusion area or neovascularization, additional laser photocoagulation was applied.

2.1. Statistics. All results are expressed as the mean ± standard deviation. Differences in genders and severity of diabetic retinopathy were analyzed by the Fisher's exact test. Comparisons of age, BCVA, CMT, timing of additional laser, and the duration of follow-up were performed using the Student's t-test. Expansion rates were analyzed using repeated measure ANOVA. The number of PRP shots was compared with Mann–Whitney U test. In all analyses, $p < 0.05$ was considered to be statistically significant. Statistics were calculated using Statcel 3 statistical software, version 3 (OMS Inc., Saitama, Japan).

3. Results

3.1. Patient Characteristics. The laser treatment was performed with the conventional laser (Novus Varia, Lumenis, Santa Clara, CA, USA) in 6 eyes and the short-pulse laser (PASCAL Streamline) in 11 eyes. Clinical characteristics of the patients are shown in Table 1. Conventional laser group included 3 PDR eyes, and short-pulse laser group included 2 PDR eyes. Although the conventional laser group included more PDR eyes, there was no statistically significant difference.

The mean age of patients was 65.8 ± 8.3 (range: 53–77) years old in the conventional laser group and 55.0 ± 14.1 (range: 34–77) years old in short-pulse laser group. The mean follow-up period was 15.5 ± 3.6 (range: 12–21) months in the conventional group and 16.6 ± 3.7 (range: 12–24) in short-pulse laser group. There were no statistically significant differences in age and follow-up period between the two groups. And all phakic patients did not receive cataract surgery during the follow-up period.

3.2. Laser Setting Parameters. Both laser methods were performed in the same spot size (200 μm) at different power to attain gray-white burn with Mainster PRP 165 contact lens (Ocular Instruments Inc., Bellevue, WA, USA). Yellow wavelength (577 nm) was used in both modalities. Sub-Tenon's triamcinolone acetonide (Kenacort; Bristol-Myers Squibb, Tokyo, Japan) injections (STTA) were performed after the first session of laser treatment (4 eyes in the conventional laser group and 2 eyes in the short-pulse laser group). The summary of the settings used in the conventional laser and the short-pulse laser was shown in Table 2. One eye in the conventional laser group was previously treated with targeted retinal photocoagulation (TRP) [20]. In the short-pulse laser group, 4 eyes were treated with TRP, and 3 eyes were previously treated with TRP. Other 4 eyes were treated with PRP. The mean PRP number of laser shots performed in the treatment-naive eye was 1798 ± 885 in the conventional laser group and 4247 ± 279 in short-pulse laser group, and there was a significant difference ($p < 0.05$, Mann–Whitney U test).

3.3. The Best-Corrected Visual Acuity. The mean BCVA (logMAR) before the conventional laser treatment was 0.64 ± 0.41 and 0.35 ± 0.44 at 12 months after treatment. The mean BCVA before the short-pulse laser treatment was −0.05 ± 0.12 and 0.00 ± 0.13 at 12 months after

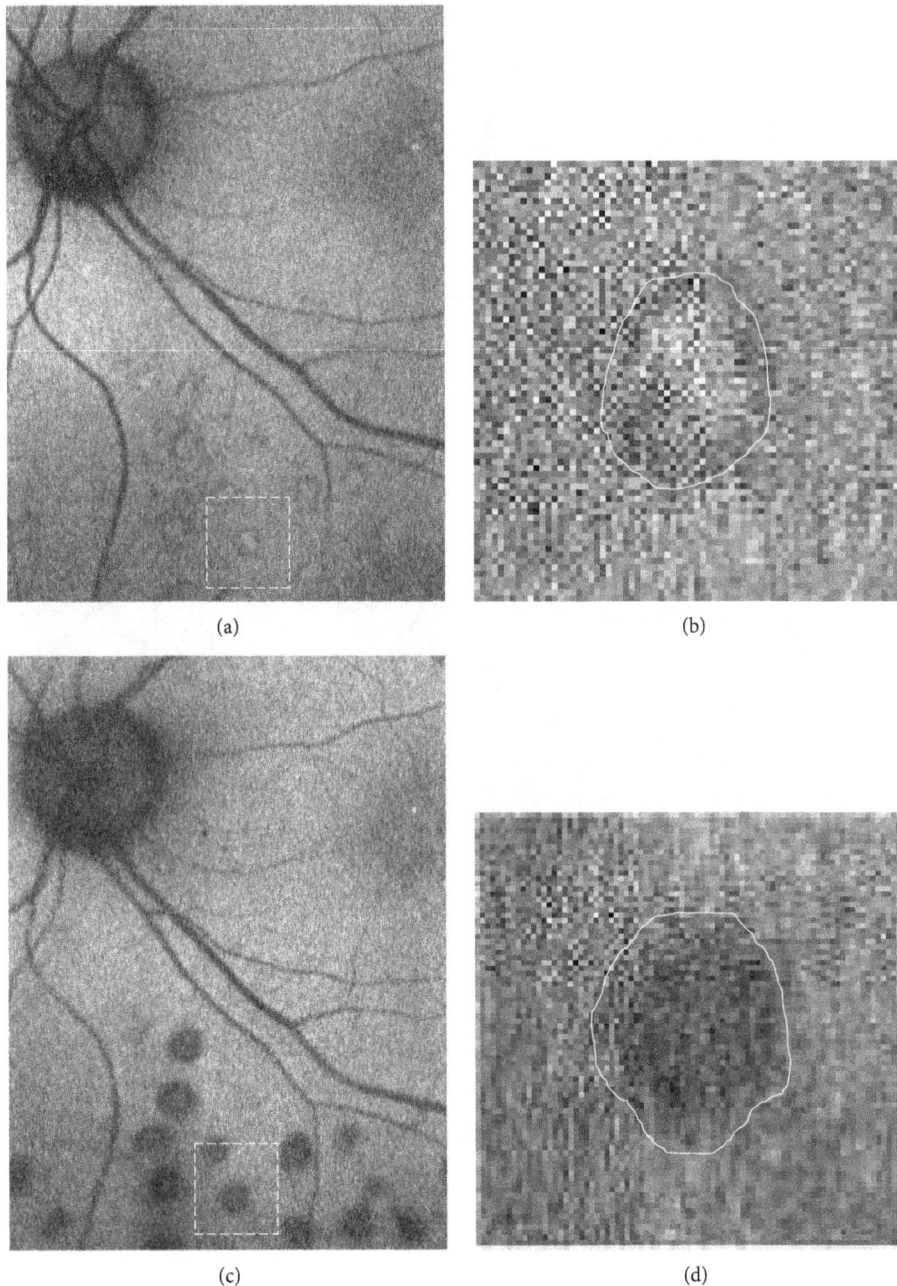

FIGURE 1: Representative images of fundus autofluorescence (FAF) in the conventional laser group. The images were taken 1 month after laser treatment (a, b) and 12 months after treatment (c, d). Twenty laser scars near the vascular arcade were measured using the digital image analysis software ImageJ on each visit. Higher magnification of the area surrounded by white-dashed line was shown in (b) and (d). White line indicated the outline of FAF laser scars for measurement (b, d). High magnification images show the changes of laser scars from hyperautofluorescent at 1 months (b) to hypoautofluorescent at 12 months after laser treatment (d).

treatment. There was no significant aggravation of BCVA 12 months after treatment in both groups.

3.4. Central Macular Thickness (CMT). The mean CMT before the conventional laser treatment was $339.6 \pm 80.0\,\mu$m, and the mean CMT at 12 months after treatment was $329.0 \pm 81.0\,\mu$m. The mean CMT before the short-pulse laser treatment was $266.5 \pm 35.4\,\mu$m and that at 12 months after treatment was $272.1 \pm 32.3\,\mu$m. There was no significant aggravation of CMT 12 months after treatment in both groups.

3.5. Disease Regression Outcomes. In the conventional laser group, two eyes (33%) required additional laser due to the residual nonperfusion area (9 or 13 months after treatment). Two eyes (33%) were treated additionally due to residual nonperfusion area and neovascularization (7 or 13 months after treatment). And one eye (14%) developed macular edema 4 months after laser treatment, and focal laser photocoagulation was performed using Navilas laser system (OD-OS GmbH, Teltow, Germany). This patient was previously treated by several injections of antivascular endothelial

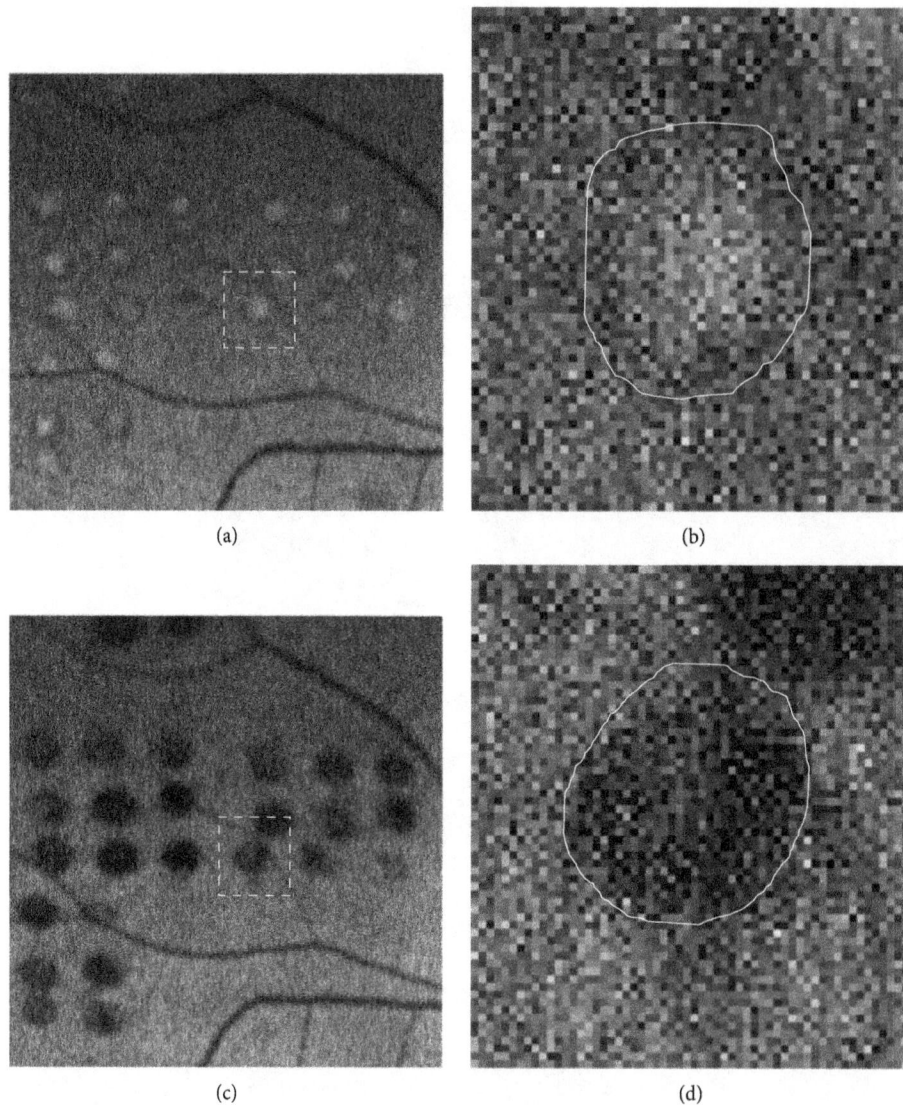

FIGURE 2: Representative images of FAF in the short-pulse laser group. The images were taken 1 month after laser treatment (a, b) and 12 months after treatment (c, d). Twenty laser scars near the vascular arcade were measured using the digital image analysis software ImageJ on each visit. Higher magnification of the area surrounded by white-dashed line was shown in (b) and (d). White line indicated the outline of FAF laser scars for measurement (b, d). High magnification images show the changes of laser scars from hyperautofluorescent at 1 month (b) to hypoautofluorescent at 12 months after laser treatment (d).

growth factor (VEGF) for diabetic macular edema (DME). At the time when PRP was given, DME was resolved, and she was not treated with STTA.

In the short-pulse laser group, 4 eyes (36%) received additional laser due to the residual nonperfusion area (6–9 months after treatment). One eye developed retinal break with posterior vitreous detachment, and the laser photocoagulation was performed around the retinal break (5 months after treatment). One eye (9%) showed recurrence of macular edema 7 months after laser treatment, and focal laser photocoagulation was performed. This patient was treated with STTA when PRP was given (4411 shots in one session).

The timing of additional laser showed no significant difference between both groups.

3.6. Photocoagulation Scar Expansion.

We measured the size of 20 laser scars near the vascular arcade on each visit and calculated the expansion rate over time. The intraclass correlation coefficient (ICC, %) was evaluated (Table 3). Based on these results, the collected data were considered to be reliable and useful for further analysis.

The expansion rates of scars with the conventional laser were 1.12 ± 0.08 (3 M), 1.27 ± 0.12 (6 M), and 1.39 ± 0.11 (12 M) (Figures 3 and 4).

On the other hand, the expansion rates of scars with the short-pulse laser against the scar size in 1 month after treatment were 1.04 ± 0.05 (3 M), 1.09 ± 0.04 (6 M), and 1.13 ± 0.05 (12 M) (Figures 3 and 4).

As a result, the expansion rates of both groups increased significantly over time ($p < 0.01$) and the expansion rates of

TABLE 1: Patient characteristics.

	Conventional laser	Short-pulse laser	p
Number of eyes	6	11	
Mean age, years	65.8 ± 8.3	55.0 ± 14.1	0.13†
Male : Female	4 : 2	5 : 3	0.65‡
NPDR : PDR	3 : 3	9 : 2	0.29‡
Duration of follow-up (months)	15.5 ± 3.6	16.6 ± 3.7	0.58†
BCVA (logMAR) pretreatment	0.64 ± 0.41	-0.05 ± 0.12	<0.01†
BCVA (logMAR) posttreatment (12 M)	0.35 ± 0.44	0.00 ± 0.13	<0.05†
Mean CMT pretreatment (μm)	339.6 ± 80.0	266.5 ± 35.4	<0.05†
Mean CMT post- treatment (μm) (12 M)	329.0 ± 81.0	272.1 ± 32.3	0.08†
Phakic eyes : pseudophakic eyes	3 : 3	10 : 1	0.10‡
Number of operators	5	5	
STTA	4	2	0.07‡

†Student's t-test; ‡Fisher's exact test. NPDR: nonproliferative diabetic retinopathy; PDR: proliferative diabetic retinopathy; BCVA: best-corrected visual acuity; CMT: central macular thickness; STTA: sub-Tenon's injections of triamcinolone acetonide.

TABLE 2: Settings of laser treatment.

	Conventional laser	Short-pulse laser	p
Power (mW)	100–260	300–500	—
Pulse duration (ms)	200	20	—
Spot size (μm)	200	20	—
Wavelength (nm)	Yellow (577)	Yellow (577)	—
Spacing (spot)	1	0.75	—
Mean number of total PRP shots (in treatment naive eyes)	1798 ± 885 (958–3505)	4247 ± 279 (3875–4600)	<0.05†

†Mann–Whitney U test. PRP: panretinal photocoagulation.

TABLE 3: Intraclass correlation coefficient.

	Conventional group		Short-pulse group	
	M1	M2	M1	M2
Mean scar area divided by disc area, month 1	0.072 ± 0.010	0.074 ± 0.009	0.037 ± 0.040	0.038 ± 0.003
Mean of M1 and M2	0.073 ± 0.009		0.037 ± 0.004	
ICC, %	81.6		79.2	
Mean scar area divided by disc area, month 3	0.081 ± 0.013	0.081 ± 0.012	0.039 ± 0.004	0.040 ± 0.004
Mean of M1 and M2	0.081 ± 0.013		0.040 ± 0.004	
ICC, %	88.3		81.1	
Mean scar area divided by disc area, month 6	0.093 ± 0.012	0.093 ± 0.011	0.041 ± 0.004	0.041 ± 0.004
Mean of M1 and M2	0.093 ± 0.011		0.041 ± 0.004	
ICC, %	87.0		87.3	
Mean scar area divided by disc area, month 12	0.102 ± 0.017	0.102 ± 0.016	0.043 ± 0.003	0.043 ± 0.003
Mean of M1 and M2	0.102 ± 0.016		0.043 ± 0.003	
ICC, %	83.5		84.1	

M1: measurement 1; M2: measurement 2. ICC: intraclass correlation coefficient.

short-pulse laser scars were significantly lower than those of conventional laser scars over time ($p < 0.01$) (Figure 3). There were 5 operators in each group, and there were no significant differences in expansion rates among operators.

3.7. FAF Findings. The conventional laser scars changed from hyperautofluorescent to hypoautofluorescent more rapidly than the short-pulse laser scars (Figure 4). All the photocoagulation scars in both groups were hyperautofluorescent at month 3 (Figures 4(a)–4(c)). The photocoagulation scars in the conventional laser group became hypoautofluorescent in 5 out of 6 eyes (83.3%) at month 6 (Figure 4(b)) and 6 out of 6 eyes (100%) at month 12. On the other hand, the photocoagulation scars in the short-pulse laser group became

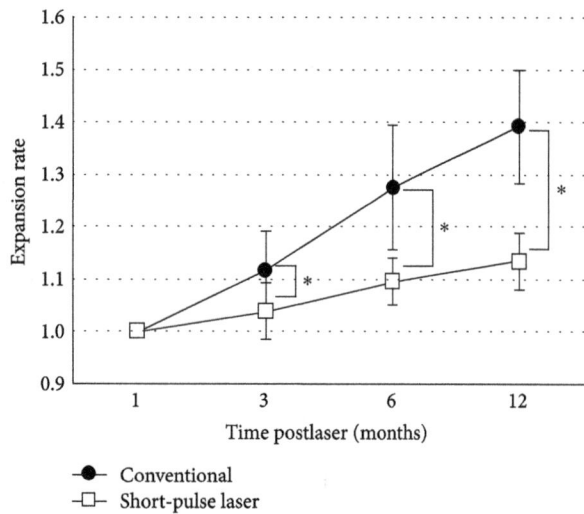

FIGURE 3: Expansion rates of laser scars with the conventional laser (closed circle) and short-pulse laser (open square) in months 3, 6, and 12 after laser treatment. Laser scars significantly expanded in both modalities, and the expansion rates of the short-pulse laser were significantly lower than those of conventional laser scars. Repeated measure ANOVA, $^*p < 0.01$.

hypoautofluorescent in 1 out of 11 eyes (9.1%) at month 6 (Figure 4(d)) and 7 out of 11 eyes (63.6%) at month 12. There was no relationship between FAF changes and laser augmentations. The FAF findings were all similar among operators.

4. Discussion

Our study showed that the laser photocoagulation scars kept growing for 12 months; however, the expansion rates of the short-pulse laser scars were significantly lower than those of the conventional laser scars during the period of observation. We used noninvasive FAF images taken by Optos 200Tx. By using FAF images, we were able to measure the sizes of photocoagulation scars easily due to their sharp outlines [15, 16].

These results were consistent with the following two previous reports. According to Nagpal et al., the expansion rate of the conventional laser was 27.2% and that of the short-pulse laser was 14.0% three months after laser treatment [8]. Shiraya et al. showed us that the expansion rate of the conventional laser was 18% and that of the short-pulse laser was 14% six months after laser photocoagulation [12].

On the other hand, some reports indicated that the 20-millisecond-pulse burns progressively reduced in size after photocoagulation [9, 15, 16, 21]. It can be surmised that the early retinal edema decreased with the lapse of time in these reports. Therefore, we set the values in one month after laser treatment as a benchmark to avoid the effect of the early retinal edema.

When the conventional laser is performed, photoreceptors usually suffer damage although the main target is RPE. Photoreceptors connect with adjacent photoreceptors through horizontal or amacrine cells. After local photoreceptors undergo necrosis, it causes apoptosis of the surrounding photoreceptors subsequently. As a consequence, photocoagulation scars expand [11, 22]. In contrast, when

the short-pulse laser is performed, the retinal damage is mostly confined to the outer retina because its pulse duration is very short (10–30 ms) [16, 21, 22]. Accordingly, photoreceptors suffer much less damage and the photocoagulation scars enlarge less than the conventional laser as a result.

In this FAF study, the short-pulse laser scars changed from hyperautofluorescent to hypoautofluorescent more slowly than the conventional laser scars. In the short-pulse laser group, all 4 eyes followed by 18 months showed hypoautofluorescent scars. This is possibly because of the chorioretinal damage by the short-pulse laser is confined to the outer retina. Conventional laser induces choriocapillaris atrophy which accelerates death of RPE and photoreceptors [23] and accelerated death of RPE and photoreceptors resulted in reduced FAF signal [19].

These results should be considered when laser photocoagulation therapy is performed for patients who have diabetic retinopathy or other retinal diseases. A report indicated that PRP performed by the short-pulse laser is less effective than that performed by the conventional argon laser in regression of neovascularization or incidence of vitreous hemorrhage within 6 months after treatment when the same number of spots was applied [5]. It is possible to deduce that the total area of PRP scars in the argon-treated patient exceeds that of the patient who underwent the short-pulse laser [10], and we should also consider the variability of photocoagulation lesions between physicians and patients [24], although there were no differences in expansion rates among operators in this study. Therefore, it is important for an operator to reconsider the settings of treatment parameters when using short-pulse laser therapy for serious retinal diseases such as high-risk PDR [5]. In this study, we set spacing as 0.75, and the total number of laser spots for PRP is significantly higher in the short-pulse laser group, and during this study follow-up period, no eye developed new vitreous hemorrhage in both groups during this study. Although the number of eyes with PDR was higher in the conventional laser group, suitable space setting (0.75) and higher number of laser spots might result in successful PRP.

As for PRP-induced macular edema, there were no significant differences in CMT before and after laser photocoagulation both in the conventional laser and short-pulse laser group in this study. STTA before PRP has been known as an effective treatment to prevent from PRP-induced macular edema [25], and we usually employ STTA when we start PRP in the eyes with already existing macular edema. However, one eye developed macular edema after PRP in the conventional laser group. She had past history of DME treated with multiple injections of anti-VEGF, but she did not receive STTA when PRP was given because macular edema was resolved at that time. But her parafoveal retinal thickness was 372 μm when PRP was initiated. Shimura et al. reported that patients whose preoperative parafoveal thickness was >300 μm had a worse visual prognosis due to PRP-induced macular edema [26]. From this background, this eye also should have been treated with STTA when PRP was given. Conversely, one eye also showed recurrence of macular edema after PRP in the short-pulse group 7 months after treatment, and he was treated with STTA when

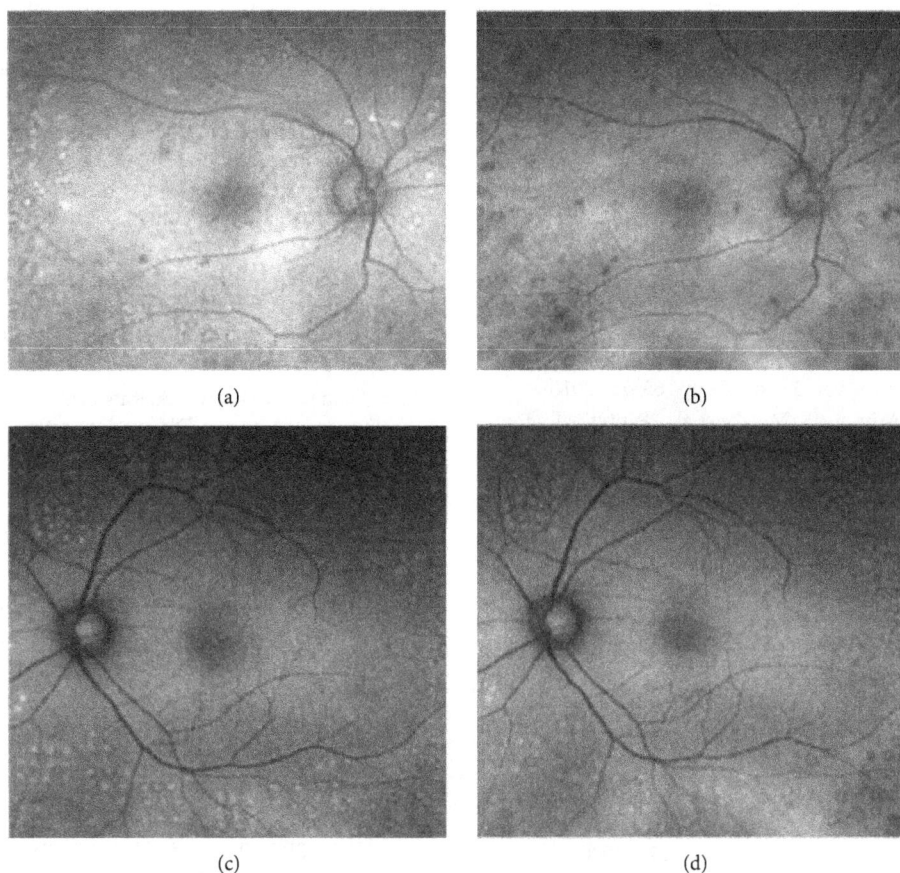

FIGURE 4: Representative images of FAF in the conventional laser group (a, b) and short-pulse laser group (c, d). The images were taken 3 months after laser treatment (a, c) and 6 months after laser treatment (b, d). Three months after laser treatment, the laser scars showed an increased level of autofluorescence (AF) surrounded by a decreased level of AF in both groups (a, c). Six months after laser treatment, the laser scars in the conventional laser group changed to hypoautofluorescent (b). However, in the short-pulse laser group, laser scars did not change to hypoautofluorescent (d).

PRP was given (4411 shots). From the overall results, there was no difference in terms of regression of retinopathy and worsening of macular edema between the conventional laser group and short-pulse laser group in our study.

There were several limitations that need to be acknowledged in our current study. First, there was a relatively small number of eyes with nonrandomized, retrospective methods. To compare the efficacy and expansion rate with the short-pulse laser and conventional laser, a large number of study with randomization will be warranted. Second, we used the wide-field imaging system, but we adopted only the postpole area. The reason was because the magnification of the posterior pole and that of midperiphery was different when using the images of Optos 200Tx [27]. Moreover, laser photocoagulation scars enlarge more in the posterior pole area than in the peripheral area [11]. Taking these differences into consideration, we decided to adopt the photocoagulation scars to evaluate only in the area of the posterior pole. Recently, the new software using stereographic projection, in which the lesion areas on ultra-wide-field images can be calculated in anatomically correct physical units (mm^2), has been developed [28]. Nevertheless, this software is not commercially available yet, we believe that the total area of laser scar

evaluation using FAF will give us more useful information of efficacy on laser photocoagulation in the future.

5. Conclusion

FAF imaging was useful to evaluate the temporal changes in the laser photocoagulation scar size. The scars with the short-pulse laser consistently showed lower expansion rates compared with those of the conventional laser. The change in CMT between the two groups was not significant.

Disclosure

A preliminary version of this paper was presented at the 9th Congress of Asia-Pacific Vitreo-retina Society meeting in Sydney, 2015.

Conflicts of Interest

The authors declare that there are no conflicts of interest regarding the publication of this article.

References

[1] J. Ding and T. Y. Wong, "Current epidemiology of diabetic retinopathy and diabetic macular edema," *Current Diabetes Reports*, vol. 12, no. 4, pp. 346–354, 2012.

[2] Diabetic retinopathy study research group, "Photocoagulation treatment of proliferative diabetic retinopathy: clinical application of diabetic retinopathy study (DRS) findings, DRS report number 8," *Ophthalmology*, vol. 88, no. 7, pp. 583–600, 1981.

[3] A. Ito, Y. Hirano, M. Nozaki, M. Ashikari, K. Sugitani, and Y. Ogura, "Short pulse laser induces less inflammatory cytokines in the murine retina after laser photocoagulation," *Ophthalmic Research*, vol. 53, no. 2, pp. 65–73, 2015.

[4] Y. Takamura, S. Arimura, S. Miyake et al., "Panretinal photocoagulation using short-pulse laser induces less inflammation and macular thickening in patients with diabetic retinopathy," *Journal of Ophthalmology*, vol. 2017, Article ID 8530261, 9 pages, 2017.

[5] A. V. Chappelow, K. Tan, N. K. Waheed, and P. K. Kaiser, "Panretinal photocoagulation for proliferative diabetic retinopathy: pattern scan laser versus argon laser," *American Journal of Ophthalmology*, vol. 153, no. 1, pp. 137–142.e2, 2012.

[6] C. Sanghvi, R. McLauchlan, C. Delgado et al., "Initial experience with the Pascal photocoagulator: a pilot study of 75 procedures," *British Journal of Ophthalmology*, vol. 92, no. 8, pp. 1061–1064, 2008.

[7] M. S. Blumenkranz, D. Yellachich, D. E. Andersen et al., "Semiautomated patterned scanning laser for retinal photocoagulation," *Retina*, vol. 26, no. 3, pp. 370–376, 2006.

[8] M. Nagpal, S. Marlecha, and K. Nagpal, "Comparison of laser photocoagulation for diabetic retinopathy using 532-nm standard laser versus multispot pattern scan laser," *Retina*, vol. 30, no. 3, pp. 452–458, 2010.

[9] A. Jain, M. S. Blumenkranz, Y. Paulus et al., "Effect of pulse duration on size and character of the lesion in retinal photocoagulation," *Archives of Ophthalmology*, vol. 126, no. 1, pp. 78–85, 2008.

[10] K. Nishida, H. Sakaguchi, M. Kamei et al., "Simulation of panretinal laser photocoagulation using geometric methods for calculating the photocoagulation index," *European Journal of Ophthalmology*, vol. 27, no. 2, pp. 205–209, 2017.

[11] K. Maeshima, N. Utsugi-Sutoh, T. Otani, and S. Kishi, "Progressive enlargement of scattered photocoagulation scars in diabetic retinopathy," *Retina*, vol. 24, no. 4, pp. 507–511, 2004.

[12] T. Shiraya, S. Kato, T. Shigeeda, T. Yamaguchi, and T. Kaiya, "Comparison of burn size after retinal photocoagulation by conventional and high-power short-duration methods," *Acta Ophthalmologica*, vol. 92, no. 7, pp. e585–e586, 2014.

[13] R. Brancato, A. Pece, P. Avanza, and E. Radrizzani, "Photocoagulation scar expansion after laser therapy for choroidal neovascularization in degenerative myopia," *Retina*, vol. 10, no. 4, pp. 239–243, 1990.

[14] H. Schatz, D. Madeira, H. McDonald, and R. N. Johnson, "Progressive enlargement of laser scars following grid laser photocoagulation for diffuse diabetic macular edema," *Archives of Ophthalmology*, vol. 109, no. 11, pp. 1549–1551, 1991.

[15] M. M. Muqit, J. C. Gray, G. R. Marcellino et al., "In vivo laser-tissue interactions and healing responses from 20- vs 100-millisecond pulse Pascal photocoagulation burns," *Archives of Ophthalmology*, vol. 128, no. 4, pp. 448–455, 2010.

[16] M. M. K. Muqit, J. C. B. Gray, G. R. Marcellino et al., "Fundus autofluorescence and Fourier-domain optical coherence tomography imaging of 10 and 20 millisecond Pascal retinal photocoagulation treatment," *British Journal of Ophthalmology*, vol. 93, no. 4, pp. 518–525, 2009.

[17] T. Suetsugu, A. Kato, M. Yoshida et al., "Evaluation of peripheral fundus autofluorescence in eyes with wet age-related macular degeneration," *Clinical Ophthalmology*, vol. 10, pp. 2497–2503, 2016.

[18] S. Ogura, T. Yasukawa, A. Kato et al., "Wide-field fundus autofluorescence imaging to evaluate retinal function in patients with retinitis pigmentosa," *American Journal of Ophthalmology*, vol. 158, no. 5, pp. 1093–1098.e3, 2014.

[19] S. Schmitz-Valckenberg, F. G. Holz, A. C. Bird, and R. F. Spaide, "Fundus autofluorescence imaging: review and perspectives," *Retina*, vol. 28, no. 3, pp. 385–409, 2008.

[20] S. Reddy, A. Hu, and S. D. Schwartz, "Ultra wide field fluorescein angiography guided targeted retinal photocoagulation (TRP)," *Seminars in Ophthalmology*, vol. 24, no. 1, pp. 9–14, 2009.

[21] Y. M. Paulus, A. Jain, R. F. Gariano et al., "Healing of retinal photocoagulation lesions," *Investigative Ophthalmology & Visual Science*, vol. 49, no. 12, pp. 5540–5545, 2008.

[22] M. M. K. Muqit, C. Sanghvi, R. McLauchlan et al., "Study of clinical applications and safety for Pascal® laser photocoagulation in retinal vascular disorders," *Acta Ophthalmologica*, vol. 90, no. 2, pp. 155–161, 2012.

[23] A. W. Stitt, T. A. Gardiner, and D. B. Archer, "Retinal and choroidal responses to panretinal photocoagulation: an ultrastructural perspective," *Graefe's Archive for Clinical and Experimental Ophthalmology*, vol. 233, no. 11, pp. 699–705, 1995.

[24] M. Saeger, J. Heckmann, K. Purtskhvanidze, A. Caliebe, J. Roider, and S. Koinzer, "Variability of panretinal photocoagulation lesions across physicians and patients. Quantification of diameter and intensity variation," *Graefe's Archive for Clinical and Experimental Ophthalmology*, vol. 255, no. 1, pp. 49–59, 2017.

[25] M. Shimura, K. Yasuda, and T. Shiono, "Posterior sub-Tenon's capsule injection of triamcinolone acetonide prevents panretinal photocoagulation-induced visual dysfunction in patients with severe diabetic retinopathy and good vision," *Ophthalmology*, vol. 113, no. 3, pp. 381–387, 2006.

[26] M. Shimura, K. Yasuda, T. Nakazawa, and M. Tamai, "Visual dysfunction after panretinal photocoagulation in patients with severe diabetic retinopathy and good vision," *American Journal of Ophthalmology*, vol. 140, no. 1, pp. 8.e1–8.e10, 2005.

[27] A. Oishi, J. Hidaka, and N. Yoshimura, "Quantification of the image obtained with a wide-field scanning ophthalmoscope," *Investigative Ophthalmology & Visual Science*, vol. 55, no. 4, pp. 2424–2431, 2014.

[28] C. S. Tan, M. C. Chew, J. van Hemert, M. A. Singer, D. Bell, and S. V. R. Sadda, "Measuring the precise area of peripheral retinal non-perfusion using ultra-widefield imaging and its correlation with the ischaemic index," *British Journal of Ophthalmology*, vol. 100, no. 2, pp. 235–239, 2016.

29

Vascular Endothelial Growth Factor (VEGF) Serological and Lacrimal Signaling in Patients Affected by Vernal Keratoconjunctivitis (VKC)

Marcella Nebbioso ⓘ,[1] **Andrea Iannaccone,**[1] **Marzia Duse,**[2] **Michele Aventaggiato,**[3] **Alice Bruscolini ⓘ,**[1] **and Anna Maria Zicari ⓘ**[2]

[1]*Department of Sense Organs, Sapienza University of Rome, p. le A. Moro 5, 00185 Rome, Italy*
[2]*Department of Pediatrics, Sapienza University of Rome, p. le A. Moro 5, 00185 Rome, Italy*
[3]*Department of Experimental Medicine, Sapienza University of Rome, p. le A. Moro 5, 00185 Rome, Italy*

Correspondence should be addressed to Marcella Nebbioso; marcella.nebbioso@uniroma1.it

Academic Editor: Tamer A. Macky

Background. Vernal keratoconjunctivitis (VKC) is a rare inflammatory disease involving the ocular surface, with seasonally exacerbated symptoms. Both type-1 and type-4 hypersensitivity reactions play a role in the development of VKC. *Purpose.* The aim of the present study was to assess the presence and evaluate the concentration of the vascular endothelial growth factor (VEGF) in tear and blood samples from patients with VKC, during the acute phase, based on the histopathological vasculostromal structure of the tarsal papillae. *Methods.* Two groups of children aged between 6 and 16 years of life were enrolled: 21 patients (16 males, 76%) affected by VKC, tarsal or mixed form, and 13 healthy children (5 males, 38%) used as controls. Blood and tear samples were obtained from all patients, in order to specifically assess the presence of VEGF. Statistical analyses were performed with one-way ANOVA, followed by post hoc comparisons with the Bonferroni tests. Pearson's correlation was chosen as statistical analysis to assess the relationship between the expression levels of VEGF in tears and blood and the clinical parameters measured. *Results.* Comparing the 2 groups for VEGF concentration, a statistically significant difference was found in tear samples: the mean value was 12.13 pg/mL ($\pm$5.54 SD) in the patient group and 7 pg/ml ($\pm$4.76 SD) in controls ($p < 0.05$). However, no statistically significant difference was found when comparing VEGF concentration in blood samples ($p > 0.05$), with a mean value of 45.17 pg/mL ($\pm$18.67 SD) in VKC patients and 38.08 pg/mL ($\pm$19.43 SD) in controls. *Conclusions.* This pilot study highlights the importance of lacrimal and vascular inflammatory biomarkers that can be detected in VKC patients during the acute phase, but not in healthy children. The small group of patients warrants additional studies on a larger sample, not only to further investigate the role of VEGF but also to evaluate the angiogenic biomarkers before and after topical treatment.

1. Introduction

Vernal keratoconjunctivitis (VKC) is a rare (<1 : 10.000), chronic, bilateral, at times asymmetrical, often severe inflammation of the ocular surface. It was first described in the ophthalmic literature as conjunctiva lymphatica more than 150 years ago. Subsequently, numerous authors referred to it using different names, each one labeling one of the various aspects of the disease [1–3]. VKC especially affects young

males, with an average age of onset of 6-7 years and a reported male-to-female ratio varying from 4 : 1 to 2 : 1, and tends to regress during or soon after puberty, disappearing in the majority of cases around 4–10 years after onset. It is more common in dry and hot climates, such as the Mediterranean area, Central Africa, West Africa, the Middle East, Japan, the Indian subcontinent, and South America [3–6]. VKC is typically characterized by seasonal exacerbations, although the most severe forms can suffer from perennial symptoms, and visual impairment may occur if the cornea is involved. According to the predominant conjunctival district involved, three forms of vernal keratoconjunctivitis have been identified and described: tarsal (palpebral), limbal (bulbar), and mixed type. In the first form, more prevalent in Europe and the Americas, large papillae (>1 mm) occur predominantly at the upper tarsus and those with a size of 7-8 mm are known as cobblestone papillae, constituting from the vasculostromal structure of collagen types I and II and proteoglycans [3–5]. The limbal form, which is more seen in Africa, is usually accompanied by limbal infiltrates and Horner–Trantas nodules; the mixed type presents intermediate characteristics between the two. A recent study has suggested an update to this classification that should include a phenotype with a predominant corneal involvement. Even though this was associated with nonspecific alterations of the corneal epithelium, relevant changes were measured by confocal microscopy and they were correlated with the degree of photophobia reported by patients. Corneal changes include punctate epithelial keratitis, epithelial macroerosions, gelatinous limbal hypertrophy, and plaque formation [3–5]. If untreated, the initial damage may lead to the onset of oval-shaped epithelial defects, known as shield ulcers, which are reported to occur in 3–11% of patients [3–6]. These undoubtedly represent the most severe signs of the disease, as they can have a heavy impact on the quality of life and even cause visual impairment or lead to astigmatism, keratoconus, corneal perforations, and scars. Although the allergic nature of VKC has been accepted for a long time, its exact aetiology and pathogenesis are still unclear. The role of hormonal factors is suggested by positive staining for oestrogen and progesterone receptors in the conjunctiva from patients, predilection for male sex, and resolution after puberty [3, 6, 7]. Genetic predisposition also contributes to the development of this disease, and although no relationship has been found yet between VKC and a particular genotype, the constant and increased presence of eosinophils in blood, tears, and conjunctival scrapings, the expression of a multitude of mediators and cytokines, and the predominance of CD4 cells locally suggest that VKC may be a phenotypic model of upregulation of the cytokine gene cluster on chromosome 5q [7–12]. In addition, multiple studies have investigated the family history of allergic diseases (asthma, rhinitis, eczema, urticaria, and dermatitis) and immunological diseases (Hashimoto's thyroiditis, type I diabetes, psoriasis, rheumatoid arthritis, and systemic lupus erythematosus), reporting such an association in roughly half of the patients diagnosed with VKC [3, 5, 6, 13, 14]. At this point, the accumulation of a large amount of immunological data has established that the pathogenesis of VKC is much more complex than a mere type 1 hypersensitivity reaction, also involving IgE-independent (type IV) mechanisms and cytokines, such as the interleukin 17 (IL-17) [7, 10, 12].

The purpose of the present study was to assess the presence and evaluate the concentration of vascular endothelial growth factor (VEGF) in tear and blood samples of patients affected by VKC, during its acute phase, comparing the results with a control group, in order to evaluate the role of VEGF in the pathogenesis of this disease.

2. Patients and Methods

The study was performed at the Department of Sense Organs of the "Policlinico Umberto I" and at the Department of Pediatrics, Division of Allergy and Immunology, Sapienza University of Rome. In accordance with the Helsinki Declaration, all parents were informed about the use of their data and informed consent was obtained. The study also fully obeyed the Good Clinical Practice guidelines and was approved by the Ethical Committee of our hospital, Sapienza University of Rome (authorization Rif. CE: 4708, 9/11/2017; Prot. Cod.: VKC06/2017).

We enrolled 21 children (16 males, 76%), aged between 6 and 16 years of life, affected by tarsal and mixed forms of VKC (Figure 1; Table 1). Thirteen healthy children (8 males, 62%) with negative skin prick test (SPT), without allergic, ocular, and systemic disease, cross-matched for sex and age with patients affected by VKC, were used as controls. At the time of enrolment, a complete hematologic and cardiologic examination was performed, systemic blood pressure was determined, and blood samples were collected. A complete ophthalmic evaluation was performed on both eyes through a detailed medical and ocular history. The eye examination included the following:

(i) Best-corrected visual acuity (BCVA) for far and near distance

(ii) Slit-lamp biomicroscopy

(iii) Intraocular pressure measurements

(iv) Dilated fundus examination

The diagnosis and follow-up were performed by an expert ophthalmologist through a score based on ocular signs such as little and/or giant papillae, conjunctival hyperemia, keratitis, and Horner–Trantas dots and on subjective ocular symptoms such as itching, photophobia, foreign body sensation, tearing, and mucous secretion according to the system described by each variable. In this score, each variable was graded as follows: 0 = absent; 1 = light; 2 = mild; 3 = moderate; and 4 = severe [3, 9]. Patients with a total score ≥10 were included in the study. Some authors subsequently expanded it by including two supplemental parameters: the duration of symptoms (0 if <1 year, 1 if >1 year, and 2 if >2 years) and the worsening of symptoms in spring and summer (0 if not present and 1 if present). Conjunctival scraping was also performed, in order to further improve the diagnosis in patients with VKC. Skin prick tests (SPTs) were performed on each patient for common inhalants and food allergens (Lofarma, Milan, Italy): *Dermatophagoides pteronyssinus* (Der P), *Dermatophagoides farinae* (Der F), dog/cat dander, *Olea europaea*, *Lolium perenne*, *Alternaria alternata*, *Parietaria officinalis*, lactalbumin, β-lactoglobulin, casein, egg white and yolk, soy, and cod fish. A positive SPT was defined by the presence of a wheal more than 3 mm respect to the wheal size of the control (saline solution). Serum was obtained from the peripheral blood samples collected from all the children included in the study to evaluate the serum level of VEGF, autoimmunity, ANA, and total IgE (Table 1). Blood samples were obtained at enrolment. In both patients and controls,

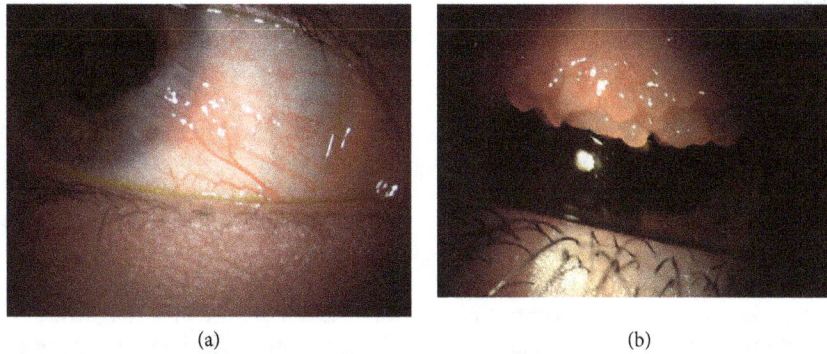

Figure 1: Patient affected from vernal keratoconjunctivitis (VKC). (a) Mixed form with cornel signs limbar neovascular and (b) tarsal papillae on the superior conjunctiva.

Table 1: Demographics and clinical grading of 21 vernal keratoconjunctivitis (VKC) patients.

Characteristics of VKC patients		
Sex	16 males (76%)	5 females (24%)
Age (from 6 to 16 years)	Mean 8.62	SD ± 2.65
VA (BCVA)	20/20	SD ± 0.0
Atopic SPT	11 positive (52.4%); major allergens: house dust and grasses	10 negative (47.6%)
Family condition	12 (57%) familiar with allergic DS	3 (14%) familiar with autoimmune DS
VKC forms	Tarsal: 13 (62%)	Mixed: 8 (38%)
Vitamin D levels (VKC vs controls) (in ng/ml)	19.8 ± 6.7 vs 24.7 ± 6.5	Lower levels if compared to controls ($p < 0.0001$)
ANA positivity	30.8%	Total IgE 4100 UI/ml	46.1%
Photophobia (grade 4)	42.3%	Secretion or tearing	28.8%
Foreign body sensation	25.4%	Itching and conjunctival hyperemia	11.5%

SD: standard deviation; VA: visual acuity; BCVA: best-corrected visual acuity for far distance; SPT: skin prick test for several common inhalants and food allergens; DS: diseases.

tear samples were obtained as follows: 20–50 μl of open eye tears was gently collected from the external canthus of the most affected eye using a capillary micropipette and avoiding the tear reflex as much as possible. The samples were placed in Eppendorf Tubes, centrifuged at $160 \times g$ for 8 min, and stored at $-80°C$. The samples were successively probed using three microwell plate arrays.

3. VEGF Level Measurement

Lacrimal and serum VEGF levels in healthy and VKC patients were determined with the VEGF EIA Kit from Enzo Life Sciences and following manufacturer's instructions. Briefly, 100 ml of samples was mixed with 100 ml of the assay buffer and placed in each well of a 96-well plate. The mix was then incubated for 18 h at 4°C. The following day, each well was rinsed with a washing buffer before adding 100 ml of an anti-VEGF antibody/well. The antibody was incubated for 30 min at 4°C. Afterward, 100 ml of a substrate solution was added and incubated for 30 minutes at room temperature (RT) in the dark. After adding a stop solution, the optical density at 450 nm was measured using the GloMax-Multi Detection System (Promega, Milan, Italy). The fluorescence intensity of the assay buffer was subtracted from each experimental sample.

4. Statistical Analysis

Data obtained were used for statistical analysis. Quantitative variables were summarized with mean and standard deviation (SD). The differences between groups were evaluated by Fisher's chi-square test or test. The correlations between clinical, demographic, and biological parameters were performed with Spearman's rho. The results are expressed as means ± SD and 95% confidence intervals (95% CIs). Statistical analyses were performed with one-way ANOVA, followed by post hoc comparisons with the Bonferroni tests. Calculation of Pearson's correlation was also chosen as statistical analysis. Values were relieved to assess the relationship between the expression levels of VEGF in tears and blood and the clinical parameters measured. A p value < 0.05 was considered statistically significant. Statistical analysis was conducted through the SPSS 18.0 software (Statistical Package of Social Sciences, Chicago, IL, USA).

5. Results

The study included 21 patients (16 males and 5 females) aged between 6 and 16 years of life (mean 8.62; SD ± 2.65), affected by tarsal and mixed forms of VKC, and thirteen healthy children (8 males and 5 females) aged between 6 and

15 years (mean 7.98; SD ± 3.2). The 2 groups for mean age and gender were not statistically significant. According to literature, VKC prevalence was higher in males than in females (76% vs 24%) in the population we studied [1, 3, 14, 15]. Allergological, serological, and lacrimal tests were normal in the control group, while 11 VKC patients (52.4%) showed positive Skin Prick Test (SPT) for several common inhalants and food allergens. Fifty-seven percent of patients were familiar with allergic diseases and 14% had a parent with autoimmune disease. Comparing the 2 groups after using the VEGF EIA kit for VEGF concentration, a statistically significant difference was found in tear samples: the mean value was 12.13 pg/mL (±5.54 SD) in the patients group and 7 pg/ml (±4.76 SD) in controls ($p < 0.05$) (Figure 2). However, no statistically significant difference was found when comparing VEGF concentration in blood samples ($p > 0.05$), with a mean value of 45.17 pg/mL (±18.67 SD) in VKC patients and 38.08 pg/ml (±19.43 SD) in controls ($p = 0.29$) (Table 2).

The correlation of Pearson revealed an r value of −0.14, −0.18, −0.15, and −0.12 between the expression levels of VEGF in tears and the clinical parameters giant papillae, foreign body, conjunctival hyperemia, and itching, respectively. Moreover, the correlation of Pearson showed an r value of −0.28, 0.01, 0.04, and −0.03 between the expression levels of VEGF in serum and the clinical parameters giant papillae, foreign body, conjunctival hyperemia, and itching, respectively. There were significant correlations between the mean values of VEGF tears and the clinical parameters ($p < 0.05$). However, the statistically significant correlation was only identified between VEGF serum and giant papillae, and there was no relationship between VEGF serum and the other clinical parameters (Table 3).

6. Discussion

The purpose of this study was to assess the presence and evaluate the concentration of VEGF in tear and blood samples of patients affected by VKC in acute phase in comparison with the control group in order to assess the pathogenic role of VEGF.

VKC is a rare, chronic ocular disease that affects children, mainly involving males over females, and usually regressing during or soon after puberty. This aspect emphasizes the role of hormonal factors in the pathogenesis of the disease, as pointed by several studies [3, 9, 15]. Although VKC has been always regarded as an IgE-mediated disease, the literature reports that roughly 50% of patients have a positive SPT or high levels of serum IgE. Our data were in line with these findings. Thus, the IgE-mast-cell-mediated process and Th1 response are not enough to explain all the mechanisms of the disease. The role of Th2 responses in VKC has been studied for a long time, and VKC is actually not regarded just as an ocular disease but as a systemic disease with a T-cell-activated response. Many studies underlined the role of single cytokines and mediators in the development of the disease, such as the IL-17 and the HMGB-1 [11–13, 15]. In the present study, we focused on the assessment and quantification of the VEGF, comparing

the concentration of such a molecule in tear and blood samples from VKC and control subjects. Tear samples are relatively easy to collect from the patients as a noninvasive diagnostic procedure that provides valuable information on differential tear cytology and levels of mediators at the site of inflammation [7, 10, 11]. The critical limitation of such a procedure is the volume of the tear sample, which ideally should be collected without stimulating the tear reflex, and the quantity of the sample obtainable, often very limited. Determination of tear mediator, cytokine, or chemokine levels is not yet used for diagnosis, but only for the study of allergic physiopathology or for the evaluation of efficacy of antiallergic agents [4, 7, 10, 11, 16]. The concentration and distribution of inflammatory mediators or inhibitors in the tear fluid have been extensively studied in ocular allergy, in an attempt to find a disease marker, to better understand the immune mechanisms involved in the ocular surface inflammation and to identify potential targets for therapeutic interventions [7, 8].

Epithelial cells, fibroblasts, and inflammatory cells including eosinophils and monocytes/macrophages are possible sources of VEGF in VKC [7, 17]. Angiogenic and growth factor pathological expression is frequently associated with the expression of matrix metalloproteases (MMPs) [7]. MMPs cause the extravasation of leukocytes through limited proteolysis of basement membranes; degradation of proteoglycans, laminin, fibronectin, and collagens; and activation of the precursor forms of other MMPs. An imbalance between MMPs and their natural tissue inhibitors (TIMP) is also probably involved in the pathogenesis of conjunctival inflammation, remodeling, and corneal changes in VKC. In fact, MMP-1, MMP-2, MMP-3, MMP-8, MMP-9, and MMP-10 are highly expressed in all forms of active VKC, consequently to the increase of proinflammatory cytokines, such as IL-1b and tumor necrosis factor-α (TNF-α) [7]. Moreover, chronic conjunctival inflammation in VKC is associated with increased expression of α3 and α6 integrin subunits' receptors, epidermal growth factor receptor (EGFR), VEGF, transforming growth factor-b (TGF-b), basic fibroblast growth factor (bFGF), and platelet-derived growth factor (PDGF), thus suggesting a possible contribution of integrins, EGFR, and growth factors in VKC conjunctival remodeling and also a role of growth factors in the expression and function of integrins [8].

On the other hand, an anti-VEGF therapy could be helpful for anterior segment eye disease as an adjunct in the treatment of allergic and immunologic eye diseases. The most important growth factor in corneal angiogenesis is VEGF, and it is upregulated during corneal neovascularization (NV). Recently, anti-VEGF therapies are one of the most important drugs used for corneal NV treatment. In fact, anti-VEGF therapies (bevacizumab, ranibizumab, and aflibercept) have shown efficacy in attenuation of corneal neovascularization in both animal models and clinical trials [22, 23]. Case reports in this area include, for example, topical bevacizumab use in a patient with longstanding ocular cicatricial pemphigoid unresponsive to steroid, but moderately responding to the treatment, a single case of ocular graft-versus-host disease that responded

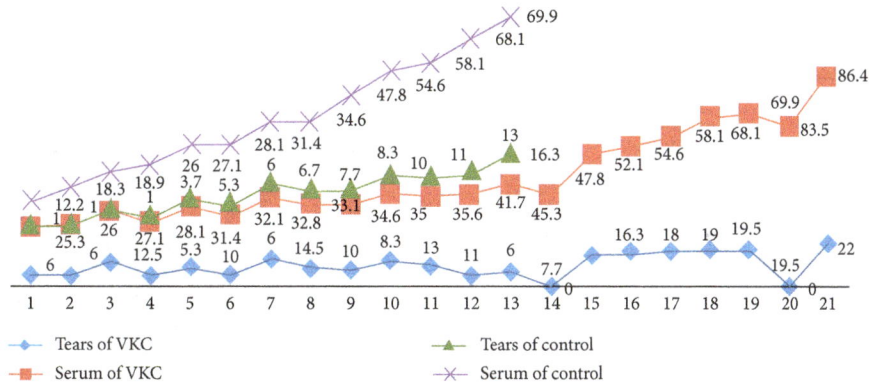

FIGURE 2: EIA values for VEGF concentration in tears and blood in control and vernal keratoconjunctivitis (VKC) groups.

TABLE 2: Comparisons of the 2 groups after using the VEGF EIA kit for vascular endothelial growth factor (VEGF) concentration.

VKC group ($N = 21$)	Control group ($N = 13$)	p value
VEGF tears in pg/mL: 12.13 ± 5.54	Tears in pg/mL: 7 ± 4.76	<0.05 (0.011)
VEGF serum in pg/mL: 45.17 ± 18.67	Serum in pg/mL: 38.08 ± 19.43	NS > 0.05 (0.29)

SD: standard deviation; NS: not statistically significant. The values are expressed as mean ± SD. A statistically significant difference was found in tear samples ($p < 0.05$). No statistically significant difference was found when comparing VEGF concentration in blood samples ($p > 0.05$).

TABLE 3: Pearson correlation coefficient (CC) results (parametric test) (statistical significance was set at $p < 0.05$).

	VKC group ($N = 21$), mean value in pg/mL (±SD)			
VEGF relationship		Clinic score	Pearson CC	p value
Tears/giant papillae	12.13 (5.54)	3.43 (0.59)	−0.14	<0.05
Tears/foreign body	12.13 (5.54)	3.24 (0.83)	−0.18	<0.05
Tears/conjunctival hyperemia	12.13 (5.54)	2.76 (0.97)	−0.15	<0.05
Tears/itching	12.13 (5.54)	2.57 (0.73)	−0.12	<0.05
Serum/giant papillae	45.17 (18.67)	3.43 (0.59)	−0.28	<0.05
Serum/foreign body	45.17 (18.67)	3.24 (0.83)	0.01	NS
Serum/conjunctival hyperemia	45.17 (18.67)	2.76 (0.97)	0.04	NS
Serum/itching	45.17 (18.67)	2.57 (0.73)	−0.03	NS

NS: not statistically significant.

partially to subconjunctival bevacizumab, and a report of topical bevacizumab application in 2 patients with Stevens–Johnson syndrome [22, 23]. Visual acuity improved in all 3 eyes, with decreased corneal NV, haze, and conjunctival injection without any serious adverse events. In conclusion, bevacizumab has partially reduced corneal NV through different routes of administrations: topical, subconjunctival, and intraocular application, while early treatment with subconjunctival administration of ranibizumab may successfully reduce corneal NV. Establishment of safe doses is highly important before these drugs can be involved in the clinical setting [22, 23].

Thus, VEGF becomes a potential marker for the disease and/or its severity. It is our aim to cover in a future study how the tear levels of such a mediator could possibly be modified before and after treatment with therapeutic ocular drops [4, 18–21]. When evaluating blood samples, the difference was not statistically significant. However, we found a statistically significant difference of the VEGF concentration in tears between VKC and control groups. Again, this finding suggests the need for further studies, which should include a larger number of patients suffering from VKC.

Then, VEGF concentration could be evaluated before and after treatment with cyclosporine or anti-VEGF ocular drops to investigation to better understand its role in the pathogenesis of the disease. In summary, it might even be seen as a potential therapeutic target.

Disclosure

This paper contains part of the results that have been presented as abstract at International Conference on Pediatrics & Neonatology (ICPN-2018). The authors have no proprietary interest in any materials or methods described within this article.

Conflicts of Interest

The authors declare that they have no conflicts of interest.

Authors' Contributions

Nebbioso M. and Zicari A.M. participated in the study design. Iannaccone A. and Bruscolini A. performed the literature search. Duse M. helped in the data interpretation. Iannaccone A. and Nebbioso M. wrote the paper. Aventaggiato M. collected data.

References

[1] L. Bielory, "Allergic and immunologic disorders of the eye. Part II: ocular allergy," *Journal of Allergy and Clinical Immunology*, vol. 106, pp. 1019–1032, 2000.

[2] M. Sacchetti, I. Abicca, A. Bruscolini, C. Cavaliere, M. Nebbioso, and A. Lambiase, "Allergic conjunctivitis: current concepts on pathogenesis and management," *Journal of Biological Regulators and Homeostatic Agents*, vol. 32, no. 1, pp. 49–60, 2018.

[3] S. Bonini, M. Coassin, S. Aronni, and A. Lambiase, "Vernal keratoconjunctivitis," *Eye*, vol. 18, no. 4, pp. 345–351, 2004.

[4] F. Mantelli, M. S. Santos, T. Petitti et al., "Systematic review and meta-analysis of randomised clinical trials on topical treatments for vernal keratoconjunctivitis," *British Journal of Ophthalmology*, vol. 91, no. 12, pp. 1656–1661, 2007.

[5] P. C. Donshik, W. H. Ehlers, and M. Ballow, "Giant papillary conjunctivitis," *Immunology and Allergy Clinics of North America*, vol. 28, no. 1, pp. 83–103, 2008.

[6] M. Nebbioso, A. M. Zicari, C. Celani, V. Lollobrigida, R. Grenga, and M. Duse, "Pathogenesis of vernal keratoconjunctivitis and associated factors," *Seminars in Ophthalmology*, vol. 30, no. 5-6, pp. 340–344, 2015.

[7] A. Leonardi, S. Sathe, M. Bortolotti, A. Beaton, and R. Sack, "Cytokines, matrix metalloproteases, angiogenic and growth factors in tears of normal subjects and vernal keratoconjunctivitis patients," *Allergy*, vol. 64, no. 5, pp. 710–717, 2009.

[8] A. M. Abu El-Asrar, S. Al-Mansouri, K. F. Tabbara, L. Missotten, and K. Geboes, "Immunopathogenesis of conjunctival remodelling in vernal keratoconjunctivitis," *Eye*, vol. 20, no. 1, pp. 71–79, 2006.

[9] S. Bonini, S. Bonini, A. Lambiase et al., "Vernal keratoconjunctivitis: a model of 5q cytokine gene cluster disease," *International Archives of Allergy and Immunology*, vol. 107, no. 1-3, pp. 95–98, 1995.

[10] N. Asano-Kato, K. Fukagawa, N. Okada et al., "TGF-beta1, IL-1beta, and Th2 cytokines stimulate vascular endothelial growth factor production from conjunctival fibroblasts," *Experimental Eye Research*, vol. 80, no. 4, pp. 555–560, 2005.

[11] A. M. Zicari, A. Zicari, M. Nebbioso et al., "High-mobility group box-1 (HMGB-1) and serum soluble receptor for advanced glycation end products (sRAGE) in children affected by vernal keratoconjunctivitis," *Pediatric Allergy and Immunology*, vol. 25, no. 1, pp. 57–63, 2014.

[12] A. M. Zicari, M. Nebbioso, A. Zicari et al., "Serum levels of IL-17 in patients with vernal keratoconjunctivitis," *European Review for Medical and Pharmacological Sciences*, vol. 17, no. 9, pp. 1242–1244, 2013.

[13] A. M. Zicari, B. Mora, V. Lollobrigida et al., "Immunogenetic investigation in vernal keratoconjunctivitis," *Pediatric Allergic and Immunology*, vol. 25, no. 5, pp. 508–510, 2014.

[14] A. M. Zicari, M. Nebbioso, V. Lollobrigida et al., "Vernal keratoconjunctivitis: atopy and autoimmunity," *European Review for Medical and Pharmacological Sciences*, vol. 17, no. 10, pp. 1419–1423, 2013.

[15] A. Leonardi, "Vernal keratoconjunctivitis: pathogenesis and treatment," *Progress in Retinal and Eye Research*, vol. 21, no. 3, pp. 319–339, 2002.

[16] D. Magaña, G. Aguilar, M. Linares et al., "Intracellular IL-4, IL-5, and IFN-γ as the main characteristic of CD4+CD30+ T cells after allergen stimulation in patients with vernal keratoconjunctivitis," *Molecular Vision*, vol. 21, pp. 443–450, 2015, eCollection 2015.

[17] N. Kumagai, K. Fukuda, Y. Fujitsu, K. Yamamoto, and T. Nishida, "Role of structural cells of the cornea and conjunctiva in the pathogenesis of vernal keratoconjunctivitis," *Progress in Retinal and Eye Research*, vol. 25, pp. 165–187, 2006.

[18] L. Spadavecchia, P. Fanelli, R. Tesse et al., "Efficacy of 1.25% and 1% topical cyclosporine in the treatment of severe vernal keratoconjunctivitis in childhood," *Pediatric Allergy and Immunology*, vol. 17, no. 7, pp. 527–532, 2006.

[19] P. Vichyanond and P. Kosrirukvongs, "Use of cyclosporine A and tacrolimus in treatment of vernal keratoconjunctivitis," *Current Allergy and Asthma Reports*, vol. 13, no. 3, pp. 308–14, 2013.

[20] M. Oray and E. Toker, "Tear cytokine levels in vernal keratoconjunctivitis: the effect of topical 0.05% cyclosporine a therapy," *Cornea*, vol. 32, no. 8, pp. 1149–1154, 2013.

[21] H. Zanjani, M. N. Aminifard, A. Ghafourian et al., "Comparative evaluation of tacrolimus versus interferon alpha-2b eye drops in the treatment of vernal keratoconjunctivitis: a randomized, double-masked study," *Cornea*, vol. 36, no. 6, pp. 675–678, 2017.

[22] H. Hosseini, M. H. Nowroozzadeh, R. Salouti, and M. Nejabat, "Anti-VEGF therapy with bevacizumab for anterior segment eye disease," *Cornea*, vol. 31, no. 3, pp. 322–334, 2012.

[23] T. Al-Debasi, A. Al-Bekairy, A. Al-Katheri, S. Al Harbi, and M. Mansour, "Topical versus subconjunctival anti-vascular endothelial growth factor therapy (bevacizumab, ranibizumab and aflibercept) for treatment of corneal neovascularization," *Saudi Journal of Ophthalmology*, vol. 31, no. 2, pp. 99–105, 2017.

30

Characterization of Soft Contact Lens Edge Fitting during Daily Wear using Ultrahigh-Resolution Optical Coherence Tomography

Lele Cui (iD),[1] Sisi Chen,[1] Weihe Zhou,[1] Kaixuan Sheng,[2] Lei Zhang,[1] Meixiao Shen (iD),[1] and Ming Li (iD)[1]

[1]*Eye Hospital and School of Ophthalmology and Optometry, Wenzhou Medical University, Wenzhou, Zhejiang, China*
[2]*Ningbo Aier Guangming Eye Hosptial, Ningbo, Zhejiang, China*

Correspondence should be addressed to Meixiao Shen; shenmxiao7@hotmail.com and Ming Li; lm@mail.eye.ac.cn

Academic Editor: Antonio Queiros

Purpose. To determine conjunctival overlap over the edge of soft contact lens and to visualize the peripheral postlens tear film (PoLTF) underneath soft contact lenses using ultrahigh-resolution optical coherence tomography (UHR-OCT). *Methods*. Twenty participants (4 males and 16 females, 23.0 ± 3.7 years) were fitted with two different types of soft contact lenses randomly. The limbus with lens was imaged with the UHR-OCT at the horizontal meridian every two hours up to 6 hours during lens wear. The conjunctival overlap was ranked as the percentage of the edge covered by the conjunctiva. The frequency of occurrence for visualized peripheral PoLTF was determined. *Results*. The average conjunctival overlaps at insertion were 49% and 73% for galyfilcon A and balafilcon A lenses and increased significantly to 84% and 90% by 6 hours of lens wear ($P < 0.001$). Lenses with rounded edges had more conjunctival overlap than the lenses with angled edges ($P = 0.014$). There were significant decreases for PoLTF on the conjunctiva ($P = 0.014$) and peripheral cornea ($P = 0.004$) over the study period compared to insertion. The percentage of subjects with PoLTF on the conjunctiva (32.5%) and peripheral cornea (36%) were greater in subjects wearing balafilcon A lenses ($P = 0.017$). *Conclusions*. Increased conjunctival overlap over the lens edges and reduced PoLTF underneath the peripheral region of soft contact lenses were shown during lens daily wear. The lens edge configuration may play a role in conjunctival response and peripheral PoLTF.

1. Introduction

When a soft contact lens, between 14 and 14.5 cm in diameter, is worn on the eye, it completely covers the cornea and overlaps approximately 2 mm on to the bulbar conjunctiva [1]. Additionally, in the course of eye movements and blinking, the lens may momentarily become displaced and overlap further onto the bulbar conjunctiva, perhaps up to 4-5 mm from the limbus. The interactions between contact lens and conjunctiva, such as the encroachment onto the lens edge, have been reported associated with conjunctival indentation and conjunctival flaps [2]. A poor-fitting contact lens may induce clinical complications of the conjunctiva, including physical irritation that results excess staining [3], deep arcuate band staining caused by pressure from the lens edge, hyperemia, and chemosis [4]. So wearing contact lens has the influence not only on the physiology of the cornea but also on the conjunctiva. The postlens tear film

(PoLTF) plays important roles in contact lens fitting. It cushions and lubricates the lens movement on the ocular surface [5–7] and provides oxygen transmission to the cornea [8]. The depletion of the PoLTF may cause lens adherence [9] and ocular surface staining [10], all of which are characteristic of contact lens-associated dry eye [11]. These complications may result in contact lens discontinuation [12]. Measurements of the central PoLTF have been the subject of several previous studies [13–15]. The central PoLTF is several micrometers in thickness, and PoLTFs decrease further after lens insertion [14]. However, not much is known about the PoLTF on the peripheral cornea and conjunctiva during lens wear.

With the advent of ultrahigh-resolution optical coherence tomography (UHR-OCT), it is possible to image the contact lens edge at the conjunctiva and visualize the PoLTF underneath the periphery of the lens [11, 16]. Evaluating the diurnal variation of conjunctival responses related to the

TABLE 1: Design parameters of contact lenses measured in the study.

	PureVision	Acuvue Advance
Manufacturer	Bausch & Lomb	Vistakon, Johnson & Johnson
Diameter (mm)	14.0	14.0
Base curvature (mm)	8.6	8.7
Power (D)	−3.00 D	−3.00 D
Material	Balafilcon A	Galyfilcon A
Modulus (MPa)	1.1	0.43
Edge shape	Rounded	Angled
Center thickness (mm)	0.09	0.07
Water content (%)	36	47

contact lens and peripheral PoLTF may provide insightful information for a better understanding of the change of the lens edge fitting. The goal of this study was to measure the conjunctival overlap over the lens edge and determine the PoLTF underneath the peripheral region of soft contact lenses during daily wear by UHR-OCT.

2. Subjects and Methods

This study was approved by the Office of Research Ethics of the Wenzhou Medical University and was conducted in accordance with the tenets of the Declaration of Helsinki. Informed consent was obtained from each participant prior to enrollment in the study. Twenty healthy subjects (4 males and 16 females; mean ± standard deviation age, 23.0 ± 3.7 years) with no previously diagnosed dry eye and with no dry eye symptoms or ocular surface disease were recruited for the study.

To observe the lens edges and interaction with the ocular surface and detect the presence of the peripheral PoLTF, a custom built, high speed, UHR-OCT instrument with 3 μm resolution was used for this study [11, 16]. Briefly, the light source was a three-module superluminescent diode (Broadlighter, T840-HP, Superlum diodes Ltd., Co., Cork, Ireland) with a center wavelength of 840 nm and a full width at half maximum bandwidth of 100 nm. The power of the incident light delivered into the anterior segment was lowered to 750 μW to ensure the safety of the eye.

All subjects were tested in a consulting room with controlled temperature (15–25°C) and humidity (30%–50%) after 10 AM to avoid the edematous cornea and sleep-induced alterations of the tear film [17]. Two eyes of each subject were fitted with two different types of soft contact lenses (Table 1). The order of these two lenses was randomized for each eye of each subject. OCT images were taken immediately after lens insertion and at 2, 4, and 6 hours during lens wear. The subjects were asked to sit in front of the instrument and look straight at an external target while an 8 mm-width scan was made on the horizontal meridian. The limbal images for the temporal side were obtained for each eye by rotating the OCT probe to target the limbus while the subject fixated on the target with the primary gaze.

Because UHR-OCT images of the contact lens edges were optically distorted due to the different refractive indices and

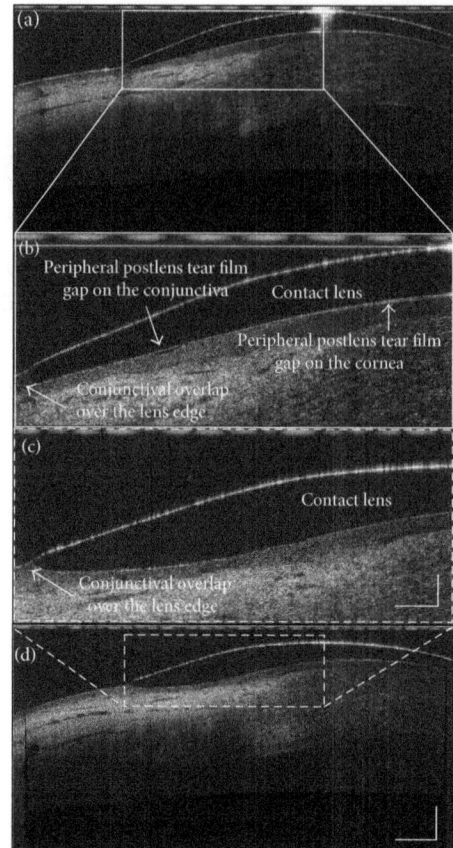

FIGURE 1: Edge conjunctival coverage and PoLTF underneath the peripheral lens. Conjunctival response to soft contact lens was characterized as an overlap of conjunctival tissue at the edge of the lens. The PoLTFs on the cornea and on the conjunctiva were clearly visualized as gaps between the lens and the ocular surfaces in (b). One was located at the peripheral cornea, and the other was located at the limbal transition to the conjunctiva. (b) and (c) were the magnified images of (a) and (d). (a) and (b) are balafilcon A lenses. (c) and (d) are galyfilcon A lenses. The bars denote 100 μm for two of the images (a) and (d) and 250 μm for the other two images (b) and (c).

curved surfaces [18, 19] custom software was used to correct the image using Fermat's principle [18]. The percentage of edge covered by the conjunctiva was categorized by an analog ranking scale of 0%, 25%, 50%, 75%, and 100% for each lens after correction for the optical distortion [17]. Images labeled as 0% edge coverage showed almost no conjunctival overlap over the temporal lens edges. Images labeled as 100% edge coverage had conjunctival overlap that covered almost the entire temporal lens edges (Figures 1(a) and 1(b)). In the OCT images, the peripheral PoLTF was visualized as a gap between the corneal or limbal surfaces and the posterior surface of the lens (Figure 1(b)). The gaps on the cornea and conjunctiva were visualized and ranked. Each image was inspected and ranked as "1" if a gap was presented on the cornea and the conjunctiva. It was ranked as "0" as the gap was absent [17]. The observer (ML) was masked to the lens types to minimize bias during evaluation of the edge coverage and PoLTF gaps.

Linear mixed model for edge ranking and generalized estimating equation (GEE) for gaps on the conjunctiva and cornea was used to estimate the contact lenses group

TABLE 2: Conjunctival response and peripheral PoLTF for two lenses during lens daily wear.

Lens	Edge conjunctival coverage ranking (%)			Peripheral postlens tear film at the limbus			Peripheral postlens tear film on the cornea		
	$\overline{x} \pm s$	F	P	n (%)	Wald χ^2	P	n (%)	Wald χ^2	P
A	68.12 ± 25.15	23.18	<0.001	7 (8.75%)	786.47	<0.001	14 (17.5%)	9.35	0.025
B	81.88 ± 17.78	8.75	0.001	26 (32.50%)	2.87	0.413	29 (36.25%)	6.49	0.09
A + B	75.00 ± 22.78	27.60[a]*	<0.001[a]*	33 (20.63%)	10.58[a]*	0.014[a]*	43 (26.88%)	13.08[a]*	0.004[a]*
Between A and B	$(F = 6.58, P = 0.014)^{b*}$			$(\chi^2 = 5.70, P = 0.017)^{b*}$			$(\chi^2 = 4.18, P = 0.041)^{b*}$		
	$(F = 3.08, P = 0.039)^{\#}$			$(\chi^2 = 6.79, P = 0.079)^{\#}$			$(\chi^2 = 2.62, P = 0.454)^{\#}$		

Lens A: galyfilcon A; lens B: balafilcon A; *F statistic and P value of the main effect (lens and time); #F statistic and P value of interaction; [a]differences over time; [b]differences between lenses.

difference and over time change of the variables. Least significant difference (LSD) was performed for post hoc comparisons between any two time points. The Wilcoxon Rank-Sum test and the chi square test were utilized for intergroup comparisons at each time point. Data analysis was performed using IBM SPSS Statistics (Version 20.0, IBM Corp., Armonk, NY, USA). $P < 0.05$ was considered significant.

3. Results

The average conjunctival overlaps at insertion were 49% and 73% for galyfilcon A and balafilcon A lenses, respectively. The values were increased significantly by 6 hours of lens wear ($F = 27.60$, $P < 0.001$; Table 2), which reached 84% and 90%. Lenses with rounded edges (balafilcon A lenses) had more conjunctival overlap than the galyfilcon A lenses with angled edges ($F = 6.58$, $P = 0.014$; Table 2). Galyfilcon A lenses had showed greater increase tendency of conjunctival overlap over time ($F = 3.08$, $P = 0.039$; Figure 2 and Table 2).

Limbal PoLTF was visualized at 15% at insertion and 5% at 6 hours for galyfilcon A lenses, and the value went from 40% to 20% for balafilcon A lenses (Wald $\chi^2 = 10.58$, $P = 0.014$; Figure 3 and Table 2). The percentage of subjects with PoLTF around the limbus was greater in subjects wearing balafilcon A (32.5%) compared to galyfilcon A lenses (7.5%) (Wald $\chi^2 = 5.70$, $P = 0.017$; Figure 3 and Table 2). There were significant decreases for PoLTF on the peripheral cornea over the study period compared to insertion (Wald $\chi^2 = 13.08$, $P = 0.004$; Figure 4 and Table 2). For 35% of eyes, the PoLTF was visualized at the peripheral cornea at insertion and in 5% after 6 hours of lens wear for galyfilcon A lenses. The PoLTF was visualized at the peripheral cornea at insertion in 50% of eyes and in 20% after 6 hours of lens wear for balafilcon A lenses. More subjects, 36% in average, wearing the balafilcon A lenses had PoLTF present at the peripheral cornea than those wearing galyfilcon A lenses (Wald $\chi^2 = 4.18$, $P = 0.041$; Figure 4 and Table 2).

4. Discussion

Evaluating the interactions between soft contact lenses and the ocular surface, especially at the interface with the limbus and conjunctiva, has been a challenge because of the

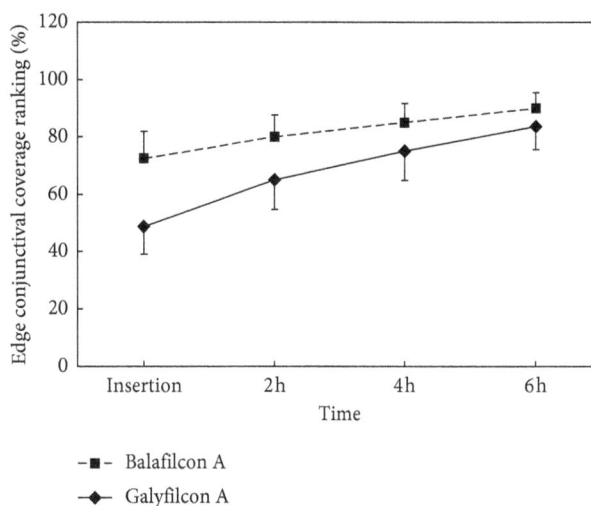

FIGURE 2: Time-dependent overlap of conjunctiva at lens edge. The average conjunctival overlap increased significantly at 6 hours after insertion. Balafilcon A lenses had more conjunctival overlap than the galyfilcon A lenses. Galyfilcon A lenses had showed greater increase in tendency of conjunctival overlap over time. Bars denote 95% confidence interval (CI).

anatomical characteristics of this tissue and the limitation of imaging techniques. Few studies have produced images of the interaction between the soft contact lens and conjunctiva due to the relatively low resolution of the OCT image. With the rapid development of OCT technology, high- or ultrahigh-resolution OCT images can now be obtained in contact lens practices [20, 21]. We previously demonstrated different contact lens edge configurations and the presence of the peripheral PoLTF by UHR-OCT [11, 16]. In the present study, we aimed at evaluating the conjunctival response to soft contact lens which was characterized as an overlap of conjunctival tissue at the edge of the lens and the presence of the peripheral PoLTF during the daily wear.

The conjunctival overlap was evident and different between two soft contact lenses investigated in this study. The difference may be because of different pressure profiles [22] produced across the ocular surface underneath each lens [23]. When a lens is fitted on the eye, it must flex to align with the ocular surface. Using finite element analysis, pressure profiles of soft contact lenses on the eye were simulated, and local pressures were projected to exist around the lens edge and midperiphery of the cornea (Evans SR, et al. IOVS 2005; 46:

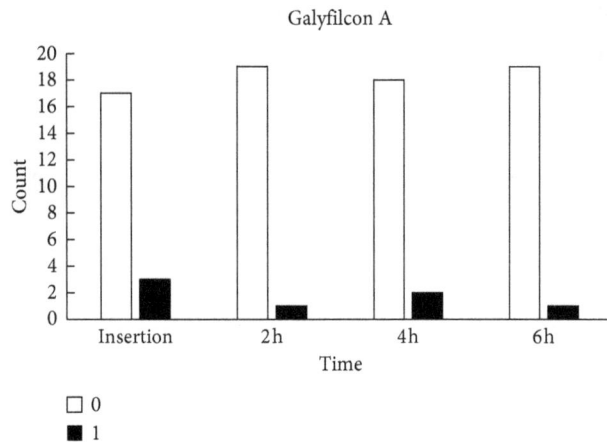

(a)

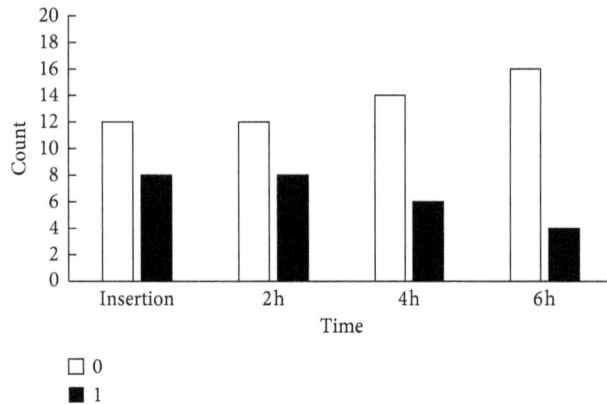

(b)

FIGURE 3: Time-dependent changes in PoLTF at the limbus. It was ranked as "1" if a gap was presented on the conjunctiva and "0" as the gap was absent. (a) Time-dependent changes in PoLTF at the limbus for galyfilcon A lenses and (b) balafilcon A lenses. Frequency of occurrence for PoLTF on the conjunctiva decreased over the study period compared to insertion.

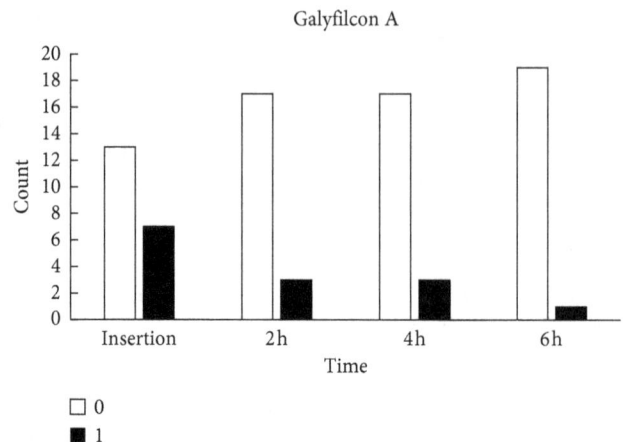

(a)

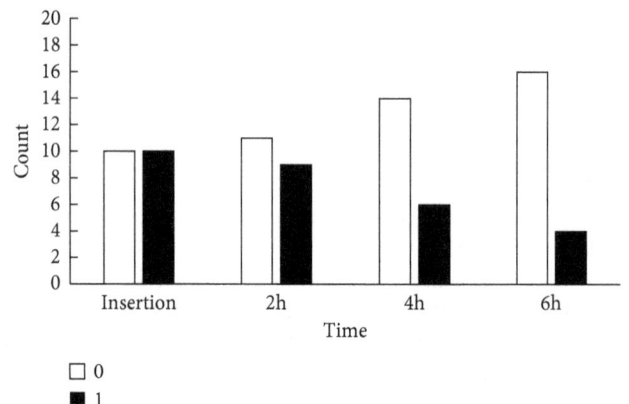

(b)

FIGURE 4: Time-dependent changes in PoLTF on the cornea. It was ranked as "1" if a gap was presented on the cornea and "0" as the gap was absent. (a) Time-dependent changes in PoLTF on the cornea for galyfilcon A lenses and (b) balafilcon A lenses. Frequency of occurrence for PoLTF on the cornea decreased over the study period compared to insertion.

ARVO E-Abstract 2059; Hofmann G, et al. IOVS 2010; 51: ARVO E-Abstract 3418). Compared to the cornea, the conjunctiva is composed of softer tissue (lower elastic modulus) which means that the conjunctiva may be easy to deform and build up around the lens edge [24]. Lens diameter, lens power, base curvature, and lens thickness profile may influence the level of local pressures [25]. In the present study, the values of central lens thickness, base curvature, diameter, and power for two lenses were very close. Contact lenses with rounded edges produced more conjunctival overlap than angled edges. Our results presented here indicate that edge shape and lens design are likely to affect lens-induced pressure and consequently affect conjunctival overlap.

The conjunctival overlap increased by six hours of lens wear, suggesting that wearing time may be another factor contributing to the overlap. Because tear meniscus volume is reduced after short-term lens wear [26, 27], especially at the end of the day, the lens may become dehydrated. Consequently, the lens dehydration or shrinkage might change the pressure profiles on

the ocular surface and increase the lens edge tip pressure, thus resulting in more conjunctival overlap.

In particular, the existence of the PoLTF at the corneal periphery or conjunctiva likely indicates the presence of higher localized pressure points. Two touch points may create a pocket or gap that contains the PoLTF. In the present study, the PoLTF at the peripheral cornea and at the limbal transition zone were clearly visualized in a portion of the subjects for up to 6 hours. Subjects wearing balafilcon A lenses with rounded edges were more likely to have a peripheral PoLTF than subjects wearing the galyfilcon A lenses with angled edged, which was similar to our previous results [16]. Besides, the shape of ocular surface affects the fit of a lens, and significant differences in the peripheral PoLTF between two different lenses also indicate that lens designs play important roles. Our results here may indicate that round edged contact lenses have higher localized pressure near the lens edge and at the midperiphery of the cornea. This could result in the persistence of the PoLTF. Lenses with a high modulus were found to have more movement [28]. More movement in a lens with a high modulus might be attributed to the difficulty of deformation and the adherence to the ocular surface that may result in a high frequency of occurrence for peripheral PoLTF.

Lens wearing time may be another factor contributing to the changes of the peripheral PoLTF. At the peripheral cornea as well as limbus, the number of subjects in which the PoLTF could be visualized decreased during the 6 h of lens wear. Over a period of time, lenses appear to deform and conform to the ocular surface [29], and lid tension during blinking may facilitate the deformation of the lens, both of which may explain the diminished peripheral PoLTF on the cornea and limbus.

There were some limitations in the present study. We did not take into account lens movement that may play a role in the conjunctival overlap. The PoLTF at the periphery was visualized but not quantified with respect to size and location. We only evaluated the conjunctival overlap and PoLTF at the horizontal meridian. As this was the first attempt to characterize the edge fitting properties of soft contact lenses during daily wear, the role of these variables will be considered in future studies. Linking the shape of the ocular surface and the lens edge fitting and three-dimensional quantitation of the size and location of the peripheral PoLTF may be necessary to fully understand the overall lens edge fitting.

In summary, evaluation by UHR-OCT of soft contact lens wear over a 6-hour period showed increased conjunctival overlap over the lens edges and reduced PoLTF underneath the peripheral region of soft contact lenses. The lens edge configuration may play a role in conjunctival response and peripheral PoLTF. UHR-OCT is well suitable for evaluating the lens edge fitting during daily soft contact lens wear.

Disclosure

Lele Cui and Sisi Chen are the first coauthors.

Conflicts of Interest

The authors have no proprietary interest in any materials or methods described within this article.

Authors' Contributions

Lele Cui, Meixiao Shen, and Ming Li were involved in designing of the study. Sisi Chen, Lele Cui, and Lei Zhang conducted the study. Sisi Chen, Lele Cui, Kaixuan Sheng, and Weihe Zhou collected data. Lele Cui and Weihe Zhou performed analysis and interpretation. Lele Cui, Meixiao Shen, and Ming Li reviewed and prepared the manuscript. Lele Cui and Sisi Chen contributed equally to this work.

Acknowledgments

This study was supported by the National Natural Science Foundation of China (81400374 to Lele Cui), Zhejiang Medical Science and Technology Program (2018KY543 to Lele Cui and 2017KY113 to Ming Li), and Wenzhou Science and Technology Program (Y20150265 to Ming Li).

References

[1] N. Efron, M. Al-Dossari, and N. Pritchard, "Confocal microscopy of the bulbar conjunctiva in contact lens wear," *Cornea*, vol. 29, no. 1, pp. 43–52, 2010.

[2] A. D. Graham, T. N. Truong, and M. C. Lin, "Conjunctival epithelial flap in continuous contact lens wear," *Optometry and Vision Science*, vol. 86, no. 4, pp. e324–e331, 2009.

[3] M. Guillon and C. Maissa, "Bulbar conjunctival staining in contact lens wearers and non lens wearers and its association with symptomatology," *Contact Lens and Anterior Eye*, vol. 28, no. 2, pp. 67–73, 2005.

[4] N. Efron, "Conjunctiva," in *Contact Lens Complications*, Edinburgh, Ed., pp. 61–86, Butterworth-Heinemann, Oxford, UK, 2004.

[5] S. A. Little and A. S. Bruce, "Postlens tear film morphology, lens movement and symptoms in hydrogel lens wearers," *Ophthalmic and Physiological Optics*, vol. 14, no. 1, pp. 65–69, 1994.

[6] S. A. Little and A. S. Bruce, "Osmotic determinants of postlens tear film morphology and hydrogel lens movement," *Ophthalmic and Physiological Optics*, vol. 15, no. 2, pp. 117–124, 1995.

[7] A. S. Bruce and J. C. Mainstone, "Lens adherence and postlens tear film changes in closed-eye wear of hydrogel lenses," *Optometry and Vision Science*, vol. 73, no. 1, pp. 28–34, 1996.

[8] L. Wagner, K. Polse, and R. Mandell, "Tear pumping and edema with soft contact lenses," *Investigative Ophthalmology and Visual Science*, vol. 19, no. 11, pp. 1397–1400, 1980.

[9] S. A. Little and A. S. Bruce, "Hydrogel (acuvue) lens movement is influenced by the postlens tear film," *Optometry and Vision Science*, vol. 71, no. 6, pp. 364–370, 1994.

[10] S. A. Little and A. S. Bruce, "Role of the post-lens tear film in the mechanism of inferior arcuate staining with ultrathin hydrogel lenses," *CLAO Journal*, vol. 21, no. 3, pp. 175–181, 1995.

[11] J. Wang, S. Jiao, M. Ruggeri, M. A. Shousha, and Q. Chen, "In situ visualization of tears on contact lens using ultra high resolution optical coherence tomography," *Eye and Contact Lens: Science and Clinical Practice*, vol. 35, no. 2, pp. 44–49, 2009.

[12] M. J. Doughty, D. Fonn, D. Richter, T. Simpson, B. Caffery, and K. Gordon, "A patient questionnaire approach to estimating the prevalence of dry eye symptoms in patients presenting to optometric practices across Canada," *Optometry and Vision Science*, vol. 74, no. 8, pp. 624–631, 1997.

[13] J. Wang, D. Fonn, T. L. Simpson, and L. Jones, "Precorneal and pre- and postlens tear film thickness measured indirectly with optical coherence tomography," *Investigative Opthalmology and Visual Science*, vol. 44, no. 6, pp. 2524–2528, 2003.

[14] Q. Chen, J. Wang, A. Tao, M. Shen, S. Jiao, and F. Lu, "Ultrahigh-resolution measurement by optical coherence tomography of dynamic tear film changes on contact lenses," *Investigative Opthalmology and Visual Science*, vol. 51, no. 4, pp. 1988–1993, 2010.

[15] J. J. Nichols, G. L. Mitchell, and P. E. King-Smith, "The impact of contact lens care solutions on the thickness of the tear film and contact lens," *Cornea*, vol. 24, no. 7, pp. 825–832, 2005.

[16] M. Shen, L. Cui, C. Riley, M. R. Wang, and J. Wang, "Characterization of soft contact lens edge fitting using ultrahigh resolution and ultra-long scan depth optical coherence

tomography," *Investigative Opthalmology and Visual Science*, vol. 52, no. 7, pp. 4091–4097, 2011.

[17] M. Shen, J. Wang, J. Qu et al., "Diurnal variation of ocular hysteresis, corneal thickness, and intraocular pressure," *Optometry and Vision Science*, vol. 85, no. 12, pp. 1185–1192, 2008.

[18] V. Westphal, A. Rollins, S. Radhakrishnan, and J. Izatt, "Correction of geometric and refractive image distortions in optical coherence tomography applying Fermat's principle," *Optics Express*, vol. 10, no. 9, pp. 397–404, 2002.

[19] L. Sorbara, T. L. Simpson, J. Maram, E. S. Song, K. Bizheva, and N. Hutchings, "Optical edge effects create conjunctival indentation thickness artefacts," *Ophthalmic and Physiological Optics*, vol. 35, no. 3, pp. 283–292, 2015.

[20] B. J. Kaluzny, J. J. Kaluzny, A. Szkulmowska et al., "Spectral optical coherence tomography: a new imaging technique in contact lens practice," *Ophthalmic and Physiological Optics*, vol. 26, no. 2, pp. 127–132, 2006.

[21] V. Christopoulos, L. Kagemann, G. Wollstein et al., "In vivo corneal high-speed, ultra high-resolution optical coherence tomography," *Archives of Ophthalmology*, vol. 125, no. 8, pp. 1027–1035, 2007.

[22] P. E. Allaire and R. D. Flack, "Squeeze forces in contact lenses with a steep base curve radius," *American Journal of Optometry and Physiological Optics*, vol. 57, no. 4, pp. 219–227, 1980.

[23] D. M. Lieberman and J. W. Grierson, "The lids influence on corneal shape," *Cornea*, vol. 19, no. 3, pp. 336–342, 2000.

[24] P. Riordan-Eva, "Anatomy and embryology of the eye," in *Vaughan & Asbury's General Ophthalmology*, R. Shelley, J. B. Peter, and R. Jim, Eds., pp. 1–29, Appleton & Lange, Stamford, CT, USA, 16th edition, 1999.

[25] D. K. Martin, J. Boulos, J. Gan, K. Gavriel, and P. Harvey, "A unifying parameter to describe the clinical mechanics of hydrogel contact lenses," *Optometry and Vision Science*, vol. 66, no. 2, pp. 87–91, 1989.

[26] Q. Chen, J. Wang, M. Shen et al., "Lower volumes of tear menisci in contact lens wearers with dry eye symptoms," *Investigative Opthalmology and Visual Science*, vol. 50, no. 7, pp. 3159–3163, 2009.

[27] Q. Le, C. Jiang, A. C. Jiang, and J. Xu, "The analysis of tear meniscus in soft contact lens wearers by spectral optical coherence tomography," *Cornea*, vol. 28, no. 8, pp. 851–855, 2009.

[28] L. Cui, M. Shen, M. R. Wang, and J. Wang, "Micrometer-scale contact lens movements imaged by ultrahigh-resolution optical coherence tomography," *American Journal of Ophthalmology*, vol. 153, no. 2, pp. 275–283, 2012.

[29] A. J. Taylor and S. D. Wilson, "Centration mechanism of soft contact lenses," *Optometry and Vision Science*, vol. 73, no. 3, pp. 215–221, 1996.

31

Treatment Efficacy and Compliance in Patients with Diabetic Macular Edema Treated with Ranibizumab in a Real-Life Setting

Anne-Laurence Best,[1] **Franck Fajnkuchen,**[1,2] **Sylvia Nghiem-Buffet** ⓘ**,**[1,2] **Typhaine Grenet,**[1,2] **Gabriel Quentel,**[2] **Corinne Delahaye-Mazza,**[2] **Salomon Y. Cohen,**[2,3] **and Audrey Giocanti-Aurégan** ⓘ[1]

[1]*Ophthalmology Department, Avicenne Hospital, DHU Vision and Handicaps, APHP, Paris 13 University, Bobigny, France*
[2]*Centre d'Imagerie et de Laser, Paris, France*
[3]*Ophthalmology Department, Centre Hospitalier Intercommunal de Créteil, Paris Est University, Créteil, France*

Correspondence should be addressed to Audrey Giocanti-Aurégan; audreygiocanti@yahoo.fr

Academic Editor: Toshinori Murata

Purpose. To assess real-life efficacy of ranibizumab and treatment compliance of patients with vision loss secondary to diabetic macular edema (DME). *Methods.* A retrospective study was conducted in DME patients treated with ranibizumab. Patients were monitored every 4 weeks for visual acuity (VA) and central retinal thickness (CRT) by SD-OCT. All patients received a loading dose of 3 monthly injections followed by retreatments on an as-needed basis. The primary endpoint was the change in VA at M12. Patient compliance to the follow-up and the correlation between the injection number and VA were also investigated. Compliance was compared to that of neovascular age-related macular degeneration (nAMD) patients. *Results.* Seventy-two eyes of 55 consecutive DME patients were included. At baseline, the mean VA was 56.5 letters and CRT was 470 μm. At M12, the mean VA was 63.4 letters ($p < 0.0001$), 31.1% of patients had a VA > 70 letters, the mean VA change was +6.9 letters, and the mean CRT was 361.9 μm ($p = 0.0001$) after a mean number of 5.33 intravitreal injections. In patients who received ≥7 injections, the VA gain and final VA were significantly higher than in patients who received <7 injections. At M12, 25.45% of DME patients were lost to follow-up versus 16.8% of nAMD patients ($n = 55$). *Discussion/Conclusion.* Our study confirms the real-life efficacy of ranibizumab in DME at M12 and the need for a large number of injections to achieve better visual outcomes. We also showed a trend to a lower compliance in diabetic versus nAMD patients.

1. Introduction

Diabetic macular edema (DME) is the leading cause of decreased vision in diabetic patients with a prevalence of 4.8% [1]. Its management has improved over the last ten years with the increased availability of therapeutic agents. Laser photocoagulation has long been the reference treatment and has led to a 50% reduction in visual acuity (VA) decrease at 3 years, but this improvement is not sustained over the long term [2]. Thereafter, intravitreal injections (IVI) of corticosteroids have shown promising results [3–6] but their side effects limit their benefits [7, 8]. Ranibizumab was the first anti-VEGF agent to show a benefit in terms of VA in the treatment of central DME [9–12] in Phase III studies. In these pivotal studies, the VA gain over the first year varies from +6.8 to +12 letters with a number of IVI ranging between 7 and 12. The visual gain and IVI number depend on the treatment regimen and follow-up strategies used.

The aim of this study was to assess the efficacy and safety of ranibizumab for the treatment of DME in a real-life setting in a French private practice.

2. Methods

All consecutive patients with vision loss secondary to DME who received their first IVI of ranibizumab 0.5 mg between June 2012 and June 2015 in a private ophthalmology center specialized in retina diseases, CIL (Center for Imaging and Laser) in Paris, were retrospectively included. This study was conducted in accordance with the tenets of the Declaration of Helsinki, and an informed consent was obtained from patients. Approval was obtained from the France Macula Federation ethics committee.

Inclusion criteria were patients ≥ 18 years old, with type 1 or 2 diabetes with vision loss due to center-involved DME. Both eyes of the same patient could be included.

Exclusion criteria were history of another vitreous or retinal pathology, presence of macular ischemia, stroke or cardiac failure ≤ 3 months before inclusion, and ocular surgery ≤ 6 months before inclusion.

For each patient, the systemic data were collected (diabetes type and duration, HbA1C, blood pressure, dyslipidemia, presence of nephropathy, macroangiopathy, sleep apnea syndrome, and type of treatment).

At baseline and during the follow-up, all patients underwent a complete ophthalmologic examination with best-corrected visual acuity (BCVA) measurement according to the ETDRS scale and slit-lamp and noncontact fundus examination (SuperField Volk). Angiography (Spectralis, Heidelberg Engineering, Heidelberg, Germany) was performed to rule out macular ischemia and to assess the stage of diabetic retinopathy (DR). Spectral-domain optical coherence tomography (SD-OCT) (Spectralis, Heidelberg Engineering, Heidelberg, Germany) was performed to measure the central macular thickness (CRT) and macular volume (MV) during the follow-up. DME was defined by a CRT ≥ 300 μm.

The treatment regimen followed the 2012 European guidelines for ranibizumab use modified in 2014 [13, 14]. Patients received 3 monthly IVI of ranibizumab during the loading phase, followed by reinjection according to a pro re nata (PRN) regimen. Patients were monitored every 4 weeks with BCVA measurement, fundus examination, and CRT measurement. A decrease in BCVA > 5 letters and/or a CRT > 300 μm were indications for retreatment. In the absence of BCVA improvement after the loading phase, treatment was discontinued. Patients with a VA gain < 5 letters or a CRT improvement < 10% from baseline values after 3 IVI were considered as nonresponders.

The primary endpoint was the change in BCVA between baseline and month 12 of follow-up (M12).

Secondary endpoints were the CRT, MV after the loading phase and at M12, number of IVI in the first year of follow-up, and the assessment of patient compliance. Compliance was assessed through 2 parameters: the prevalence of patients lost to follow-up, that is, patients who stopped their follow-up before the end of the first year, and the prevalence of patients with an irregular follow-up, that is, patients who did not attend the required appointments and missed their examination between M12 and M14, but continued their treatment. The compliance of DME patients was compared to that of a series of consecutive neovascular age-related macular degeneration (nAMD) patients treated with ranibizumab for one year in the same center, during the same period.

2.1. Statistical Analysis. A matched Student parametric test was used for statistical analysis, and a p value < 0.05 was considered significant. For prevalence comparison, a Fisher's exact test was performed. The statistical analysis was carried out using Prism 7 software.

3. Results

Seventy-two eyes of 55 patients treated with ranibizumab injections were included. Seventeen patients (30.9%) had bilateral DME, and 38 patients (69.1%) had unilateral DME. The mean DME duration before the first injection was 20.2 months.

The mean follow-up duration after the first IVI was 19.6 months (±11.39 months), with a median of 17.87 months. Baseline patient characteristics are presented in Table 1.

Diabetic retinopathy (DR) was mild nonproliferative DR (NPDR) in 5 eyes (7%), moderate NPDR in 18 eyes (25%), severe NPDR in 20 eyes (27.8%), and proliferative DR in 8 eyes (11.1%). Laser photocoagulation had been previously performed in 21 eyes (29.1%).

Twenty-seven eyes (37.5%) were not treatment naive: 26 eyes had received macular laser therapy and 1 eye had been treated with IVI of triamcinolone in 2004 prior to inclusion. Forty-five eyes (62.5%) were treatment naive (Table 2).

3.1. Functional Outcomes. The mean baseline BCVA was 56.5 ± 11.9 ETDRS (±SD) letters. Five out of the 72 (6.9%) eyes had a baseline BCVA score > 70 ETDRS (Table 3, Figure 1).

The mean BCVA gain was +6.4 ± 7.3 letters at M3 ($p < 0.0001$), +6.1 ± 16.7 letters at M6 ($p < 0.0001$), +6.5 ± 8.5 letters at M9 ($p < 0.0001$), and +6.9 ± 10.2 ETDRS letters at M12 ($p < 0.0001$). After one year of treatment, 37.8% (17/45) of patients had a VA gain ≥ 10 letters and 22.2% (10/45) had ≥15 letters and 31.1% (14/45) had reached the BCVA threshold of >70 letters versus only 6.9% at baseline.

At the end of the first year of follow-up, 2 eyes had lost ≥10 letters.

3.2. Anatomical Outcomes. The mean baseline CRT was 470 μm (±134.5). The mean CRT change was −148 μm (±177) at M3 and −108.1 μm (±176) at M12 (Table 3, Figure 2). CRT was <300 μm in 40% (18/45) of eyes at M12.

The baseline MV was 13.2 mm^3. The mean change in MV was −2 ± 1.6 mm^3 at M3 and −1.6 ± 1.6 mm^3 at M12 (Table 3, Figure 3).

3.3. Number of Intravitreal Injections. 55 patients (72 eyes) received a mean number of 5.33 ± 2.1 injections of ranibizumab over the first year. Nineteen eyes had a follow-up of two years with a mean number of 10.84 IVI.

3.4. Compliance with Treatment. Nine (16.4%) and 14 (25.45%) patients (10 and 16 eyes) were lost to follow-up at M6 and M12, respectively. As a result, 41 patients (56 eyes) had at least 12 months of follow-up, but only 33 out of the 55 patients (60%, 45 eyes) attended the control consultation scheduled between the 12th and 14th month, the others were seen later (i.e., 8 patients—14.5%—had an irregular follow-up).

TABLE 1: Baseline characteristics of patients.

Patient number	$n = 55$
Sex	
Men	$n = 34$ (61.8%)
Women	$n = 21$ (38.2%)
Type of diabetes	
Type 1	$n = 8$ (15.5%)
Type 2	$n = 47$ (85.5%)
Age (years), mean ($\pm$SD*)	66.7 ($\pm$9.59)
Duration of diabetes (years), mean ($\pm$SD)	18.1 ($\pm$13.29)
HbA1c, mean ($\pm$SD)	7.4% ($\pm$1.25)
Insulinotherapy	$n = 20$ (36%)
High blood pressure	$n = 34$ (61.8%)
Dyslipidemia	$n = 14$ (25%)
Nephropathy	$n = 15$ (27%)
Macroangiopathy	$n = 2$ (3.6%)
Sleep apnea syndrome	$n = 2$ (3.6%)

*SD: standard deviation.

TABLE 2: Baseline features of retinopathy, maculopathy, and ophthalmologic history.

Eye number	$n = 72$
NPDR	
Mild	5 (7%)
Moderate	18 (25%)
Severe	20 (27.7%)
PDR	8 (11.1%)
Laser photocoagulation	
PRP	
Ongoing	22 (30.5%)
Completed	21 (29.1%)
Focal/grid	26 (36.1%)
Intravitreal injection history	
Corticosteroids	1 (1.3%)
DME duration (months): mean ($\pm$SD)	20.2 ($\pm$25.13)
Pseudophakic	18 (25%)
Vitreomacular surgery	4 (5.6%)
Epiretinal membrane	10 (13.8%)
High intraocular pressure history	4 (5.5%)

NPRD: nonproliferative diabetic retinopathy; PDR: proliferative diabetic retinopathy; PRP: panretinal photocoagulation; SD: standard deviation; n: number of eyes.

3.5. Baseline Characteristics and Compliance of nAMD Patients.

Fifty-five consecutive patients with nAMD seen in the same private practice and requiring ranibizumab IVI since January 2013 and followed over 12 months were also included. We included 41 women and 14 men with a mean age of 85.3 ($\pm$6.3). The mean baseline visual acuity was 61.6 ($\pm$13.5) letters.

A mean number of 7.38 consultations were carried out over one year. A mean number of 4.5 IVI were administered over the first year. Only 16.8% of patients were lost to follow-up at one year.

3.6. Subgroup Analysis

3.6.1. Subanalysis according to the Number of IVI at 1 Year.

Two subgroups of patients were defined based on the number of IVI administered during the first year: one group received <7 IVI ($n = 30$ eyes) and one received $\geq$7 IVI ($n = 15$ eyes). Patients who received <7 IVT had a baseline BCVA of 55.5 letters and a visual gain of +5.43 letters versus a baseline BCVA of 57.1 letters ($p = 0.09$) and a visual gain of +11.19 letters for patients who received $\geq$7 IVT. At one year, a mean BCVA of 60.96 $\pm$ 15.66 letters was achieved in the group that received <7 IVT versus 68.26 $\pm$ 6.99 letters in the group with $\geq$7 IVT ($p = 0.04$).

3.6.2. Functional Response Subanalysis at 1 Year.

Two subgroups were defined according to the functional response after one year of treatment. A subgroup of good responders ($n = 8$ eyes) was defined as a BCVA gain > 15 letters at 1 year, and a subgroup of poorer responders was defined by a BCVA gain $\leq$ 15 letters. The group of poorer responders received fewer IVI than the group of good responders (mean IVI number: 5.59 versus 6.5) over the first year ($p = 0.03$). In the good responder group, the baseline BCVA was 46.9 letters and 58.2 letters in the poorer responders ($p = 0.047$).

3.7. Safety.

No case of endophthalmitis was reported during the follow-up. One patient with type 2 diabetes had a stroke 6 weeks after the last IVI. This patient subsequently underwent a complete ophthalmologic evaluation, and the decision was made to discontinue IVI.

4. Discussion

The results of our study confirm the efficacy of ranibizumab for the treatment of DME responsible for vision loss in a real-life setting with a VA gain of +6.9 $\pm$ 10.2 letters after a mean number of 5.33 IVT over the first year of follow-up.

However, our functional results at 1 year are slightly lower than those reported in pivotal [10] and http://drcr.net studies [8, 12, 15] which show a gain from +6.5 to +12 letters at M12. This discrepancy could probably be due to an insufficient number of injections in our real-life series. Indeed, in our study, patients received 5.33 IVI with a mean annual number of 7.68 consultations, compared to 7–9.4 IVI in pivotal and DRCR.net studies with a number of consultations generally higher than that of our patients.

In the RISE and RIDE studies [11], patients were injected monthly for 36 months. In this case, the VA gains ranged from +11.9 to +12 letters [16] after one year of follow-up. In Europe, in the RESTORE study [10], with a strict monthly monitoring, the visual gain was +6.8 letters at the end of the first year of treatment with a mean number of 7 IVI. Patients were treated according to a PRN regimen, and the retreatment criterion was strictly functional.

TABLE 3: Best-corrected visual acuity (BCVA), central retinal thickness (CRT), and macular volume (MV) over the first year of follow-up.

	Baseline	Month 3	Month 6	Month 9	Month 12
Number of eyes	$n = 72$	$n = 60$	$n = 58$	$n = 52$	$n = 45$
BCVA (ETDRS letters $\pm$ SD)	56.5 ± 11.9	62.9 ± 12.4	62.6 ± 13.0	63.0 ± 12.2	63.4 ± 13.8
CRT (μm $\pm$ SD)	470 ± 134.5	322 ± 97.8	344.7 ± 122.8	350.5 ± 99	361.9 ± 124.8
MV (mm^3 $\pm$ SD)	13.2 ± 2.4	11.2 ± 1.5	11.4 ± 1.7	11.6 ± 1.7	11.6 ± 1.6
BCVA > 70 letters	5 (6.9%)	22 (36.6%)	18 (31%)	16 (30.7%)	14 (31.1%)
		0–3 months	0–6 months	0–9 months	0–12 months
Number of eyes	$n = 72$	$n = 60$	$n = 58$	$n = 52$	$n = 45$
BCVA gain (ETDRS letters $\pm$ SD)		$+6.4 \pm 7.3^*$	$+6.1 \pm 16.7^*$	$+6.5 \pm 8.5^*$	$+6.9 \pm 10.2^*$
Change in CRT (μm $\pm$ SD)		-148 ± 177	-125.3 ± 177	-119.5 ± 143	-108.1 ± 176
Change in MV (mm^3 $\pm$ SD)		-2 ± 1.6	-1.8 ± 1.8	-1.7 ± 1.4	-1.6 ± 1.6
Gain $\geq$ 10 letters		22 (30.5%)	19 (26.3%)	18 (25%)	17 (37.8%)
Gain $\geq$ 15 letters		9 (12.5%)	11 (15.2%)	5 (6.9%)	10 (22.2%)
Loss $\geq$ 10 letters		1 (1.3%)	6 (8.3%)	2 (2.7%)	3 (4.1%)
Loss $\geq$ 15 letters		0	3 (4.1%)	0	2 (2.7%)

$^*p < 0.0001$.

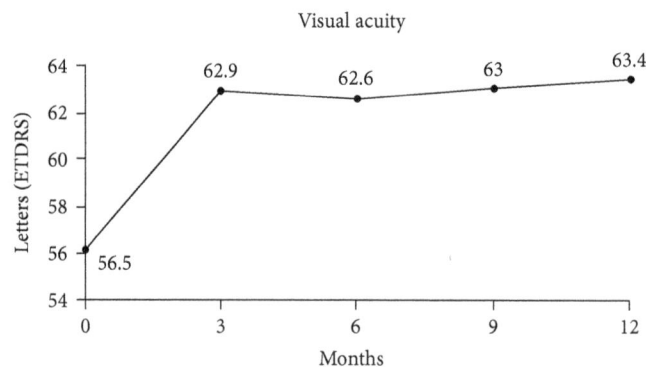

FIGURE 1: Mean change in best-corrected visual acuity over the first year of follow-up.

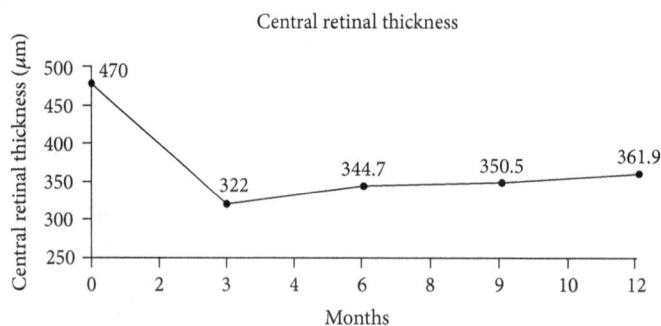

FIGURE 2: Mean change in central retinal thickness over the first year of follow-up.

In the DRCR.net studies [8, 12, 15], ranibizumab IVI were administrated according to a PRN regimen with retreatment based on functional and anatomical outcomes with severe retreatment criteria during the first 6 months to achieve a VA of 20/20 or a dry retina. Thus, patients usually received 5 or 6 injections during the first 24 weeks. With this type of treatment and monitoring every 4 weeks, a gain of +9 letters after 9 IVI was observed with protocol I and +11.2 letters after 10 IVI with protocol T. However, in our study, despite consultations scheduled every 4 weeks, the time between each consultation was longer than 4 weeks in patients who completed the one-year follow-up since they only attended a mean number of 7.68 visits over 12 months.

A clear difference in terms of visual outcomes between the real-life setting and pivotal studies has already been observed in nAMD patients treated with ranibizumab. In

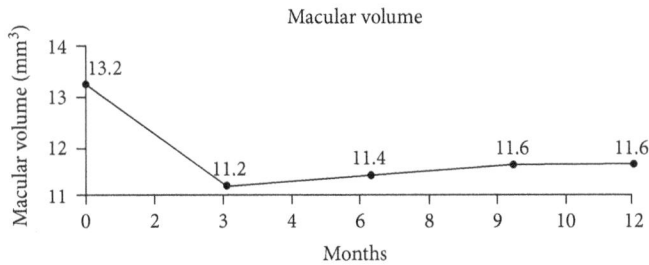

FIGURE 3: Mean change in macular volume over the first year of follow-up.

nAMD, the MARINA [17] and ANCHOR [18] pivotal studies have shown VA gains ranging between +7.2 and +11.3 letters at one year. The PrONTO study [19] has shown a sustained VA improvement with a personalized PRN regimen and retreatment based on functional and anatomical outcomes allowing a gain of +9.3 letters at one year with twice fewer injections but with a proper monthly follow-up. Real-life studies have shown a smaller improvement with a gain of +4.4 letters at one year for the LUMINOUS [20] study. Another real-life study conducted in our center has shown an even lower visual gain of +0.7 letter after 3.79 IVI and 8.06 consultations over the first year under a PRN regimen, and the authors have concluded on the need for a more regular follow-up with a strict 4-week interval between each consultation. These real-life studies have stressed that there could be a difference in terms of functional outcomes between data from randomized studies with a strict monitoring and treatment protocols and the real-life conditions.

In DME, differences in functional outcomes seem less significant than in nAMD between pivotal and real-life results. The ADMOR real-life study [21] has investigated the efficacy of ranibizumab in patients with DME in South Asia. The results showed a gain of +8.5 letters at 1 year with a mean number of 7 ± 2 IVI over the first year. In this study, patients were not strictly monitored every 4 weeks and attended a mean number of 10 ± 2 visits during their follow-up. Patients in the ADMOR study had a more severe DME, with an initial VA less than ours (55.3 ± 13.4 letters), and a higher baseline CRT ($532 \pm 129 \mu$m). Another real-life study by Hrarat et al. [22] has reported a gain of +10.7 ± 16.9 letters after 12 months of treatment with a mean number of 5.4 ± 1.9 IVI and 8.8 ± 2.5 visits during the follow-up. The mean baseline VA was 48.3 ± 17 letters, and the baseline CRT was $519.7 \pm 157.3 \mu$m. This very low baseline VA could explain their high VA gain [16]. A Swedish real-life study by Granström et al. [23] assessing the efficacy of a 12-month treatment with ranibizumab in DME, retrospectively conducted in two ophthalmic departments using a PRN regimen, has reported a gain of +5.2 letters after 12 months of treatment, but the mean number of injections was not specified. Patients had an initial VA greater than ours (65.0 ± 12.1 letters) with a lower initial CRT: $403 \pm 122 \mu$m.

In our study, with a stricter follow-up and treatment regimen, the VA gains could have probably been greater. This finding is reinforced by a statistically significant correlation between the VA gain and the number of IVI in our study. Patients with more than 7 IVI had a higher VA gain than those who received less than 7 IVI ($p < 0.04$). In addition, the number of injections was greater in the group of patients who had a gain greater than 15 letters compared to the group that did not exceed this threshold ($p < 0.03$).

These results encourage us to adopt a strict follow-up and highlight the need for a regular follow-up by providing appropriate information to patients. Appropriate information is indeed important as the compliance of diabetic patients may be low. Thus, in our series, it should be noted that a significant number of patients were lost to follow-up (25.45% of patients), suggesting that some diabetic patients are poorly compliant. The small percentage of patients (60%) who attended the 12-month consultation supports this hypothesis. This discrepancy between real-life and pivotal studies stresses that real-life studies are necessary to assess the true efficacy of a treatment and to understand the factors limiting efficacy.

The treatment regimen of DME represents a real burden for patients and their family, and diabetic patients must also attend different medical consultations with several specialists and this may be a barrier to a monthly follow-up. Thus, this burden of consultations not only with ophthalmologists could contribute to the lower compliance of diabetic patients compared to that of nAMD patients. Indeed, we assessed in the same private practice 55 consecutive patients with nAMD requiring ranibizumab IVI and followed them over 12 months. They attended a mean number of 7.38 consultations and received a mean number of 4.5 IVI over the first year. Only 16.8% of patients were lost to follow-up at one year versus 25.45% in our series of diabetic patients ($p = 0.6$).

Different assumptions may be made regarding the lower compliance of diabetic patients compared to AMD patients: the fact that (i) DME is part of a chronic extraophthalmological disease, diabetes, which, because of its chronicity, may lead to a lassitude with regard to the disease; (ii) the loss of vision is progressive in DME compared to the sudden and often deeper vision loss in nAMD; (iii) diabetic patients are younger and often in the working age, making them less available than nAMD patients who are often retired; and (iv) the cost of the treatment, which may also be a barrier, in particular in a private center where patients must advance the cost. Other studies are needed to confirm the lower compliance of DME patients compared to nAMD patients.

Based on our findings and the results of the literature [24], it seems essential to adopt the treatment regimen to specificities of the diabetic population and to patient availability and preferences after information and, in the case of patients who cannot follow a strict monthly regimen to choose the appropriate treatment, for instance, a treat-and-extend regimen, providing the same visual outcomes with a lower number of consultations [24] and thus, even despite a possible overtreatment for a few patients.

In conclusion, our real-life study shows a VA improvement in patients with DME, with however a slightly lower gain than that found in pivotal studies after a lower number of IVI. This discrepancy between results obtained in a real-life setting and pivotal studies is not as important as in nAMD despite a higher compliance of nAMD patients in a real-life setting.

This study also shows that the visual outcomes correlate with the number of IVI, and that a strict monthly follow-up is challenging in the real life.

Disclosure

This study was presented as a paper at the French Society of Ophthalmology in Paris by May 2016 and as a poster at ARVO Meeting in Seattle by May 2016.

Conflicts of Interest

Dr. Audrey Giocanti-Aurégan reports personal fees from Allergan, Alimera, Bayer, Novartis, and Optos plc outside the submitted work. Dr. Franck Fajnkuchen and Dr. Typhaine Grenet report personal fees from Allergan, Bayer, and Novartis outside the submitted work. Dr. Sylvia Nghiem-Buffet reports personal fees from Allergan, Bayer, Novartis, and Zeiss outside the submitted work. Dr. Corinne Delahaye-Mazza and Dr. Anne-Laurence Best have nothing to disclose. Dr. Gabriel Quentel reports personal fees from Novartis outside the submitted work. Professor Salomon Y. Cohen reports personal fees from Novartis, Bayer, Allergan, Alcon, and Thea outside the submitted work.

Acknowledgments

This work was supported by an unrestricted grant from AVOPH (Bobigny, France), an association for research and education, and CIL-ASSOC (association for research—Centre d'Imagerie et de Laser, Paris, France).

References

[1] C. Delcourt, P. Massin, and M. Rosilio, "Epidemiology of diabetic retinopathy: expected *vs* reported prevalence of cases in the French population," *Diabetes & Metabolism*, vol. 35, no. 6, pp. 431–438, 2009.

[2] "Photocoagulation for diabetic macular edema. Early Treatment Diabetic Retinopathy Study report number 1," *Archives of Ophthalmology*, vol. 103, no. 12, pp. 1796–1806, 1985.

[3] J. A. Haller, B. D. Kuppermann, M. S. Blumenkranz et al., "Randomized controlled trial of an intravitreous dexamethasone drug delivery system in patients with diabetic macular edema," *Archives of Ophthalmology*, vol. 128, no. 3, pp. 289–296, 2010.

[4] Diabetic Retinopathy Clinical Research Network, "A randomized trial comparing intravitreal triamcinolone acetonide and focal/grid photocoagulation for diabetic macular edema," *Ophthalmology*, vol. 115, no. 9, pp. 1447–1459.e10, 2008.

[5] M. C. Gillies, F. K. P. Sutter, J. M. Simpson, J. Larsson, H. Ali, and M. Zhu, "Intravitreal triamcinolone for refractory diabetic macular edema: two-year results of a double-masked, placebo-controlled, randomized clinical trial," *Ophthalmology*, vol. 113, no. 9, pp. 1533–1538, 2006.

[6] M. C. Gillies, I. L. McAllister, M. Zhu et al., "Intravitreal triamcinolone prior to laser treatment of diabetic macular edema: 24-month results of a randomized controlled trial," *Ophthalmology*, vol. 118, no. 5, pp. 866–872, 2011.

[7] M. C. Gillies, J. M. Simpson, C. Gaston et al., "Five-year results of a randomized trial with open-label extension of triamcinolone acetonide for refractory diabetic macular edema," *Ophthalmology*, vol. 116, no. 11, pp. 2182–2187, 2009.

[8] M. C. Gillies, L. L. Lim, A. Campain et al., "A randomized clinical trial of intravitreal bevacizumab versus intravitreal dexamethasone for diabetic macular edema: the BEVORDEX study," *Ophthalmology*, vol. 121, no. 12, pp. 2473–2481, 2014.

[9] P. Massin, F. Bandello, J. G. Garweg et al., "Safety and efficacy of ranibizumab in diabetic macular edema (RESOLVE study): a 12-month, randomized, controlled, double-masked, multi-center phase II study," *Diabetes Care*, vol. 33, no. 11, pp. 2399–2405, 2010.

[10] P. Mitchell, P. Massin, S. Bressler et al., "Three-year patient-reported visual function outcomes in diabetic macular edema managed with ranibizumab: the RESTORE extension study," *Current Medical Research and Opinion*, vol. 31, no. 11, pp. 1967–1975, 2015.

[11] Q. D. Nguyen, D. M. Brown, D. M. Marcus et al., "Ranibizumab for diabetic macular edema: results from 2 phase III randomized trials: RISE and RIDE," *Ophthalmology*, vol. 119, no. 4, pp. 789–801, 2012.

[12] M. J. Elman, A. Ayala, N. M. Bressler et al., "Intravitreal ranibizumab for diabetic macular edema with prompt versus deferred laser treatment: 5-year randomized trial results," *Ophthalmology*, vol. 122, no. 2, pp. 375–381, 2015.

[13] Haute Autorité de Santé, "Commission de la transparence Avis," Janvier 2015, https://www.has-sante.fr/portail/upload/docs/evamed/CT-14433_LUCENTIS_PIS_ETUDE_LUEUR_Avis1_CT14433.pdf.

[14] F. Bandello, J. Cunha-Vaz, N. V. Chong et al., "New approaches for the treatment of diabetic macular oedema: recommendations by an expert panel," *Eye*, vol. 26, no. 4, pp. 485–493, 2012.

[15] Diabetic Retinopathy Clinical Research Network, Writing Committee, M. J. Elman et al., "Expanded 2-year follow-up of ranibizumab plus prompt or deferred laser or triamcinolone plus prompt laser for diabetic macular edema," *Ophthalmology*, vol. 118, no. 4, pp. 609–614, 2011.

[16] P. U. Dugel, J. Hillenkamp, S. Sivaprasad et al., "Baseline visual acuity strongly predicts visual acuity gain in patients with diabetic macular edema following anti-vascular endothelial growth factor treatment across trials," *Clinical Ophthalmology*, vol. 10, pp. 1103–1110, 2016.

[17] P. J. Rosenfeld, D. M. Brown, J. S. Heier et al., "Ranibizumab for neovascular age-related macular degeneration," *The New England Journal of Medicine*, vol. 355, no. 14, pp. 1419–1431, 2006.

[18] D. M. Brown, M. Michels, P. K. Kaiser, J. S. Heier, J. P. Sy, and T. Ianchulev, "Ranibizumab versus verteporfin photodynamic

therapy for neovascular age-related macular degeneration: two-year results of the ANCHOR study," *Ophthalmology*, vol. 116, no. 1, pp. 57–65.e5, 2009.

[19] G. A. Lalwani, P. J. Rosenfeld, A. E. Fung et al., "A variable-dosing regimen with intravitreal ranibizumab for neovascular age-related macular degeneration: year 2 of the PrONTO Study," *American Journal of Ophthalmology*, vol. 148, no. 1, pp. 43–58.e1, 2009.

[20] F. G. Holz, F. Bandello, M. Gillies et al., "Safety of ranibizumab in routine clinical practice: 1-year retrospective pooled analysis of four European neovascular AMD registries within the LUMINOUS programme," *British Journal of Ophthalmology*, vol. 97, no. 9, pp. 1161–1167, 2013.

[21] F. Ghanchi and C. A. Hazel, "South Asian diabetic macular oedema treated with ranibizumab (ADMOR)—real-life experience," *Eye*, vol. 30, no. 1, pp. 133–138, 2016.

[22] L. Hrarat, F. Fajnkuchen, M. Boubaya et al., "Outcomes after a 1-year treatment with ranibizumab for diabetic macular edema in a clinical setting," *Ophthalmologica*, vol. 236, no. 4, pp. 207–214, 2016.

[23] T. Granström, H. Forsman, A. Lindholm Olinder et al., "Patient-reported outcomes and visual acuity after 12 months of anti-VEGF-treatment for sight-threatening diabetic macular edema in a real world setting," *Diabetes Research and Clinical Practice*, vol. 121, pp. 157–165, 2016.

[24] C. Prünte, F. Fajnkuchen, S. Mahmood et al., "Ranibizumab 0.5 mg treat-and-extend regimen for diabetic macular oedema: the RETAIN study," *British Journal of Ophthalmology*, vol. 100, no. 6, pp. 787–795, 2016.

Permissions

All chapters in this book were first published in JO, by Hindawi Publishing Corporation; hereby published with permission under the Creative Commons Attribution License or equivalent. Every chapter published in this book has been scrutinized by our experts. Their significance has been extensively debated. The topics covered herein carry significant findings which will fuel the growth of the discipline. They may even be implemented as practical applications or may be referred to as a beginning point for another development.

The contributors of this book come from diverse backgrounds, making this book a truly international effort. This book will bring forth new frontiers with its revolutionizing research information and detailed analysis of the nascent developments around the world.

We would like to thank all the contributing authors for lending their expertise to make the book truly unique. They have played a crucial role in the development of this book. Without their invaluable contributions this book wouldn't have been possible. They have made vital efforts to compile up to date information on the varied aspects of this subject to make this book a valuable addition to the collection of many professionals and students.

This book was conceptualized with the vision of imparting up-to-date information and advanced data in this field. To ensure the same, a matchless editorial board was set up. Every individual on the board went through rigorous rounds of assessment to prove their worth. After which they invested a large part of their time researching and compiling the most relevant data for our readers.

The editorial board has been involved in producing this book since its inception. They have spent rigorous hours researching and exploring the diverse topics which have resulted in the successful publishing of this book. They have passed on their knowledge of decades through this book. To expedite this challenging task, the publisher supported the team at every step. A small team of assistant editors was also appointed to further simplify the editing procedure and attain best results for the readers.

Apart from the editorial board, the designing team has also invested a significant amount of their time in understanding the subject and creating the most relevant covers. They scrutinized every image to scout for the most suitable representation of the subject and create an appropriate cover for the book.

The publishing team has been an ardent support to the editorial, designing and production team. Their endless efforts to recruit the best for this project, has resulted in the accomplishment of this book. They are a veteran in the field of academics and their pool of knowledge is as vast as their experience in printing. Their expertise and guidance has proved useful at every step. Their uncompromising quality standards have made this book an exceptional effort. Their encouragement from time to time has been an inspiration for everyone.

The publisher and the editorial board hope that this book will prove to be a valuable piece of knowledge for researchers, students, practitioners and scholars across the globe.

List of Contributors

Marcella Nebbioso, Marta Sacchetti, Guia Bianchi, Paola Del Regno and Alessandro Lambiase
Department of Sense Organs, Sapienza University of Rome, p. le A. Moro 5, 00185 Rome, Italy

Anna Maria Zicari and Marzia Duse
Department of Pediatrics, Faculty of Medicine and Odontology, Sapienza University of Rome, p. le A. Moro 5, 00185 Rome, Italy

Fan Lu, Aizhu Tao, Yinu Hu and Ping Lu
School of Ophthalmology and Optometry, Wenzhou Medical University, Wenzhou, Zhejiang, China

Weiwei Tao
First Affiliated Hospital of Wenzhou Medical University, Wenzhou, Zhejiang, China

Jianqing Li, Jiayi Xu, Yiyi Chen, Jiaju Zhang, Yihong Cao and Peirong Lu
Department of Ophthalmology, e First Affiliated Hospital of Soochow University, 188 Shizi Street, Suzhou 215006, China

Daisuke Nagasato, Hitoshi Tabuchi, Hideharu Ohsugi, Hiroki Masumoto, Naofumi Ishitobi, Tomoaki Sonobe and Masahiro Kameoka
Department of Ophthalmology, Tsukazaki Hospital, Himeji, Japan

Hiroki Enno
Rist Inc., Tokyo, Japan

Masanori Niki and Yoshinori Mitamura
Department of Ophthalmology, Institute of Biomedical Sciences, Tokushima University Graduate School, Tokushima, Japan

Ken Hayashi
Hayashi Eye Hospital, Fukuoka, Japan

Maria Satue, Miriam Idoipe, Antonio Mateo, Elena Garcia-Martin, Alejandro Blasco-Martinez and Antonio Sanchez-Perez
IIS-Aragon, Aragon Institute for Health Research (IIS Arag´on), Zaragoza, Spain
Ophthalmology Department, Miguel Servet University Hospital, Zaragoza, Spain

Alicia Gavin and Maria Romero-Sanz
Ophthalmology Department, Miguel Servet University Hospital, Zaragoza, Spain

Vasilios S. Liarakos
Ophthalmology Department, Naval Hospital, Athens, Greece

LakshmiPriya Rangaraju, J. Jason McAnany, Michael R. Tan, Justin Wanek, Norman P. Blair and Jennifer I. Lim
Department of Ophthalmology and Visual Sciences, University of Illinois at Chicago, Chicago, IL, USA

Xuejuan Jiang and Mahnaz Shahidi
Department of Ophthalmology, University of Southern California, Los Angeles, CA, USA

Erkut Küçük and Kürsad Ramazan Zor
Ophthalmology Department, Niğdë Omer Halisdemir University, Faculty of Medicine, 51240 Niğde, Turkey

Uğur Yılmaz
Ophthalmology Department, Pamukkale University Faculty of Medicine, 20160 Denizli, Turkey

Ying Sun
The First Hospital of Jilin University, Changchun, China

Huang Wu
The Second Hospital of Jilin University, Changchun, China

Yinghong Qiu and Zhiqiang Yue
Ophthalmology Hospital of Hebei Province, Hebei, China

Yushuo Gao, Yisheng Zhong, Yanji Zhu, Yujuan Cai, Qing Lu, Xi Shen and Bing Xie
Department of Ophthalmology, Ruijin Hospital, Shanghai Jiao Tong University School of Medicine, 197, Ruijin Er Road, Shanghai 200025, China

Anna M. Demetriades
Department of Ophthalmology, NewYork-Presbyterian Hospital-Cornell, New York, NY, USA

Jikui Shen
Departments of Ophthalmology and Neuroscience, The Johns Hopkins University School of Medicine, Maumenee 719, 600 N. Wolfe Street, Baltimore, MD, USA

Xiuping Chen and Fei Yuan
Department of Ophthalmology, Zhongshan Hospital of Fudan University, Shanghai, China

Xiaoshan Min and Lingyan Shi
Department of Ophthalmology, Xiangya Hospital, Central South University, Changsha, Hunan Province, China

Hui Jiang
Department of Ophthalmology, e Second Affiliated Hospital of Hunan University of Chinese Medicine, Changsha, Hunan Province, China

C. Kern, C. Wertheimer, O. Nilmayer, M. Dirisamer, S. Priglinger and W. J. Mayer
Department of Ophthalmology, University Hospital LMU, Munich, Germany

K. Kortuem
Department of Ophthalmology, University Hospital LMU, Munich, Germany
Moorfields Eye Hospital, London, UK

Sadık Görkem Çevik
Department of Ophthalmology, Yüksek Ihtisas Research and Training Hospital, Bursa, Turkey

Sami Yılmaz and Remzi Avcı
Retina Eye Hospital, Bursa, Turkey

Mediha Tok Çevik
Sisli Hamidiye Etfal Research and Training Hospital, İstanbul, Turkey

Fatma Düriye Akalp
Department of Ophthalmology, Acıbadem Hospital, Bursa, Turkey

Fanglin He, Zhanlin Zhao, Yan Liu, Linna Lu and Yao Fu
Department of Ophthalmology, Shanghai Ninth People's Hospital, Shanghai Jiaotong University School of Medicine, Shanghai, China
Shanghai Key Laboratory of Orbital Disease and Ocular Oncology, Shanghai, China

Maged Maher Salib Roshdy, Sherine Shafik Wahba and Rania Serag Elkitkat
Ophthalmology Department, Ain Shams University, Cairo, Egypt
Al Watany Eye Hospital, Cairo, Egypt

Amira Maurice Hakim
Al Watany Eye Hospital, Cairo, Egypt

Ramy Riad Fikry
Al Watany Eye Hospital, Cairo, Egypt
Ophthalmology Department, Cairo University, Cairo, Egypt

Monika Wipf and Anja Palmowski-Wolfe
University Eye Hospital, University of Basel, Mittlere Strasse 91, 4031 Basel, Switzerland

Britt-Isabelle Berg
Department of Cranio-Maxillofacial Surgery, University of Basel, Spitalstrasse 21, 4031 Basel, Switzerland
Division of Oral and Maxillofacial Radiology, Columbia University Medical Center, 622 W.168th St., New York, NY 10032, USA

Ailee Laham
Department of Ophthalmology, University of Cincinnati College of Medicine, Cincinnati, OH, USA

Robert A. Sisk
Department of Ophthalmology, University of Cincinnati College of Medicine, Cincinnati, OH, USA
Cincinnati Eye Institute, Cincinnati, OH, USA
Division of Pediatric Ophthalmology, Cincinnati Children's Hospital Medical Center, Cincinnati, OH, USA

Robert B. Hufnagel
Division of Human Genetics, Cincinnati Children's Hospital Medical Center, Cincinnati, OH, USA

Elizabeth S. Wohler and Nara Sobreira
McKusick-Nathans Institute of Genetic Medicine, Johns Hopkins University School of Medicine, Baltimore, MD, USA

Zubair M. Ahmed
Department of Otorhinolaryngology, School of Medicine, University of Maryland, Baltimore, MD, USA

Ying Dong
Department of Ophthalmology, e First Affiliated Hospital, Chinese PLA General Hospital, Beijing 100048, China
Department of Dermatology, Northwestern University, Chicago, IL 60611, USA

Han Peng and Robert M. Lavker
Department of Dermatology, Northwestern University, Chicago, IL 60611, USA

Aisha Mohammed Alemam
College of Medicine, Taiba University, Medina, Saudi Arabia

Mohammed Hamad Aldebasi
College of Medicine, Al Imam Mohammad Ibn Saud Islamic University (IMSIU), Riyadh, Saudi Arabia

Abdulkarem Rehmatullah
MCPS, FICO(Lond), FRCSG, Paediatric Ophthalmologist, Ohud Hospital, Medina, Saudi Arabia

Rami Alsaidi
Msc, Ohud Hospital Medina, Saudi Arabia

Ishraq Tashkandi
MD, FRCSEdn, Consultant Pediatric Ophthalmologist, RTPD Ophthalmology Program, Ohud Hospital, Madina, Saudi Arabia

Fusae Kato, Miho Nozaki, Aki Kato, Norio Hasegawa, Hiroshi Morita, Munenori Yoshida and Yuichiro Ogura
Department of Ophthalmology and Visual Science, Nagoya City University Graduate School of Medical Sciences, 1-Kawasumi, Mizuho-ku, Nagoya 467-8601, Japan

Yi Sun, Xiuhua Jia, Shiqi Ling and Juan Deng
Department of Ophthalmology, ird Affiliated Hospital of Sun Yat-Sen University, Guangzhou 510630, China

Bowen Zhang
Surgical Department, The First Affiliated Hospital of Guangzhou Medical University, Guangzhou 510120, China

Hao-ChenGuo, Wan-Qing Jin, An-Peng Pan, Qin-Mei Wang, Jia Qu and A-YongYu
The Eye Hospital of Wenzhou Medical University, Wenzhou, Zhejiang, China

Jose Garcia-Arumi
Hospital Universitari Vall d'Hebron, Barcelona, Spain

Francisco Gómez-Ulla
Instituto Oftalmológico Gómez-Ulla, Complejo Hospitalario Universitario de Santiago de Compostela, A Coruña, Spain

Navea Amparo
FISABIO-Oftalmología Médica, Valencia, Spain

Enrique Cervera
Hospital General de Valencia, Valencia, Spain

Jaume Crespí
Hospital de la Santa Creu i Sant Pau, Barcelona, Spain

Roberto Gallego
Unidad de Mácula, Clínica OFTALVIST, Valencia, Spain

Ali Demircan, Zeynep Alkin, Ceren Yesilkaya, Gokhan Demir and Burcu Kemer
Beyoglu Eye Research and Training Hospital, Istanbul, Turkey

Sylvia Nghiem-Buffet
Centre Ophtalmologique d'Imagerie et de Laser, 11 Rue Antoine Bourdelle, Paris, France
Ophthalmology Department, DHU Vision and Handicaps, APHP, Avicenne Hospital, Paris 13 University, 125 Rue de Stalingrad, Bobigny, France

Salomon Y. Cohen
Centre Ophtalmologique d'Imagerie et de Laser, 11 Rue Antoine Bourdelle, Paris, France
Department of Ophthalmology, Centre Hospitalier Intercommunal, Universit´e Paris-Est-Créteil, Paris 12 University, 40 Avenue de Verdun, 91000 Créteil, France

Audrey Giocanti-Auregan
Ophthalmology Department, DHU Vision and Handicaps, APHP, Avicenne Hospital, Paris 13 University, 125 Rue de Stalingrad, Bobigny, France

Agnès Glacet-Bernard, Manar Addou-Regnard and Eric H. Souied
Department of Ophthalmology, Centre Hospitalier Intercommunal, Université Paris-Est-Créteil, Paris 12 University, 40 Avenue de Verdun, 91000 Créteil, France

João Beirão and Pedro Menéres
Instituto de Ciências Biomédicas Abel Salazar, Universidade do Porto, Porto, Portugal

Vasco Miranda, João Coelho and Maria-João Menéres
Centro Hospitalar Porto, Porto, Portugal

Beatriz Pinheiro-Torres
Alimera Sciences, Alpharetta, USA

Kata Miháltz
Department of Ophthalmology, Hietzing Hospital, Wolkersbergenstrasse 1, Vienna, Austria

Birgit Weingessel, Florian Sulzbacher, Christopher Schütze and Pia V. Vécsei-Marlovits
Department of Ophthalmology, Hietzing Hospital, Wolkersbergenstrasse 1, Vienna, Austria
Karl Landsteiner Institute for Process Optimization and Quality Management in Cataract Surgery, Wolkersbergenstrasse 1, Vienna, Austria

Andreas Gleiss
Center for Medical Statistics, Informatics and Intelligent Systems, Medical University of Vienna, Vienna, Austria

Masahiko Iigaki, Miho Nozaki, Munenori Yoshida and Yuichiro Ogura
Department of Ophthalmology and Visual Science, Nagoya City University Graduate School of Medical Sciences, Nagoya 467-8601, Japan

Marcella Nebbioso, Andrea Iannaccone and Alice Bruscolini
Department of Sense Organs, Sapienza University of Rome, p. le A. Moro 5, 00185 Rome, Italy

Marzia Duse and Anna Maria Zicari
Department of Pediatrics, Sapienza University of Rome, p. le A. Moro 5, 00185 Rome, Italy

Michele Aventaggiato
Department of Experimental Medicine, Sapienza University of Rome, p. le A. Moro 5, 00185 Rome, Italy

Lele Cui, Sisi Chen, Weihe Zhou, Lei Zhang, Meixiao Shen and Ming Li
Eye Hospital and School of Ophthalmology and Optometry, Wenzhou Medical University, Wenzhou, Zhejiang, China

Kaixuan Sheng
Ningbo Aier Guangming Eye Hosptial, Ningbo, Zhejiang, China

Anne-Laurence Best and Audrey Giocanti-Aurégan
Ophthalmology Department, Avicenne Hospital, DHU Vision and Handicaps, APHP, Paris 13 University, Bobigny, France

Franck Fajnkuchen, Sylvia Nghiem-Buffet and Typhaine Grenet
Ophthalmology Department, Avicenne Hospital, DHU Vision and Handicaps, APHP, Paris 13 University, Bobigny, France
Centre d'Imagerie et de Laser, Paris, France

Gabriel Quentel and Corinne Delahaye-Mazza
Centre d'Imagerie et de Laser, Paris, France

Salomon Y. Cohen
Centre d'Imagerie et de Laser, Paris, France
Ophthalmology Department, Centre Hospitalier Intercommunal de Créteil, Paris Est University, Créteil, France

Index

www.ingramcontent.com/pod-product-compliance
Lightning Source LLC
Chambersburg PA
CBHW080509200326
41458CB00012B/4148